MEDICINE
MORNING REPORT
Beyond the Pearls

MEDICINE MORNING REPORT

Beyond the Pearls

RAJ DASGUPTA, MD, FACP, FCCP, FAASM
Assistant Professor of Clinical Medicine
Division of Pulmonary/Critical Care/Sleep Medicine
Associate Program Director of the Sleep Medicine Fellowship
Assistant Program Director of the Internal Medicine Residency
Keck School of Medicine of the University of Southern California
Los Angeles, CA

R. MICHELLE KOOLAEE, DO, CCD
Assistant Professor of Clinical Medicine
Division of Rheumatology
Keck School of Medicine of the University of Southern California
Los Angeles, CA

ELSEVIER

ELSEVIER

1600 John F. Kennedy Blvd.
Ste 1800
Philadelphia, PA 19103-2899

Notices

Knowledge and best practice in this field are constantly changing. As new research and experience broaden our understanding, changes in research methods, professional practices, or medical treatment may become necessary.

Practitioners and researchers must always rely on their own experience and knowledge in evaluating and using any information, methods, compounds, or experiments described herein. In using such information or methods they should be mindful of their own safety and the safety of others, including parties for whom they have a professional responsibility.

With respect to any drug or pharmaceutical products identified, readers are advised to check the most current information provided (i) on procedures featured or (ii) by the manufacturer of each product to be administered, to verify the recommended dose or formula, the method and duration of administration, and contraindications. It is the responsibility of practitioners, relying on their own experience and knowledge of their patients, to make diagnoses, to determine dosages and the best treatment for each individual patient, and to take all appropriate safety precautions.

To the fullest extent of the law, neither the Publisher nor the authors, contributors, or editors, assume any liability for any injury and/or damage to persons or property as a matter of products liability, negligence or otherwise, or from any use or operation of any methods, products, instructions, or ideas contained in the material herein.

Library of Congress Cataloging-in-Publication Data

Names: Dasgupta, Raj, editor. | Koolaee, R. Michelle, editor.
Title: Medicine morning report : beyond the pearls / [edited by] Raj Dasgupta, R. Michelle Koolaee.
Description: Philadelphia, PA : Elsevier, [2017] | Includes bibliographical references and index.
Identifiers: LCCN 2016010074 | ISBN 9780323358095 (pbk. : alk. paper)
Subjects: | MESH: Clinical Medicine | Evidence-Based Medicine | Case Reports
Classification: LCC RC46 | NLM WB 293 | DDC 616—dc23
LC record available at http://lccn.loc.gov/2016010074

Executive Content Strategist: James Merritt
Content Development Specialist: Amy Meros
Publishing Services Manager: Catherine Jackson
Senior Project Manager: Daniel Fitzgerald
Designer: Ashley Miner

Printed in China

Last digit is the print number: 9 8 7 6 5 4 3 2

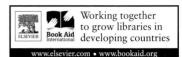

Working together
to grow libraries in
developing countries

www.elsevier.com • www.bookaid.org

*I would like to dedicate this book to my mother,
Tita Reyes Dasgupta, for all her hard work and sacrifices
she has made for her family throughout her life. Even now she helps
my wife and me by being the best grandmother to our two
beautiful children, Mina and Aiden. I must thank my
most patient and understanding wife, without whom
this book would never have been completed.*

It is with great pleasure that we present to you *Medicine Morning Report: Beyond the Pearls*, First Edition. Writing the "perfect" review text has been a dream of mine ever since I was a first-year medical student. Dr. Koolaee and I envisioned a text that incorporates United States Medical Licensing Examination (USMLE) Steps 1, 2, and 3 along with up-to-date evidence-based clinical medicine. We wanted the platform of the text to be drawn from a traditional theme, such as the "morning report" format that many of us are familiar with from residency. This book is geared toward a wide audience, from medical students to attending physicians practicing general internal medicine. Each case has been carefully chosen and covers scenarios and questions frequently encountered on the medical wards and integrates both basic science and clinical pearls.

We would like to sincerely thank all of the many contributors who have helped to create this text. Your insightful work will be a valuable tool for medical students and physicians in order to gain an in-depth understanding of internal medicine. It should be noted that while a variety of clinical cases in internal medicine were selected for this book, it is not meant to substitute a comprehensive medical reference.

CONTRIBUTORS

Joseph Abdelmalek, MD
Assistant Professor of Clinical Medicine
Division of Nephrology
University of California, San Diego
Veterans Affairs Hospital San Diego
San Diego, CA

Ahmet Baydur, MD, FACP, FCCP
Professor of Clinical Medicine
Division of Pulmonary, Critical Care and
Sleep Medicine
Keck School of Medicine of the University of
Southern California
Los Angeles, CA

Monisha Bhanote, MD, FCAP, FASCP
Medical Director, Surgical Pathology
Anatomic and Clinical Pathology,
Cytopathology
SoCal Pathologist Medical Group
San Diego, CA

John D. Carmichael, MD
Associate Professor of Clinical Medicine
Co-Director, USC Pituitary Center
Keck School of Medicine of the University of
Southern California
Los Angeles, CA

Andrea Censullo, MD
Fellow—Infectious Diseases
Cedars-Sinai/UCLA
Multicampus Program in Infectious Diseases
Los Angeles, CA

Wen Chen, MD
Internal Medicine
Keck School of Medicine of the University of
Southern California
Los Angeles, CA

Walter Chou, MD
Fellow Physician
Division of Pulmonary, Critical Care and
Sleep Medicine
Keck School of Medicine of the University of
Southern California
Los Angeles, CA

Joe Crocetti, MD
Associate Physician
Division of Pulmonary
Abington Jefferson Health
Rydal, PA

Raj Dasgupta, MD, FACP, FCCP, FAASM
Assistant Professor of Clinical Medicine
Division of Pulmonary/Critical Care/Sleep
Medicine
Associate Program Director of the Sleep
Medicine Fellowship
Assistant Program Director of the Internal
Medicine Residency
Keck School of Medicine of the University of
Southern California
Los Angeles, CA

Brian K. Do, MD
Fellow
Uveitis & Ocular Immunology
Department of Ophthalmology
The New York Eye & Ear Infirmary of
Mount Sinai
New York, NY

Emily S. Gillett, MD, PhD, FAAP
Clinical Fellow
Division of Pediatric Pulmonology and Sleep
Medicine
Children's Hospital Los Angeles
Los Angeles, CA

Christopher J. Graber, MD, MPH
Associate Clinical Professor of Medicine
Infectious Diseases Section
VA Greater Los Angeles Healthcare System
Los Angeles, CA

Nida Hamiduzzaman, MD
Assistant Professor of Clinical Medicine
Associate Program Director, Internal
Medicine Residency
Keck School of Medicine of the University of
Southern California
Los Angeles, CA

Eric Hsieh, MD
Program Director, Internal Medicine
Residency
Keck School of Medicine of the University of
Southern California
Los Angeles, CA

Albert Huang, MD
Attending Physician
Physical Medicine and Rehabilitation
Los Angeles, CA

Arzhang Cyrus Javan, MD, DTM&H
Clinical Instructor of Medicine
David Geffen School of Medicine at UCLA
Division of Infectious Diseases
Olive View-UCLA Medical Center
Sylmar, CA
Clinical Instructor of Medicine
Division of Infectious Diseases
Cedars-Sinai Medical Center
Los Angeles, CA

Arthur Jeng, MD
Associate Clinical Professor of Medicine
David Geffen School of Medicine at UCLA
Division of Infectious Diseases
Olive View-UCLA Medical Center
Sylmar, CA

John Khoury, MD
Neurology
Abington Neurological Associates
Willow Grove, PA
Associate Director
Sleep Disorders Center
Abington Memorial Hospital
Abington, PA

R. Michelle Koolaee, DO, CCD
Assistant Professor of Clinical Medicine
Division of Rheumatology
Keck School of Medicine of the University of
Southern California
Los Angeles, CA

Ravi Lakdawala, MD
Fellow Physician
Division of Nephrology and Hypertension
Keck School of Medicine of the University of
Southern California
Los Angeles, CA

Nicholas Landsman, MD
Resident Physician
Internal Medicine
Keck School of Medicine of the University of
Southern California
Los Angeles, CA

Carla LoPinto-Khoury, MD
Assistant Professor
Neurology
Drexel College of Medicine
Philadelphia, PA

Patricia Lorenzo, MD
Fellow Physician
Division of Endocrinology
Keck School of Medicine of the University of
Southern California
Los Angeles, CA

Ted Lyu, MD
Clinical Instructor
Ophthalmology
Icahn School of Medicine at Mount Sinai
New York, NY

Daniel Martinez, MD
Assistant Professor of Clinical Medicine
Keck School of Medicine of the University of
Southern California
Los Angeles, CA

Joseph Meouchy, MD
Fellow, Division of Nephrology and
Hypertension
Keck School of Medicine of the University of
Southern California
Los Angeles, CA

Brandon A. Miller, MD
Assistant Professor of Clinical Medicine
Keck School of Medicine of the University of
Southern California
Los Angeles, CA

Aarti Chawla Mittal, DO
Assistant Professor of Clinical Medicine
Associate Program Director, Pulmonary and
Critical Care Fellowship
Loma Linda University School of Medicine
Assistant Professor of Clinical Medicine
University of California, Riverside School of
Medicine
Riverside, CA

Andrew Morado, MD
Chief Pulmonary Fellow
Division of Pulmonary, Critical Care and
Sleep Medicine
Keck School of Medicine of the University of
Southern California
Los Angeles, CA

Steven M. Naids, MD
Ophthalmology
Icahn School of Medicine at Mount Sinai
New York, NY

Emily Omura, BA, MD
Fellow, Division of Endocrinology
Keck School of Medicine of the University of
Southern California
Los Angeles, CA

Nirav Patel, MD
Chief Medical Officer (Interim)
Infection Control Officer
Director of Antibiotic Stewardship
SSM Health Saint Louis University Hospital
Assistant Professor of Internal Medicine
Division of Infectious Diseases, Allergy and
Immunology (Primary)
Division of Pulmonary, Critical Care and
Sleep Medicine (Secondary)
Saint Louis University School of Medicine
St. Louis, MO

Dawn Piarulli, MD
Clinical Fellow
Division of Rheumatology
Keck School of Medicine of the University of
Southern California
Los Angeles, CA

Seth Politano, DO, FACP
Assistant Professor of Clinical Medicine
Associate Program Director, Internal
Medicine Residency
Keck School of Medicine of the University of
Southern California
Los Angeles, CA

Rachel Ramirez, MD
Associate Program Director
Department of Medicine
Abington Hospital
Abington, PA
Assistant Professor of Clinical Medicine
Drexel University College of Medicine
Philadelphia, PA

Caitlin Reed, MD, MPH
Medical Director, Inpatient Tuberculosis Unit
Olive View-UCLA Medical Center
Assistant Clinical Professor of Medicine
Division of Infectious Diseases
David Geffen School of Medicine at UCLA
Los Angeles, CA

Mark Riley, MS
Medical Student
Ohio University Heritage College of
Osteopathic Medicine
Dublin, OH

Gina Rossetti, MD
Assistant Professor of Clinical Medicine
Associate Program Director, Internal
Medicine Residency
Keck School of Medicine of the University of
Southern California
Los Angeles, CA

Joshua Sapkin, MD
Assistant Professor of Clinical Medicine
Associate Program Director, Internal
Medicine Residency
Keck School of Medicine of the University of
Southern California
Los Angeles, CA

Patrick E. Sarte, MD, MS, FAAP, FACP
Assistant Professor of Clinical Medicine
Associate Director, Internal Medicine
Residency Program
Keck School of Medicine of the University of
Southern California
Los Angeles, CA

Stanley Silverman, MD
Associate Physician
Pulmonary
Abington Jefferson Health
Rydal, PA

Mark Sims, MD
Resident, PGY-3
Medicine-Pediatrics
LAC+USC Medical Center
Los Angeles, CA

Richard Snyder, MD, FACP, FCCP
Associate Chief Medical Officer
Abington Hospital Jefferson Health
Abington, PA

Kelly Walsma, MD
Fellow Physician
Division of Pulmonary, Critical Care and
Sleep Medicine
Keck School of Medicine of the University of
Southern California
Los Angeles, CA

CONTENTS

Albert Huang ■ John Khoury

A 63-Year-Old Female With Change in Mental Status and Slurred Speech

A 63-year-old female presents to the emergency department (ED) with sudden onset of difficulty speaking. The symptoms began approximately 1 hour earlier during dinner with family when her speech became slurred and incomprehensible. Due to her difficulty speaking in the ED, she is unable to provide additional information. Per her husband, her past medical history is notable for coronary artery disease, prior heart attack, diabetes mellitus, hypertension, breast cancer, and low back pain.

What is the first step in evaluating acute neurologic changes?
In this emergent situation, her presentation with new onset dysarthria is concerning for an acute ischemic cerebrovascular accident (CVA), and the evaluation must be expedited because treatment with the intravenous thrombolytic recombinant tissue plasminogen activator (rt-PA) is time sensitive. In addition to assessing for an acute ischemic stroke, other possible etiologies that could present with an acute change in neurologic status need to be considered, such as hypoglycemia, hyperglycemia, migraine with aura (complex migraine), hemorrhagic stroke, Todd's paralysis, cerebral neoplasm, and head trauma.

In suspecting an ischemic stroke, what initial history element is critical to obtain?
A timeline beginning with the onset of symptoms must be established. The window to treat an ischemic infarction is under 3 to 4.5 hours* from the onset of symptoms. Thus, the evaluation must be conducted in an expedited fashion and is best performed in a team setting where multiple members can attend to different tasks at the same time. Time is brain and, similar to a myocardial infarction treatment, treatment should not be delayed simply because there is a 3- to 4.5-hour window to treat. Studies have shown that patients treated earlier with rt-PA have better outcomes.

CLINICAL PEARL   **STEP 2/3**

The time of onset is unreliable if the patient is found unconscious or wakes from sleep with the new symptoms. The onset of symptoms is defined as the time when the patient was last awake and symptom-free or considered neurologically "normal." In the event the patient awoke from sleep with new neurologic deficits, he or she is not eligible for acute treatment with rt-PA because the exact time of onset cannot be definitively determined.

---

*Treatment of an acute stroke from 3 to 4.5 hours is dependent on review of additional exclusion criteria as recommended by the American Heart Association/American Stroke Association.

TABLE 1.1 ■ Exclusion Criteria for Treatment With rt-PA Within 3 Hours of Symptom Onset per FDA Prescribing Information

Absolute Exclusion Criteria
- Active internal bleeding
- Recent intracranial or intraspinal surgery or serious head trauma
- Intracranial conditions that may increase the risk of bleeding
- Bleeding diathesis
- Current severe uncontrolled hypertension
- Current intracranial hemorrhage
- Subarachnoid hemorrhage

What questions should be asked to exclude other possible diagnoses related to decreased cognition and slurred speech?

Alternative conditions could resemble an acute stroke and therefore must be considered. Hypoglycemia warrants questions regarding diabetes and glucose control. If the patient has had similar symptoms in the past associated with a proceeding aura, he or she may be suffering from a migraine with aura. History of cancer may signal the presence of a brain tumor, potentially metastasis. A history of alcoholism could indicate Wernicke's encephalopathy (which classically causes ophthalmoplegia, ataxia, and confusion), and fever could suggest the presence of an abscess or systemic infection. Home medications should be reviewed for possible drug toxicities (e.g. lithium, phenytoin, and carbamazepine) and the possibility of a postictal period warrants questions regarding a seizure prior to the onset of symptoms.

In preparation for treatment with rt-PA for an ischemic stroke, additional questions must be asked to determine whether the patient is a candidate for therapy. A targeted history should be elicited to evaluate for exclusion criteria that would rule out the possibility of treating with rt-PA (Table 1.1).

Regarding the patient's history of cancer, it is important to know how long ago it was treated and whether it is still active. A cerebral metastatic lesion could mimic the symptoms of an ischemic stroke. Newly discovered cerebral lesions and recent intracranial surgery (within 3 months) have an increased risk for intracranial bleeding with use of rt-PA. Because her husband noted that she suffered from low back pain, questions regarding surgical treatment, such as a lumbar fusion, are important because recent intraspinal surgery is also a contraindication.

Upon further questioning, the family notes the patient's breast cancer was managed with a lumpectomy over 10 years ago and without evidence of spread. Her back pain was treated with injections, the last one a year ago.

On exam, her temperature is 37.1 °C (98.8 °F), pulse rate is 92/min, respiration rate is 22/min, and oxygen saturation is 94% on room air. She is unable to form intelligible words. There is a noticeable slur to her speech, and exam reveals a dense right-sided facial droop that involves the forehead. She is able to move all extremities, though the right arm strength is 4–/5 and the right leg strength 4+/5. Auscultation of the heart reveals a regular rate and rhythm without a murmur.

Considering the time-sensitive nature of the initial assessment, how should the exam be focused?

Airway, breathing, and circulation must be assessed first to determine whether emergent treatment is necessary for airway protection. In addition to the initial vital signs, a bedside glucose check should be obtained to assess for acute hypoglycemia as it can often mimic a stroke. In an urgent and especially an emergent setting, it can be considered the fourth vital sign. Because a stroke is suspected, a computed tomography (CT) scan is urgently needed to evaluate for the presence or absence of an intracranial hemorrhage.

The neurological exam is paramount and needs to be performed to understand the deficits, localize the lesion, and for documentation to monitor subsequent measurements of improvement. Although a thorough neurologic exam is necessary to assess for deficits that will need to be treated prior to returning home, a brief exam is sufficient to determine progression of the stroke and whether the patient is a candidate for rt-PA. Many standardized scales are available for use. One common scale is the National Institutes of Health Stroke Scale (NIHSS). The NIHSS is a focused neurological assessment that includes an evaluation of consciousness, cranial nerves, and gross motor, sensory, and cerebellar deficits. It has been validated for prediction of lesion size and can be used as a prognostic indicator of eventual outcome.

What signs or symptoms are highly predictive for an ischemic stroke?

Because early identification of an acute ischemic stroke is important to initiate protocols for further diagnostic studies and possible treatment with rt-PA, a simplified assessment was developed and validated for use by first responders. The Cincinnati Prehospital Stroke Scale is a modified version of the NIHSS that assesses facial droop, arm drift, and presence of aphasia. When any one of these abnormalities is identified by a physician, there is a sensitivity of 66% and specificity of 87% in identifying the presence of an ischemic stroke. When used by prehospital responders, there is excellent interrater correlation.

During the reevaluation, the patient is responsive and able to follow commands. Her facial droop and aphasia remain unchanged, and she continues to have difficulty forming words. Although she demonstrated an initial drift when holding up her right arm, the weakness has worsened and she has difficulty holding her arm up against gravity.

What additional neurologic deficits are commonly seen in a cerebrovascular accident?

In addition to these exam findings, ischemic strokes can lead to any number of neurologic deficits. The anatomic location of the damaged brain tissue will dictate the neurologic deficits. The middle cerebral artery (MCA) supplies blood to the lateral frontal, parietal, and temporal lobes. Involvement of the MCA can lead to contralateral hemiparesis. Typically the pattern of weakness is face weakness > arm weakness > leg weakness, and additional deficits may include sensory loss, dysarthria, and homonymous hemianopia. Involvement of the dominant hemisphere, most commonly the left side of the brain, can lead to loss of language skills such as aphasia, alexia, apraxia, and acalculia. Involvement of the nondominant hemisphere can result in neglect of the contralateral side, loss of smell, and loss in prosody of speech. See Figure 1.1 for CT images of an MCA stroke.

The anterior cerebral artery supplies blood to the medial frontal lobe and can lead to contralateral hemiparesis where leg weakness is worse than arm weakness with relative sparing of the face due to its lateral location on the motor homunculus. Involvement of the frontal lobe can lead to disinhibition and behavioral changes. Patients with anterior cerebral artery lesions can also demonstrate increased spontaneity and distractibility.

Involvement of the vertebrobasilar arteries affects the medulla and pons. Two associated syndromes are Wallenberg syndrome (involvement of the lateral medullary) and Weber syndrome (involvement of the midbrain, descending corticospinal pathway). Wallenberg syndrome causes

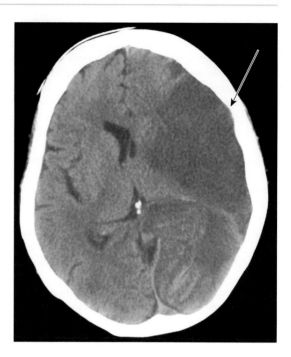

Figure 1.1 Computed tomography scan of the head revealing a subacute left hemisphere middle cerebral artery (MCA) ischemic stroke as indicated by the arrow. *(Courtesy of* https://commons .wikimedia.org/wiki/File:EartlyrtMC Astroke3dlatter.png*)*

alternating hemianesthesia (ipsilateral loss of pain and temperature sensation of the face with contralateral loss of pain and temperature sensation of the body), ipsilateral Horner syndrome, dysarthria, dysphonia, dysphagia, nausea, nystagmus, vertigo, and ataxia. Weber syndrome can lead to an ipsilateral third nerve palsy and paralysis of the contralateral arm and leg.

Strokes related to posterior circulation can affect the midbrain, occipital, and occipito-parietal cortices. Deficits include visual field loss, balance and proprioceptive deficits, prosopagnosia, and memory impairments. Due to collateral circulation from the posterior cerebral artery via the posterior communicating artery to the middle cerebral artery, there may also be deficits related to the MCA, such as hemiparesis and sensory loss.

BASIC SCIENCE/CLINICAL PEARL   **STEP 1/2/3**

Bell's palsy is caused by dysfunction or injury of the facial nerve lower motor neurons. This can often be confused with an ischemic stroke (upper motor neuron injury). In stroke patients, the injury to the seventh cranial nerve (CN 7) leads to paralysis of the lower half of the face with sparing of the muscles in the forehead due to contralateral innervations of the frontalis and orbicularis oculi muscles. In Bell's palsy, injury to peripheral CN 7 results in contralateral weakness of the upper and lower face, including the inability to fully close the patient's eyelid.

In addition to an initial set of vital signs, a bedside glucose is obtained and is 112 mg/dL (normal). A 12-lead electrocardiogram (ECG) reveals a rate of 95/min. Initial laboratory studies (Table 1.2) and a CT scan of her head (Fig. 1.1) are available for review.

TABLE 1.2 ■ **Initial Laboratory Tests**

White blood count (4.0-11.0)	5.0 K/μL
Hemoglobin (12.0-16.0)	12.7 g/dL
Hematocrit (35.0-47.0)	38.5%
Platelets (140-440)	186 K/μL
aPTT (24-37)	20
International normalized ratio (0.90-1.10)	0.98
Complete metabolic panel	Normal
Thyroid-stimulating hormone (0.3-5.0)	4.8 μU/mL

aPTT, Activated partial thromboplastin time.

Diagnosis: Left middle cerebral artery ischemic stroke

CLINICAL PEARL   **STEP 2/3**

4 to 6% of patients who receive rt-PA suffer hemorrhagic conversion of the ischemic stroke. Although the original trial demonstrated and increased incidence of hemorrhage in rt-PA patients when compared to placebo, the mortality rates were similar when compared at 3 months.

In this case, there are no contraindications, and both the patient and her family agree to treatment with rt-PA, which is started immediately. She is transferred to the Neuro Intensive Care Unit (NICU) where her blood pressure is closely monitored and serial neurologic checks are preformed hourly.

What additional diagnostic studies can be performed in the evaluation of an ischemic stroke?

Following the initial acute management and initiation of antithrombolytic therapy (if indicated and agreed upon by the patient and family members), additional studies are necessary to assess for a possible source of the ischemic stroke. A magnetic resonance angiogram (MRA) of the head and neck evaluates for carotid and intracranial stenosis. If carotid stenosis is identified, treatment may be pursued with a carotid endarterectomy or carotid artery stenting. An echocardiogram with bubble study can assess for the presence of an embolic etiology, valvular vegetations, or left-to-right shunt. If negative and there is still high clinical suspicion for embolic disease, then a transesophageal echocardiogram may be performed as well to look for vegetations or aortic arch plaque. In the event the initial CT scan of the head is unrevealing for a cause of neurologic deficits, a magnetic resonance imaging (MRI) scan with diffusion-weighted images (DWI) is more sensitive in identifying ischemic lesions. Laboratory studies include a lipid profile, fasting glucose levels, and hemoglobin A1C for evaluation of secondary stroke prevention.

Upon transfer to an intensive care unit, close monitoring is continued with telemetry and hourly neurologic checks. In addition, blood pressure must be followed closely. Although hypertensive management is important for long-term prevention, permissive hypertension is utilized during the immediate subacute phase to allow for increased perfusion to affected cerebral tissue. An exception to acute treatment of hypertension is in the setting of a hypertensive emergency where the systolic pressure is greater than 220 mm Hg or the diastolic pressure is greater than 120 mm Hg and there is evidence of end-organ damage.

CLINICAL PEARL	STEP 2/3

In the setting of a hypertensive crisis, blood pressure should be lowered gradually, ideally no more than 15% within several hours. Decreasing the blood pressure any quicker could lead to significantly decreased perfusion pressure and the potential for end-organ damage.

What treatments can be started for secondary prevention of stroke?
To prevent hemorrhagic conversion, anticoagulation or antiplatelet medications should be held within the first 24 hours, following the initiation of antithrombolytic therapy. However, there is strong evidence demonstrating the benefit of stroke prevention with antiplatelet medications including clopidogrel (Plavix) and aspirin either alone or as a combination medication with dipyridamole. Anticoagulation with warfarin is indicated only when utilized for concurrent treatment of atrial fibrillation.

BASIC SCIENCE/CLINICAL PEARL	STEP 1/2/3

Antiplatelet treatment is a mainstay of stroke prevention. Clopidogrel works by inhibiting the adenosine diphosphate (ADP) receptor on platelets and prevents activation. On the other hand, aspirin inhibits thromboxane A2, which is secreted by activated platelets and causes activation of new platelets and platelet aggregation.

In addition, modifiable risk factors should be addressed. Due to the life-changing implications of a stroke, the patient may become more motivated to stop smoking, and cessation techniques should be discussed. A lipid profile can help direct the need for statin therapy. Diabetes and hypertension are both significant risk factors, and efforts must be taken for improved control. There is a high prevalence of obstructive sleep apnea (OSA) in patients who have a stroke, so it is important to screen for OSA in these patients.

What nonpharmacologic treatments or assessments are important prior to discharge from the hospital?
In addition to medical management, disposition will be in question depending upon residual neurologic deficits. Patients who suffer significant weakness or loss of coordination can have trouble with simple tasks such as moving from a sitting to standing position or walking. Everyday activities such as dressing and toileting become more difficult. Aphasia can make simple communication impossible. Thus, assessments by physical, occupational, and speech therapists are important to determine whether the patient is safe to return home. Often, individuals were previously independent with their everyday activities but following the onset of stroke are no long able to complete even simple tasks without assistance. This therapy should be initiated soon after admission to the hospital but can continue long after discharge. If the deficits are severe and the patient requires a great deal of assistance with walking and other tasks, an inpatient rehabilitation facility or skilled nursing facility may be considered. If the deficits are minimal but present, the discharge home with home therapy may be reasonable.

CLINICAL PEARL	STEP 2/3

If there is any suspicion of dysphagia, such as the presence of slurred speech or facial droop, the patient should be restricted to nothing by mouth (NPO) and a speech therapy consultation requested to assess swallowing function. Dysphagia can often go unnoticed, described as silent aspiration, and increases the risk for aspiration of solids and liquids, which can result in an aspiration pneumonia.

Following treatment with rt-PA, the patient's neurologic deficits improve but remain persistent. She continues to have difficulty communicating secondary to the aphasia. Despite improvement of her right-sided weakness, she demonstrates continued trouble with walking and coordinating fine motor skills, which made dressing and eating difficult. Thus, after an inpatient consultation by a physiatrist, she is accepted for acute inpatient rehabilitation.

BEYOND THE PEARLS

- Recent studies show that rt-PA may be given up to 4.5 hours from the onset of symptoms for the treatment of stroke. This guideline is based on the European Cooperative Acute Stroke Study [ECASS] III. The FDA approval allows for treatment within 3 hours of onset, but the American Academy of Neurology (AAN)/American Heart Association (AHA)/American Stroke Association (ASA) recommend treatment up to 4.5 hours (Class B evidence) despite the fact that this is technically off-label use in the United States. Treatment between the 3- and 4.5-hour window can be beneficial for a smaller group of individuals and requires consideration of additional exclusion criteria.
- Current exclusion criteria/contraindications for treatment with rt-PA are still being discussed and revised between the FDA and AHA/ASA for treatment within 3 hours.
- Rapid resolution of neurologic symptoms is an exclusion criteria, although recent studies have shown when these patients are not treated with rt-PA, they can still suffer from a poor stroke outcome. Thrombolytic therapy has been given to patients on an off-label basis, though treating in this scenario is not formally recommended and warrants further study.
- Another symptom occasionally associated with Bell's palsy is loss of taste. This impairment is caused by dysfunction of the chorda tympani innervating taste on the tongue.
- The visual field loss pattern can provide insight into the site and size of the cerebral tissue affected. Although homonymous hemianopia can be caused by a large MCA stroke or an isolated occipital lesion, the former can be differentiated by corresponding hemiparesis. In addition, smaller MCA strokes with involvement of optic radiations will lead to quandrantinopia.
- Diagnostically, the presence of an acute ischemic stroke can be made based on clinical features, and confirmation with CT and additional advanced imaging is not necessary. However, it is common practice to perform an MRI for additional characterization of the stroke and angiography to evaluate for vascular malformations.
- The major concern regarding treatment with rt-PA for ischemic stroke remains intracranial hemorrhage. Although the original trial demonstrated an increased incidence of hemorrhage in rt-PA patients when compared to placebo, the mortality rates were similar when compared at 3 months.

References

Genentech. 2015. *Activase prescribing information.* Available at <http://www.gene.com/download/pdf/activase_prescribing.pdf>. Accessed 07.12.15.

Hacke W, Kaste M, Bluhmki E, et al. Thrombolysis with alteplase 3 to 4.5 hours after acute ischemic stroke. *N Engl J Med.* 2008;359(13):1317-1329.

Jauch EC, Saver JL, Adams HP Jr, et al. Guidelines for the early management of patient with early ischemic stroke: a guideline for healthcare professionals from the American Heart Association/American Stroke Association. *Stroke.* 2013;44:870-947.

Kothari RU, Pancioli A, Liu T, Brott T, Broderick J. Cincinnati Prehospital Stroke Scale: reproducibility and validity. *Ann Emerg Med.* 1999;33(4):373-378.

The Stroke Prevention by Aggressive Reduction in Cholesterol Levels (SPARCL) Investigators. High-dose atorvastatin after stroke or transient ischemic attack. *N Engl J Med.* 2006;355(6):349-359.

CASE 2

Monisha Bhanote

A 61-Year-Old Male With Constipation

A 61-year-old male presents to his primary care doctor with complaints of alternating constipation and diarrhea. He is on no known medications. He does receive an annual flu shot at his local pharmacy, but other than that, he has not been evaluated by a doctor in a very long time.

His physical exam shows some abdominal distension and left lower quadrant tenderness but is otherwise essentially unremarkable. He has no significant smoking or drinking history. He is a divorced construction worker and claims to eat a double cheeseburger on most days at his job. His initial panel of blood work shows mild anemia and an unremarkable chemistry panel. His in-office blood pressure and temperature are within normal limits. His guaiac stool exam is positive.

What are the preventative medical guidelines for adults?
It is recommended that adults get a health evaluation every 1 to 3 years, depending on their risk factors, and then annually after age 50. Male patients can be screened for prostate cancer after the age of 50, with appropriate patient education. Female patients are evaluated for cervical cancer at age 21 or earlier if indicated via a Pap test. In addition, females should be aware of breast cancer screening as early as age 18, with clinical breast exams and then mammography by the age of 40, unless the patient has risk factors, in which case imaging can start earlier. Colorectal carcinoma is evaluated at age 50 in both male and female patients, with a colonoscopy at age 50, then every 10 years, or an annual fecal occult blood test (FOBT) plus sigmoidoscopy every 5 years, or annual FOBT.

CLINICAL PEARL	STEP 2/3

High-sensitivity FOBT, sigmoidoscopy with FOBT, and colonoscopy are effective in decreasing colorectal cancer mortality.

What are some screening tests that could be recommended to this patient based on his age and symptoms?
Because this patient has not been seen by a doctor in a long time, he needs a health evaluation that includes history (including family history of disease), preventative screenings and counseling, updated immunization, and an age-appropriate physical exam. General counseling regarding diet, exercise, and substance use is recommended at every age. His pertinent evaluation in reference to his symptoms includes a colonoscopy.

The patient is referred to a gastroenterologist for a colonoscopy. His colonoscopy reveals four small polypoid lesions throughout his colon as well as a reddish irregular craterlike lesion in his rectum. The four polypoid lesions are removed entirely and the rectal lesion is biopsied.

TABLE 2.1 ▓ Polyps of the Large Intestine

Inflammatory Polyps	Hamartomatous Polyps	Epithelial Polyps	Mesenchymal Polyps
Inflammatory pseudopolyp	Juvenile polyp	Hyperplastic polyp	Neurofibroma
Prolapse type polyp	Peutz-Jeghers polyp	Sessile serrated polyp/adenoma	Granular cell tumor
Inflammatory myoglandular polyp		Conventional adenoma	Fibroblastic polyp

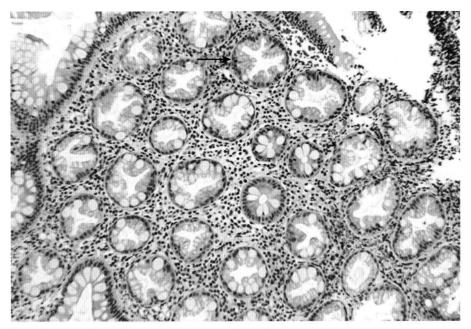

Figure 2.1 Hyperplastic polyp showing star-shaped glands with bland morphology as indicated by the arrow (haematoxylin and eosin [H&E] stain).

What kinds of polyps occur in the colorectal region?

The large intestine can have a multitude of different types of polyps (see Table 2.1). The patient was found to have three tubular adenomas and one hyperplastic polyp. Hyperplastic polyps are generally <5 mm and show a bland cytology with well-formed, elongated glands and crypts with serrated (saw tooth) or star-shaped appearance (see Fig. 2.1). Adenomas can be tubular, tubulovillous, villous, serrated, or flat. This patient had three traditional adenomas, which were all tubular. Tubular adenomas have at least low-grade dysplasia with the presence of architecturally noncomplex crypts with nuclei that are stratified or pseudostratified and remain at the lower half of the cytoplasm (see Fig. 2.2).

CLINICAL PEARL   **STEP 2/3**

Hyperplastic polyps are the most common type of polyp in the colon.

TABLE 2.2 ■ Risk Factors for the Development of Colorectal Carcinoma

Constitutional	Environmental
Family history (first-degree relative)	Physical inactivity (<3 hours per week)
Inflammatory bowel disease (Crohn's, ulcerative colitis)	Obesity
Colon polyps (polyposis syndromes, etc.)	Red meat consumption/ diet high in animal fat
Age (middle-aged to elderly)	Smoking
Race (African Americans have higher risk)	Alcohol use
	Low-fiber/low-vegetable/ low-fruit diet

CLINICAL PEARL   **STEP 2/3**

Adenomas are the most common neoplasm of the large intestine and are defined as dysplastic clonal proliferations of colonic epithelium.

In addition to his four polyps, the ulcerated lesion in his rectum turns out to be an invasive adenocarcinoma (Fig. 2.3).

Diagnosis: Invasive adenocarcinoma

What are the risk factors for development of colorectal carcinoma?

The risk of developing colorectal carcinoma is affected by multiple factors, which can be constitutional or environmental (see Table 2.2). Family history of a first-degree relative and inflammatory bowel disease is a significant endogenous risk factor. Physical inactivity, obesity, red meat consumption, smoking, and alcohol use are all risk factors linked to colorectal carcinoma that are preventable.

CLINICAL PEARL   **STEP 2/3**

High-fat diets may increase the anaerobic gut flora, leading to a higher concentration of secondary bile acids, which may be carcinogens.

CLINICAL PEARL   **STEP 2/3**

High folate intake is associated with a decreased risk of colorectal carcinoma.

CLINICAL PEARL   **STEP 2/3**

Colorectal cancer is the second leading cause of cancer-related deaths in the United States and the third most common cancer in men and in women.

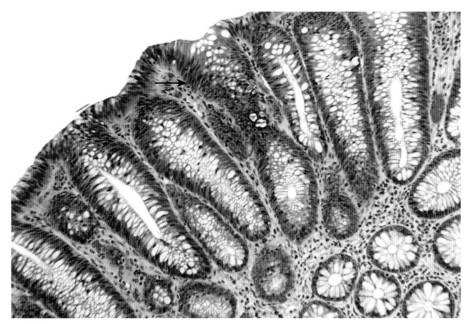

Figure 2.2 Tubular adenoma showing pseudostratified nuclei arranged in a predominant tubular architecture as indicated by the arrow (H&E stain).

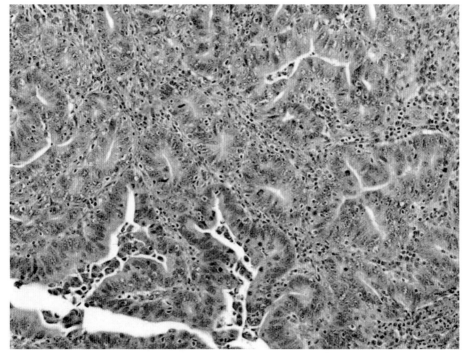

Figure 2.3 Rectal biopsy shows back-to-back glands with a complex architecture, loss of polarity, pseudostratification, nuclear hyperchromasia, and brisk mitotic activity (H&E stain).

What are the symptoms associated with left-sided versus right-sided colorectal carcinomas?
Most patients have general symptoms that include a change in bowel habit, abdominal distension, hematochezia, and constipation. Other symptoms that are not specific to colorectal carcinoma, but that are seen in many cancers, include weight loss, malaise, fever, and anemia. Left-sided carcinomas are more often associated with rectal bleeding, tenesmus, and alternating diarrhea and constipation, whereas right-sided carcinomas may have vague abdominal pain and anemia due to blood loss from ulceration of the tumor.

What is the mechanism for development of colorectal carcinoma?
Colorectal carcinoma begins as a benign adenomatous polyp (low-grade dysplasia), which then progresses to high-grade dysplasia, and eventually to an invasive carcinoma. The development of carcinoma is caused by the acquisition of multiple tumor-associated mutations causing genomic instability. Chromosomal instability, which is the loss of heterozygosity at APC, TP53, and SMAD4, is the most common genomic instability in colorectal cancer. It is characteristic of 80 to 85% of sporadic colorectal cancers. Another cause of genomic instability is DNA repair defects. This inactivation of genes required for repair of base–base mismatches can be inherited, as in hereditary nonpolyposis colorectal cancer (HNPCC)/Lynch syndrome, or acquired in sporadic colorectal cancers. Aberrant DNA methylation is another mechanism of gene inactivation in patients with colorectal carcinoma.
   Oncogenes RAS and BRAF, which activate the mitogen-activated protein kinase (MAPK) signaling pathway, also occur in colorectal carcinomas.

What are syndromes associated with development of colorectal carcinoma?
Less than half a percent of colorectal carcinomas are associated with genetic syndromes such as familial adenomatous polyposis (FAP), juvenile polyposis syndrome, Peutz-Jeghers syndrome, and Cowden syndrome. However, hereditary nonpolyposis forms are associated with a 2 to 3% incidence. The most common of these is Lynch syndrome, also known as HNPCC.

CLINICAL PEARL	STEP 2/3

Familial polyposis syndrome (FAP) is associated with >100 colon polyps (mostly tubular adenomas), mutation in APC gene, and either an epidermoid cyst, osteoma, or desmoid tumor.

CLINICAL PEARL	STEP 2/3

Peutz-Jeghers syndrome is associated with Peutz-Jegher–type polyps, melanotic mucocutaneous pigmentation, and sex cord tumors of the ovaries/testes.

CLINICAL PEARL	STEP 2/3

Cowden's syndrome is associated with facial tricholemmomas, acral keratosis, oral mucosal papillomas, and colorectal polyps.

What is the management of colorectal carcinoma?
The management of colorectal carcinoma depends primarily on the stage of the cancer. Stage I is managed with surgical resection alone. Stage II management varies depending on the location of the cancer and may include surgery and/or chemotherapy/radiation. Stage III and IV patients may receive chemotherapy. Radiation may be useful in rectal cancers, although it is not often used in other parts of the colon, as those parts are not radiosensitive.

The patient is admitted to the hospital and prepped for surgery. He receives a rectosigmoid resection (see Fig. 2.4). Microscopically, the tumor appears to invade the muscularis propria (see Fig. 2.5). The surgical margins are negative, and there are 12 negative lymph nodes.

CLINICAL PEARL   STEP 2/3

The most common sites of colorectal cancer recurrence are the liver and lungs.

Pathologic staging of colorectal carcinoma depends on the depth of invasion of the bowel wall and surrounding structures, lymph node involvement, and distant metastasis. His final pathologic stage is T2N0M0 and clinical stage is I. He recovers quite well postoperatively and is sent home after 2 days.

What is the prognosis of colorectal carcinoma?

Survival is related to the stage of the disease. Patients with an invasive carcinoma into the submucosa (T1) or muscularis propria (T2) have a 5-year survival rate of 90%. Patients with tumors that invade into the pericolorectal tissues (T3) or visceral peritoneum (T4) without positive lymph nodes have a 5-year survival rate of 70%. When patients have positive lymph nodes with any T stage, their 5-year survival rate decreases to approximately 40%. Metastatic disease decreases the 5-year survival rate even further to 5%.

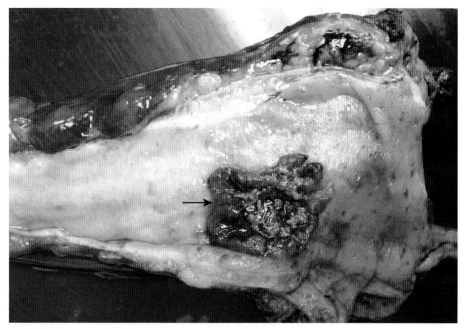

Figure 2.4 Portion of rectosigmoid resection showing a craterlike reddish lesion with heaped up irregular borders as indicated by the arrow. Adjacent bluish green discoloration in mucosa due to tattooing during colonoscopy (Gross photograph).

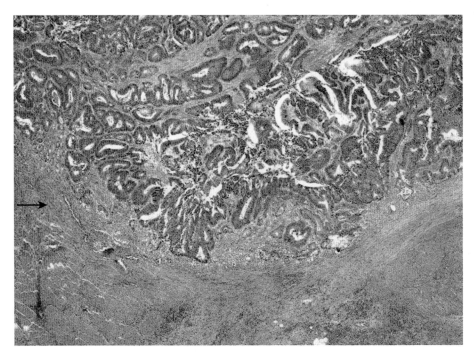

Figure 2.5 Invasive adenocarcinoma, moderately differentiated, invading into the muscularis propria as indicated by the arrow (H&E stain).

What kind of follow-up is recommended following treatment of colorectal carcinoma?

Medical history and physical exam should be performed every 3 to 6 months for 5 years. Carcinoembryonic antigen (CEA) levels should follow the same timing but only in patients with T2 or greater disease. An abdominal and chest computed tomography (CT) scan is recommended annually for 3 years. Additionally, when the tumor is located in the rectum, a pelvic CT scan is recommended.

A colonoscopy should be performed 1 year after surgery and then every 5 years. There is no recommendation for routine positron emission tomography (PET) scans, chest radiographs, or complete blood counts or liver function tests. Secondary therapy includes exercise, which maintains an appropriate body weight.

CLINICAL PEARL   **STEP 2/3**

CEA is an antigen produced by many colon cancers. It should not be used as a screening tool, However, it can be used preoperatively to follow the course of disease. CEA may be elevated prior to surgery but should return to normal 30 days postoperatively. If it remains elevated, it could be an indicator of recurrent disease.

BEYOND THE PEARLS

- Ninety percent of colorectal cancer deaths are preventable.
- Polypectomy can prevent colorectal carcinoma.
- It generally takes 10 to 15 years for an adenoma to become a carcinoma.
- Patients with familial adenomatous polyposis (FAP) may benefit from a preventative total proctocolectomy because of their increased risk of development of colorectal carcinoma.

BEYOND THE PEARLS—cont'd

- Although patients with Cowden syndrome have an increased number of colorectal polyps, they are mostly hamartomatous; therefore, they have a low rate of colorectal carcinoma.
- *MACC1* is a gene that has been isolated as a potential contributor to metastatic disease in colorectal carcinoma.
- HNPCC is associated with multiple primary colorectal cancers, accelerated tumor progression, and increased risk of endometrial, gastric, and urothelial tumors.
- HNPCC is usually a poorly differentiated carcinoma with a marked lymphocytic infiltration.
- Patients with mismatch repair genes do not benefit from chemotherapy.
- 5-Fluorouracil is a potent inhibitor of thymidylate synthase. Without thymidylate synthase, tumor cells cannot form dTMP (a precursor of DNA synthesis).
- 5-Fluorouracil side effects include myelosuppression, angina, mucositis, hyperpigmentation, and cerebellar ataxia.

References

Ballard-Barbash R, Friedenreich CM, Courneya KS, et al. Physical activity, biomarkers, and disease outcomes in cancer survivors: a systematic review. *J Natl Cancer Inst*. 2012;104(11):815-840.

Markowitz SD, Bertagnolli M. Molecular origins of cancer: molecular basis of colorectal cancer. *N Engl J Med*. 2009;361(25):2449-2460.

Meyerhardt JA, Mangu PB, Flynn PJ, et al. Follow-up care, surveillance protocol, and secondary prevention measures for survivors of colorectal cancer: American Society of Clinical Oncology clinical practice guideline endorsement. *J Clin Oncol*. 2013;31(35):4465-4470.

Odze RD. *Surgical Pathology of the GI Tract, Liver, Biliary Tract, and Pancreas*. 2nd ed. Philadelphia: Elsevier; 2009.

Park L. *Preventive care in adults: recommendations*. In: Fletcher RH, ed. Available at <www.uptodate.com>. Accessed 04.02.16.

Stein U, Walther W, Arlt F, et al. MACC1, a newly identified key regulator of HGF-MET signaling, predicts colon cancer metastasis. *Nat Med*. 2008;15(1):59-67.

Monisha Bhanote

A 37-Year-Old Female With a Palpable Breast Mass

A 37-year-old female presents to her primary care physician with a palpable breast mass. She says she felt the mass about 2 weeks ago while taking a shower. She did not note any pain or change in the size of the mass during her last menstruation. She is married and without children and has no significant medical or surgical history.

How is a female breast examined?

Breast exams should be performed first with the patient sitting and then with the patient supine. The axillary and supraclavicular lymph nodes should also be checked. The breasts should be inspected with the patient's arms at the side, above the head, and on the hips to flex the pectoralis muscles. The skin should be examined for changes, such as erythema, rash, and edema. The mass should be palpated for size, tenderness, and consistency.

CLINICAL PEARL	STEP 1
Most breast masses are not cancer.	

Upon exam, a grape-sized mobile mass is noted in the upper outer quadrant of the patient's left breast. No other masses are noted. The patient has no palpable axillary or supraclavicular adenopathy. She has no known significant family history of breast or gynecologic carcinoma.

What are some other questions you may want to ask the patient?

The patient should be asked whether she has noticed any nipple discharge and whether the discharge is clear, milky, or bloody. Other symptoms associated with many types of carcinoma, such as weight loss, malaise, or bone pain, should also be noted.

What are the most common causes of breast masses or lumps?

Not all breast masses or lumps are cancer. Breast lumps can be seen in the normal breast, with infections or injuries, in fibrocystic change, as well as benign and malignant neoplasms. Fibrocystic change in the breast can be subclassified as nonproliferative fibrocystic change and proliferative fibrocystic change (see Table 3.1).

CLINICAL PEARL	STEP 1
The relative risk of developing breast cancer with nonproliferative fibrocystic change is zero. The relative risk of developing breast cancer with proliferative fibrocystic change is 1.5 to 2×, while the risk increases to 4 to 5× with atypical ductal hyperplasia and atypical lobular hyperplasia.	

TABLE 3.1 ▥ **Fibrocystic Changes**

Nonproliferative	Proliferative
Fibrosis	Ductal hyperplasia (usual and atypical)
Microcysts	Sclerosing adenosis
Apocrine metaplasia	Small duct papilloma
Calcifications	Radial scar
Duct ectasia	

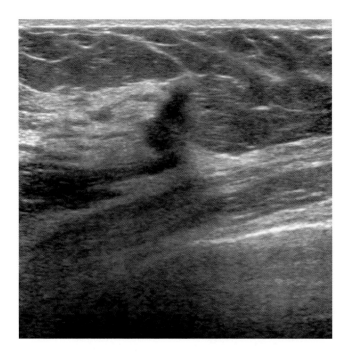

Figure 3.1 Ultrasound image showing the lesion to be taller in the vertical direction than it is wide in the horizontal direction. *(Dabbs D.* Breast Pathology. *Philadelphia: Elsevier Saunders; 2012.)*

What are some clinical features that may distinguish fibrocystic change from cancer?
Fibrocystic change tends to be bilateral, and patients can have multiple nodules or lumps. Menstrual variation is common with cyclical pain. These lumps can regress during pregnancy. Breast cancer, on the other hand, is most often unilateral with a single mass and shows no changes during menstruation.

The patient undergoes an ultrasound, which shows a noncompressible nodule that is taller than it is wide. The lesion measures approximately 24 mm and is solid with focal spiculations and without any significant cyst fluid (see Fig. 3.1 and Table 3.2). The patient admits to noticing minimal nipple discharge, which was blood tinged one day. The nipple discharge is sampled and submitted for cytology (see Fig. 3.2).

TABLE 3.2 ▮ **Ultrasound Findings Suspicious for Malignancy**

- Spiculation
- Taller than wide
- Angular margins
- Shadowing
- Branching pattern
- Hypoechogenicity
- Calcifications
- Duct extension
- Branching pattern
- Microlobulations

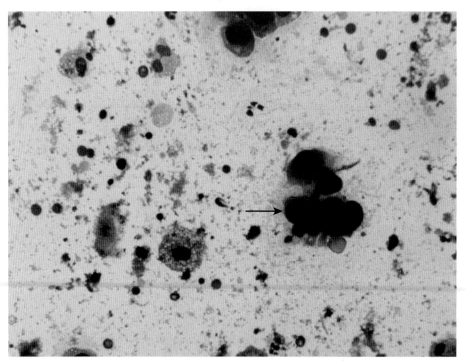

Figure 3.2 Nipple discharge sample showing large purple cells with high nuclear:cytoplasmic ratios as indicated by the arrow, suspicious for malignancy (Diff-Quik stain).

What are identifiable risk factors for breast carcinoma?

The incidence of breast carcinoma increases with age. History of a first-degree relative with breast cancer is a risk factor. There is a greater risk with a long reproductive life (with early menarche and late menopause). Proliferative fibrocystic change has an increased risk, whereas nonproliferative fibrocystic change has no increased risk. Other factors associated with breast carcinoma include obesity, nulliparity, previous breast cancer in the opposite breast, and a history of endometrial or ovarian carcinoma.

CLINICAL PEARL   **STEP 2/3**

Five to 10 percent of breast cancers are associated with *BRCA* genes:
- *BRCA1* is found on chromosome 17q21
- *BRCA2* is found on chromosome 13q12-13

BRCA1 accounts for a large number of familial cancer occurring at an early age.

What are some clinical findings of breast carcinoma?

Breast carcinoma can present as a solitary painless mass. Sometimes nipple retraction or skin dimpling can occur. In later stages, the mass can affix to the chest wall. Mammographic findings that are worrisome include microcalcifications and architectural distortion.

CLINICAL PEARL   **STEP 2/3**

Most breast cancers are found in the upper outer quadrant of the breast.

Because the patient's ultrasound shows a solid mass and her nipple discharge is highly suspicious for malignancy, the patient undergoes an ultrasound-guided core biopsy, which confirms the presence of an invasive carcinoma. She opts to undergo a needle localization lumpectomy, which shows a solid tan mass that measures approximately 2.4 cm in greatest dimension (see Fig. 3.3).

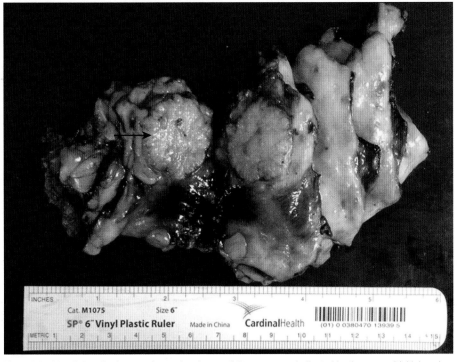

Figure 3.3 Needle localization specimen showing a solid tan mass as indicated by the arrow. Multiple colors of ink designate different surgical margins.

TABLE 3.3 ▦ Neoplasms of the Breast

Benign Neoplasms	Fibroadenoma
	Phyllodes tumor
	Intraductal papilloma
Malignant Neoplasms	Ductal carcinoma in situ
	Lobular carcinoma in situ
	Invasive ductal carcinoma
	Invasive lobular carcinoma
	Mucinous (colloid) carcinoma
	Tubular carcinoma
	Medullary carcinoma
	Inflammatory carcinoma

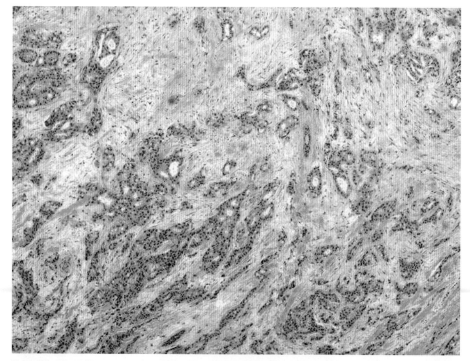

Figure 3.4 Histologic section of patient's tumor showing some tubule formation, consistent with a diagnosis of invasive ductal carcinoma (haematoxylin and eosin [H&E] stain).

Diagnosis: Invasive ductal carcinoma, moderately differentiated

What are the most common neoplasms of the breast?

Breast neoplasms can be benign or malignant (see Table 3.3). Malignant neoplasms are broadly divided into ductal or lobular origin. Ductal carcinomas can then be further subdivided based on specific morphologic features, thereby making numerous variants. The patient's breast mass showed an invasive ductal carcinoma (see Fig. 3.4). Invasive lobular carcinoma, a type of breast

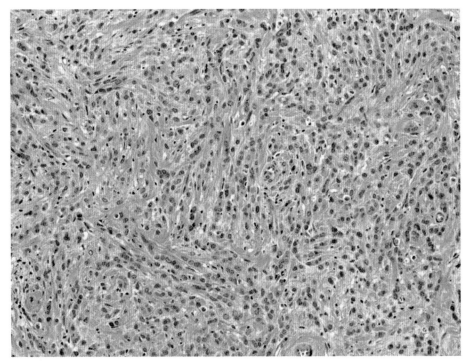

Figure 3.5 Histologic section of invasive lobular carcinoma showing single-file growth of tumor cells (H&E stain).

cancer that does not make tubules, is subdivided into two variants: classic and pleomorphic. Invasive lobular carcinoma tumor cells tend to be noncohesive and have a single-file linear pattern of growth (see Fig. 3.5).

What findings affect the prognosis of breast cancer?

Breast cancer prognosis is affected by the size of the tumor, lymph node status, histologic type and grade of tumor, estrogen and progesterone receptor status, and overexpression of c-erbB2 (HER2/neu). Histologic grading is a powerful indicator of prognosis. The most common grading system used in the United States is the Scarff-Bloom-Richardson (SBR) system. This grading system is based on three morphologic features: formation of tubular/glandular structures, nuclear pleomorphism, and mitotic activity. Seven possible scores are then condensed into three SBR grades, which translate into well, moderately, or poorly differentiated carcinomas.

Based on this scoring system, the patient's tumor is moderately differentiated. Her tumor receptor status is estrogen and progesterone receptor positive with overexpression of HER2/neu 2+ by immunohistochemistry, which was then confirmed negative with fluorescence in situ hybridization (FISH)/fluorescent in situ hybridization (see Figs. 3.6A-C).

CLINICAL PEARL   **STEP 2/3**

More favorable breast carcinomas include pure colloid (mucinous) carcinoma, medullary carcinoma, and tubular carcinoma.

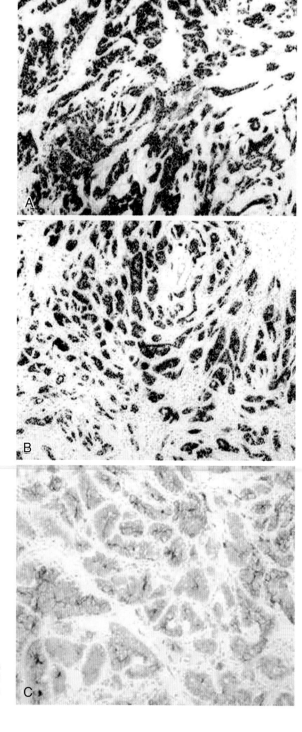

Figure 3.6 Immunoperoxidase stains for **(A)** ER (nuclear stain), **(B)** PR (nuclear stain), and **(C)** HER2/neu (membranous stain), respectively.

CLINICAL PEARL STEP 2/3

HER2/neu overexpression is associated with more aggressive behavior. HER2/neu immunoperoxidase stain is scored as 1+, 2+, or 3+ based on the amount of membranous staining in the tumor cells. 1+ is considered negative, 2+ is considered equivocal, and 3+ is considered positive. A 2+ score can be reflexed to fluorescent in situ hybridization.

What are the patient's treatment options?

Treatment options vary based on the type of tumor and other factors related to the tumor. Treatment can include surgery, radiation, chemotherapy and hormone therapy in any one or more combinations. The patient was stage 2a (T2, N0, Mx). Her treatment included surgery as well as chemotherapy and hormonal therapy.

CLINICAL PEARL STEP 2/3

Estrogen and progesterone receptors are considered positive if there is at least 1% positive tumor nuclei in the tumor sample. Both estrogen and progesterone show nuclear staining patterns.

What is the recommended frequency of screening for breast cancer?

The American Cancer Society recommends an annual breast exam and mammogram for women age 50 and above. For women under 50, a breast exam is recommended every 3 years between the ages of 20 and 40 and annually between the ages of 40 and 50. A baseline mammogram can be performed between 35 and 40 years of age and then every 1 to 2 years between the ages of 40 and 50.

CLINICAL PEARL STEP 3

Women who are at high risk for breast cancer should get an MRI and a mammogram every year. These include:

- Women with a lifetime risk of breast cancer of 20 to 25% or greater
- Women with a known *BRCA1/BRCA2* mutation
- Women with a first-degree relative (parent, sibling, or child) with *BRCA1* or *BRCA2* who have not had testing themselves
- Women who have undergone any radiation to the chest between the ages of 10 and 30 years
- Women who have Li-Fraumeni syndrome, Cowden syndrome, or Bannayan-Riley-Ruvalcaba syndrome, or a first-degree relative with one of these syndromes

BEYOND THE PEARLS

- Fibroadenomas are the most common benign neoplasm in the female breast.
- Ductal carcinoma in situ (DCIS) is a precursor lesion for invasive ductal carcinoma.
- Although rare, breast cancer can occur in men and is most often an invasive ductal carcinoma.
- E-cadherin is a member of transmembrane glycoproteins responsible for the calcium-dependent cell–cell adhesion mechanism.

Continued

BEYOND THE PEARLS—cont'd

- E-cadherin immunoperoxidase stain shows diffuse membrane expression in ductal carcinomas and is negative in lobular carcinomas.
- Invasive lobular carcinoma is the number one entity for false-negative mammographic imaging.
- The American Society of Clinical Oncology and the College of American Pathologists recommend that estrogen and progesterone status be determined on all invasive breast cancers and breast cancer recurrences.
- Trastuzumab was approved by the U.S. Food and Drug Administration in 1998 for use in HER2-positive metastatic tumors.
- HER2 status generally remains unchanged after therapy and in metastatic tumors.

References

Acs G, Lawton TJ, Rebbeck TR, LiVolsi VA, Zhang PJ. Differential expression of E-cadherin in lobular and ductal neoplasms of the breast and its biologic and diagnostic implications. *Am J Clin Pathol.* 2001;115:85-98.

American Cancer Society. *Detailed Guide: Breast Cancer. 2014.* Available at <http://www.cancer.org>. Accessed 08.12.15.

Dabbs D. *Breast Pathology.* Philadelphia: Elsevier Saunders; 2012.

Gokhale S. Ultrasound characterization of breast masses. *Indian J Radiol Imaging.* 2009;19(3):242-247.

Hammond ME, Hayes DF, Dowsett M, et al. American Society of Clinical Oncology/College of American Pathologists guideline recommendations for immunohistochemical testing of estrogen and progesterone receptors in breast cancer. *J Clin Oncol.* 2010;28:2784-2795.

Nida Hamiduzzaman ▧ Joshua Sapkin ▧ Seth Politano ▧ Patrick E. Sarte

A 65-Year-Old Male With Acute Chest Pain

A 65-year-old male with a history of cigarette smoking and essential hypertension presents with chest pain that began 4 hours earlier when he was walking from his office to his car, a distance of two city blocks. The pain improved after he arrived at his car but has persisted since then. It worsened significantly in intensity when he attempted to walk his dog after dinner, and this prompted him to seek medical attention at the emergency department of his local hospital.

What is the differential diagnosis of a patient presenting with acute chest pain?

The main organ systems to consider when an individual presents with acute chest pain include cardiovascular, pulmonary, gastrointestinal, musculoskeletal, and psychiatric. Table 4.1 summarizes the most common causes of acute chest pain as well as their associated symptoms and clinical findings. Differentiating between ischemic and nonischemic causes of acute chest pain is difficult. As such, an ischemic cause of chest pain should be considered unless an alternative diagnosis is apparent. A 12-lead electrocardiogram (ECG) is the appropriate test to look for ST-segment changes, new-onset left bundle branch block, presence of Q waves, and new-onset T-wave inversions.

Clinicians should have a higher suspicion for cardiac ischemia in patients who have identifiable risk factors for coronary artery disease. These risk factors are shown in Table 4.2.

What is angina?

Angina is a manifestation of coronary artery disease that results from an imbalance between myocardial oxygen supply and demand.

This patient presents with typical anginal chest pain. How do you define typical angina?

Typical angina is defined as:
1. Substernal chest discomfort
2. A characteristic quality and duration that is provoked by exertion or emotional stress
3. Relieved by rest or nitroglycerin

Atypical angina meets two of the above characteristics, whereas noncardiac chest pain meets one or none of the typical angina characteristics.

What is unstable angina?

Unstable angina is angina that occurs with longer duration, increasing intensity, or is precipitated by less physical exertion or occurring at rest.

TABLE 4.1 ▓ **Causes of Acute Chest Pain**

Cardiovascular
Acute myocardial infarction
Acute pericarditis
Thoracic aortic dissection
Heart failure

Pulmonary
Pulmonary embolus
Pleurisy
Pneumonitis
Pneumothorax

Gastrointestinal
Gastroesophageal reflux disease
Esophageal spasm
Biliary colic
Acute pancreatitis

Musculoskeletal
Chest wall pain
Costochondritis

Psychiatric
Anxiety states
Panic disorder

TABLE 4.2 ▓ **Risk Factors for Coronary Artery Disease**

- Age: male ≥45; female ≥55
- Family history of premature coronary heart disease (CHD) (either myocardial infarction or sudden death) before age 55 years in a male first-degree relative or before age 65 in a female first-degree relative. Symptomatic cerebrovascular disease (transient ischemic attack [TIA] or cerebrovascular accident [CVA]), aortic aneurysm, and peripheral arterial disease are CHD equivalent states.
- Current cigarette smoking
- Hypertension: blood pressure >140/90 mm Hg or prescribed an antihypertensive medication
- Dyslipidemia: LDL cholesterol >130 mg/dL or HDL cholesterol <40 mg/dL in men or <50 mg/dL in women
- Diabetes
- Obesity
- Sedentary lifestyle

Which aspects of the history and physical exam should be included when evaluating a patient suspected of having an acute myocardial infarction?

The history should include the onset, duration, severity, quality, and radiation of the chest pain. Associated symptoms including nausea, vomiting, diaphoresis, dizziness, and dyspnea should be elicited. To ensure there are no contraindications to therapies that can precipitate intracerebral and gastrointestinal bleeding, inquiries about recent symptoms that could be attributed to a transient ischemic attack, stroke, peptic ulcer, or gastrointestinal bleeding should be made. Careful attention to the vital signs is important to recognize or anticipate complications, including cardiogenic shock. This is most often due to left ventricular dysfunction but can also be due to conduction abnormalities leading to an inappropriately low pulse rate. A thorough cardiopulmonary exam should be performed, looking for signs of heart failure (elevated jugular venous pressure, S3 gallop, inspiratory rales, peripheral edema). A focused neurologic exam should be performed to screen for evidence of a prior stroke.

On physical exam, temperature is 37 °C (98.6 °F), blood pressure is 160/85 mm Hg in bilateral arms, pulse rate is 112/min, and respiration rate is 22/min. The patient appears diaphoretic and in mild distress. The radial and pedal pulses are normal. No jugular venous distention is noted. Cardiac exam reveals tachycardia without murmurs, rubs, or gallops. Lungs are clear to auscultation bilaterally.

Which therapies should this patient receive upon presentation?

Unless there are compelling contraindications, all patients presenting with suspected ischemic chest pain and a presumed acute coronary syndrome should be given supplemental oxygen, aspirin, beta blockers, and nitrates. An initial dose of 325 mg of aspirin should be given, and patients are instructed to chew the aspirin tablet in order to rapidly achieve therapeutic blood levels. Sublingual nitroglycerin 0.4 mg is administered every 5 minutes until alleviation of chest pain. If chest pain is not relieved by sublingual nitroglycerin, nitroglycerin by continuous intravenous infusion may be initiated. Opiate analgesics are also employed as necessary to alleviate chest pain, which decreases the sympathetic response. Beta blockade is achieved by administering 5 mg of metoprolol tartrate intravenously over 3 to 5 minutes for a recommended total dose of 15 mg.

Laboratory results show:
Alanine aminotransferase 75 units/L
Aspartate aminotransferase 90 units/L
Creatinine: 1.0 mg/dL
Troponin: 0.2 ng/mL
The patient's ECG is shown in Figure 4.1.

Diagnosis: ST elevation myocardial infarction

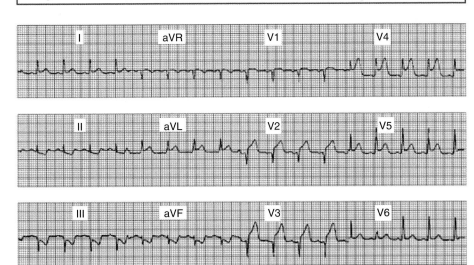

Figure 4.1 ST elevation in a patient with acute myocardial infarction. There are 3 to 4 mm of ST elevation in the anterior leads (V2 through V4), with lesser degrees of ST elevation in the lateral leads (I, aVL, V5, V6). *(From Levine GN. ST segment elevation myocardial infarction. In: Levine GN, ed. Cardiology Secrets. 4th ed. W.B. Saunders: Philadelphia; 2014:135-142.)*

BASIC SCIENCE/CLINICAL PEARL	STEP 1/2/3

In absence of left ventricular hypertrophy (LVH) and left bundle branch block (LBBB): New ST elevation at the J point in ≥2 contiguous leads of ≥2 mm (0.2 mV) in men or ≥1.5 mm (0.15 mV) in women in leads V2-V3 and/or of ≥1 mm (0.1 mV) in other contiguous chest leads or the limb leads.

The J point is the junction between the end of the QRS and the beginning of the ST segment.

CLINICAL PEARL	STEP 2/3

A new LBBB is considered a STEMI equivalent in a patient presenting with symptoms that can be attributed to cardiac ischemia.

How do you manage a patient with an ST-segment elevation myocardial infarction (STEMI)?

In patients with STEMI, reperfusion by primary percutaneous coronary intervention (PCI) is the preferred treatment, as the outcomes are superior to intravenous fibrinolytic therapy. Patients with a STEMI should be treated with PCI within 90 minutes of presentation, the "door to balloon time." If the anticipated wait time from the first medical contact to PCI is anticipated to be greater than 2 hours, intravenous fibrinolytic therapy is the recommended treatment. After receiving primary fibrinolytic therapy, patients should be transferred to a facility capable of performing PCI within 3 to 24 hours.

CLINICAL PEARL	STEP 2/3

Complications of PCI include hematoma, arterial pseudoaneurysm, arteriovenous fistula, and retroperitoneal bleeding.

What medical therapies are used to treat patients with STEMI and why?

In addition to reperfusion therapy, medical therapy for STEMI can be remembered by the mnemonic MONABASH:

M: morphine or analgesics
O: oxygen
N: nitrates
A: antiplatelet agents (aspirin + P2Y12 receptor inhibitors)
B: beta blockers
A: angiotensin-converting enzyme (ACE) inhibitors
S: statin
H: heparin

CLINICAL PEARL	STEP 2/3

The addition of a loading dose of a $P2Y_{12}$ receptor inhibitor (either 600 mg of clopidogrel, 60 mg of prasugrel, or 180 mg of tricagrelor) prior to percutaneous intervention further reduces cardiovascular events. Prasugrel should not be administered to patients with a history of prior transient ischemic attack or stroke due to the increased risk for cerebral hemorrhage.

- Morphine and other opiate analgesics alleviate pain, thereby decreasing the sympathetic nervous system response.
- Oxygen ensures adequate partial pressure of oxygen in the blood.
- Nitrates reduce preload by increasing venous capacitance and improve coronary blood flow by coronary vasodilation.

BASIC SCIENCE/CLINICAL PEARL   **STEP 1/2/3**

Sublingual nitroglycerin should not be given to patients with an inferior wall STEMI or isolated right ventricular infarction due to the increased risk of hypotension. The right ventricle is dependent on preload due to impaired contractility during a STEMI.

- Aspirin inhibits platelet aggregation and improves mortality.
- Beta blockers reduce myocardial oxygen demand and reduce mortality and should be given to all patients. Beta blockers should be held only in patients with new-onset heart failure, systolic blood pressure below 90 mm Hg, bradycardia (<50/min), or second-degree atrioventricular block.
- ACE inhibitors inhibit post myocardial infarction remodeling and help to preserve ventricular function. For patients intolerant of an ACE inhibitor due to cough, an angiotensin receptor blocker should be considered.
- Administer unfractionated heparin in addition to a GP IIb/IIIa receptor antagonist or bivalirudin monotherapy for individuals who are at high risk of bleeding.
- Statins reduce vascular inflammation and stabilize atherosclerotic plaques.

Thrombolytic therapy with fibrin-specific agents is used. The main side effect of thrombolytic therapy is bleeding complications such as intracerebral hemorrhage, bruising at venous puncture sites, hematuria, or gastrointestinal bleeding.

CLINICAL PEARL   **STEP 2/3**

Risk factors for intracerebral hemorrhage include older age, lower body weight, female sex, previous stroke, and systolic blood pressure above 160 mm Hg at presentation.

What are contraindications to thrombolytic therapy?
Contraindications to thrombolytic therapy are shown in Table 4.3 and Table 4.4.

The patient is given oxygen, nitroglycerin 0.4 mg sublingual, and morphine 2 mg for relief of pain. He also is started on a beta blocker and an ACE inhibitor to decrease mortality. In addition, he is given statin, heparin, and GP IIb/IIIa receptor antagonist. He is taken for a PCI within 60 minutes of presentation.

TABLE 4.3 ■ **Absolute Contraindications to Thrombolytic Therapy**

- Any previous intracerebral hemorrhage
- Ischemic stroke within 3 months
- Suspected aortic dissection
- Active bleeding
- Significant closed head or facial trauma within 3 months
- Known cerebrovascular lesion

TABLE 4.4 ▓ **Relative Contraindications to Thrombolytic Therapy**

- History of poorly controlled hypertension
- Active peptic ulcer disease
- Pregnancy
- Current use of anticoagulants
- Recent internal bleeding within 2 to 4 weeks
- History of ischemic stroke more than 3 months ago
- Systolic blood pressure >180 mm Hg or diastolic blood pressure >110 mm Hg on presentation

What complications can occur following STEMI?

Complications that may occur include arrhythmias, heart failure, and vascular complications related to arterial access from PCI. Other complications that may occur include ventricular septal defect, papillary muscle rupture with secondary severe mitral regurgitation, left ventricular free wall rupture, and left ventricular thrombus.

Acute: arrhythmias, hypokinesis or akinesis of one or several ventricular walls, ventricular septal rupture, papillary muscle rupture with severe mitral regurgitation, left ventricular free wall rupture, pericarditis (Dressler's syndrome)

Chronic: ventricular dilation, ventricular thrombus, ventricular aneurysm, arrhythmias (more common with low ejection fraction)

What long-term medical therapies are indicated for individuals who have survived a STEMI?

Aspirin should be continued indefinitely, but the dose can be reduced to 81 mg/day after 4 weeks. Beta blockers and ACE inhibitors should be continued indefinitely unless patients have contra-indications. Patients should receive high-intensity statin therapy (i.e., atorvastatin 40-80 mg or rosuvastatin 20-40 mg daily) following a STEMI. For patients with a drug-eluting or bare metal stent, a P2Y12 receptor inhibitor (either clopidogrel or prasugrel) should also be continued for at least 1 year.

BEYOND THE PEARLS

- In most cases of a new LBBB, prior ECGs are unavailable for comparison, and hence the LBBB is presumed new.
- The presence of Q waves does not distinguish between transmural and nontransmural myocardial infarction.
- Q waves indicate abnormal electrical activity but are not simultaneous with irreversible myocardial damage.
- Posterior STEMI ECGs are often missed and diagnosed as an NSTEMI. Suspicion should be raised when an ECG demonstrates ST depression in leads V1 to V4.
- Isolated right ventricular myocardial infarctions are very rare. They usually occur in conjunction with an inferior wall STEMI. Right ventricular infarction is confirmed by the presence of ST elevation in the right-sided leads (V3R to V6R).
- During an ST-segment elevation myocardial infarction, transthoracic ECG will invariably detect a hypokinesis or akinesis of one or several walls of the ventricles. This finding would be absent in benign early repolarization.

References

Kushner FG, Hand M, Smith SC Jr, et al. Focused updates: ACC/AHA guidelines for the management of patients with ST-elevation myocardial infarction (updating the 2004 guideline and 2007 focused update) and ACC/AHA/SCAI guidelines on percutaneous coronary intervention (updating the 2005 guideline and 2007 focused update): a report of the American College of Cardiology Foundation/American Heart Association Task Force on Practice Guidelines. *Circulation*. 2009;120(22):2271-2306.

O'Gara PT, Kushner FG, Ascheim DD, et al. ACCF/AHA guideline for the management of ST-elevation myocardial infarction: executive summary: a report of the American College of Cardiology Foundation/American Heart Association Task Force on Practice Guidelines. *Circulation*. 2013;127:529-555.

Mark Sims ■ Raj Dasgupta

A 31-Year-Old Male With Human Immunodeficiency Virus, Cough, and Shortness of Breath

A 31-year-old male with a past medical history significant for human immunodeficiency virus (HIV) presents with 2 months of worsening cough and dyspnea on exertion. He was previously diagnosed with community-acquired pneumonia and treated with a 5-day course of azithromycin without improvement.

How is a cough characterized?

Cough is broadly characterized on the basis of duration. Acute cough lasts for less than 3 weeks, subacute cough lasts for 3 to 8 weeks, and chronic cough lasts more than 8 weeks. These designations are helpful, especially in an outpatient setting, as they can focus our differential diagnosis. Acute cough is typically infectious, with upper and lower respiratory tract infections being the most common causes. Subacute and chronic cough have a broader differential. The most common causes of chronic cough are actually benign. These are gastroesophageal reflux disease, cough variant asthma, and upper airway cough syndrome (previously known as postnasal drip). A thorough history and physical exam should elucidate these causes and rule out other more serious underlying disease. The presence of fever, constitutional symptoms, dyspnea on exertion, or hemoptysis should trigger expanded evaluation as these indicate potentially serious pathology. Finally, the age and underlying comorbidities that may alter the differential should be considered.

HIV was diagnosed 4 months prior to admission. The patient takes efavirenz/emtricitabine/tenofovir (Atripla) once a day, trimethoprim/sulfamethoxazole once a day, and azithromycin once a week.

BASIC SCIENCE PEARL	STEP 1

HIV is a single-stranded, positive-sense RNA virus that infects human dendritic cells in the anogenital epithelium. The HIV envelope protein, glycoprotein 120, binds to CD4 and CCR5 or CXCR4 coreceptors to infect helper T cells.

Based on this drug regimen, what can one presume about the patient's HIV status?
As a clinician it is important to be familiar with the indications and uses of prophylactic regimens in HIV patients. Bactrim is used as primary prophylaxis for *Pneumocystis jirovecii* pneumonia (PCP) when the CD4 count is less than 200 and for *Toxoplasmosis gondii* when the CD4 count is less than 100. Azithromycin is used as primary prophylaxis for mycobacterium avium complex when the CD4 count is less than 50. Therefore, one can assume the patient's CD4 count was less than 50 at the time of diagnosis and that he is profoundly immunosuppressed. It is important to note that in certain endemic or resource-limited regions, screening for tuberculosis, histoplasmosis, coccidiomycosis, and cryptococcosis may be necessary.

> The patient denies any other medical or surgical history. He lives in an apartment and recently emigrated from Mexico. He has smoked three cigarettes a day for 10 years, drinks one beer a day, denies intravenous drug use, and is sexually active with multiple male partners. A review of systems is negative.

CLINICAL PEARL   **STEP 2/3**

Certain fungal infections are endemic to geographic locations: coccidiomycosis to southern Arizona and California, blastomycosis to the Mississippi and Ohio River valleys, and histoplasmosis to the midwestern and southeastern United States.

> Physical exam reveals a thin-appearing male in mild distress who is intermittently coughing during exam. The cardiopulmonary exam is normal. Throughout his skin, most notably on his nose and forehead, are raised, violaceous, bulbous plaques. CD4 count performed at diagnosis is 20.

What is the skin lesion pictured in Figure 5.1?
Kaposi sarcoma (KS) is found in advanced HIV. It is a neoplastic, vascular lesion. Initial treatment for this disease is highly active antiretroviral therapy (HAART). However, progression on HAART may necessitate the use of cytotoxic chemotherapy.

What other skin lesion mimics KS?
Bacillary angiomatosis is characterized by similar smaller, red to violet, pedunculated papules. It is caused by *Bartonella* spp. and treated with antibiotic therapy. Definitive diagnosis is by skin biopsy with Warthin–Starry stain showing clumps of tangled, dark bacilli. The skin lesions tend to be faster growing, more numerous, less erythematous, and smaller. Especially if cytotoxic chemotherapy is being considered, this diagnosis should be excluded with skin biopsy.

> A chest radiograph (CXR) is performed.

Describe the findings on the CXR (shown in Fig. 5.2).
The CXR reveals bilateral, scattered, patchy pulmonary infiltrates. There is a predominant mass located in the left lower lobe or lingula of the upper lobe. A lobar infiltrate can be more accurately located. An upper lobe infiltrate will obscure the left heart border and a lower lobe infiltrate will obscure the diaphragm. The same concept is true for the right middle lobe and lower lobe obscuring the right heart border and diaphragm, respectively.

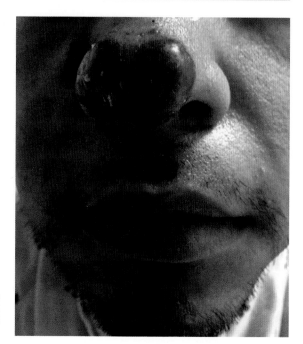

Figure 5.1 Skin lesion on patient's nose. Similar smaller lesions are seen throughout the upper extremity and trunk.

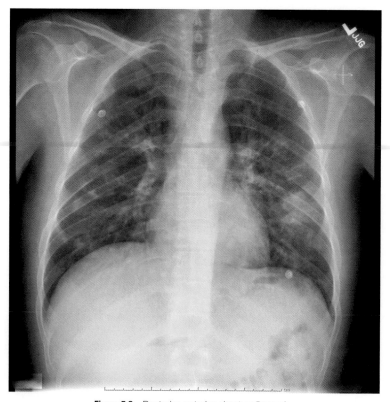

Figure 5.2   Posterior-anterior chest radiograph.

What is the next appropriate step in management?

This patient should be placed in airborne respiratory isolation given the high risk of active pulmonary tuberculosis. The risk of tuberculosis doubles within the first year of diagnosis of HIV. The risk of activation increases with declining immunity such that 1 out of 10 new diagnoses of tuberculosis occur in those with HIV. Respiratory isolation is defined as a single patient, negative pressure room with a double door. All contacts should be trained in the use of an N-95 mask respirator. The "95" refers to the percentage of filtration capacity and is only effective when both the mouth and nose are covered. Whenever the patient is outside of the room for procedures or tests, he or she should wear a surgical mask, and exposure to other patients should be minimized.

CLINICAL PEARL   **STEP 2/3**

Airborne precautions are required for tuberculosis, influenza, measles, varicella, and rubeola. An N-95 mask respirator and negative pressure room are required.

How do you evaluate for and manage a potential case of active tuberculosis?

Tuberculosis in the HIV patient is more likely to present as an acute disease in contrast to the typical chronic course in immunocompetent individuals. Evaluation for active tuberculosis involves the collection of sputum for microscopic evaluation and culture. The Infectious Disease Society of America recommends that three early morning sputum specimens be collected for evaluation. However, as the CD4 count decreases, the yield of sputum for microscopic evaluation decreases and the risk of extrapulmonary tuberculosis increases. Therefore, physicians should have a low suspicion to treat for smear-negative tuberculosis as well as evaluate other sites of involvement for tuberculosis in the HIV patient. Presumptive treatment for tuberculosis may be necessary when a patient is critically ill or when the site of involvement is remote. Remember, there is no utility to either tuberculin skin test *or* interferon gamma release assay in the diagnosis of active tuberculosis. These tests assess for latent tuberculosis in the asymptomatic patient.

> Given the CXR findings, the patient is placed in respiratory isolation to rule out active tuberculosis. Induced sputum for acid-fast bacilli is performed and is negative. Blood cultures are negative. Sputum cultures for typical organisms are negative.

What is the next best step in management?

A computed tomography (CT) scan of the chest with and without contrast is the next best step in management. The results of further imaging can better characterize findings on CXR. There may be subcentimeter or diffuse findings within the lung parenchyma that are not appreciated on CXR. In the immunosuppressed patient, you should have a low threshold for CT of the chest as such patients are more susceptible to atypical infections. Finally, if there is a need for therapeutic or diagnostic intervention, the CT imaging may be used for planning and determination of feasibility.

> Results of CT scan of the chest (see Fig. 5.3) reveal a lesion in the left lingula of the upper lobe as well as numerous pulmonary nodules in the right and left lobes, predominantly in the lower lobes.

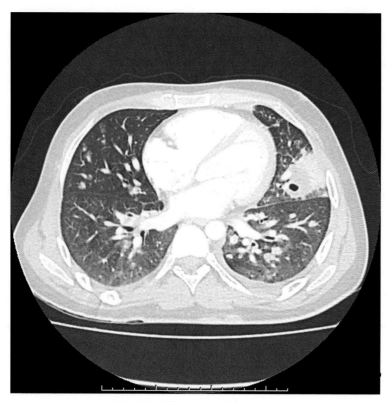

Figure 5.3   CT of chest with contrast.

Describe the lung lesion you see in the left lingula. How does this alter the differential?
The left lingula contains a cavitary lesion suggesting a necrotic lung process. Although bacterial causes are the most common cause of lobar pneumonia in HIV-positive patients (including *Streptococcus pneumoniae,* nontypeable *Haemophilus influenzae,* and *Moraxella catarrhalis*) these are less likely to cavitate. Of the bacterial causes, *Staphylococcus aureus* and *Klebsiella pneumoniae* can cause a cavitary lesion. Given the patient's presumed CD4 count, atypical, fungal, and noninfectious causes should be considered. *Coccidioides immitis, Cryptococcus neoformans, Histoplasma capsulatum, Aspergillus fumigatus, Mycobacterium tuberculosis, Mycobacterium avium* complex, and *Nocardia* spp. should be considered in this patient. In order to evaluate and appropriately treat this patient, it is essential to perform bronchoscopy with biopsy and culture of the cavitary lesion.

During the bronchoscopy, the lesions shown in Figure 5.4 are seen throughout right and left mainstem bronchi.

What are these lesions?
The violaceous, raised lesions seen during bronchoscopy are characteristic of systemic involvement of KS. Caution must be taken during bronchoscopy as these lesions bleed easily given their vascular origin. Acquired immunodeficiency syndrome (AIDS) associated KS can be divided into visceral and cutaneous disease. Visceral disease often involves the oral cavity on the hard palate

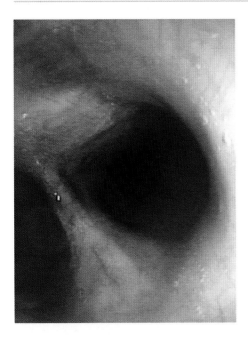

Figure 5.4 Bronchoscopy image at the carina. Similar violaceous lesions were seen throughout the right and left mainstem bronchi.

but can involve other organ systems, including the respiratory tract. Pulmonary involvement in KS may result in dyspnea, hemoptysis, or chest pain or may be asymptomatic.

CLINICAL PEARL   **STEP 2/3**

Gastrointestinal manifestations of KS are not uncommon and may include weight loss, abdominal pain, nausea and vomiting, gastrointestinal bleeding, malabsorption, intestinal obstruction, and diarrhea.

Does this patient require systemic treatment for KS?

This patient meets the clinical criteria for systemic treatment including
- KS mucocutaneous disease
- Compatible features on chest CT
- Endobronchial lesions characteristic of KS

Cytotoxic chemotherapy is used in the treatment of KS only when there is confirmed systemic involvement and no response or progression on HAART therapy.

Skin punch biopsy is performed on a cutaneous lesion.

What confirmatory stain for KS is seen in the pathology slide shown in Figure 5.5?

Human herpesvirus (HHV) 8 immunohistochemical stain is seen in Figure 5.5. HHV-8 is the causative agent in KS. Additionally one sees whorls of spindle-shaped cells with leukocytic infiltration and neovascularization with aberrant proliferation of small blood vessels typical for this neoplastic lesion.

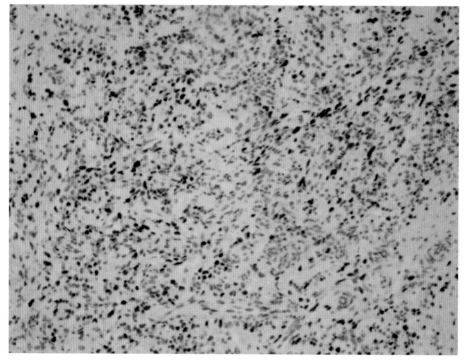

Figure 5.5   Skin punch biopsy of the cutaneous lesion.

BASIC SCIENCE PEARL   **STEP 1**

Vascular endothelial growth factor (VEGF) is a potent mediator of angiogenesis and is implicated in tumor growth, including KS and renal cell carcinoma. Monoclonal antibodies to the VEGF receptor including bevacizumab are used in many chemotherapeutic regimens to prevent tumor angiogenesis.

Does the presence of pulmonary KS in this patient adequately explain his symptoms? What other diagnostic testing can be done during bronchoscopy?

The patient with HIV should be evaluated broadly for infectious agents, neoplasm, and treatment-related complications. These patients are at much higher risk for opportunistic infections, and the presentation and symptoms are not easily distinguished from one another. During bronchoscopy, bronchoalveolar lavage should be performed and sent for cultures. Any suspicious lesions should be biopsied with either endobronchial or transcutaneous approach, especially when the diagnosis is in question or the patient is not responding to therapy.

Bronchoalveolar lavage is performed for fungal, mycobacterial, and aerobic/anaerobic culture. Fungal stain, acid-fast bacilli (AFB) stain and PCP stain are performed. Transbronchial biopsy is performed, the results of which are shown in Figure 5.6.

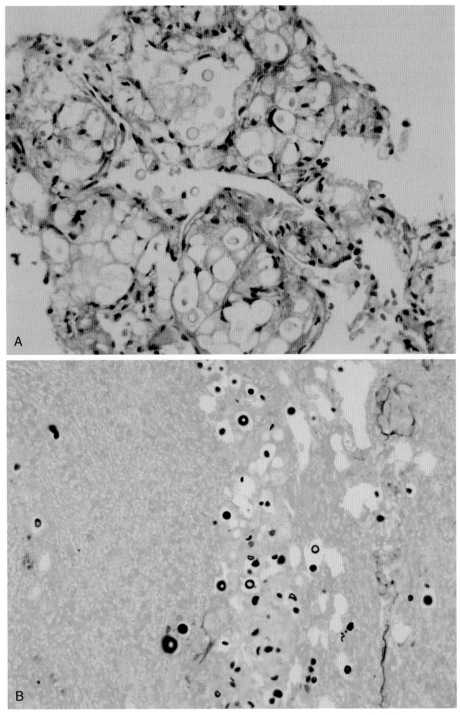

Figure 5.6 A, B, Transbronchial biopsy specimen taken from the left upper lobe lesion.

Interpret the pathology slides.

Figure 5.6A is a hematoxylin and eosin (H&E) stain. The underlying structure of the alveoli and terminal bronchioles reveals inflammatory infiltrate and thickening of the alveolar walls, which are normally one to two cell layers in width. Within the tissue there are multiple yeast forms with a thick and prominent capsule. Figure 5.6B is a Grocott's methenamine silver (GMS) stain. Although the GMS stain is nonspecific for *Cryptococcus*, it does stain the thick cell wall, which is typical for this organism. Confirmatory staining with mucicarmine is done when the morphologic identification is unclear.

Confirmatory fungal culture grows *Cryptococcus neoformans*.

Diagnosis: Kaposi sarcoma with systemic involvement and disseminated *Cryptococcus*

What is the treatment for *Cryptococcus neoformans* pneumonia? What further diagnostic testing is essential prior to initiation of antifungal therapy?

Pulmonary cryptococcosis is more common in immunosuppressed patients, and treatment must address the high rate of progression to disseminated disease. For mild disease, one can consider fluconazole monotherapy with monitoring for dissemination. However, for moderate to severe pulmonary disease, induction therapy with amphotericin B and flucytosine is necessary. This regimen is identical to that used in cryptococcal meningoencephalitis even in the absence of central nervous system disease. Prior to initiating treatment in the immunosuppressed patient, invasive disease must be ruled out with lumbar puncture. Prior to lumbar puncture, neuroimaging should be considered as increased intracranial pressure will contraindicate lumbar puncture.

CLINICAL PEARL   **STEP 2/3**

The side effects of amphotericin ("ampho-terrible") include fever, chills, acute kidney injury, hypokalemia, hypomagnesemia, and acidosis such that it is typically administered with fluids, antihistamines, and antipyretic medications. Closely monitor electrolytes and kidney function when using this potent antifungal.

BASIC SCIENCE PEARL   **STEP 1**

The side effects of amphotericin B are ameliorated by using a liposomal formulation of the parent drug. Decreased binding of the drug to host cellular membranes results in increased bioavailability and reduced toxicity.

A lumbar puncture is performed and is suggestive of cryptococcal meningitis with a positive India ink stain. Subsequent cryptococcal antigen and culture was positive. The patient did well with treatment for both disseminated cryptococcal disease with flucytosine and amphotericin B. He was started on doxorubicin in addition to HAART for AIDS-associated KS.

BEYOND THE PEARLS

- Adherence to highly active antiretroviral therapy (HAART) is essential to avoid developing viral resistance. When testing HIV patients for viral resistance, the patients must be adherent to therapy or the results will show no resistance. Without selective pressure (i.e., HAART) the HIV virus will revert to the wild type.
- High-risk patient populations, including men who have sex with men, serodiscordant partners, injection drug users, and those with a history of multiple sexually transmitted infections, should be offered preexposure prophylaxis (PREP). PREP, usually in the form of Truvada (tenofovir/emtricitabine) daily therapy, can greatly reduce the risk of acquiring HIV.
- *Nocardia* is notoriously difficult to culture but may be recognized by its weak acid-fast staining. It is often confused with its cousin, *Actinomyces*. Think of *Nocardia* infection in transplant, chronic glucocorticoid therapy, and malignancy patients with atypical pulmonary, central nervous system, and skin manifestations.
- HHV-8 is the causative agent of two other rare entities aside from KS. Primary effusion lymphoma presents in advanced HIV with pleural, pericardial, or peritoneal malignancy. Multicentric Castleman's disease presents with diffuse lymphadenopathy, constitutional symptoms, immune thrombocytopenia, autoimmune hemolytic anemia, acquired factor VIII deficiency, and, not uncommonly, KS.
- *Cryptococcus gattii* is a distinct species apart from *neoformans* and more commonly causes cryptococcal meningitis in immunocompetent hosts. These patients may have a severe clinical course marked by treatment failure. Most microbiology laboratories, however, are unable to distinguish the two species in routine fungal culture.
- Cardiotoxicity is a well-known adverse effect of doxorubicin and anthracycline-based chemotherapy. Although age, concomitant radiation therapy, and prior cardiac disease are risk factors, the single most important risk factor is a cumulative dose >500 mg/m^2. Pretreatment assessment of cardiac function should be considered in patients receiving this medication.

References

Gbabe OF, Okwundu CI, Dedicoat M, Freeman EE. Treatment of severe or progressive Kaposi's sarcoma in HIV-infected adults. *Cochrane Database Syst Rev*. 2014;(8):CD003256, doi: 10.1002/14651858. CD003256.pub2.

Guidelines for Prevention and Treatment of Opportunistic Infections in HIV-Infected Adults and Adolescents. Recommendations from the Centers for Disease Control and Prevention, the National Institutes of Health, and the HIV Medicine Association of the Infectious Diseases Society of America. *Updated April 16, 2015*. Available at <http://aidsinfo.nih.gov/guidelines>. Accessed 08.12.15.

Lin CY, Sun HY, Chen MY, et al. Aetiology of cavitary lung lesions in patients with HIV infection. *HIV Med*. 2009;10:191-198.

Perfect JR, Dismukes WE, Dromer F, et al. Clinical practice guidelines for the management of cryptococcal disease: 2010 update by the infectious diseases society of america. *Clin Infect Dis*. 2010;50:291-322.

World Health Organization. *International Standards for Tuberculosis Care (Endorsed by IDSA) Web site*. Available at <http://www.idsociety.org/Organism/#HIV/AIDS>; January 2006. Accessed 08.12.15.

Albert Huang ■ John Khoury

A 54-Year-Old Male With Worsening Weakness

A 54-year-old male presents with weakness that has been worsening over the past several days. He first noticed trouble with walking and was frequently tripping earlier in the week. Since then, there has been noticeable weakness in his legs. He also noticed increased weakness in his hands and has been dropping objects more frequently. This morning, he awoke unable to get out of bed or stand. His wife called 911 and emergency medical services transported him to this hospital. He has never had issues with weakness or walking in the past and suffers from high blood pressure, which is currently managed with metoprolol.

In evaluating worsening lower extremity weakness, what types of questions are important to ask first?

The causes of lower extremity weakness can be broad, and it is important to be aware of conditions that necessitate emergency management. Traumatic spinal cord injury can result in myelopathy, pararparesis, and bowel and bladder symptoms. The patient should be asked of any recent falls or accidents, history of low back pain and vertebral disc herniation, as well as new bowel or bladder symptoms. If the injury is due to a vertebral fracture or dislocation, immediate neurosurgical management may be needed for decompression and possible fusion of the involved vertebrae.

Onset and timing of the weakness can assist in narrowing down the possible causes. Sudden and severe weakness suggests an associated trauma resulting in acute spinal cord compression. It could also suggest a vascular etiology such as an acute infarction, arteriovenous (AV) malformation, or acute hemorrhage involving the spinal cord. A gradual onset and subacute course of weakness can suggest an inflammatory cause (multiple sclerosis, transverse myelitis, or Guillain-Barré syndrome), spinal abscess, neoplasm, or compressive disc herniation. A slow and insidious progression of weakness can indicate a metabolic process associated with peripheral neuropathy such as diabetes, vitamin B12 deficiency, or a paraneoplastic process.

Determining if and when sensation is affected can provide further insight into the etiology of the weakness. A pure myopathic process should not present with associated sensory symptoms. Conditions that affect the neuromuscular junction, such as botulism and myasthenia gravis, would also lack sensory impairment. Numbness or decreased sensation preceding weakness suggests a neuropathic process such as diabetic neuropathy because sensory nerve fibers tend to be smaller and more prone to metabolic damage before larger nerve fibers that innervate muscles. Decreased or absent sensation occurring simultaneously with severe weakness may indicate a concurrent process affecting a similar system such as an upper motor neuron process involving the brain or spinal cord.

BASIC SCIENCE/CLINICAL PEARL   **STEP 1/2/3**

The time of year can add potential diagnoses not otherwise considered. For example, summer months bring mosquitos and specifically ones that can transmit West Nile virus (WNV). This arbovirus is capable of causing neurologic impairments including weakness and should be considered in the differential depending on the time of year as well as areas where WNV is prevalent, such as the west and central parts of the continental United States.

Upon further questioning, the patient denies additional medical history or surgeries. He is an architect and travels often to construction sites. On the review of systems, he notes a recent gastrointestinal (GI) illness 2 weeks prior when he was unable to keep down food for 2 days. He denies recent changes in weight, fever, rashes, chest pain, shortness of breath, abdominal pain, nausea, vomiting, and back pain. He also denies any recent falls or traumatic injuries.

What questions on the review of systems are also important to note in this case?
Considering the severe and progressive nature of the patient's weakness, respiratory status must be noted. Symptoms that would be concerning for respiratory compromise include impaired swallowing and difficulty coughing. Fever and other signs of infection can point toward the presence of a spinal abscess. Unexplained weight loss and increased fatigue can point toward a neoplastic process such as a tumor or metastatic lesions. The presence of a rash, muscular pain, or viral symptoms could suggest an autoimmune cause for weakness, such as dermatomyositis, polymyositis, or polymyalgia rheumatica.

On exam, the patient's oral temperature is 36.8 °C (98.3 °F), pulse rate is 95/min, blood pressure is 134/90 mm Hg, and respiration rate is 18/min. The head/eyes/ear/nose/throat exam is unremarkable. The cardiac exam is S1/S2 without additional sounds. The pulmonary exam is clear to auscultation bilaterally. His abdomen is soft and palpation is negative for tenderness or masses. The strength in his arms is 4+/5 on abduction of shoulders, 4/5 on elbow flexion, and his grip strength is 3/5. Strength in his legs is 3/5 on hip flexion, 2/5 on knee extension, and 0/5 on ankle plantar flexion. Reflexes are absent at the wrist and Achilles tendons, and Babinski's sign is absent. Sensation is symmetric to light touch but slightly diminished throughout his arms and legs when compared to his face.

BASIC SCIENCE/CLINICAL PEARL   **STEP 1/2/3**

When testing sensation, it is important to establish a normal reference point. For example, a high cervical spinal cord lesion could affect sensation in both upper and lower extremities equally and make mild paresthesia difficult to detect if each arm or leg is compared against another one. If there is reasonable concern that sensation is affected, an alternative reference point can be used such as the chest or face.

How is muscle strength assessed and graded on physical exam?
Muscle strength is graded from 0 to 5 and uses examiner-provided resistance and then gravity as references. A 5 is given for full and normal muscle strength, which the examiner is unable to break. A grade of 4 represents muscle strength where the patient is able to partially resist the examiner. Grade 3 is when the patient is unable to resist the examiner but able to move the limb against gravity through a full range of motion. A grade of 2 represents full range of motion with

gravity eliminated. An example of grade 2 is movement along the plane of a bed, but not up and off of it. A grade of 1 is given to trace muscle movement or contractions, and a grade of 0 is when no muscle contractions are detectable. A + or − may also be added to the numerical grade and represents strength slightly greater or less than the associated numerical grade.

What signs are concerning for respiratory compromise in acute neuromuscular disease?
When evaluating worsening or rapidly progressive neuromuscular disease, it is important to determine whether the muscles of respiration are involved. They can be grouped into the upper airway muscles, muscles of inspiration, and muscles of expiration. A bulbar palsy can lead to impaired swallowing, and weakness involving the muscles of expiration can result in difficulty clearing secretions. Both of these conditions put a patient at risk for an aspiration pneumonia. Issues with inspiratory muscles can result in impaired lung expansion, ventilation/perfusion mismatch, and difficulty with adequate oxygenation. Symptoms to be aware of include severe and rapidly worsening generalized weakness, dysphagia, dysphonia, new dyspnea with exertion or rest, and trouble swallowing. Signs signaling the need for admission to a monitored setting include rapid and shallow breathing, tachycardia, accessory muscle use, and orthopnea. Although patients can be monitored with telemetry, the rapid nature of neuromuscular disease easily warrants care in an intensive care unit (ICU) should there be any concern regarding the patient's breathing.

What is the differential diagnosis at this point?
This patient presents with progressive, symmetric muscle weakness, associated with depressed reflexes and sensory deficits. The involvement of the sensory systems rules out causes isolated to the neuromuscular junction, such as myasthenia gravis, botulism, and Lambert-Eaton myasthenic syndrome, or to the muscle, such as a drug-induced myopathy, dermatomyositis, or polymyositis. Knowing the motor symptoms are more severe than the sensory symptoms, potential conditions include an acute inflammatory demyelinating polyneuropathy (AIDP or Guillain-Barré syndrome), chronic inflammatory demyelinating polyneuropathy (CIDP), acquired immunodeficiency syndrome (AIDS), neuroinvasive form of a West Nile virus infection, and lead poisoning. Looking at spinal causes, weakness affecting primarily the legs suggest involvement of the thoracic or lumbar cord. Upper and lower extremity weakness makes involvement of the cervical levels more likely. Possible diagnoses include transverse myelitis, neoplasm (primary or metastatic), abscess, traumatic spinal artery infarction, or severe disc herniation. Cerebral causes of weakness include embolic ischemia with bilateral involvement and acute hydrocephalus.

Initial laboratory studies are presented in Table 6.1. A computed tomography (CT) scan of the patient's head is unremarkable. Magnetic resonance imaging (MRI) of the patient's head along with his cervical, thoracic, lumbar, and sacral spine is also unremarkable. A lumbar puncture is performed and the opening pressure is recorded as 172 mm H_2O. A sample of the patient's cerebrospinal fluid (CSF) is sent for analysis and presented in Table 6.2. An electromyography/nerve conduction study (EMG/NCS) reveals evidence of acute demyelinating lesions affecting both arms and legs.

BASIC SCIENCE/CLINICAL PEARL   **STEP 1/2/3**

When ordering diagnostic imaging of the spine to evaluate for lower extremity symptoms, do not forget to include thoracic imaging in addition to lumbar imaging if there is concern for an upper motor neuron lesion. If the patient has upper extremity symptoms, the cervical spine should be imaged as well.

TABLE 6.1 ■ Initial Laboratory Tests

White blood count (4.0-11.0)	6200/μL
Hemaglobin (12.0-16.0)	14.5 g/dL
Hematocrit (35.0-47.0)	43.5%
Platelets (140-440)	311,000/μL
aPTT (24-37)	32
International normalized ratio (0.90-1.10)	0.92
Complete metabolic panel	Normal

aPTT, Activated partial thromboplastin time.

TABLE 6.2 ■ Cerebral Spinal Fluid Laboratory Results

Appearance (clear)	Clear
RBC count (<1 cell/μL)	0 cells/μL
WBC count (0-5 cells/μL)	0 cells/μL
Glucose (>60% of serum glucose)	Normal
Protein (<45 mg/dL)	105 mg/dL
Bacterial and viral cultures (negative)	Pending

How should interpretation of the CSF be approached?
A lumbar puncture for spinal fluid provides diagnostic information starting from the opening pressure to visual characterization of the spinal fluid in addition to laboratory analysis. In adults, a normal pressure can be as high as 200 mm H_2O, and if the patient is obese 250 mm H_2O. Elevated CSF pressures can indicate the presence of tumor or infection. Xanthochromia, which is discoloration of normally clear CSF, can also be concerning for pathology. A pink or orange color suggests the presence of blood products related to either intracranial hemorrhage or a traumatic tap. Yellowish discoloration can suggest the presence of blood as well as increased protein levels. Standard laboratory tests include cell counts with white cell differential, protein level, and ratio of the glucose in the CSF compared to serum. An elevated white cell count can indicate the presence of infection. Counts less than 100 per mm^3 can be associated with viral infection, whereas counts above 1000 per mm^3 are typically associated with bacterial infections. On the other hand, fungal CSF infection can present with variable counts and can complicate interpretation. For definite diagnosis of an infection, a positive culture is necessary. An elevated protein level is a nonspecific indicator of a neoplasm, inflammation, demyelination, spinal block, or infection. The introduction of blood, whether by traumatic tap or hemorrhage, can also elevate the protein level and requires correction. Additional tests can be ordered for culture or polymerase chain reaction (PCR) to detect the presence of a bacterial, viral, or fungal infection.

What objective studies can be performed to assess the need for intubation?
Several studies can be performed at the bedside to closely monitor for pulmonary failure and the potential need for intubation and mechanical ventilation. The vital capacity (VC) is the volume of air the patient is able to move in and out of the body. A normal VC is approximately 60 to 70 mL/kg. Although a volume of 15 mL/kg is considered the absolute value for mechanical ventilation, it is reasonable to intubate at 20 mL/kg due to the rapid progression of neuromuscular

diseases. The maximum inspiratory (P_{Imax}) and expiratory (P_{Emax}) pressures can also provide objective evidence for the need to intubate. A P_{Imax} greater than −30 cm H_2O and P_{Emax} less than 40 cm H_2O can indicate whether intubation and mechanical ventilation will be necessary.

BASIC SCIENCE/CLINICAL PEARL   **STEP 1/2/3**

The decision to intubate should typically be made earlier than later to allow for a controlled environment and avoidance of complications. Specific to the neuromuscular disease Guillain-Barré syndrome (GBS), patients who are severe enough to require intubation typically have associated dysautonomic symptoms such as bradycardia, changes in blood pressure, and anesthesia-related hypotension.

Diagnosis: Acute inflammatory demyelinating polyneuropathy—Guillain-Barré syndrome

---

How is Guillain-Barré syndrome (GBS) characterized?

The classic description of GBS is an ascending paralysis that is symmetric and progressive. It is accompanied by significantly depressed or absent reflexes and generally lacks notable sensory deficits. The symptoms progress quickly and reach their peak around 2 to 4 weeks. It is typically described as an ascending weakness starting in the legs and then up through the arms. In severe cases, it can affect the respiratory and bulbar musculature. Different forms can result in asymmetrical weakness and varying levels of sensory loss.

In the past, different presentations of GBS have been thought of as varied forms with similar pathology. It is currently known as an autoimmune condition in which each variant is caused by a different set of antibodies. Three notable forms are inflammatory demyelinating polyneuropathy, axonal neuropathy, and Miller Fisher syndrome (MFS). Acute inflammatory demyelinating polyneuropathy (AIDP) and the chronic form (CIDP) are more commonly seen in the United States and Europe. GBS primarily affects the myelin sheath of the motor neuron. An axonal form of destruction has been termed acute motor axonal neuropathy (AMAN) and its more severe counterpart acute motor sensory axonal neuropathy (AMSAN). This form is more commonly seen in Northern China and Japan. The third presentation, MFS, consists of the triad of ophthalmoplegia, ataxia, and areflexia. MFS can be associated with weakness of the limbs, although it is not necessary for diagnosis.

CLINICAL PEARL   **STEP 2/3**

A common feature associated with GBS is back, radicular, and neuropathic pain, which can mistakenly suggest a spinal cause of weakness such as severe disc herniation. Other associated features include urinary retention and gastrointestinal dysfunction, which may initially be attributed to cauda equine or a spinal cord lesion.

What are the expected diagnostic findings associated with GBS?

Because GBS primarily affects the peripheral nerves, the initial studies can be unremarkable. Laboratory studies and diagnostic imaging with CT and MRI may be relatively normal. At best, there may be a slight elevation in creatinine kinase. The notable hallmark is albuminocytologic dissociation seen in the CSF fluid with significantly elevated protein levels and normal white blood cell count. Electrodiagnostic studies can identify the presence of demyelination characteristic of AIDP or axonal damage consistent with AMAN or AMSAN.

What infections have been associated with GBS?

Although many instances of GBS lack a preceding cause, a viral illness, either respiratory or gastrointestinal, can occur prior to the onset of weakness. Epstein-Barr virus and cytomegalovirus have been previously identified as a precursor, and *Campylobacter jejuni (C. jejuni)* is typically associated with AMAN or AMSAN. Patients with initial *C. jejuni* gastroenteritis usually develop symptoms of GBS over a week later. Although stool cultures may be negative at the time of presentation, serum studies will still show evidence of recent infection.

How is acute treatment approached?

There are two options for direct management of GBS. Plasmapheresis was the first treatment shown to be effective in reducing time required on mechanical ventilation. It has also been shown to improve recovery time and increase functional muscle strength sooner as patients are able to walk earlier. The treatment consists of removing the patient's plasma and replacing it with fresh albumin or fresh frozen plasma. Due to the large volume that is replaced, there is the potential for blood pressure shifts and hypotension. Care must be taken when performing plasmapheresis in patients with GBS due to the presence of autonomic dysfunction and risk for labile blood pressure and orthostatic hypotension.

More recently, treatment with intravenous immunoglobulin (IVIG) has demonstrated equivalent efficacy to plasmapheresis with similar outcomes. It can be administered over the course of 2 to 5 days and does not require the resources necessary for plasmapheresis. Thus, IVIG can be provided in smaller hospitals and is more widely available. In addition, it is better tolerated, and complications related to dysautonomia and plasmapheresis are not a concern because a large volume of plasma does not need to be exchanged.

Close monitoring may be necessary to assess for impending respiratory failure. It is important to place the patient in a bed with telemetry or in the ICU, especially if intubation is anticipated. Older age, rapid progression of symptoms, and infection with *C. jejuni* are indicators of poor prognosis. Symptoms of dysphagia or a hoarse and changed voice suggest bulbar involvement. Monitoring of vital capacity and maximum inspiratory and expiratory pressures as discussed above are objective measures that can signal the need for intubation.

Only a small percentage of people die from complications related to GBS, and prognosis can be good with close monitoring, supportive care, and treatment with IVIG or plasmapheresis. Despite severe quadraparesis, the need for mechanical ventilation, and even tracheostomy, patients can still make excellent recoveries and eventually return home with assistance and potentially achieve independent function again.

How does CIDP compare to AIDP?

CIDP is part of a temporal continuum with AIDP. With AIDP, the nadir or peak severity of weakness usually occurs around 2 to 4 weeks after onset. If it continues to worsen beyond 8 weeks, it is considered CIDP. Between 4 and 8 weeks, it is in a subacute inflammatory stage. Unlike AIDP, which presents as an isolated event, CIDP can have a relapsing/remitting-type progression typically seen in younger individuals or a slow and progressive course more common in older individuals. The slower progression can make misdiagnosis more common, particularly in providers unfamiliar with the chronic form of this polyneuropathy. When seen under microscopy, the nerves of a relapsing/remitting form of CIDP may display an onion-bulb appearance similar to other neuropathies that demonstrate a demyelinating/remyelinating course.

How should rehabilitation be approached?

As previously discussed, patients with severe symptoms can make excellent recoveries and potentially walk and become functionally independent. Thus, it is important to initiate early preventive measures. Because quadraparesis can limit a patient's bed mobility and ability to roll in bed, it is important to initiate measures to prevent pressure ulcers. An appropriate pressure relief mattress should be ordered and nursing instructed to turn the patient at least every 2 hours. Physical and occupational therapy (PT and OT) can provide additional services at the bedside such as passive range of motion to prevent tendon shortening and splinting to avoid nerve compression injuries, both of which can limit the ability to transfer and walk when strength returns.

Once the patient begins to show increasing signs of mobility, bedside PT and OT can continue for early mobility training. Upon discharge from the acute care hospital, an inpatient rehabilitation facility (IRF) should be strongly considered for postacute care in severe cases where the patient can receive a coordinated multidisciplinary approach to their care. Furthermore, a physician with rehabilitation expertise provides additional oversight and frequently assesses for common comorbid conditions such as persistent pain, depression, and fatigue.

The patient is admitted to the ICU where he is closely monitored for respiratory compromise. A course of IVIG is started. His paralysis worsens with involvement of his arms and results in quadraparesis. An appropriate pressure relief mattress is ordered and nursing is instructed to turn him every 2 hours for prevention of decubitus ulcers. Bedside PT and OT is ordered for splinting and range of motion as tolerated by the patient. Due to worsening respiratory function, he is intubated and requires a short course of mechanical ventilation. He eventually recovers over the course of 3 to 4 weeks and is discharged to an acute IRF to continue his functional recovery.

BEYOND THE PEARLS

- Because muscle strength grading depends on examiner strength, it is relative and subjective. A petite individual as compared to a stronger individual would provide varied levels of resistance, thus making the grading from 5 and 4 relative.
- The presence of an intracranial mass or increased pressure from hydrocephalus typically prompts concern for uncal herniation when performing a lumbar puncture. A CT of the head is typically recommended prior to a lumbar puncture to assess for intracranial pathology, which can increase the risk for herniation, particularly when evaluating for a central cause of infection. However, opinions vary regarding the true risk due to reevaluation of the literature, which includes retrospective review autopsies that failed to show the presence of cerebral herniation as a cause of death in patients who died following a lumbar puncture.
- Although the act of drawing three consecutive tubes when performing a lumbar puncture is a commonplace method to evaluate for a traumatic tap, literature does not support the presence of diminishing red blood cell count as absolute evidence of a traumatic tap. If bleeding is still a concern, clear CSF fluid obtained one level above the first can confirm the first was traumatic.
- One proposed mechanism for GBS is that the initial viral infection leads to production of antibodies, which cross-react with the components of the nerve relative to the variant of GBS, such as the myelin sheath, axon, or possibly the spinal roots. Despite similarities among the different variants of GBS, a common antibody has yet to be discovered, and different antibodies attack different gangliosides in each form.

BEYOND THE PEARLS—cont'd

- In addition to viral infections, GBS has been identified following vaccinations. The first instance was during the administration of swine flu vaccine in 1976. There was also an increase in GBS cases following influenza immunizations in the 1990s and H1N1 in late 2000. However, considering the rare incidence and risk of GBS following these vaccinations and the benefit of immunizations, vaccination is still generally recommended. Epidemiological studies assessing the incidence of GBS following influenza vaccination found approximately 1 GBS case per 1 million vaccinations, but cause and effect is not well established. Furthermore, some studies suggest no association between GBS and influenza vaccinations.
- The sural nerve is commonly identified for biopsy to diagnose CIDP. However, it may not be affected in all cases of CIDP. Care should be given in determining whether the sural nerve is adequately affected or in selecting a nerve that is affected but still functional as evidenced by electrodiagnostic testing. Other potential nerve biopsy candidates include the superficial peroneal and superficial radial nerves.

References

Alshekhlee A, Hussain Z, Sultan B, Katirji B. Guillain-Barré syndrome: incidence and mortality rates in US hospitals. *Neurology.* 2008;70(18):1608.

Baxter R, Lewis N, Bakshi N, et al; CISA Network. Recurrent Guillain-Barré syndrome following vaccination. *Clin Infect Dis.* 2012;54:800.

Dimachkie MM, Barohn RJ. Guillain-Barré syndrome and variants. *Neurol Clin.* 2013;31(2):491-510.

Edlow JA, Caplan LR. Avoiding pitfalls in the diagnosis of subarachnoid hemorrhage. *N Engl J Med.* 2000;342(1):29-36.

Hughes RA, Charlton J, Latinovic R, Gulliford MC. No association between immunization and Guillain-Barré syndrome in the United Kingdom, 1992 to 2000. *Arch Intern Med.* 2006;66:1301.

Hughes RA, Cornblath DR. Guillain-Barré syndrome. *Lancet.* 2005;366(9497):1653-1666.

Lasky T, Terracciano GJ, Magder L, et al. The Guillain-Barré syndrome and the 1992-1993 and 1993-1994 influenza vaccines. *N Engl J Med.* 1998;339(25):1797-1802.

Mehta S. Neuromuscular disease causing acute respiratory failure. *Respir Care.* 2006;51(9):1016-1021.

Meythaler JM. Rehabilitation of Guillain-Barré syndrome. *Arch Phys Med Rehabil.* 1997;78:872-879.

Orlikowski D, Prigent H, Sharshar T, Lofaso F, Raphael JC. Respiratory dysfunction in Guillain-Barré syndrome. *Neurocrit Care.* 2004;1(4):412-422.

Roos KL, Tunkel AR, eds. *Handbook of Clinical Neurology.* 3rd series. Vol. 96. Elsevier; 2010.

Ryerson LZ, Herbert J, Howard J, Kister I. Adult-onset spastic paraparesis: an approach to diagnostic work-up. *J Neurol Sci.* 2014;346:43-50.

Welch H, Hasbun R. Lumbar puncture and cerebrospinal fluid analysis. In: Aminoff MJ, Boller F, Swaab DF, eds. *Bacterial Infections of the Central Nervous System.* Edinburgh, London: Elsevier; 2010.

Arthur Jeng ▪ Arzhang Cyrus Javan

A 56-Year-Old Male With 3 Weeks of Fever

A 56-year-old male presents to the emergency room with complaints of fevers and chills for the past 3 weeks. Otherwise, his review of systems is negative for headache, cough, shortness of breath, abdominal pain, dysuria, urinary frequency or urgency, or back/flank pain. Vital signs reveal his temperature is 39.1 °C (102.4 °F), pulse rate is 118/min, blood pressure is 154/80 mm Hg, and respiration rate is 17/min. Physical exam is normal, with a cardiac exam showing tachycardia but otherwise regular rhythm and no rubs or murmurs. His laboratory data are shown in Table 7.1. The emergency room physician admits the patient for pyelonephritis based on the abnormal urinalysis (UA).

What do you think about his admission diagnosis?

This patient has fevers but a paucity of other symptoms. Although pyelonephritis can cause fevers, he does not have any symptoms of either pyelonephritis (flank pain, nausea) or lower urinary tract infection (UTI) (dysuria, urinary frequency/urgency). Additionally, the UA does not demonstrate significant pyuria. Therefore, despite being labeled with the diagnosis of pyelonephritis, it is unlikely the reason for his fevers, and additional investigation needs to be performed.

What is the differential diagnosis?

The differential diagnoses should include causes of subacute chronic fevers with a paucity of symptoms. This would include subacute bacterial endocarditis, indolent infections such as extrapulmonary tuberculosis, brucellosis (undulant fever), Q fever, typhoid fever, typhus (from *Rickettsia*), certain cancers (especially lymphoma, leukemia, and renal cell carcinoma), and autoimmune diseases. Human immunodeficiency virus (HIV)/acquired immunodeficiency syndrome (AIDS) can allow opportunistic organisms, such as *Cryptococcus,* cytomegalovirus (CMV), and *Mycobacterium avium* complex to cause fever with no localizing symptoms. It may also predispose patients to febrile noninfectious processes such as multicentric Castleman's disease and lymphoma.

Which other tests should be ordered?

- **Blood culture:** Two or more sets of blood cultures are essential for the initial evaluation of fever of uncertain origin. Blood cultures are the key diagnostic study for infective endocarditis, and they can also diagnose less common infections that one may not be considering, such as *Brucella* and *Cryptococcus.*
- **Computed tomography (CT) scans:** If all workup, including cultures, have been unrevealing, CT scans of the body (chest, abdomen, pelvis) are indicated, as these scans can evaluate for occult infections (e.g., abscesses of the liver, intestinal region, adnexa in women and prostate in men, evidence of tuberculosis), masses concerning for malignancy (lymph node enlargement, liver/kidney masses, bony metastases), and signs of collagen vascular diseases (inflammation of the lungs and serosal linings).

TABLE 7.1 ▓ Initial Laboratory Tests

Leukocyte count	9000/µL
Hemoglobin	14.2 g/dL
Platelet count	476,000/µL
Leukocyte differential	75% neutrophils, 20% lymphocytes, 5% monocytes
Serum creatinine	0.6 mg/dL
Liver function tests	Normal
Sedimentation rate	78 (elevated)
Urinalysis	pH 6.5, 1+leukocyte esterase, 10 white blood cells

- **HIV test:** The Centers for Disease Control and Prevention (CDC) recommends that all patients in the health care system have an HIV screen. This screening test is even more critical in patients who have fever of uncertain origin, as opportunistic infections need to be evaluated if they are found to have HIV.

On hospital day 2, the urine culture demonstrates 50,000 colony forming units (cfu)/mL of *Streptococcus viridans* group. Someone from your team sees this result and comments that your patient has a UTI with *S. viridans* as the pathogen.

What do you think about this diagnosis?
To diagnose a UTI, three factors need to be satisfied:
1. Symptoms consistent with a UTI
2. Significant pyuria
3. Significant bacteriuria with a bacteria that causes UTIs
Because *S. viridans* does not cause UTIs and the patient does not have UTI symptoms, this is not the diagnosis. The bacteriuria is either a contaminant, or it is reflecting bacteremia (the nephrons filter the blood, often leading to pathogens leaking from blood into the urine).

CLINICAL PEARL	**STEP 2/3**

The other bacteria where this mistake is commonly made is *Staphylococcus aureus (S. aureus)*. When *S. aureus* is found in the urine, it is unlikely to represent an *S. aureus* UTI, as these bacteria do not commonly cause UTIs (in the absence of a urinary catheter or other prostheses in the urinary tract). It should prompt the clinician to evaluate for bacteremia with *S. aureus,* with subsequent leakage from blood to urine, as in this case.

Later that day, the microbiology lab technician calls you and reports that four of four blood culture bottles are growing gram-positive cocci in chains. The bacteria are subsequently identified as being in the *S. viridans* group.

What is the likely diagnosis now, and what other tests should you order?
The microbiology data show significant bacteremia within *S. viridans* group, making subacute bacterial endocarditis the most likely diagnosis.

CLINICAL PEARL   **STEP 2/3**

Subacute bacterial endocarditis, which can progress for weeks or months before the patient seeks medical care, is most commonly caused by *S. viridans* group, followed by *Enterococcus* and other streptococci (e.g., *Streptococcus gallolyticus*). These pathogens prefer to adhere to previously damaged or abnormal valves (e.g., rheumatic, prosthetic, congenitally or acquired abnormal valves), primarily through bacteremia from endogenous tissue disruption/manipulation (e.g., odontogenic procedures or intestinal mucosal breach). In contrast, *S. aureus* can cause acute infective endocarditis, with clinical progression over days, and it is associated with rapid valve destruction and/or development of complications. Although *S. aureus* does have a predilection to infect previously abnormal/damaged valves, it is also well known to adhere to normal valves. Especially in industrialized societies, *S. aureus* has become the most common cause of infective endocarditis, either as a result of intravenous drug use or through secondary bacteremia from venous catheters (e.g., central venous lines, PermCath dialysis catheters).

As such, the patient needs an echocardiogram to evaluate for cardiac vegetations and any complications, including valvular dehiscence and/or myocardial/perivalvular abscess. In most hospitals, the initial echocardiogram to obtain is the transthoracic echocardiogram (TTE), as this is a noninvasive study that can be obtained very quickly. The modified Duke criteria can be used to assist in the evaluation and diagnosis of infective endocarditis (Table 7.2). A list of typical organisms that cause infective endocarditis is shown in Table 7.3. When a patient has infective endocarditis but the blood cultures do not grow any organisms, it is called culture-negative infective endocarditis. These pathogens are uncommon causes of infective endocarditis (Table 7.4) and require further evaluation through serology or PCR to establish a microbiological diagnosis. Detailed history-taking may uncover epidemiologic risk factors for acquiring one of these pathogens.

CLINICAL PEARL   **STEP 2/3**

Culture-negative infective endocarditis is most commonly caused by antibiotic administration prior to blood culture collection, either from the patient's self-administration or from the emergency department. True culture-negative infective endocarditis with nonculturable bacteria is not common.

A medical student who heard about the case comments that it is unbelievable that the patient may have infective endocarditis because he does not have a murmur or any signs of emboli on exam.

How do you respond?
Studies have shown that the only reliable symptom of infective endocarditis is fever, which is seen in 95% of such patients. Murmur attributable to infective endocarditis is only heard in 31% of patients, CHF appreciated in 22%, Janeway lesions in 6%, skin petechiae/splinter hemorrhages in 9%, and conjunctival lesions in 3%. Therefore, the absence of a murmur or signs of emboli on exam should not decrease the suspicion for infective endocarditis in the right clinical scenario.

TABLE 7.2 ■ Modified Duke Criteria

(Need two major criteria or one major + three minor criteria or five minor criteria)

Major Criteria	**Blood Culture Criteria**
	• Typical microorganisms consistent with infective endocarditis from two separate blood cultures: viridans streptococci, *Streptococcus bovis,* HACEK group, *Staphylococcus aureus;* or community-acquired enterococci in the absence of a primary focus; or
	• Microorganisms consistent with infective endocarditis from persistently positive blood cultures defined as follows: At least two positive cultures of blood samples drawn >12 hours apart; or all of three or a majority of four or more separate blood cultures (with first and last sample drawn at least 1 hour apart); or
	• Single positive blood culture for *Coxiella burnetii* or anti–phase 1 IgG antibody titer >1:800
	Endocardial Involvement Criteria
	Echocardiogram positive for infective endocarditis defined as follows: oscillating intracardiac mass on valve or supporting structures, in the path of regurgitant jets, or on implanted material in the absence of an alternative anatomic explanation; or abscess; or new partial dehiscence of prosthetic valve; new valvular regurgitation (worsening or changing or preexisting murmur not sufficient)
Minor Criteria	Predisposition, predisposing heart condition, or injection drug use
	Fever, temperature >38 °C (100.4 °F)
	Vascular phenomena: major arterial emboli, septic pulmonary infarcts, mycotic aneurysm, intracranial hemorrhage, conjunctival hemorrhages, and Janeway lesions
	Immunologic phenomena: glomerulonephritis, Osler's nodes, Roth's spots, and rheumatoid factor
	Microbiological evidence: positive blood culture but does not meet a major criterion as noted above or serological evidence of active infection with organism consistent with infective endocarditis

HACEK, A grouping of gram-negative bacilli: *Haemophilus* species (*Haemophilus parainfluenzae, Haemophilus aphrophilus, Haemophilus paraphrophilus*), *Actinobacillus actinomycetemcomitans, Cardiobacterium hominis, Eikenella corrodens,* and *Kingella* species.

TABLE 7.3 ■ Bacteria That Cause Infective Endocarditis and Prevalence From International Collaboration on Endocarditis (ICE) Prospective Cohort Study

Staphylococci	*Cases (%) from ICE Cohort*
Staphylococcus aureus	31.6
Coagulase-negative staphylococci	10.5
Streptococci	
Viridans group streptococci	18
Streptococcus gallolyticus (bovis)	6.5
Other streptococci (β-hemolytic streptococci, nutritionally variant streptococci)	5.1
Enterococcus	10.6
HACEK Group	1.7
Haemophilus species (*Haemophilus parainfluenzae, Haemophilus aphrophilus, Haemophilus paraphrophilus*), *Actinobacillus actinomycetemcomitans, Cardiobacterium hominis, Eikenella corrodens,* and *Kingella* species	
Gram-Negative Bacteria (Non-HACEK)	2.1
Fungi (e.g., Candida)	1.8
Culture-Negative	8.1

TABLE 7.4 ■ Most Common Organisms Causing Culture-Negative Endocarditis

Bartonella spp. *(B. henselae, B. quintana)*	Most common cause of culture-negative infective endocarditis in United States *B. henselae:* exposure to cats and fleas *B. quintana:* louse transmission, homeless shelters, and alcohol abuse
Brucella spp.	Unpasteurized milk/dairy products, livestock contact; blood cultures will be positive in 80% with extended incubation time
Chlamydia psittaci *Chlamydophila psittaci*	Psittacine bird exposure (parrots, parakeets)
Coxiella burnetii (Q fever)	Most common cause of culture-negative infective endocarditis in many parts of Europe; high titers Ab to both phase 1 and 2 antigens
Legionella spp.	Contaminated water exposure
Tropheryma whipplei	Whipple's disease agent (diarrhea, weight loss, arthralgias, abdominal pain, lymphadenopathy, central nervous system involvement)

CLINICAL PEARL   **STEP 2/3**

Although cardiac auscultation is commonly used to rule out infective endocarditis, the murmur attributable to infective endocarditis is frequently not heard. This murmur only occurs when the infection has caused enough valvular destruction to allow blood regurgitation. Thus, the murmur of infective endocarditis is a regurgitant one, either holosystolic for mitral/tricuspid regurgitation or diastolic decrescendo for aortic/pulmonic insufficiency. Sometimes a murmur from a preexisting valvular abnormality that predisposes a patient to having infective endocarditis can be heard, such as aortic stenosis, but this is not the actual murmur of infective endocarditis. Therefore, the lack of a murmur does not rule out infective endocarditis, nor should it decrease one's suspicion for infective endocarditis in a patient who otherwise has compatible laboratory or clinical data.

A TTE is performed, and it does not demonstrate any valvular vegetations.

Does this rule out infective endocarditis? What should you do now?
A TTE does not rule out infective endocarditis, as it is relatively insensitive for visualizing cardiac vegetations, especially on the left side of the heart. Studies have shown that the sensitivity of a TTE to diagnose endocarditis is lower (by 30 to 50%) compared to use of a transesophageal echocardiogram (TEE). Thus, a TEE needs to be performed next.

CLINICAL PEARL   **STEP 2/3**

Even if a TTE does demonstrate a cardiac vegetation, thereby clinching the diagnosis of infective endocarditis, in most cases patients will still need a TEE. This is because the TTE is very poor at visualizing the complications of infective endocarditis, such as myocardial/perivalvular abscesses or early valve dehiscence, especially on the left side. These complications need surgical management and not mere antibiotics alone.

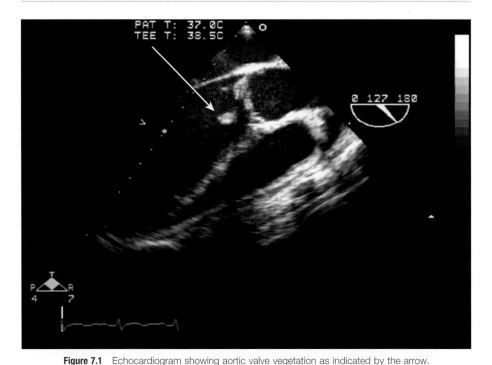

Figure 7.1   Echocardiogram showing aortic valve vegetation as indicated by the arrow.

CLINICAL PEARL   **STEP 2/3**

Even if a TEE does not show vegetations, the patient may still have infective endocarditis if the microbiologic data are consistent with this diagnosis (e.g., persistent bacteremia with a typical bacteria of infective endocarditis in the absence of an alternative source). The TEE's sensitivity is not 100%, so it cannot rule out infective endocarditis; its sensitivity ranges 82 to 95%, with false negatives seen in cases where the vegetations are too small to visualize or where they have already embolized.

A TEE is performed by the cardiologists and demonstrates a 0.5 cm vegetation on the aortic valve. No abscesses are appreciated, and aortic regurgitation is mild (Fig. 7.1).

Diagnosis: Aortic valve infective endocarditis with *S. viridans* group

---

What are some of the complications to worry about?
Because the vegetation is on a left-sided valve, the worry is for systemic embolization. With arterial embolization, cerebral strokes, kidney abscess/infarction, mycotic aneurysms (especially in the cerebral vessels), splenic infarcts, liver abscesses, skin emboli (Janeway lesions), eye emboli (causing endophthalmitis), and spinal osteomyelitis/abscess can be seen. Local disease extension, such as abscess erosion into the conduction pathway causing heart block and valvular dehiscence causing acute congestive heart failure, can lead to sudden death. Immune-complex disease, such as glomerulonephritis, Osler's nodes of the skin, and Roth's spots of the retina, can also occur, especially when infective endocarditis is more subacute.

CLINICAL PEARL   **STEP 2/3**

It is prudent to place a patient with left-sided infective endocarditis on telemetry to monitor for arrhythmias and to regularly check electrocardiograms (ECGs) in order to closely monitor for PR interval prolongation as a sign of myocardial abscess development and extension into the conduction pathway.

Does this patient need valve replacement surgery?

The indications for surgical intervention and valve replacement include:

- Acute congestive heart failure unresponsive to medical therapy and/or valve dehiscence/perforation/rupture seen on echocardiogram
- Perivalvular and myocardial abscess or fistula formation
- ≥1 emboli while on appropriate antibiotics during first 2 weeks
- Failure of antibiotic therapy (uncontrolled infection) including persistently positive blood cultures and/or fever and/or persistent emboli
- Fungal (e.g., candida) endocarditis and other virulent or antibiotic-resistant organisms (gram-negative bacteria, vancomycin-resistant enterococci)
- Most cases of prosthetic valve infective endocarditis
- Mycotic aneurysms that need resection
  The following are conditions where surgery should be strongly considered:
- Large (>1 cm) anterior mitral valve vegetation
- Increase in vegetation size after appropriate antibiotic therapy

This patient does not have any criteria (at the moment) to require valve replacement surgery.

CLINICAL PEARL   **STEP 2/3**

Although historically cardiothoracic surgeons often delayed valve surgery until the patient received a long course of antibiotics or unless a complication warranted it, recent prospective, randomized trial data has shown that early valve surgery (<48 hours of admission) is associated with decreased mortality and embolic events when compared with standard care (3% vs. 28%, respectively) in patients with infective endocarditis.

You had empirically started the antibiotics vancomycin and ceftriaxone on the day of admission after the cultures were obtained. The microbiology lab has now reported the antibiotic susceptibilities for the *S. viridans* group, showing the following minimum inhibitory concentrations (MICs): penicillin 0.05 mcg/mL, ceftriaxone 0.1 mcg/mL, and vancomycin 0.5 mcg/mL.

Which antibiotic regimen would you now use?

The mainstay of treatment for infective endocarditis is a prolonged (4- to 6-week) bactericidal regimen with intravenous antibiotics. The MIC refers to the minimum concentration of antibiotic necessary to inhibit or kill the bacteria, and the Clinical and Laboratory Standards Institute (CLSI) has established the antibiotic concentration cutoff level at or below which the microbiology laboratory can label the bacteria as "susceptible" or "resistant" to the drug tested. Looking at the bacteria's MIC to the antibiotics, this *S. viridans* isolate is susceptible to all the antibiotics tested. Therefore, the vancomycin should be stopped immediately, as this drug is not needed and can be nephrotoxic with prolonged exposure. Either penicillin or ceftriaxone could be used to treat this susceptible bacteria, although the former antibiotic has a much narrower spectrum (thus causing less collateral damage), whereas the latter is easier to dose (once daily). Table 7.5 lists suggested antibiotics for the different bacteria that cause infective endocarditis.

TABLE 7.5 ■ Treatment for Infective Endocarditis by Pathogens

Methicillin-Susceptible Staphylococcus aureus **(MSSA)**

Native valve	Naf/Oxacillin 2 g IV q4 h × 6 wks or Cefazolin 2 g IV q8 h × 6 wks Uncomplicated right sided: × 2 wks
Prosthetic valve	Naf/Oxacillin 2 g IV q4 h × ≥6 wks + Gentamicin 1 mg/kg IV q8 h × 2 wks + Rifampin 300 g PO/IV q8 h × ≥6 wks

Methicillin-Resistant Staphylococcus aureus **(MRSA)**

Native valve	Vancomycin 15 mg/kg IV q12 h × 6 wks or Daptomycin >8 mg/kg IV q24 h × 6 wks
Prosthetic valve	Vancomycin 15 mg/kg IV q12 h × ≥6 wks Gentamicin 1 mg/kg IV q8 h × 2 wks + Rifampin 300 g PO/IV q8 h × ≥6 wks

Coagulase-Negative Staphylococci

Native valve	Vancomycin 15-20 mg/kg IV q8-12 h × 6 wks
Prosthetic valve	Vancomycin 15-20 mg/kg IV q8-12 h × ≥6 wks + Gentamicin 1 mg/kg IV q8 h × 2 wks + Rifampin 300 mg PO/IV q8 h × ≥6 wks
Penicillin-susceptible viridans streptococci (mean inhibitory concentration ≤0.12 mcg/mL)	Penicillin 2-3 million units IV q4 h × 4 wks or Ceftriaxone 2 g IV q daily × 4 wks
Relatively penicillin-resistant viridans streptococci (mean inhibitory concentration >0.12-<0.5 mcg/mL)	Penicillin 4 million units IV q4 h × 4 wks + Gentamicin 3 mg/kg IV q24 h ×2 wks or Vancomycin 15 mg/kg IV q12 h × 4 wks
Penicillin-resistant viridans (mean inhibitory concentration ≥0.5 mcg/mL) and Nutritionally Variant Streptococci (Abiotrophia & Granulicatella spp)	Pencillin 3-5 million units IV q4 h or Ceftriaxone 2 g IV q24 h+ Gentamicin 3 mg/kg IV q24 h × ≥4 wks or Vancomycin 15 mg/kg IV q12 h × ≥4 wks
Enterococci Ampicillin-susceptible enterococci	Ampicillin 2 g IV q4 h + Gentamicin 1 mg/kg IV q8 h × 4-6 wks
Ampicillin-resistant enterococci	Vancomycin 15 mg/kg IV q12 h + Gentamicin 1 mg/kg IV q8 h × 6 wks
HACEK bacteria	Ceftriaxone 2 g IV q daily × 4 wks or Ciprofloxacin 500 mg PO q12 h × 4 wks (if intolerant to beta-lactam)

HACEK, A grouping of gram-negative bacilli: *Haemophilus* species (*Haemophilus parainfluenzae, Haemophilus aphrophilus, Haemophilus paraphrophilus), Actinobacillus actinomycetemcomitans, Cardiobacterium hominis, Eikenella corrodens,* and *Kingella* species.

You change the antibiotics to penicillin G, 3 million units intravenous (IV) every 4 hours. The patient has become afebrile and stable and does not meet any valve surgery criteria during hospitalization. You decide to discharge him on the penicillin G regimen for 4 weeks via a pump. He has a peripherally inserted central catheter (PICC) line placed for long-term access. On follow-up, after completion of therapy, the patient has done well, and you discontinue the antibiotic and PICC line. He is worried about his risk of getting infective endocarditis again and asks you what to do about antibiotic prophylaxis for dental procedures.

How should you advise him?

Although historically oral antibiotics were given for many high-risk cardiac conditions (e.g., aortic stenosis/regurgitation, mitral stenosis/regurgitation, ventricular septal defect, hypertrophic cardiomyopathy) when receiving major dental procedures (e.g., manipulation of gingival tissue or the periapical region of teeth or perforation of the oral mucosa), the current recommendation is to give such prophylaxis for the following cardiac conditions only:
- Previous infective endocarditis
- Prosthetic valves or prosthetic material on valve repair
- Congenital heart disease that has not been adequately repaired
- Cardiac transplant recipient with subsequent valvulopathy

As this patient has had an episode of infective endocarditis, he would need amoxicillin, 2 g prophylaxis, 30 to 60 minutes prior to major dental procedures.

BEYOND THE PEARLS

- Infective endocarditis should be part of the differential diagnosis when patients have subacute to chronic fevers with a paucity of localizing symptoms.
- Like other endovascular infections (e.g., septic thrombophlebitis, catheter-related blood stream infections), infective endocarditis is characterized by near continuous bacteremia, and therefore the key to diagnosis is obtaining several sets of blood cultures prior to antibiotic administration.
- Bacteriuria with organisms that do not typically cause UTIs but that do cause infective endocarditis (e.g., *S. aureus* or *S. viridans* group) should prompt investigation for bacteremia and infective endocarditis due to that organism.
- Fever is the only reliable symptom of infective endocarditis. Lack of murmur or embolic phenomena should not decrease one's suspicion for infective endocarditis.
- Clearance of blood cultures after 1 day of antibiotic therapy should not decrease clinical suspicion for infective endocarditis. Many bacteria are exquisitely susceptible to antibiotics (e.g., streptococci) and thus cannot be recovered in blood cultures after initial antibiotic administration, even if the vegetation still harbors a large load of bacteria. This may not be true of highly antibiotic-resistant strains (e.g., vancomycin-resistant enterococci). However, negative follow-up blood cultures in the absence of antibiotic administration does make infective endocarditis a less likely diagnosis.
- Aside from blood cultures, the echocardiogram is important for the diagnosis of infective endocarditis. However, neither the transthoracic echocardiogram nor the transesophageal echocardiogram rules out infective endocarditis in the right clinical scenario (e.g., unexplained and/or persistent bacteremia with a bacterium typical for infective endocarditis).
- The term *endocarditis* does not necessarily equate to an infection of the endocardium. The suffix -itis only refers to inflammation. As such, endocarditis refers to inflammation of the endocardium, including the heart valves. Therefore, endocarditis can be noninfective, such as in marantic endocarditis (associated with the prothrombotic states of malignancy) and Libman-Sacks endocarditis (associated with systemic lupus erythematosus).
- *Streptococcus gallolyticus,* formerly known as *Streptococcus bovis,* bacteremia and endocarditis should prompt concern for and workup of colon cancer (with colonoscopy). Bacteremia with this streptococcus is often a harbinger for colonic malignancy.
- Gram-negative bacteria (non-HACEK) are distinctly uncommon causes of infective endocarditis (<2% of cases). Historically these bacteria were seen in injection drug users. More recently, health care contact has been the more frequent risk factor, especially if

the patient has a prosthetic valve or implanted endovascular device. *Escherichia coli*, *Pseudomonas aeruginosa*, and *Salmonella* spp. are most commonly reported.

- Alternative, nonnephrotoxic antibiotics have been studied for the treatment of methicillin-resistant *Staphylococcus aureus* (MRSA) bacteremia and infective endocarditis. Daptomycin is a cyclic lipopeptide antibiotic that damages the bacterial cell membrane, is bactericidal for gram-positive bacteria, and has been shown to be effective for treatment of MRSA bacteremia and right-sided endocarditis. Ceftaroline is a novel bactericidal cephalosporin that can kill MRSA and has been shown in smaller studies to also be effective in the treatment of MRSA bacteremia and endocarditis.

- Few options exist for vancomycin-resistant enterococcus (VRE) infective endocarditis due to a paucity of antibiotics active against this bacteria. Daptomycin is one option, given its bactericidal activity, but it may need to be used at higher than approved doses (10 to 12 mg/kg/day). However, VRE can develop nonsusceptibility to this antibiotic. Synergistic combinations will need to be studied clinically (e.g., combining daptomycin with ampicillin) as they seem to hold promise in vitro. Linezolid is another antibiotic with activity against VRE, but its bacteriostatic properties make it a less desirable option.

References

Abraham J, Mansour C, Veledar E, Khan B, Lerakis S. *Staphylococcus aureus* bacteremia and endocarditis: the Grady Memorial Hospital experience with methicillin-sensitive *S aureus* and methicillin-resistant *S aureus* bacteremia. *Am Heart J.* 2004;147(3):536-539.

Baddour LM, Wilson WR, Bayer AS, et al. Infective endocarditis: diagnosis, antimicrobial therapy, and management of complications: a statement for healthcare professionals from the Committee on Rheumatic Fever, Endocarditis, and Kawasaki Disease, Council on Cardiovascular Disease in the Young, and the Councils on Clinical Cardiology, Stroke, and Cardiovascular Surgery and Anesthesia, American Heart Association: endorsed by the Infectious Diseases Society of America. *Circulation.* 2005;111(23):e394-e434.

Baddour LM, Wilson WR, Bayer AS, et al; American Heart Association Committee on Rheumatic Fever, Endocarditis, and Kawasaki Disease of the Council on Cardiovascular Disease in the Young, Council on Clinical Cardiology, Council on Cardiovascular Surgery and Anesthesia, and Stroke Council. Infective Endocarditis in Adults: Diagnosis, Antimicrobial Therapy, and Management of Complications: A Scientific Statement for Healthcare Professionals From the American Heart Association. *Circulation.* 2015;132(15):1435-1486.

Fowler VG Jr, Boucher HW, Corey GR, et al. Daptomycin versus standard therapy for bacteremia and endocarditis caused by *Staphylococcus aureus*. *N Engl J Med.* 2006;355(7):653-665.

Fowler VG Jr, Li J, Corey GR, et al. Role of echocardiography in evaluation of patients with *Staphylococcus aureus* bacteremia: experience in 103 patients. *J Am Coll Cardiol.* 1997;30(4):1072-1078.

Fowler VG Jr, Miro JM, Hoen B, et al. *Staphylococcus aureus* endocarditis throughout the world: a consequence of medical progress. The International Collaboration on Endocarditis Prospective Cohort Study. *JAMA.* 2005;29:3012-3021.

Fu J, Ye X, Chen C, Chen S. The efficacy and safety of linezolid and glycopeptides in the treatment of *Staphylococcus aureus* infections. *PLoS ONE.* 2013;8(3):e58240.

Ho TT, Cadena J, Childs LM, Gonzalez-Velex M, Lewis JS 2nd. Methicillin-resistant *Staph.aureus* bacteremia and endocarditis treated with ceftaroline salvage therapy. *J Antimicrob Chemother.* 2012;67:1267-1270.

Kang D, Kim YJ, Kim SH, et al. Early surgery versus conventional treatment for infective endocarditis. *N Engl J Med.* 2012;366:2466-2473.

Li JS, Sexton DJ, Mick N, et al. Proposed modifications to the Duke criteria for the diagnosis of infective endocarditis. *Clin Infect Dis.* 2000;30:633-638.

Røder BL, Wandall DA, Frimodt-Møller N, et al. Clinical features of *Staph.aureus* endocarditis: a 10 year experience in Denmark. *Arch Int Med.* 1999;159(5):462-469.

Sakoulas G, Bayer AS, Pogliano J, et al. Ampicillin enhances daptomycin- and cationic host defense peptide-mediated killing of ampicillin- and vancomycin-resistant *Enterococcus faecium*. *Antimicrob Agents Chemother.* 2012;56(2):838-844.

Sullenberger AL, Avedissian LS, Kent SM. Importance of transesophageal echocardiography in the evaluation of *Staphylococcus aureus* bacteremia. *J Heart Valve Dis.* 2005;14(1):23-28.

Gina Rossetti ■ Eric Hsieh

A 25-Year-Old Female With Polyuria and Polydipsia

A 25-year-old Caucasian female with a history of type 1 diabetes presents to the emergency department with 3 days of polyuria, polydipsia, and dysuria. The morning of presentation she also developed a fever, nausea, and abdominal pain. She has no shortness of breath, cough, chest pain, or diarrhea. Because of her nausea, she has not been eating and has stopped taking her insulin to avoid hypoglycemia. She comes to your medical intensive care unit (ICU) for further management.

How does the history help narrow your differential diagnosis?

This is a 25-year-old female with a history of diabetes now presenting with urinary symptoms suggestive of a urinary tract infection (UTI). Diabetic ketoacidosis must be considered in diabetic patients who have infections, abdominal catastrophes, medication noncompliance, and myocardial infarctions.

On physical exam, the patient's temperature is 39.1 °C (102.3 °F). Her pulse rate is 136/min, her blood pressure is 106/58 mm Hg, and her respiration rate is 26/min. She is alert and oriented but is breathing rapidly and has a fruity odor on her breath. Her pupils are equal, round and reactive to light, and extraocular eye movements are intact. Her tympanic membranes are clear and she has no tenderness on palpation of her sinuses. Her neck is supple with no lymphadenopathy or jugular venous pulsation. Her breath sounds are clear to auscultation. Her cardiovascular exam is significant for tachycardia; however, she has a regular rate and rhythm with no murmurs, rubs, or gallops. Her abdominal exam is significant for tenderness to palpation in all four quadrants as well as right costovertebral angle tenderness. Her extremities are warm with no cyanosis, clubbing, or edema. Her neurologic exam is intact. Her serum glucose is 440 mg/dL. The basic metabolic panel (BMP) is significant for a sodium of 126 mEq/L, a potassium of 4.8 mEq/L, a chloride of 86 mEq/L, a bicarbonate of 12 mEq/L, a blood urea nitrogen of 32 mg/dL, and a creatinine of 1.4 mg/dL. The phosphorus is 6.0 mg/dL. The complete blood count (CBC) is significant for a leukocytosis of 18,000 μL. The arterial blood gas shows a pH of 7.2, a partial pressure of carbon dioxide (pCO_2) of 32 mm Hg and a bicarbonate (HCO_3) of 14 mEq/L.

What is your differential diagnosis?

Considering the patient's elevated glucose, anion gap of 28, acidosis, and precipitating UTI, she likely has diabetic ketoacidosis (DKA).

Urinalysis reveals 4+ glucose, 30 white blood cells (WBCs), large bacteria, and positive nitrites.

> **Diagnosis:** Diabetic ketoacidosis precipitated by a urinary tract infection

What is the definition of diabetic ketoacidosis?

Although there is no consensus on the definition of DKA, the diagnosis requires the presence of an anion gap, metabolic acidosis, and ketonemia. Although they are usually hyperglycemic, 1 to 7% of patients may have a glucose level less than 200 mg/dL. In other words, you have to have the D (diabetes), the K (ketonemia), and the A (acidosis) to call it DKA.

What are the most common precipitating factors of DKA?

The most common precipitating factor is infection. A UTI and pneumonia are the two most common sources, although it is important to consider a less obvious source such as bacteremia, cellulitis, occult sinusitis, tooth abscess, or perirectal abscess. Other common precipitating factors include a new diagnosis of diabetes and lack of insulin compliance. Patients can also present with an abdominal catastrophe such as cholecystitis, pancreatitis, appendicitis, diverticulitis, perforated viscus, or acute ischemic bowel. Less common causes include myocardial infarction, pregnancy, drugs (glucocorticoid, β-agonists, cocaine, pentamidine), and stroke. Many times, however, no precipitating factor is identified.

CLINICAL PEARL   **STEP 2/3**

Rhinocerebral mucormycosis is associated with DKA. It is important to consider this diagnosis in the presence of facial pain, facial numbness, orbital swelling, proptosis, visual changes, or bloody nasal discharge.

BASIC SCIENCE PEARL   **STEP 1**

Physical stress and infection in the setting of decreased insulin leads to the release of hormones such as cortisol, catecholamines, and glucagon. These hormones act upon the liver to increase gluconeogenesis, glycogenolysis, and conversion of free fatty acids to ketone bodies. In addition, decreased insulin and increased glucagon act to stimulate the muscle cells to release amino acids and the fat cells to release glycerol and free fatty acids. These act as additional substrates for the liver to produce ketones and glucose, which are then released into the blood stream.

What clinical manifestations in the history and physical exam would make you concerned about a diagnosis of DKA?

Signs and symptoms of DKA are often nonspecific. Classically, patients will present with polyuria, polydipsia, nausea, vomiting, weakness, air hunger, and altered sensorium. The severity of altered mental status can range from fully alert to obtunded. Obtundation correlates well with a high plasma osmolality (>340 mOsm/L). Body temperature is often below normal; thus, lack of a fever does not exclude infection. Tachycardia is common; however, blood pressure is usually maintained unless there is an underlying process such as severe sepsis or cardiogenic shock. Kussmaul respirations (deep breathing with air hunger) usually indicate a blood pH less than 7.2, although shallow respirations may reflect a more severe acidosis. Patients often have a fruity odor to their breath due to the production of acetone. Abdominal pain will be present in 30% of cases and may be due to an underlying abdominal process or the DKA itself.

BASIC SCIENCE/CLINICAL PEARL	STEP 1/2/3

Calculate the serum osmolality in obtunded patients. If the value is less than 330 mosm/kg, look for other causes of altered sensorium. To calculate serum osmolality, do not include the blood urea nitrogen (BUN) as urea has less osmotic activity. The formula is as follows:

$$\text{Serum osm} = 2[Na^+] + [\text{Glucose}]/18$$

CLINICAL PEARL	STEP 2/3

It is extremely important to perform a thorough physical exam to look for any precipitating factors or signs of infection. Many of these diagnoses are life threatening if not identified and treated early in the clinical course.

What laboratory abnormalities would you expect in this patient?

There are many laboratory abnormalities classically associated with DKA. The serum glucose is typically elevated but at times can be less than 200, particularly in the setting of prolonged fasting, which accelerates ketogenesis and suppresses glycogenolysis. The average initial glucose is 450 to 650 mg/dL. The serum sodium concentration may vary but patients have a total body sodium deficit. The serum sodium may be transiently low due to the osmotic activity of glucose, which draws water into the extracellular space and dilutes the sodium.

The initial serum potassium is typically normal or elevated due to acidosis; however, total body potassium is usually depleted due to cellular shifts from hyperosmolality and acidosis, diminished cellular uptake due to lack of insulin, and renal losses. The potassium is usually depleted by 3 to 5 mEq/kg. Similar to the potassium, the initial phosphorus concentration may be normal or high, but total body phosphorus is usually depleted. The BUN and the creatinine both often increase due to prerenal azotemia secondary to osmotic diuresis or vomiting. A leukocytosis is common and does not necessarily indicate infection; hematocrit and mean corpuscular volume (MCV) may be elevated because of osmotic swelling, as glucose is an osmole that freely distributes across red blood cell (RBC) membranes.

BASIC SCIENCE PEARL	STEP 1

To correct the serum sodium for the serum glucose, use the following formula:

$$\text{Corrected } [Na] = [Na] + 1.6 \,(\text{Glucose} - 100)/100.$$

CLINICAL PEARL	STEP 2/3

Serum and urine ketones should be used to confirm the diagnosis but not to monitor therapy. Instead, the anion gap should be followed.

CLINICAL PEARL	STEP 2/3

It is important to consider other causes of anion gap metabolic acidosis, including lactic acidosis, uremia, salicylates, methanol, and ethylene glycol. Patients with DKA can have other causes for their acidosis that can precipitate the DKA episode and need to be corrected.

What is your initial management?

The overall goals of care for any patient in DKA are to improve circulatory volume and tissue perfusion, normalize blood glucose, correct acidosis and eliminate ketonemia, correct electrolyte imbalances, and prevent complications. Additionally, the precipitating cause should be sought out and treated.

Intravenous (IV) Fluids: In order to improve circulatory volume and tissue perfusion, the first step is to start IV fluids. The average fluid deficit is 3 to 5 L. IV fluids are important for maintaining cardiac output, renal perfusion, reducing blood glucose/plasma osmolality, and decreasing concentrations of counterregulatory hormones. Initial fluid therapy should consist of isotonic saline (normal saline) as volume deficit should be corrected before any free water deficit. A reasonable goal is to use normal saline to replenish the volume deficit over 12 to 24 hours. Normal saline at a rate of 1 L/hour for the initial hour should be followed by 500 cc/hour during the next 4 hours and then 250 cc/hour. After the initial period of volume replacement, you may switch to half normal saline at half the rate to replete the free water deficit. Dextrose should be added once the blood glucose has decreased to 200 mg/dL to avoid hypoglycemia and allow insulin therapy of adequate duration to eliminate ketogenesis.

CLINICAL PEARL   **STEP 2/3**

The key is to adjust the fluids (dextrose concentration and rate), not the insulin drip, when addressing blood sugars.

Insulin: This is the only intervention that will reverse the ketogenesis. Therapy should begin with an IV bolus of regular insulin (0.1 unit/Kg) followed by an infusion of 0.1 unit/kg/hour. For example, a 70-Kg person would receive a 7-unit regular insulin bolus followed by 7 units per hour of regular insulin drip. The anion gap should be monitored along with serum bicarbonate and electrolytes. The insulin drip can be discontinued once the anion gap has resolved, the bicarbonate has increased, and the patient is tolerating a diet. Subcutaneous insulin must be overlapped with IV insulin to allow the subcutaneous insulin to take effect.

Potassium: Potassium deficiency can be a fatal complication and must be avoided. Since insulin therapy and resolving acidosis will shift potassium back into cells, serum potassium levels should be monitored frequently and replaced aggressively. Be careful, however, of overrepletion of potassium in patients who have renal failure or oliguria.

CLINICAL PEARL   **STEP 2/3**

Infusion of potassium too quickly may result in fatal complications such as cardiac arrhythmias. This is particularly important to note when replacement is given intravenously.

CLINICAL PEARL   **STEP 2/3**

There are two situations in which insulin should not be given first: hypokalemia and hypotension. In hypokalemia, insulin administration prior to adequate restoration of potassium will lead to potassium influx into cells, further dropping extracellular potassium levels, and can precipitate cardiac arrhythmias. In hypotension, the influx of glucose into cells, followed by water, can lead to further collapse of extravascular space and worsening of hypotension.

How do you monitor therapy?

Glucose should be measured hourly initially and adjusted to every 2 to 4 hours depending on blood sugar and clinical course. The goal of close monitoring is to prevent hypoglycemia by adjusting IV fluids while maintaining insulin drip. A basic metabolic panel should be checked every 2-4 hours initially. Serum magnesium and phosphorus levels should be monitored if clinically indicated. Plasma and urine ketones are helpful in making the diagnosis but not in monitoring therapy. Follow the anion gap and bicarbarbonate to monitor response to therapy.

How do you complete your therapy?

When the anion gap closes and bicarbonate rises, the DKA is resolving and the patient may be ready to start eating. Chemistries should be followed frequently at the time of conversion to subcutaneous insulin to ensure the patient does not slip back into ketogenesis. DKA patients should receive a complete educational program regarding diet, exercise, insulin dosage, glucose monitoring and follow-up care with the diabetic educators and clinics.

CLINICAL PEARL   **STEP 2/3**

It is critical that the insulin drip not be discontinued until the subcutaneous insulin is well into its effect (~1 hour). A reasonable approach is to determine the daily insulin requirement based on the patient's weight. Insulin can be dosed at 0.5-0.8 units/kg/day. There are a variety of insulin regimens to consider, which may vary based on the patient's weight, renal function, and dietary restrictions. One possible regimen may include starting a once-daily long-acting insulin, such as glargine, and covering with a sliding scale of short-acting insulin with meals.

BEYOND THE PEARLS

- There is no clear benefit to bicarbonate replacement. However, it has been considered in patients with pH <6.9 and impending cardiovascular collapse, lactic acidosis, or severe hyperkalemia.
- Severe phosphorus depletion can result in respiratory depression, muscle weakness, hemolytic anemia, and cardiac dysfunction. Excessive replacement can lead to hypocalcemia and soft tissue complications. Phosphorus should be checked within 6 to 8 hours and repleted if <1 to 2 mg/dL.
- Acetoacetate and β-hydroxybutyrate are the primary ketones that cause the anion gap acidosis. The nitroprusside test for ketone detection in serum or urine measures acetone and acetoacetate but not β-hydroxybutyrate.

References

Ilag LL, Kronick S, Ernst RD, et al. Impact of a critical pathway on inpatient management of diabetic ketoacidosis. *Diabetes Res Clin Pract.* 2003;62:23-32.

Kitabchi AE, Umpierrez GE, Murphy MB, et al. Management of hyperglycemic crises in patients with diabetes. *Diabetes Care.* 2001;24:131-153.

Kitabchi AE, Umpierrez GE, Murphy MB, et al. Hyperglycemic crises in diabetes. *Diabetes Care.* 2004;27(suppl 1):S94-S102.

Pinhas-Hamiel O, Dolan LM, Zeitler PS. Diabetic ketoacidosis among obese African-American adolescents with NIDDM. *Diabetes Care.* 1997;20:484-486.

Trachtenbarg DE. Diabetic ketoacidosis. *Am Fam Physician.* 2005;71(9):1705-1714.

Dawn Piarulli ■ R. Michelle Koolaee

A 22-Year-Old Female With Joint Pain

A 22-year-old female with no significant past medical history presents to an urgent care center reporting 3.5 months of worsening joint pain and swelling. She states that both her hands, her right knee, and her left ankle have been bothering her and are swollen at times.

Why is the duration of this patient's joint pain important?

Table 9.1 summarizes the etiologies of inflammatory arthritis based on symptom duration. The duration of joint symptoms can implicate certain diagnoses over others. When the arthritis is acute (lasting a few days or less), one must immediately consider septic arthritis or crystal-induced arthritis (i.e., gout, pseudogout). Septic arthritis can occur secondary to organisms of bacterial, viral, or fungal origin. An arthrocentesis should be immediately performed to rule out this possibility as well as to evaluate for crystal-induced arthritis. See Case 47 for more information about septic and crystal-induced arthritis.

When symptoms have been present for more than a few days but less than 6 to 8 weeks, one should consider subacute types of infectious or parainfectious arthritides such as poststreptococcal arthritis or viral arthritis such as parvovirus B19 arthritis. Another differential diagnosis to consider is reactive arthritis. Reactive arthritis (formally known as Reiter's syndrome) is an acute inflammatory arthritis that can occur after genitourinary infections (i.e., *Chlamydia*) or after gastrointestinal infections like *Yersinia, Salmonella, Shigella, Campylobacter,* or *Clostridium difficile.*

CLINICAL PEARL   **STEP 2/3**

One mnemonic for reactive arthritis is "Can't see, can't pee, can't climb a tree" for conjunctivitis, urethritis, and arthritis of reactive arthritis. The entire triad does not need to be present in order to consider this diagnosis.

In a patient who presents with chronic arthritis (more than 6 to 8 weeks), it is reasonable to consider autoimmune illnesses, which include systemic lupus erythematosus (SLE), rheumatoid arthritis (RA), or the seronegative spondyloarthropathies (SpAs), to name a few. Be mindful that arthritis due to tuberculous or fungal infections may fall into the chronic category if not detected early on.

TABLE 9.1 ▨ Differential Diagnosis for Inflammatory Arthritis Based on Duration of Symptoms

Duration	Differential Diagnoses to Consider
A few days or less	Septic arthritis (bacterial, fungal, or tuberculous), crystal-induced arthritis (gout/pseudogout)
More than a few days but less than 6 to 8 weeks	Viral arthritis (especially parvovirus B19), poststreptococcal arthritis, bacterial arthritis (bacterial, fungal, or tuberculous), reactive arthritis (which follows gastrointestinal or genitourinary infections)
Chronic/more than 8 weeks	Rheumatoid arthritis, systemic lupus erythematosus, scleroderma, sarcoidosis, Sjögren's syndrome, chronic infections (tuberculous arthritis, fungal arthritis, Lyme disease)

TABLE 9.2 ▨ Differential Diagnosis for Inflammatory Arthritis According to the Number of Joints Involved

Number of Joints	Differential Diagnoses to Consider
Monoarthritis (1 joint)	Infectious causes: septic arthritis (bacterial, TB, fungal), gonococcal arthritis, Lyme arthritis Rheumatologic causes: reactive arthritis, less commonly systemic diseases (i.e., RA, SLE, seronegative SpA) present as monoarthritis Malignancy: metastatic cancer, primary bone tumors (osteoid osteoma) Other: crystal-induced arthritis, OA, trauma (fracture, hemarthrosis, ligamentous, or tendinous injury), PVNS
Oligoarthritis (≤4 joints)	Infectious causes: septic/Lyme arthritis (less commonly oligoarticular; usually are monoarticular), gonococcal arthritis Rheumatologic causes: reactive arthritis, commonly systemic diseases (i.e., RA, SLE, seronegative SpA) Other: crystal-induced arthritis, OA
Polyarthritis (≥5 joints)	Infectious causes: gonococcal arthritis, viral arthritis (parvovirus B19 especially) Rheumatologic causes are common: reactive arthritis, systemic diseases (i.e., RA, SLE, seronegative SpA) Other: crystal-induced arthritis, OA

IBD, Inflammatory bowel disease; *OA,* osteoarthritis; *PVNS,* pigmented villonodular synovitis; *RA,* rheumatoid arthritis; *SLE,* systemic lupus erythematosus; *SpA,* spondyloarthropathy; *TB,* tubercular.

What is meant by the term *oligoarthritis*, and why is the number of joints involved in arthritis important?

Arthritis is usually categorized into monoarthritis, oligoarthritis, or polyarthritis. These terms refer to the number of joints involved in arthritis. Oligoarthritis refers to ≤4 affected joints, whereas polyarthritis refers to five or more affected joints. The number of joints involved is important because the differential diagnosis for each class of arthritis is a bit different (although there can be overlap). Table 9.2 highlights the differential diagnosis according to the number of joints involved.

On further questioning, the patient reports a history of pain, stiffness, and swelling worst at her second through fourth metacarpophalangeal (MCP) and proximal interphalangeal (PIP) joints bilaterally. She reports 2 hours of morning stiffness and has been having trouble opening jars and closing buttons on her clothes. Exercising has been difficult because of her joint swelling. Her mother's sister was diagnosed with arthritis in her 30s; she has not kept in close contact with her and is not sure what type of arthritis. She has not had any recent infections. She denies diarrhea, rashes, or back pain.

Why is it important to ask about the duration of morning stiffness?

When trying to determine what is causing chronic arthritis, it is important to determine whether a patient is suffering from an inflammatory arthritis or a noninflammatory arthritis. Inflammatory arthritis is associated with at least 30 minutes and often greater than 1 hour of morning stiffness. Patients with osteoarthritis can also have morning stiffness, but it usually lasts less than 20 minutes.

The patient's exam reveals an afebrile, well-nourished, well-developed young female with normal heart, lung, and abdominal exam. She has no clubbing, cyanosis, or edema. However, on musculoskeletal exam, there is synovitis of both wrists, several MCPs, and several PIPs. The right knee has a moderate effusion, and there is synovitis at the left tibiotalar joint. At the affected joints, she has decreased range of motion secondary to pain. There are no contractures on exam. Her skin reveals no rashes.

What is the definition of *synovitis* and what does it indicate?

Synovitis is the physical exam term used to indicate the finding of active inflammatory arthritis. A joint with synovitis may have bogginess, swelling, tenderness, and may or may not have a palpable effusion. Synovitis is not specific to any particular type of inflammatory arthritis; any type may have this finding. When an effusion is present with synovitis and no diagnosis has been made, arthrocentesis is critical to perform to help establish a diagnosis. See Case 47 for discussion on synovial fluid analysis. Table 9.3 summarizes ways in which inflammatory and noninflammatory arthritis differ.

CLINICAL PEARL   **STEP 2/3**

The presence of a joint effusion is not always a definitive sign of inflammatory arthritis (i.e., patients with knee osteoarthritis very commonly present with knee effusions). In this case, arthrocentesis may be necessary to differentiate inflammatory versus noninflammatory arthritis.

CLINICAL PEARL   **STEP 2/3**

When evaluating for synovitis, check range of motion by having the patient make a fist. A patient with severe inflammatory arthritis will have difficulty making a complete fist (this is a particularly helpful finding in someone with an equivocal exam for synovitis [i.e., obese patients]).

TABLE 9.3 ▦ **Distinguishing Inflammatory Versus Noninflammatory Arthritis**

Feature	Noninflammatory (Osteoarthritis)	Inflammatory (Rheumatoid)
Age of onset	Typically older patients (usually >50)	Any age
Morning stiffness	Morning stiffness <30 minutes	Morning stiffness >1 hour
Joint involvement	DIPs, first CMC, hips, knees, spine Asymmetric involvement of joints	PIPs, MCPs, wrists, radiohumeral joint, glenohumeral joint, MTPs Symmetric involvement of joints
Radiographic findings	Subchondral sclerosis and cysts Osteophytes Asymmetric narrowing (within one joint)	Periarticular osteopenia Erosions Symmetric narrowing (within one joint)
Effusions on exam	Occasionally	Frequently
Physical exam findings	Bony enlargement Heberden's/Bouchard's nodes	Synovitis Rheumatoid nodules in advanced disease

CMC, Carpometacarpal; *DIP,* distal interphalangeal; *MCP,* metacarpophalangeal; *MTP,* metatarsophalangeal; *PIP,* proximal interphalangeal.

How would you summarize the findings and the most likely differential diagnoses?

In summary, this is a young female who presents with a chronic, polyarticular, symmetric arthritis affecting both small and large joints.

RA is a likely diagnosis, given the involvement of bilateral small joints in conjunction with symptom duration of greater than 6 to 8 weeks. Other possibilities include SpA with peripheral joint involvement such as ankylosing spondylitis (AS), psoriatic arthritis (PsA), or reactive arthritis. Peripheral joint involvement refers to joints of the extremities (such as shoulders, elbows, wrists, MCPs, PIPs, distal interphalangeal joints [DIPs], knees, ankles, or metatarsal interphalangeal joints [MTPs]). Axial joint involvement refers to spinal or sacroiliac joint involvement, which the patient does not have. She has no rash, so PsA is less likely (although 10% of the time the arthritic symptoms may precede the rash). With no history of recent infections, reactive arthritis is less likely. Patients with Sjögren's syndrome may also present with polyarticular inflammatory arthritis; however, she does not have any symptoms of keratoconjunctivitis sicca (dry eye) or xerostomia (dry mouth). Given the chronicity of her symptoms, an infectious cause of her arthritis would be very unlikely.

What are other physical exam findings in RA?

There are several physical exam findings in RA aside from synovitis; these are more typical in patients with advanced disease. One finding is rheumatoid nodules, which are located on the extensor surfaces of the extremities, often near the elbows, or sometimes on the fingers. Patients may also present with deformities, which include ulnar deviation of the digits, as well as swan neck, boutonnière, or Z thumb deformities. Flexion contractures at the elbows or knees are seen too. Although it is not unusual to encounter a patient with these deformities, therapy for RA has advanced so considerably over the last two decades that patients compliant with newer therapies (i.e., biologic drugs) should generally not develop such crippling deformities. Figures 9.1 through 9.4 demonstrate some of these exam findings.

Laboratory testing is significant for an elevated erythrocyte sedimentation rate (ESR) at 75 mm/hr, positive rheumatoid factor (RF), and strongly positive anti-cyclic citrullinated peptide (anti-CCP) antibodies. Radiographs of the hands and wrists demonstrate periarticular osteopenia, moderate radiocarpal joint space narrowing, as well as erosions of several MCP joints.

Diagnosis: Rheumatoid arthritis

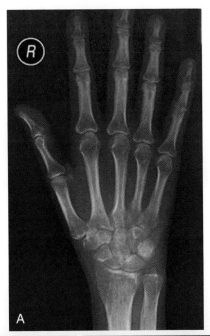

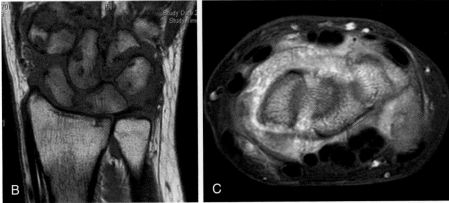

Figure 9.1 Early RA changes on x-ray demonstrate **(A)** periarticular osteopenia and no erosions. **(B, C)** Magnetic resonance imaging (MRI), which is more sensitive than plain films, shows erosions and marrow edema. *(From Campbell RSD. Rheumatoid arthritis of the wrist. In Waldman SD, ed. Imaging of Pain. Philadelphia: W.B. Saunders; 2011:299-301.)*

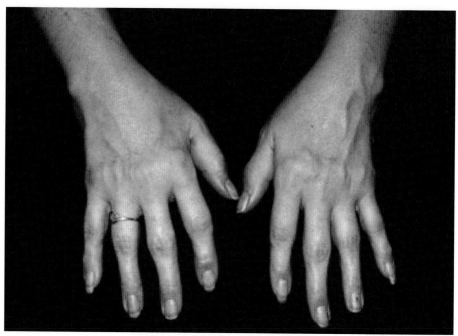

Figure 9.2   Early RA changes with synovitis of MCPs, PIPs, and wrists. *(From Posalski J, Weisman MH. Articular and periarticular manifestations of established rheumatoid arthritis. In Hochberg MC, Silman AJ, Smolen JS, Weinblatt ME, Weisman MH, eds.* Rheumatoid Arthritis. *Philadelphia: Mosby; 2009:49-61.)*

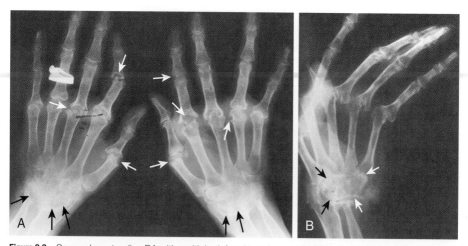

Figure 9.3   Severe, longstanding RA with multiple deformities. **A,** Longstanding rheumatoid arthritis. Erosions *(arrows)* at MCP and PIP joints and at the wrists bilaterally. Note soft tissue swelling around all MCP joints and joint space narrowing at all affected joints. **B,** Advanced rheumatoid arthritis with ulnar deviation and subluxation at MCP joints of all digits. Bony ankylosis involves the intercarpal bones *(arrows)* and ulnar translation of the carpus is present. *(From Peh WCG, Gilula LA. Radiologic examination of the hand. In Weinzweig J, ed.* Plastic Surgery Secrets Plus. *2nd ed. Philadelphia: Mosby; 2010;755-759.)*

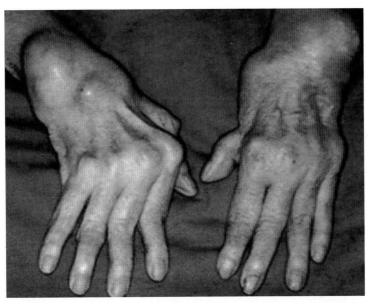

Figure 9.4 Longstanding RA on exam. Severe advanced RA of the hands. Massive tendon swelling over the dorsal surface of both wrists, severe muscle wasting, ulnar deviation of the metacarpophalangeal joints, and swan-neck deformity of the fingers. *(From Forbes CD, Jackson WF.* Color Atlas and Text of Clinical Medicine. *3rd ed. London: Mosby; 2003.)*

What are RFs and how should one interpret positive anti-CCP antibodies?

RFs are circulating immunoglobulin M (IgM) antibodies against the fragment crystallizable (Fc) portions of immunoglobulin G (IgG). They are not specific in regard to their affinity, can react to different antigenic sites of IgG, and can react with different tissue antigens depending on the person. Their function is unknown, and although not specific, they do serve as a biomarker for RA, as they are present in 26 to 90% of RA patients.

CLINICAL PEARL   **STEP 2/3**

Some other common reasons for a positive RF besides RA include advanced age (this is very common), other connective tissue diseases (i.e., SLE, mixed connective tissue disease, Sjögren's syndrome), mixed cryoglobulinemia types II and III, smoking, or chronic hepatitis C (HCV) infection.

A patient can be considered to have seropositive disease if RF is positive or if they are positive for anti-CCP antibodies (or both). The presence of anti-CCP antibodies has a specificity of >90% for RA and is associated with a more aggressive, destructive arthritis. Furthermore, RA patients with a positive anti-CCP antibody are more likely to develop extraarticular manifestations such as interstitial lung disease (ILD), pericardial effusions/pericarditis, or vasculitis than patients who are anti-CCP antibody negative.

CLINICAL PEARL   **STEP 2/3**

Periarticular osteopenia is one of the earliest radiographic findings in the hands in RA.

CLINICAL PEARL   **STEP 2/3**

Two musculoskeletal exam findings that are almost always due to longstanding, aggressive inflammatory arthritis include flexion contractures at the elbows (patients cannot fully straighten their arms) and limited extension at the wrists (this is due to severe joint space narrowing at the radiocarpal joint). Other causes of the elbow contractures include a history of fracture of the elbow or as a result of severe immobility (i.e., stroke, cerebral palsy).

CLINICAL PEARL   **STEP 2/3**

Leflunomide can also cause hepatotoxicity, so pay particular attention to liver tests when combining methotrexate with leflunomide.

What is the recommended initial treatment for RA?

The accepted first-line therapy for RA is the traditional disease-modifying antirheumatic drug (DMARD) methotrexate (MTX), which is dosed weekly, either via oral or subcutaneous route of administration. Gastrointestinal intolerance and liver toxicity are not infrequent side effects and can sometimes limit therapy. Other well-described side effects include hair loss, oral ulcers, skin nodules, and rarely a hypersensitivity pneumonitis. In RA, MTX is used in much lower doses than it is in malignancies when used as a chemotherapy agent, and is contraindicated in pregnancy.

What therapies are available if the patient does not respond to or has intolerance to MTX?

Other DMARDs commonly used include hydroxychloroquine (the mildest), sulfasalazine, and leflunomide. MTX can be combined with any of the other traditional DMARDs to better control disease.

BASIC SCIENCE PEARL   **STEP 1**

MTX irreversibly binds to dihydrofolate reductase, which inhibits purine synthesis and therefore inhibits DNA synthesis. It is specific to the S phase of the cell cycle. Because of its irreversible binding, it is very effective in decreasing cell division (especially in rapidly dividing cells like hair follicles). Thus, MTX can cause hair loss. (Folic acid is given to prevent such side effects.)

MTX additionally increases adenosine production at inflamed sites. Adenosine is a purine nucleoside shown to have an antiinflammatory effect in vivo. (It diminishes leukocyte accumulation in an in vivo model of inflammation.)

CLINICAL PEARL   **STEP 2/3**

Biologic therapies are very costly (approximately $1000/month), so the decision to initiate biologic therapy should be a thoughtful one. Efforts should be made to optimize DMARD therapy when possible before initiating biologic drugs.

When should biologic therapy be considered for RA?

Biologic therapies for RA include tumor necrosis factor (TNF) alpha inhibitors (fusion proteins like etanercept and monoclonal antibodies like infliximab and adalimumab), cytotoxic T lymphocyte-associated antigen 4 (CTLA-4) costimulatory molecule inhibitors (abatacept), monoclonal antibodies to the CD20 receptor (rituximab), or monoclonal antibodies against interleukin-6 (tocilizumab). The newest therapeutic option is the small-molecule DMARD tofacitinib (a Janus kinase inhibitor). Biologic therapies should be considered in patients whom have failed or have contraindications to traditional DMARDs or those with very rapidly progressive and destructive RA. This young patient has evidence of moderate radiographic damage with only a few months of arthritic symptoms, so biologics could be considered. If a patient presents with extraarticular manifestations (i.e., ILD), it would also be a reason to institute biologic therapy.

See Table 9.4 for a detailed description of the biologic agents for RA.

CLINICAL PEARL	**STEP 2/3**

Traditional DMARDs and biologic therapies can prevent additional joint destruction but cannot reverse any joint damage that has already been done.

CLINICAL PEARL	**STEP 2/3**

The risk of fulminant liver failure with biologics is much higher in patients with hepatitis B and carries a high morbidity and mortality. These patients should be comanaged with a hepatologist. If the biologic is necessary, careful liver function monitoring is required. (These patients often receive concomitant antiviral therapy.)

What are the side effects and risks of the biologic medications?

Because these are immunosuppressive medications, there is an increased risk of infections (viral, bacterial, tubercular, and fungal) in general. In particular, there can be reactivation of latent tuberculosis (TB), which can lead to significant morbidity; therefore, all patients receive either a purified protein derivative (PPD) or QuantiFERON gold screening test prior to initiating therapy. In patients with hepatitis B, there is a risk of fulminant liver failure in patients who are on biologics, particularly the TNF-alpha inhibitors. There is also a risk of fulminant liver failure in patients with hepatitis C (although the risk is much lower than with hepatitis B). Due to these risks, testing for both hepatitis B and C should be performed prior to starting biologic therapy. Additionally, patients should not be vaccinated with live vaccines while on a biologic. TNF-alpha inhibitors have also been associated with development of anti-double-stranded DNA (anti-dsDNA) antibodies and even drug-induced lupus in some patients with RA. Table 9.5 highlights the most significant side effects of DMARDs and biologic therapies.

BASIC SCIENCE PEARL	**STEP 1**

TNF alpha is necessary for production of granulomas in the body. For this reason, in patients treated with TNF-alpha inhibitors, tuberculosis can present with many (or any) different findings on chest radiograph. The typical granulomatous upper lobe findings will not necessarily be present.

The patient is not sexually active and does not plan on having children any time soon, so MTX therapy is initiated. She is titrated gradually to a maximum dose of 25 mg weekly. At that time, there is significant improvement in her synovitis; however, she still has over an hour of morning stiffness and several swollen MCP joints on exam. Hydroxychloroquine and sulfasalazine are initiated, and after 4 months, her synovitis is improved, morning stiffness of the joints is minimal, and she is functionally back to normal. Her ESR has decreased to 11 mm/hr.

TABLE 9.4 ■ DMARDs, Biologics, and Small Molecule Therapies for RA

Class	Type	Drug	Mechanism	Route
DMARD (traditional)	Antimetabolite	methotrexate	DHFR inhibitor (inhibitor of purine synthesis); increases adenosine release at inflamed sites*	Oral, SC, IM
DMARD (traditional)	Antibiotic/ antiinflammatory	sulfasalazine	Poorly understood (has antibiotic and antiinflammatory effects)	Oral
DMARD (traditional)	Antimalarial	hydroxychloroquine	Incompletely understood, possibly modulation of innate immunity through toll-like receptors	Oral
DMARD (traditional)	Antimetabolite	leflunomide	Inhibits mitochondrial enzyme dihydroorotate dehydrogenase (inhibitor of pyrimidine synthesis)	Oral
Biologic	TNF-alpha inhibitor (fusion protein)	etanercept	Fusion protein of TNF receptor to Fc portion of IgG1 (decoy receptor for TNF thereby decreasing effect of circulating TNF)	SC
Biologic	TNF-alpha inhibitor (monoclonal antibody)	infliximab, adalimumab, certolizumab pegol, golimumab	Monoclonal antibody against soluble and membrane bound TNF, thereby decreasing its effects	IV or SC depending on agent
Biologic	CTLA-4/ Costimulation inhibitor	abatacept	Inhibits antigen-presenting cells' costimulatory signal thereby decreasing T-cell activation	SC or IV
Biologic	CD20 inhibitor	rituximab	Down-regulates B-cell function/number and decreases antibody production	IV
Biologic	IL-6 inhibitor	tocilizumab	Binds to soluble and membrane-bound IL-6 decreasing its inflammatory effects	IV
DMARD (new, small molecule type)	Janus kinase inhibitor	tofacitinib	Inhibits JAK1 and JAK3 production of inflammation via STAT1-dependent gene suppression	Oral

*Adenosine is a purine nucleoside shown to have an antiinflammatory effect in vivo (diminishes leukocyte accumulation in an in vivo model of inflammation).

CTLA-4, Cytotoxic T-lymphocyte-associated protein 4; DHFR, dihydrofolate reductase; DMARD, disease-modifying antirheumatic drug; IM, intramuscular; IV, intravenous; JAK, Janus kinase; SC, subcutaneous; STAT1, Signal Transducers and Activators of Transcription 1; TNF, tumor necrosis factor

TABLE 9.5 ■ Common Side Effects of DMARDs and Biologics in RA

Drug	Side Effects	Caution in Patients With:
Methotrexate	Hepatotoxicity Hypersensitivity pneumonitis Hair loss Nausea	Liver and lung disease
Sulfasalazine	Myelosuppression	—
Hydroxychloroquine	Maculopathy (eye toxicity) Rare myopathy including cardiomyopathy Rare hyperpigmentation of skin	Retinal disease
Leflunomide	Hepatotoxicity Diarrhea Weight loss Hair loss	Liver and lung disease
TNF-alpha inhibitors (i.e., etanercept, infliximab, adalimumab, certolizumab pegol, golimumab)	Reactivation of TB and/or hepatitis B Heart failure Drug-induced lupus Increased risk of infection	Heart failure TB or hepatitis B History of malignancy
Abatacept	Increased risk of infection	COPD
Rituximab	Reactivation of hepatitis B and/or TB Infusion reactions Demyelinating neuropathy rarely	TB or hepatitis B
Tocilizumab	Lipid elevation Myelosuppression Bowel rupture Infusion reactions Renal, liver toxicity	CBC, CMP, and lipid monitoring
Tofacitinib	Lipid elevation Myelosuppression Bowel rupture Renal, liver toxicity	CBC, CMP, and lipid monitoring

CBC, Complete blood count; *CMP,* comprehensive metabolic panel; *COPD,* chronic obstructive pulmonary disease; *TB,* tuberculosis; *TNF,* tumor necrosis factor

BEYOND THE PEARLS

- A late manifestation of RA is extensor tendon rupture that can lead to swan neck and boutonnière deformities (Fig. 9.5).
- Prior to surgery it is recommended that RA patients have cervical spine films with flexion and extension views to evaluate for atlantoaxial subluxation, a very dangerous sequelae of the disease.
- Felty's syndrome is a very common triad of (usually seropositive) RA, neutropenia, and splenomegaly. It is not generally seen because of the more effective RA treatments available today.
- Tofacitinib is one of the newest therapies for RA and is the first oral new class of small-molecule DMARDs.

Continued

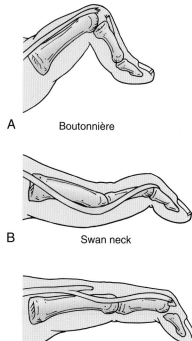

A   Boutonnière

B   Swan neck

Figure 9.5 **(A)** Boutonnière deformity (PIP flexion and DIP hyperextension). **(B)** Swan neck deformity (PIP hyperextension and DIP flexion). **(C)** Mallet finger (DIP flexion and loss of active extension). *(From The occupational therapy process: implementation of interventions. In Mosby's Field Guide to Occupational Therapy for Physical Dysfunction. St. Louis: Mosby. 2013:211-244.)*

C   Mallet

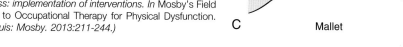

BEYOND THE PEARLS—cont'd

- Prior to instituting a TNF-alpha inhibitor, it is standard practice to screen for hepatitis B, C, and latent TB (either using PPD or QuantiFERON gold assay). Untreated hepatitis B in a patient on TNF-alpha inhibitors can lead to fulminant liver failure, with a high risk of morbidity and mortality. (The risk is less for patients with hepatitis C.) There are case reports of patients who are hepatitis B core IgG/IgM positive having liver failure while on TNF-alpha inhibitors; although less common, one should also screen for hepatitis B core IgG/IgM.
- MTX can actually exacerbate rheumatoid nodules in some individuals.
- In pregnancy, it is considered safe to use prednisone in doses <15 mg daily, sulfasalazine, hydroxychloroquine, azathioprine (although this is a weak agent for RA), and possibly biologic therapies (this is not confirmed and the decision for therapy is individualized).
- Tarsal tunnel syndrome (posterior tibial neuralgia) is not uncommon is RA; it presents as numbness and tingling along the medial ankle, radiating to the toes and plantar foot.

References

Baker D, Schumacher HR. Acute monoarthritis. *N Engl J Med.* 1993;329(14):1013-1020.

Brown AK. How to interpret plain radiographs in clinical practice. *Best Pract Res Clin Rheumatol.* 2013;27(2):249-269.

Campbell RSD, Waldman SD. Rheumatoid arthritis of the wrist. In: Waldman SD, ed. *Imaging of Pain.* Philadelphia: Saunders; 2011:299-301.

Favalli EG, Bugatti S, Biggioggero M, Caporali R. Treatment comparison in rheumatoid arthritis: head-to-head trials and innovative study designs. *Biomed Res Int*. 2014;2014:831603. doi: 10.1155/2014/831603.

Forbes CD, Jackson WF. *Color Atlas and Text of Clinical Medicine*. 3rd ed. London: Mosby; 2003.

Ghoreschi K, Jesson MI, Li X, et al. Modulation of innate and adaptive immune responses by tofacitinib (CP-690,550). *J Immunol*. 2011;186(7):4234-4243.

Joaquim A, Appenzeller S. Cervical spine involvement in rheumatoid arthritis—a systematic review. *Autoimmun Rev*. 2014;13:1195-1202.

Peh WCG, Gilula LA. Radiologic examination of the hand. In: Weinzweig J, ed. *Plastic Surgery Secrets Plus*. 2nd ed. Philadelphia: Mosby; 2010:755-759.

Posalski J, Weisman MH. Articular and periarticular Manifestations of established rheumatoid arthritis. In: Hochberg MC, Silman AJ, Smolen JS, Weinblatt ME, Weisman MH, eds. *Rheumatoid Arthritis*. Philadelphia: Mosby; 2009:49-61.

Rantalaiho V, Kautiainen H, Korpela M, et al. Targeted treatment with a combination of traditional DMARDs produces excellent clinical and radiographic long-term outcomes in early rheumatoid arthritis regardless of initial infliximab. The 5-year follow-up results of a randomized clinical trial, the NEO-RACo trial. *Ann Rheum Dis*. 2014;73:1954-1961.

Singh JA, Furst DE, Bharat A, et al. 2012 Update of the 2008 American College of Rheumatology (ACR) Recommendations for the Use of Disease-Modifying Anti-Rheumatic Drugs and Biologics in the Treatment of Rheumatoid Arthritis. *Arthritis Care Res*. 2012;64(5):625-639.

Soubrier M, Chamoux NB, Tatar Z, et al. Cardiovascular risk in rheumatoid arthritis. *Joint Bone Spine*. 2014;81:298-302.

Takeda K, Kaisho T, Akira S. Toll-like receptors. *Annu Rev Immunol*. 2003;21:335-376.

The occupational therapy process: implementation of interventions. In: *Mosby's Field Guide to Occupational Therapy for Physical Dysfunction*. St. Louis: Mosby; 2013:211-244.

Monisha Bhanote ■ Daniel Martinez

A 62-Year-Old Female With Epigastric Pain and Nausea

A 62-year-old female presents to her primary care doctor for a 2-month history of dull epigastric pain. The pain is 5/10, lasts about an hour, occasionally radiates to her chest, wakes her from sleep, and is improved with over-the-counter antacids. She has no significant past medical or surgical history, but she does take nonsteroidal antiinflammatory drugs (NSAIDs) (ibuprofen) frequently for chronic low back pain. She denies any illicit drug use, but she reports smoking and alcohol use throughout her life. She works as a stockbroker and says that the recent economic recession has made her work very stressful. She denies weight loss, nausea, vomiting, dysphagia, odynophagia, melena, hematochezia, diarrhea, or constipation.

On physical exam, her temperature is 37 °C (98.6 °F), blood pressure is 133/86 mm Hg, pulse rate is 85/min, respiration rate is 12/min, and oxygen saturation is 99% on room air. Her body mass index (BMI) is 30. She is nonjaundiced, well nourished, and well developed with normal heart and lung sounds. Her abdomen is soft, mildly tender to deep palpation, nondistended, with no hepatosplenomegaly, masses, rebound or guarding. No cervical, axillary, or inguinal lymphadenopathy is appreciated.

What pathologies should you be thinking about in this patient? How should you proceed?

The clinical vignette is a classic setup for peptic ulcer disease/gastritis or gastroesophageal reflux disease (GERD) given the description of the pain and following risk factors: older age, chronic NSAID use, alcohol/tobacco use, and stress. Another reasonable common pathology to consider is biliary colic given the description of a recurrent dull epigastric pain.

Because of her age, an astute clinician would also consider other pathologies such as a gastric malignancy (adenocarcinoma or mucosa-associated lymphoid tissue [MALT] lymphoma) or a pancreatic head mass. However, these are less likely given that she has no red flags such as a concerning family history, weight loss, jaundice, or lymphadenopathy.

Given her classic symptoms and lack of red flags, empiric treatment with a proton pump inhibitor (PPI) such as omeprazole is appropriate at this time.

She is prescribed omeprazole 20 mg orally once daily and instructed to return in 2 months. She returns and reports only a mild improvement in her symptoms. A right upper quadrant ultrasound is then ordered, which shows no evidence of gallstones or biliary ductal dilatation; this comfortably rules out biliary colic. Because of her older age and because she failed empiric therapy, she is referred to a gastroenterologist for an esophagogastroduodenoscopy (EGD).

When is an EGD indicated?

Endoscopy is commonly performed first when the patient is over 45 years old and has weight loss, anemia, or heme-positive stools. Upper endoscopy can help find causes of unexplained symptoms such as heartburn, nausea, vomiting, and problems swallowing. It can also help with abnormal lab results such anemia and nutritional deficiencies.

She arrives at her gastroenterologist and an EGD is scheduled. She tolerates the procedure well; after the procedure, her gastroenterologist explains that visually her esophagus and duodenum are unremarkable. However, her stomach did show areas of erythema (Fig. 10.1), which suggests gastritis, and biopsies were taken to confirm. He advises her to return for a follow-up and explanation of the biopsy results.

What are common visual findings of gastritis on EGD?
Findings commonly see in abnormal endoscopy are erosions, antral nodularity, thickened gastric folds, and visible submucosal vessels. Although these findings are not specific for a particular type of gastritis, the presence of a mosaic pattern in the corpus of the stomach may suggest a *Helicobacter*-type gastritis.

The patient returns to her gastroenterologist for follow-up, and he informs her that the biopsies were positive for *Helicobacter pylori* infection. Specifically, the pathology revealed an active gastritis with expansion of the lamina propria with inflammatory cells such as lymphocytes, plasma cells, and neutrophils as well as numerous small curved organisms identified in the intercellular spaces of the foveolar cells. They are seen in the hematoxylin and eosin (H&E) stain but are better appreciated with a Giemsa stain (Figs. 10.2 and 10.3). The patient was confirmed to have a *H. pylori* gastritis with the biopsy.

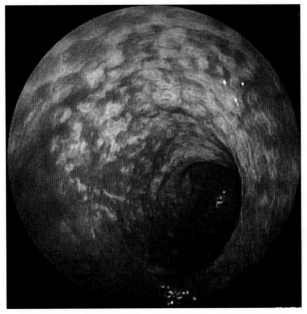

Figure 10.1 Endoscopy of the stomach with chronic gastritis induced by *H. pylori* infection. Acetate stained and Fuji Intelligent Color Enhancement (FICE) enhanced image. *(From* https://commons.wikimedia.org/wiki/File:Helicobacter_gastritis_2.jpg*)*

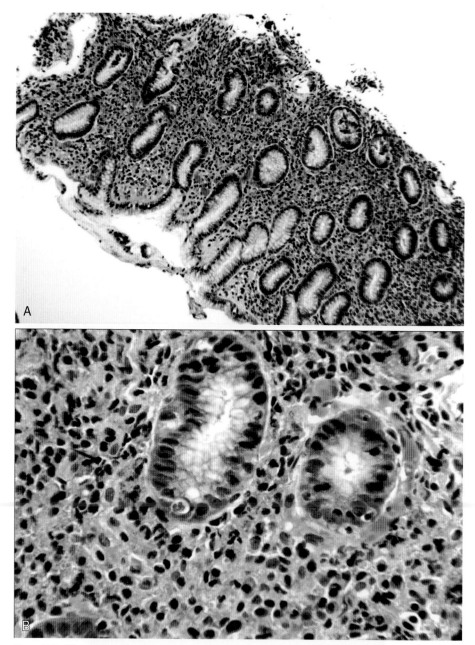

Figure 10.2   Histologic section from patient's gastric biopsy showing expansion of the lamina propria with lymphocytes, plasma cells, and neutrophils. **(A)** Low-power H&E stain, **(B)** high-power H&E stain.

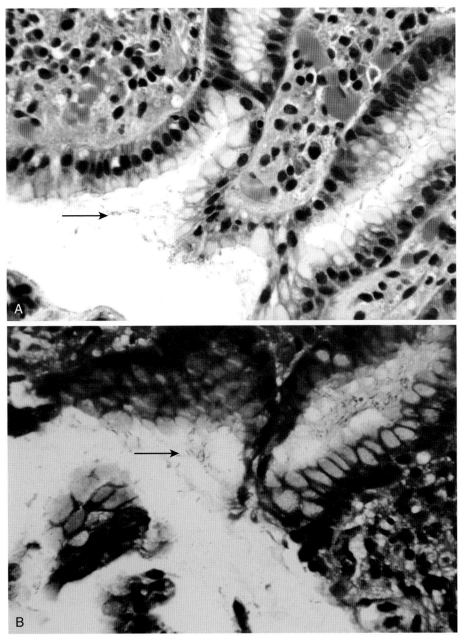

Figure 10.3 Higher-power image of the patient's biopsy showing innumerable curved-shaped organisms *(arrows)* within the intercellular spaces of the foveolar cells. **(A)** H&E stain, **(B)** Giemsa stain.

How is *Helicobacter pylori* infection diagnosed?

H. pylori is a curved, gram-negative rod bacterium that produces urease. It is an infection that is normally acquired in childhood. Colonization with this bacterium is not a disease in itself; however, it is associated with a number of disorders in the upper gastrointestinal tract. *H. pylori* infection can be diagnosed with serology, stool antigen testing, urea breath test, and biopsy.

Serology can be positive up to 18 months after eradication. The most reliable method, however, is with biopsy and histologic exam combined with either a rapid urease test or microbial culture.

Stool antigen testing is a common way of evaluating for infection in patients with typical symptoms and no red flags. If the patient were young, testing for stool antigen would have been the next step in management after she failed the trial of omeprazole.

CLINICAL PEARL   **STEP 2/3**

A urea breath test is a noninvasive diagnostic procedure in which the patient takes either radioactive carbon-14 or nonradioactive carbon-13, which the bacteria then metabolizes to produce labeled carbon dioxide that is detected in the breath.

CLINICAL PEARL   **STEP 2/3**

A stool antigen test is an enzyme immunoassay to measure anti-*H. pylori* antibodies. A positive result (antigen detected) is indicative of *H. pylori* presence. A negative result (antigen not detected) indicates absence of *H. pylori* or an antigenic level below the assay limit of detection. The test has a sensitivity and specificity of 96% for detecting *H. pylori* infection. It is recommended to not take antibiotics or medicine containing bismuth for 1 month prior to testing and to stop PPIs 2 weeks before testing to prevent false-negative testing.

Because the patient was diagnosed with *H. pylori* infection from the biopsies taken during her upper endoscopy, the gastroenterologist discusses treatment options with her.

Diagnosis: *H. pylori* infection

What are the recommendations for management of *H. pylori* infection?

H. pylori eradication is an appropriate option in patients infected with *H. pylori* and investigated nonulcer dyspepsia. For patients with dyspepsia of unclear etiology, it is reasonable to test for *H. pylori*. A positive stool antigen or rapid urease test is sufficient to initiate treatment. It is appropriate to start with triple therapy: PPI, amoxicillin, and clarithromycin for 7 to 14 days.

The patient is started on a standard triple therapy. She is also advised to adhere to a healthy and balanced diet, to stop smoking, and to limit her alcohol and ibuprofen intake. She is also to return in 1 month for a follow-up of her symptoms.

CLINICAL PEARL   **STEP 2/3**

H. pylori eradication should be confirmed at least 4 weeks after treatment. The rapid urease test is recommended and has a sensitivity of 94% and a specificity of 95% for *H. pylori* infection. However, if the rapid urease test not available, stool antigen testing can be used, although it has a lower sensitivity.

What are some complications of *H. pylori* infection?

H. pylori infections can cause peptic ulcer disease. About 10% of patients will develop gastric or duodenal ulcers (duodenal ulcers are more common than gastric). *H. pylori* infection alone does not cause ulcer formation. Other contributing factors include NSAID use, cigarette smoking, hereditary tendency, and acid hypersecretion.

H. pylori has also been associated with malignancies such as MALT lymphoma and gastric carcinoma. There is less than a 1% risk of developing MALT lymphoma, while the lifetime risk of developing gastric carcinoma is 1 to 2%. The association is with both intestinal type and diffuse type gastric carcinoma.

CLINICAL PEARL   **STEP 2/3**

Gastric cancer develops in patients with *H. pylori* infection. Patients with severe gastric atrophy, corpus-predominant gastritis, or intestinal metaplasia are at increased risk. Patients with nonulcer dyspepsia, gastric ulcers, or gastric hyperplastic polyps are also at risk. Duodenal ulcers do not pose a risk for gastric cancer.

CLINICAL PEARL   **STEP 2/3**

Gastric cancer spreads via the lymphatic system. Left supraclavicular adenopathy (also known as Virchow's node) is the most common physical finding of metastatic disease.

CLINICAL PEARL   **STEP 2/3**

Since the association of gastric MALT lymphoma with *H. pylori* infection, it was established that early-stage disease could be cured by *H. pylori* eradication, which is now the mainstay of therapy.

The patient stops taking her triple therapy medications because they gave her an upset stomach and she believed they were not helping. Work has also been much more stressful than usual, and she develops severe tension headaches. She goes to an urgent care center that gives her high-dose naproxen for her headaches. She also continues to take ibuprofen for back pain. Her abdominal symptoms resolve, and she does not follow up because she figures everything is OK.

Six months later, she appears at the emergency room complaining of a sharp 10/10 abdominal pain associated with black, tarry, foul-smelling stools. On physical exam, her temperature is 37 °C (98.6 °F), blood pressure is 90/50 mm Hg, pulse rate is 135/min, respiration rate is 22/min, and oxygen saturation is 99% on room air. She is anxious-appearing and diaphoretic with pale conjunctiva. She has a systolic ejection murmur but lungs are clear to auscultation. Her abdomen is soft but with significant epigastric tenderness to palpation and moderate guarding.

Two large-bore IVs are started and she is given 2 L normal saline bolus with mild improvement in her blood pressure and tachycardia. Labs are ordered revealing a hemoglobin of 6 g/dL, platelets of 100,000/µL, and leukocytosis of 12,000/µL. Given her history of gastritis, melena, and NSAID use in the context of hemodynamic instability and new anemia, a bleeding gastric ulcer is suspected. She receives 3 units of packed red blood cells in the emergency room, is started on a pantoprazole drip, and is admitted to the medical ICU. She responds appropriately to the transfusion: her blood pressure is 110/70 mm Hg and pulse rate is 95/min. Her hemoglobin is now 8.5 g/dL and she remains stable overnight. Gastroenterology is consulted and she is scheduled for an EGD in the morning.

What is the etiology of peptic ulcer disease?

Peptic ulcer disease, as mentioned before, is associated with *H. pylori* infection. It is also associated with NSAID use (the leading cause of bleeding ulcers), Crohn's disease, and Zollinger-Ellison syndrome (1% of cases).

CLINICAL PEARL   **STEP 2/3**

Zollinger–Ellison syndrome is caused by a gastrin-secreting tumor in the pancreas that stimulates the parietal cells in the stomach to produce acid and then mucosal ulcerations. It can be seen sporadically or as part of multiple endocrine neoplasia type I (MEN 1 = parathyroid, pituitary, and pancreatic neoplasms).

What are some complications associated with peptic ulcer disease?

Complications of peptic ulcer disease include upper gastrointestinal tract bleeding, perforation, penetration, and gastric outlet obstruction.

The patient undergoes an upper endoscopy in the morning, and a peptic ulcer is noted. It is injected and clipped to stop the bleeding. Additional biopsies are taken at that time to rule out a malignancy. She is started on quadruple therapy of omeprazole, bismuth, metronidazole, and tetracycline in the hospital. The next day she continues to have melena with worsening pain and a drop in her hemoglobin to 6.5 g/dL. She is transfused 3 additional units of packed red blood cells and surgery is consulted.

What are the major indications for peptic ulcer surgery?

The five major indications for peptic ulcer surgery are intractability, hemorrhage, perforation, penetration, and obstruction. Intractability relates to the patient's symptoms, not to delayed healing. Patients who require large volume blood transfusions to correct losses because of continuous hemorrhage or who have rebleeding episodes should undergo surgery. Perforation requires immediate surgery. Penetration indicates erosion of the ulcer through the entire thickness of the wall of the stomach without leakage of contents into the peritoneal cavity. Obstruction occurs in 2% of ulcer patients and can be managed by endoscopic balloon dilation.

The patient's hemoglobin does not improve with the additional transfusion, and she develops progressive tachycardia and hypotension. She is then emergently taken to the operating room for surgical repair because she is unstable and failed medical therapy. A partial gastrectomy is performed to remove the bleeding ulcer (Fig. 10.4).

The surgery goes well and the remainder of her hospital course is unremarkable. She is discharged with a prescription for completion of her quadruple therapy. She follows up with her primary care doctor in 2 weeks. She reports adherence to her medical therapy and that her symptoms have now resolved. The doctor reassures her that if she continues to adhere to medical recommendations, she is unlikely to have future bleeding complications. However, the doctor does indicate that there are certain risk factors for recurrent ulcers even though she has undergone surgical resection.

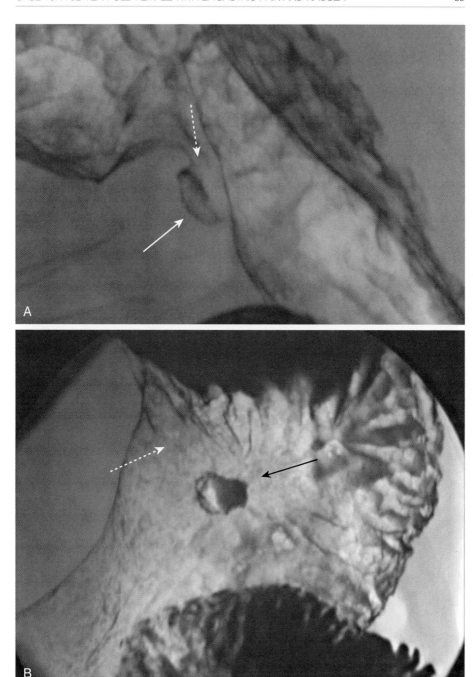

Figure 10.4 Benign lesser curvature gastric ulcer. **A,** Seen in profile there is a large collection of barium that protrudes beyond the expected contour of the normal body of the stomach along the lesser curvature, representing a gastric ulcer *(solid white arrow)*. This ulcer collection was present on multiple views (an important characteristic of an ulcer called persistence). There is a mound of edematous tissue that surrounds the ulcer *(dotted white arrow)* called an ulcer collar. **B,** Seen en face there are numerous gastric folds *(dashed white arrow)*, which all radiate to the ulcer margin and a central collection *(black arrow)* representing the ulcer itself. This was a benign gastric ulcer. *(From Herring W. Learning Radiology. 3rd ed. Philadelphia: Saunders; 2016:182-203.)*

What are causes for recurrent ulcers in patients who have undergone previous ulcer surgery?

Recurrent ulcers can be seen in untreated *H. pylori* infection, NSAID use, incomplete vagotomy, "retained antrum" syndrome, antral G-cell hyperplasia, Zollinger-Ellison syndrome, and gastric cancer. Secondary causes may include smoking, bile acid, and primary hyperparathyroidism. She is once again advised to limit her alcohol use and smoking and to decrease the use of NSAIDs.

CLINICAL PEARL   **STEP 2/3**

"Retained antrum" syndrome can be seen after a partial gastrectomy in the Billroth II operation, when antral tissue is left behind. The lack of usual acid-secreting gastric glands means that the antral segment is continually exposed to the alkaline environment of the duodenum, which causes it to secrete excessive acid and to be prone to form ulcers.

BEYOND THE PEARLS

- In patients who receive long-term NSAIDs and who have peptic ulcer disease, PPI maintenance treatment is better than *H. pylori* eradiation in preventing ulcer recurrence and/or bleeding.
- Antibiotics may cause *H. pylori* bacterium to change from their usual curved rod shape to a coccoid shape.
- The cagA gene codes for one of *H. pylori's* virulence factors, and the bacterial strains that are associated with this gene have the ability to cause ulcers. Determining cagA status may confer additional benefit in identifying populations at greater risk of developing gastric cancer.
- *Helicobacter* has more than 50 species. After *H. pylori*, the most common species to cause gastritis in humans is *H. heilmannii*, which is a slightly longer organism with five to seven spirals. It tends to cause a patchy milder gastritis and is more common in children.
- Studies suggest that *H. pylori* infection is associated with iron-deficiency anemia. Mechanisms of involvement may include occult blood loss secondary to chronic erosive gastritis, decreased iron absorption secondary to chronic gastritis, and increased iron uptake by the bacteria. *H. pylori* eradication reverses iron-deficiency anemia in patients with asymptomatic gastritis and improves oral iron absorption.
- There is a higher prevalence of *H. pylori* infection in patients with idiopathic thrombocytopenic purpura (ITP). It has been confirmed that eradication therapy induces a significant positive platelet response in patients with ITP.
- The risk of gastric cancer development depends on bacterial virulence factors and host genetic factors.
- Eradication of *H. pylori* has the potential to reduce the risk of gastric cancer development by preventing the development of preneoplastic changes such as atrophic gastritis and intestinal metaplasia.
- A t(11;18)(q21;q21) chromosomal translocation, giving rise to an API2-MLT fusion gene, in MALT lymphoma is predictive of poor response to eradication therapy.

References

Cho J-Y, Chang, YW, Jang, JY, et al. Close observation of gastric mucosal pattern by standard endoscopy can predict *Helicobacter pylori* infection status. *J Gastroenterol Hepatol.* 2013;28(2):279-284.

Malfertheiner P, Megraud F, O'Morain C, et al. Current concepts in the management of *Helicobacter pylori* infection: the Maastricht III Consensus Report. *Gut.* 2007;56:772-781.

Odze, RD, Goldbum, JR. *Surgical Pathology of the GI Tract, Liver, Biliary Tract, and Pancreas.* 2nd ed. Philadelphia: Saunders/Elsevier; 2009.

Uemura N, Okamoto S, Yamamoto S, et al. *Helicobacter pylori* infection and the development of gastric cancer. *N Engl J Med.* 2001;245(11):784-789.

Brandon A. Miller

A 69-Year-Old Male With "Congestive Heart Failure"

A 69-year-old male presents to your office for a 1-week posthospital discharge follow-up. He is seen at your practice for the management of hypertension, hyperlipidemia, and prediabetes. He has a family history significant for coronary artery disease (CAD) in both of his parents. He has been occasionally adherent with his medication regimen and lifestyle modifications, at times seeming motivated while at other times missing appointments for up to 2 years (during which time he has not called in medication refills). Recently he has been experiencing swelling in his legs and shortness of breath with exertion, which led to an emergency room visit and subsequent hospital admission. He was told at the hospital that he had "congestive heart failure" and states that he was started on "a whole bunch of new meds," which he has listed on his discharge paperwork. They include aspirin, clopidogrel, lisinopril, carvedilol, atorvastatin, and furosemide.

Why is it unsatisfactory to accept a diagnosis of "congestive heart failure" at face value? Why should you never simply put "congestive heart failure" in the problem list of your patient's chart?

Congestive heart failure (CHF) is a very nonspecific term that refers to a failure of the heart to pump blood forward as well as it normally does. This leads to signs and symptoms related to back flow (or congestion) of blood, either to the lungs or the venous system. The term CHF is considered oversimplified and not reflective of the underlying etiology of pump failure. In the United States, the most common cause of CHF is coronary artery disease (CAD); however, there are many different causes of CHF, and it is important to the note the cause in your patient in order to best determine a treatment plan.

When charting on your patient with this clinical syndrome, it is important to note a few things. First, make sure to indicate the patient's ejection fraction (EF) and the date of his or her most recent echocardiogram. Remember, not all patients with CHF have a depressed EF. In fact, approximately half of patients with CHF have a preserved EF and are classified as having heart failure with persevered EF (HFpEF). (The other broad category of CHF is heart failure with reduced EF [HFrEF]). Second, if known, make sure to specify the etiology of the heart failure. Third, note the functional capacity of the patient using the New York Heart Association (NYHA) classification (heart.org). All of these notations in the chart have implications on the treatment, either medical or surgical, of your patient. Charting can no doubt seem cumbersome at times; however, it remains a powerful tool in explaining your medical decision making and communicating with other providers that will be reading it. This is ultimately of most benefit to your patients.

CLINICAL PEARL	**STEP 2/3**

A normal ejection fraction ranges between 55 and 70%.

What symptoms are suggestive of CHF?

The symptoms that a patient with CHF reports will depend on the underlying etiology and the side of the heart that is failing. Shortness of breath is the main symptom reported in CHF due to left-sided heart disease. Shortness of breath initially occurs with exertion, and as the disease becomes more severe can be present at rest. As blood backs up due to poor forward flow and congests the pulmonary vasculature, pressure inside the intrapulmonary capillaries is exceeded, and fluid leaks into the interstitial and alveolar spaces. On a related note, orthopnea, which is defined as shortness of breath from pulmonary edema when lying flat, is caused by redistribution of blood from the lower extremities and splanchnic vessels to the vena cava when recumbent. Remember to ask your patients how many pillows they need to prop themselves up on at night to prevent shortness of breath. If this number has increased recently, this can be a clue to worsening or exacerbated CHF. Also due to similar pathophysiology, coughing and wheezing at night (cardiac asthma), are often overlooked symptoms of CHF that can be mistakenly attributed to other conditions (such as asthma, gastroesophageal reflux, or infection). Paroxysmal nocturnal dyspnea (PND) is the sudden, intense sensation of shortness of breath that causes patients to wake up in the middle of the night gasping for air and is also related to pulmonary edema in the recumbent position. The main symptom of right-sided heart failure is lower extremity swelling, which is due to leaked fluid from increased capillary pressure in the extremities from venous congestion. Other nonspecific symptoms that can be attributed to CHF are fatigue, nausea, vomiting, and early satiety due to bowel wall edema.

CLINICAL PEARL   **STEP 2/3**

The most common cause of right-sided heart failure is left-sided heart failure. The congestion due to backflow of blood into the lungs causes an increase intrapulmonary pressure, which in turn forces the right side of the heart to work harder to pump blood into the lungs. If only right-sided symptoms are present (peripheral pitting edema) and the workup reveals a normal left side of the heart, suspect a primary pulmonary process such as pulmonary hypertension. This condition is called "cor pulmonale" or right-sided heart failure due to a pulmonary process.

What signs are seen in CHF?

The signs of CHF depend on the underlying etiology and the severity of the disease. In general, patients with mild or well-controlled CHF will appear normal at rest but can appear tachypneic with exertion. Upon exam of the lungs, crackles or rales are indicative of intraalveolar fluid and decreased breath sounds are due to pleural effusions. Rales and decreased breath sounds are often bilateral, but patients can have unilateral pleural effusions, usually in the right hemithorax.

The heart exam can vary widely and often sounds normal. Make sure to feel for lifts and thrills and to palpate for the point of maximal impulse (PMI), which if displaced can signify an enlarged heart. Gallops are extra heart sounds (in addition to the normal S1 and S2) that can be heard in CHF patients, but their absence does not mean a patient does not have CHF. S3 is a third heart sound that occurs after S1 and before S2 and is caused by blood sloshing around in dilated ventricles. S4, or the fourth heart sound, occurs before S1 and represents blood being forcefully ejected into a noncompliant or "stiff" ventricle (which one may have with left ventricular hypertrophy, hypertrophic cardiomyopathy, or restrictive heart disease of any cause).

The exam of the extremities can reveal pitting edema in the feet, ankles, or legs caused by interstitial fluid that has leaked out of the capillaries from venous congestion due to right-sided heart failure. The term *pitting* refers to indentations (or pits) that form when pressure is applied to a swollen extremity.

BASIC SCIENCE PEARL   STEP 1

S1 and S2 are the normal heart sounds that occur from closing of the atrioventricular (mitral/tricuspid) and semilunar (aortic/pulmonic) valves, respectively. In the normal cardiac cycle, the atrioventricular valves close when the pressure in the ventricles increases, causing the atrioventricular valves to snap shut. As the pressure in the ventricles starts to decrease, the semilunar valves close to prevent backflow of blood. The increased pressure just described is otherwise known as systole, which occurs between S1 and S2.

CLINICAL PEARL   STEP 2/3

Knowing that systole occurs between S1 and S2 makes it a bit easier to understand and identify the extra heart sounds (S3 and S4). S3 occurs between S1 and S2 during systole because the contraction of a dilated left ventricle is what causes blood to "slosh around" in it. S4 occurs before S1, during diastole, when blood is ejected from the atria in stiff ventricles.

How is examining the jugular veins used to determine volume status? How do you examine for jugular venous distention?

Determining the jugular venous pressure (JVP) is important in patients with CHF because it can help determine a patient's volume status and should regularly be assessed. If the JVP is elevated, the patient is volume overloaded and will benefit from diuresis. Be aware, however, that determining JVP is difficult, and its absence does not mean your patient is not volume overloaded. In this instance, you must use other signs and symptoms to make a determination of volume status. The JVP can be elevated either as a result of right-sided or left-sided heart failure due to pulmonary vascular congestion.

To determine the JVP, lay your patient down and raise the head of the bed or examining table to a 45-degree angle. Ask the patient to look to the left so you can examine the right internal jugular vein. Shine a bright light at an oblique angle and look along the sternocleidomastoid muscle for the jugular venous waves. Look for biphasic or fluttering waves as opposed to the monophonic or pulsating waves of the carotid. If you are unsure, you can always palpate for a pulse or press on the patient's liver to look for a rise in the jugular venous column (hepatojugular reflex).

The landmark used to measure the JVP is the sternal angle. With the patient at a 45-degree angle, look for the highest point on the patient's neck that the jugular venous waves can be seen. If you do not see it on the neck, it can sometimes be seen at the angle of the jaw or near the ear if the venous pressure is really elevated. Imagine a line parallel to the floor extending out from the highest point of the jugular venous waves. This line will intersect with an imaginary line that is perpendicular to the floor coming straight up through the sternal angle. Measure the height from the sternal angle to the intersection of these lines and add 5 cm (the distance from sternal angle to the right atrium). If this sounds confusing, look at Figure 11.1. Values above 8 cm are considered abnormally elevated.

BASIC SCIENCE PEARL   STEP 1

The sensitivity of JVD is low, approximately 50% or lower in some studies, with low interobserver reliability. However, the specificity for JVD is approximately 100%, meaning that if it is present, there is almost always elevated right atrial pressure. This also means that if JVD is not seen, it is still possible that there is elevated pressure.

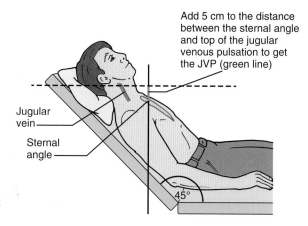

Add 5 cm to the distance
between the sternal angle
and top of the jugular
venous pulsation to get
the JVP (green line)

Jugular
vein

Sternal
angle

45°

Figure 11.1 JVP measurement
diagram.

Your patient does not know much about his hospital course but states that he had some sort of heart procedure that found "blockages in my heart." He gives you permission to obtain his hospital records, and your staff is able to obtain a discharge summary. His echocardiogram results are contained in the discharge summary and reveal the following findings: Severely dilated left ventricle with diffuse akinesis, left ventricular ejection fraction of 30%, mild-to-moderate mitral regurgitation, and elevated systolic pulmonary artery pressure estimated at 55 mm Hg.

Diagnosis: Ischemic cardiomyopathy with systolic congestive heart failure with an ejection fraction of 30%

What is the differential diagnosis of dilated cardiomyopathy?

In dilated cardiomyopathy, one or more of the ventricles is thinned and dilated. The differential diagnosis is broad and, as with any patient, a thorough history and physical exam is a necessary first step in elucidating the etiology. Be aware, however, that an estimated 30 to 50% of cases are idiopathic, and there is no obvious diagnosis after an exhaustive history and physical and diagnostic workup. The general categories to consider in dilated cardiomyopathy are ischemic (due to CAD), infectious (due to viral myocarditis or Chagas disease), stress induced, toxin mediated (due to excessive alcohol, cocaine, or methamphetamine), medication mediated (due to chemotherapeutic agents such as doxorubicin or HER2/neu receptor antagonists), peripartum or postpartum, inherited (as in inherited muscular dystrophies, hypertrophic cardiomyopathy, hereditary hemochromatosis), tachycardia mediated (due to uncontrolled atrial arrhythmia like A-fib/flutter, hyperthyroidism), nutritional deficiencies (due to thiamine ["wet beri-beri"] or selenium deficiency), and autoimmune mediated (due to systemic lupus erythematosus, rheumatoid arthritis, or dermatomyositis).

Your patient lives in the United States (with its high prevalence of CAD) and, given his risk factors and lack of other past medical history, ischemic cardiomyopathy is a reasonable place to start.

CLINICAL PEARL	STEP 2/3

Pulmonary hypertension has numerous causes and is classified by the World Health Organization into five groups. Group 2 is pulmonary hypertension due to left-sided heart disease. Be careful when interpreting pulmonary artery pressures from echocardiograms, as

---

CLINICAL PEARL—cont'd

the reported pressure will be affected by the volume status at the time of the study. For patients without left-sided heart disease on echocardiogram who have elevated pulmonary artery pressures, the diagnosis is made using a mean pulmonary artery pressure of >25 mm Hg on right heart catheterization.

The doctors who took care of your patient at the hospital were also concerned for ischemic cardiomyopathy given his risk factors, and he was taken for cardiac catheterization, which revealed an 80% stenosed lesion of the left anterior descending artery (LAD) that was treated with overlapping drug-eluting stents. There was mild disease in his other main coronary arteries (left main, right main, left circumflex) that were not intervened upon. Following the procedure, he was started on the medications as listed on his discharge paperwork (see above).

What medications are shown to have a mortality benefit in systolic heart failure? What medications that are sometimes used in patients with systolic heart failure do not have a mortality benefit? What medications should be avoided?

A beta blocker and either an angiotensin-converting enzyme (ACE) inhibitor or angiotensin II receptor blocker (ARB) should be started in all patients with systolic heart failure, regardless of cause, due to their mortality benefit. When the ejection fraction decreases and less blood is delivered to vital organs such as the kidneys, the body's natural responses are to increase sympathetic activity and to increase the production of renin, angiotensin, and aldosterone. The increased sympathetic activity causes the pulse rate to increase, which increases myocardial oxygen demand. Needless to say, this is not the best-case scenario for an already weak heart. The increased renin levels cause vasoconstriction and hypertension, which cause further strain on the heart by way of increased afterload. Beta blockers and ACE inhibitors/ARBs help to counteract these harmful and unwanted compensatory responses.

The specific beta blockers that are recommended to decrease mortality are carvedilol, bisoprolol, and the long-acting form of metoprolol, metoprolol succinate. Any ACE inhibitor or ARB will do, just do not prescribe both an ACE inhibitor *and* an ARB, as this combination has been shown to cause harm. The aldosterone-receptor antagonist spironolactone has been shown to have a mortality benefit in patients with an EF less than 35% and NYHA class II to IV symptoms. Finally, for patients who self-identify as African American with NYHA class III or IV symptoms optimized on a beta blocker and either an ACE inhibitor or ARB, the combination of hydralazine (reduces afterload) and nitrates (reduces preload) has been shown to improve mortality.

Several medications commonly used in patients with systolic heart failure can improve symptoms but have not been shown to decrease mortality. Loop diuretics such as furosemide or bumetanide are indicated in patients with volume overload but have not been shown to decrease mortality. Digoxin, which has an inotropic effect on the heart, is another medication that is sometimes used as an adjunct to improve symptoms but has no mortality benefit. Although both aspirin and statins are of benefit for secondary prevention of heart disease in ischemic cardiomyopathy, they have not been shown to improve mortality in patients with heart failure from other causes.

Due to their negative inotropic effects, nondihydropyridine calcium channel blockers (e.g., verapamil, diltiazem) are contraindicated in systolic heart failure patients. If a patient's blood pressure is uncontrolled with optimal doses of several other classes of blood pressure–lowering medications (including both an ACE inhibitor or ARB and a beta blocker), the dihydropyridine calcium channel blocker amlodipine has an overall neutral effect on mortality and can be safely used. Other medications that should be avoided include nonsteroidal antiinflammatory drugs (NSAIDs), with the exception of aspirin in ischemic cardiomyopathy (due to impairment of renal function), as well as thiazolidinediones, which cause fluid retention.

BASIC SCIENCE PEARL   **STEP 1**

Of the beta blockers with a studied mortality benefit in patients with HFrEF, metoprolol succinate is the only one that is "cardioselective," which means it works only on beta-1 receptors on the heart that are responsible for increasing the pulse rate.

CLINICAL PEARL   **STEP 2/3**

Use metoprolol succinate in a patient with chronic obstructive pulmonary disease (COPD) or asthma as the other "nonselective" beta blockers block the action of beta-2 receptors, which can cause bronchoconstriction.

CLINICAL PEARL   **STEP 2/3**

When working up ischemic cardiomyopathy, perform a stress test if your patient is at intermediate risk for CAD. If the stress test is positive with a large suspected area of ischemia, the patient will need a cardiac catheterization. Consider skipping the stress test and going straight to catheterization in patients at very high risk for CAD.

Your patient wants to know if his heart failure as defined by his EF will ever improve. You tell him that patients often recover some function, especially with revascularization; however, it is difficult to predict. You recommend a repeat echo in 3 months to evaluate, and his ejection fraction at that time remains at 30%. You classify him as having NYHA class II failure. His baseline electrocardiogram has a QRS duration of 130 ms.

Which nonpharmacologic treatments are indicated in patients with an EF of 35% or less? Which of these are indicated in your patient?

Devices such as implantable cardiac defibrillators (ICDs) and biventricular pacemakers have been shown to have a mortality and morbidity benefit in patients with heart failure and an EF of 35% or less. The basis for ICD placement is that in damaged or stretched myocardium, normal ventricular electrical activity is disrupted and patients are prone to fatal ventricular arrhythmias such as ventricular tachycardia and fibrillation. The basis for biventricular pacemaker placement is that in poorly functional ventricles, the left and right ventricles may be dyssynchronous (i.e., ejecting blood at slightly different times). This delay between right and left ventricular contraction can lead to further congestion and symptoms of heart failure. Both of these devices are indicated only if a patient's life expectancy is greater than 1 year and he or she is on an appropriate medication regimen for heart failure. Neither of these devices is implanted at the time of diagnosis, and a period of at least 2 to 3 months should pass to allow for potential recovery of heart muscle function before they are even considered.

In general, an ICD is placed for an EF of 35% or less with NYHA class II to IV symptoms and a biventricular pacemaker is placed for an EF of 35% or less with NYHA class III or IV symptoms and a QRS duration of greater than 150 ms. It would be appropriate to consider an ICD in your patient, but given his NYHA class and QRS duration, a biventricular pacemaker is not indicated at this time.

It is important to realize that the decision to implant these devices is nuanced and best determined by a cardiologist. For a full list of evidence-based recommendations pertaining to the management of heart failure, refer to the American College of Cardiology Foundation/American Heart Association (ACCF/AHA) practice guidelines, which can be found online.

BASIC SCIENCE PEARL   **STEP 1**

Primary prevention, like the placement of an ICD in a patient with systolic heart failure with an EF less than 35%, refers to preventing a disease before it ever occurs. *Secondary prevention,* like starting aspirin in patients with known CAD, refers to reducing the impact of a disease that has already occurred.

CLINICAL PEARL   **STEP 2/3**

In general, remember to start thinking of additional heart failure interventions (i.e., spironolactone, hydralazine/isosorbide mononitrate for African Americans, ICD and biventricular pacemaker placement) if the EF is less than 35% and the patient is optimized on the standard regimen.

BEYOND THE PEARLS

- Fluid restriction in heart failure is recommended for patients who are considered advanced/end stage and for those with hyponatremia. In patients with less severe heart failure, sodium restriction is more important.
- Patients with HFpEF/diastolic heart failure are dependent on adequate ventricular filling. Atrial fibrillation, in which the normal coordinated atrial contraction is replaced by ineffective quivering of the aria, can cause a rapid onset of heart failure symptoms due to this loss of "atrial kick."
- Patients with a history of heart failure should always be admitted for syncope.
- For patients with HFrEF who remain symptomatic despite optimal treatment, one option is a left ventricular assist device (LVAD), which mechanically forces blood out of the left ventricle. LVADs are considered a bridge to cardiac transplant and not as a definitive therapy.
- Don't be afraid to diurese hospitalized patients with heart failure and an elevated creatinine. It may seem counterintuitive, but these patients need diuretics to help relieve renal venous congestion.
- Platypnea is the opposite of orthopnea. Patients with platypnea feel short of breath when sitting up and better when lying flat. Conditions that cause platypnea include atrial septal defects and the hepatopulmonary syndrome.
- Bedside ultrasound is becoming more prevalent, and some clinicians believe it is the "stethoscope of the future." One can estimate intravascular volume status by looking at the inferior vena cava (IVC) as it passes through the liver. In general, the patient is volume overloaded if the IVC is not compressible. Compressibility refers to a decrease in IVC diameter with inspiration (as blood is returned to the heart from the decreased intrathoracic pressure caused by inspiration), *not* mechanical compression from pressing harder with the ultrasound probe.

References

Leblond RF, Brown DD, DeGowin RL. *DeGowin's Diagnostic Examination.* 9th ed. New York: McGraw Hill; 2009 [chapter 8].

Mann DL, Chakinala M. *Harrison's Principles of Internal Medicine.* 18th ed. New York: McGraw Hill; 2012 [chapter 24].

McMurray JJ. Clinical practice: systolic heart failure. *N Engl J Med.* 2010;362(3):228-238.

Yancy CW, Jessup M, Bozkurt B, et al. 2013 ACCF/AHA guideline for the management of heart failure: executive summary: a report of the American College of Cardiology Foundation/American Heart Association Task Force on practice guidelines. *Circulation.* 2013;128(16):1810-1852.

Rachel Ramirez ■ Daniel Martinez

A 68-Year-Old Male With Weakness and Fatigue

A 68-year-old male is brought by his wife for worsening weakness and malaise for the past few weeks. He states that he began to feel weak, fatigued, and lightheaded with associated muscle cramps. His wife notes he has been slightly less attentive over the past 10 days, especially when extended family members were visiting. He denies any sick contacts or recent travel.

What are some things to think about when someone complains of weakness and malaise?
Generalized weakness and malaise are very common complaints in the primary care setting, and, unfortunately, the differential diagnosis for these symptoms is very broad. A "shotgun" approach by testing everything is not medically appropriate, and, instead, a thorough history, physical exam, and placing the patient's symptoms in clinical context are of utmost importance in proceeding with an evaluation. However, you should keep the broad differential diagnosis in the back of your mind while proceeding with the history and physical so as to make sure you do not miss a significant pathology. The following Table 12.1 lists a comprehensive list of the causes of weakness and malaise.

The patient has a past medical history of hypertension and dyslipidemia, and he takes lisinopril, atorvastatin, and aspirin. He has never been screened for any sort of cancer because he would "rather not know." He denies any drug allergies and does not take any herbal supplements or vitamins. His past surgical history includes an appendectomy in 1965. He is a retired computer engineer who has been married for 40 years. He drinks "two fingers" of scotch on Friday nights. He has a 30-pack-year smoking history with a quit date 15 years ago. He is a Vietnam War veteran and received a blood transfusion due to a combat-related injury in 1971. He has three adult children, three grandchildren, and two dogs. His hobbies include golfing, sailing, and coin collecting. On review of systems, he reports a slight cough that he attributes to the change of seasons and a recent low-grade temperature. His wife notes an approximate 15-pound weight loss. When this is commented upon, he states that this is probably because he stopped eating ice cream for dessert a few weeks ago.

What pathologies should you be considering based on this history?
There are many classic "buzz words" that can be observed when taking a history that should lead you to consider certain pathologies. The more you take a detailed history, the more they and their associated pathologies will become second nature. In this case, Table 12.2 lists some of these buzz words and the associated pathologic consideration.

TABLE 12.1 ■ Causes of Fatigue

System Involved	Specific Conditions
Endocrine	Disorders of the thyroid, adrenal, or pancreatic endocrine glands. In this case, you would look for weight gain and constipation (hypothyroidism); weight loss, diarrhea, palpitations, and insomnia (hyperthyroidism); weight loss despite polyphagia, polydipsia, and polyuria (new-onset type 2 diabetes); or weight loss, anorexia, skin color changes, polydipsia, and salt cravings (adrenal insufficiency).
Neurologic	Disorders of the nerves and muscles can cause weakness such as myositis (autoimmune), neuromuscular blockade (Eaton-Lambert, myasthenia gravis), and demyelinating disorders (Guillain-Barré syndrome, multiple sclerosis). Normal pressure hydrocephalus can cause mental status changes, gait instability, and urinary incontinence. Stroke (ischemic) is usually associated with focal complaints ("my face is numb on one side").
Electrolyte disturbances	These include hyponatremia, hypokalemia, and hypercalcemia. Asking about bone pain, muscle cramps, or inability to stand helps rule in or out some of these problems. Progressive renal failure with elevation of the blood urea nitrogen causes anorexia, fatigue, nausea, and muscle cramps.
Cardiac	Any cardiac disease (structural or electrical) that reduces cardiac output will cause weakness and malaise. Congestive heart failure (CHF) and atrial or ventricular arrhythmias are examples, so you should inquire about palpitations, chest pain, shortness of breath, and lower extremity edema. It is also important to ask about prior coronary artery disease (CAD). Valvular heart disease, like aortic stenosis or aortic insufficiency, mitral valve stenosis, or prolapse, reduces cardiac output and shifts the cardiac pressures in the wrong direction (backward toward the lungs), so shortness of breath may be an important clue.
Infectious	Chronic or subacute infections can contribute to malaise and weakness. Tuberculosis is a chronically progressive infection that also has cough, weight loss, and night sweats as components. Subacute bacterial endocarditis (SBE) often causes a host of nonspecific complaints, but fevers and night sweats are common. Chronic viral infections such as hepatitis B or C can cause fatigue. Historical data acquired should include past blood transfusions, past intravenous drug use, sexual history, and tattoo acquisition. Infectious mononucleosis (IM) is notorious for causing fatigue. Antecedent pharyngitis and swollen lymph nodes are important features of IM. Human immunodeficiency virus (HIV) infection, in the acute phase, can cause fatigue but is often associated with fever, pharyngitis, and adenopathy.
Hematologic and malignant conditions	Anemia of any cause can manifest as fatigue. Careful history about blood loss via stool or urine, as well as iron and other nutrient intake, is important. Hematologic malignancies like leukemia and lymphoma also cause fatigue. Associated fever, night sweats, bruising, or adenopathy are clues.
Gastrointestinal disorders	Cirrhosis and inflammatory bowel disease can cause fatigue. Make sure to look for abdominal pain, blood in the stool, and weight loss.

TABLE 12.2 ■ Key Buzz Words in This Case and How They May Contribute to the Clinical Assessment

Buzz Words	Pathologic Consideration
"weeks"	Indicates a relatively new-onset, but not immediate, constellation of symptoms.
"less attentive"	Translate as "change in mental status." This indicates the issue has begun to affect his mental acuity.
"muscle cramps"	His are diffuse and not limited to one muscle group and can suggest a metabolic derangement.
"hypertension" and "dyslipidemia"	Increases his risk for CAD and cerebral vascular disease.
"lisinopril"	Can cause hyperkalemia, acute kidney injury, and a dry cough.
"atorvastatin"	Most statins can cause muscle cramps and weakness.
"aspirin"	Can cause gastrointestinal ulcers and bleeding. This can lead to anemia and fatigue.
"cough"	Consider pulmonary process like tumor, tuberculosis, chronic obstructive lung disease, interstitial lung disease, or a medication side effect.
"low-grade temperatures" and "weight loss"	Consider malignancy, infection, and autoimmune disorders.

CAD, Coronary artery disease.

The patient's blood pressure is 128/75 mm Hg, pulse rate is 82/min, respiration rate is 12/min, body mass index is 18. He appears unwell and slightly undernourished, but he is in no acute distress. He is awake and oriented to person, place, time, and purpose. His cranial nerves are intact, and he has pink conjunctiva with moist mucus membranes. There is no jugular venous distension, lymphadenopathy, or bruits in the neck. His heart has a regular rate and rhythm without extra heart sounds, murmurs, clicks, or rubs. He does not have a barrel chest, and his lungs sounds are clear to auscultation bilaterally. His abdomen is soft with no evidence of hepatosplenomegaly or masses. On rectal exam, he has soft brown stool, a normal sized and smooth prostate, with no abnormal masses. His skin has no tenting, bruising, or rashes. His joints have full range of motion and are without erythema or swelling. He is able to get out of a chair without use of his arm, and he has no motor, sensory, or coordination deficits. He has no peripheral edema. He has clubbing of his nails, but no dilation of the capillary beds.

How does this change your differential diagnosis?
His normal vital signs point away from an infectious process, but this is not completely excluded yet. He appears undernourished and given his age and weight loss history, malignancy is now higher on the differential. However, the lack of diffuse lymphadenopathy and normal prostate exam are reassuring at least from a diffusely metastatic disease or prostate cancer standpoint. The pink conjunctiva make anemia unlikely. His moist mucus membranes and lack of skin tenting make dehydration unlikely. His normal cardiac and pulmonary exam and lack of jugular venous distension (JVD) or peripheral edema make heart failure, chronic obstructive pulmonary disease, and interstitial lung disease unlikely. His normal musculoskeletal exam, lack of skin rash, friction rub, or decreased breath sounds (pleural effusion) make a rheumatologic disease less likely. His good muscle strength and normal sensation and coordination make a neurologic disease very unlikely. And lastly, his nail clubbing in light of his history of smoking and weight loss makes lung cancer a distinct possibility.

TABLE 12.3 ■ Laboratory Data Obtained the Day of the Visit

Glucose	98 mg/dL
Blood urea nitrogen	10 mg/dL
Creatinine	0.8 mg/dL
Sodium	125 mEq/L
Potassium	4.1 mEq/L
Chloride	95 mEq/L
Bicarbonate	22 mEq/L
Calcium	9.5 mg/dL
Alanine aminotransferase	60 U/L
Aspartate aminotransferase	45 U/L
Total protein	7.8 g/dL
Albumin	4.2 g/dL
Alkaline phosphatase	55 U/L
Total bilirubin	0.8 mg/dL
Thyroid stimulating hormone	2.125 mIU/L

What labs should you order next?

At this point, his history and physical exam point to some sort of malignancy. Given his specific clinical scenario, he is at greatest risk for lung or colon cancer. But since he has no lymphadenopathy, unlikely significantly anemic, and he is not severely cachectic, it is unlikely that just the malignancy itself is very advanced to the point of causing his symptom of fatigue and malaise.

At this point, lung cancer is known to have many metabolic derangements associated with it, so getting a basic metabolic panel is warranted. Since colon cancer is reasonably on the differential, it might be metastatic to the liver, so ordering a liver profile is appropriate as well (see Table 12.3).

You review the labs and appreciate that his sodium level is very low which can explain his chief complaints. You suspected a metabolic derangement before the labs, and this confirms your diagnosis. You tell the patient that his fatigue and malaise are likely due to a low sodium concentration in his body and would like to admit him to the hospital for further work-up and treatment.

What are the initial steps in evaluating hyponatremia?

Traditionally, it is important to order a serum osmolality to confirm the patient truly has a hypotonic hyponatremia. This confirms that the hyponatremia is not a laboratory artifact (such as in hyperproteinemia or hyperlipidemia) or due to an excess of another osmole (mannitol or glucose). However, these situations are rarely the case.

Generally speaking, hypotonic hyponatremia is most commonly caused by the action of antidiuretic hormone (ADH) on the kidneys by increasing free water reabsorption. This increases the ratio of free water to sodium in the body and causes hyponatremia. Therefore, the first step in the work-up of hyponatremia is to confirm that ADH is the cause of the hyponatremia and the kidneys are actually actively reabsorbing free water. This is done by measuring serum and urine osmolality. When ADH is acting on the kidneys, the urine osmolality should increase and be greater than the serum osmolality. This confirms the kidneys are actively concentrating the urine via the action of ADH.

However, if the urine osmolality is lower than the serum osmolality, then ADH is not involved in the pathophysiology of hyponatremia in the patient. In this case, there are two alternative causes for hyponatremia. First, the patient can *acutely* drink so much water that it overcomes the kidney's ability to secrete the free water; this results in an excess of free water relative to sodium and the patient becomes hyponatremic. This is called primary polydipsia and is generally psychogenic. Secondly, the patient can *chronically* be eating very little sodium each day. The kidneys have to excrete a certain very small amount of sodium each day in order to produce urine. However, if the daily input of sodium is less than this, then there is a paucity of sodium relative to free water and the patient becomes hyponatremic. This is classically seen with a "tea and toast" or "beer potomania" diet where very little sodium is eaten each day.

Obviously, the work-up does not stop with confirming that the urine is concentrated and ADH is acting on the kidneys. However, you will commonly see people stop the work-up at this point and declare that a patient has the syndrome of inappropriate ADH (SIADH). Doing that, in fact, is medically inappropriate. An astute clinical will go on to evaluate why ADH is being released and, if it is appropriate, given the other possible underlying pathologies happening with the patient.

Lastly, interpreting urine studies only make sense when the kidneys are actually functioning. If a patient has severe chronic kidney disease, end stage renal disease, or is in acute kidney injury, then it becomes difficult to interpret urine studies accurately. And generally speaking, if a patient does have severe renal failure, then the renal failure is likely the cause of the hyponatremia anyways.

BASIC SCIENCE/CLINICAL PEARL   **STEP 1/2/3**

The most common cause of hyponatremia is hypovolemia or dehydration.

CLINICAL PEARL   **STEP 3**

Symptoms of hyponatremia vary by rapidity of derangement. The symptoms primarily result from the varying degrees of cerebral edema. Chronically or mildly low sodium (125 to 135 mEq/L) produces symptoms, as with our patient in this chapter, of nausea, fatigue, and malaise. Acute drops or severe derangements of sodium (<120 mEq/L) cause marked symptoms such as headache, lethargy, obtundation, and eventually seizures, coma, and respiratory arrest.

CLINICAL PEARL   **STEP 3**

Women who take ecstasy (MDMA) are much more likely to suffer from severe hyponatremia than are men.

Once the patient is in the hospital, you decide to measure the serum and urine osmolality. The serum osmolality is 260 mmol/kg, and this confirms that the patient is truly having a hypotonic hyponatremia. The urine osmolality is 600 mOsm/kg, and this confirms that ADH is actively being secreted by the brain and that it is involved in the pathophysiology of hyponatremia in the patient. You can now comfortably rule out both primary polydipsia and a "tea and toast" diet as a cause for his hyponatremia.

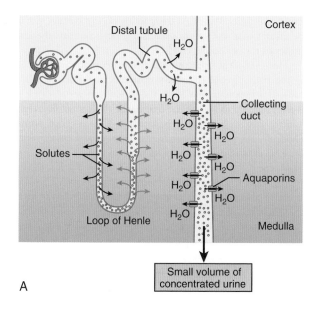

A

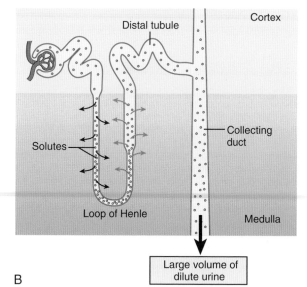

B

Figure 12.1 Diagram depicting interaction between kidney and ADH. **(A)** ADH present: Collecting duct is highly permeable to water. **(B)** No ADH present: Collecting duct is not permeable to water.

How can we understand ADH effects?

ADH affects the V2 receptors of the kidney, activating adenylyl cyclase. In turn, this causes the transport of the water channels to the luminal membrane of the cells of the collecting tubule. Water is reabsorbed, causing urine osmolality to increase up to 1000 to 1200 mOsm/kg. In the absence of ADH, water is not reabsorbed in the collecting tubules and the urine osmolality can reach down to 30 to 50 mOsm/kg . ADH also acts in a minor way to increase systemic vascular resistance by stimulating V1 receptors, hence its name vasopressin. Figure 12.1 illustrates the interaction between the kidney and ADH.

What controls the release of ADH?

ADH is most commonly released by the posterior pituitary when the osmoreceptors in the hypothalamus sense a hyperosmolar state of increased osmotic pressure. This is seen when a patient is hypernatremic, and ADH is consequently released in order to reabsorb free water in the kidneys and correct the hypernatremia. Conversely, the release of ADH is suppressed when the osmoreceptors in the hypothalamus sense a hypo-osmolar state of decreased osmotic pressure. This happens when a patient is hyponatremic; ADH is suppressed, and the kidneys are now free to excrete free water and correct the hyponatremia. See Figure 12.2 for a summary of the regulation of ADH.

Secondly, independent of the osmolar state of the serum, ADH can be released by any cause of a low effective arterial volume (EAV). A low EAV is any state where the body senses and acts *as if* the volume is low in the arterial vessels; this includes an actual state of low arterial volume (like hemorrhage) or other pathologic states that can mimic a low arterial volume (CHF, sepsis, third spacing). Pressure receptors in the body's vessel will sense the low EAV and stimulate ADH secretion. Renin and angiotensin II are also typically released during a low EAV state, and this also stimulates ADH secretion. This pathophysiology is a very common cause of hyponatremia in a hospitalized patient where a low EAV is also common.

Thirdly, ADH can be secreted when a patient is experiencing either adrenal insufficiency or hypothyroidism; this happens by multiple mechanisms which we will not get into. Again, this also can override the normal tonicity control exerted by osmoreceptors in the hypothalamus.

Lastly, ADH can simply be inappropriately released (which is a diagnosis of exclusion) in conditions such as lung cancer, a "reset osmotat," or several medications (carbamazepine, chlorpromazine, selective serotonin reuptake inhibitors, amiodarone, or ecstasy to name a few).

BASIC SCIENCE PEARL	STEP 1

ADH is also known as arginine vasopressin (human form). ADH is synthesized in the supraoptic and paraventricular nuclei of the hypothalamus. Secretory granules containing ADH migrate down the axons of those neurons (supraopticohypophysial tract) to be stored in the posterior pituitary.

CLINICAL PEARL	STEP 2/3

Alcohol inhibits ADH production, causing the typical diuresis associated with imbibing alcoholic beverages.

BASIC SCIENCE PEARL	STEP 1

ADH acts via the generation of cyclic adenosine monophosphate (cAMP) to increase collecting tubule water permeability to allow water to be passively reabsorbed.

What are the next steps in evaluating the patient's hyponatremia?

When someone is hyponatremic, the typical action of the osmoreceptors in the hypothalamus is overtaken, and as was previously discussed, this is commonly due to a low EAV state in a hospitalized patient. Alternatively, it can be due to adrenal insufficiency, hypothyroidism, or SIADH, which are less common. A systematic evaluation is simple when a patient has only one single cause of hyponatremia. Unfortunately, most patients have multiple reasons for having hyponatremia. Hospitalized patients tend to have reasons for a low EAV state (hypovolemia, CHF, sepsis, or on an excessive diuretic), and this can happen concurrently with hypothyroidism, adrenal

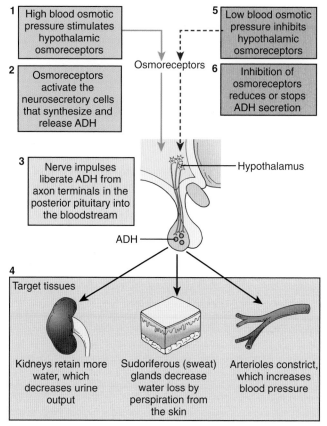

1 High blood osmotic pressure stimulates hypothalamic osmoreceptors

5 Low blood osmotic pressure inhibits hypothalamic osmoreceptors

Osmoreceptors

2 Osmoreceptors activate the neurosecretory cells that synthesize and release ADH

6 Inhibition of osmoreceptors reduces or stops ADH secretion

3 Nerve impulses liberate ADH from axon terminals in the posterior pituitary into the bloodstream

Hypothalamus

ADH

4 Target tissues

Kidneys retain more water, which decreases urine output

Sudoriferous (sweat) glands decrease water loss by perspiration from the skin

Arterioles constrict, which increases blood pressure

Figure 12.2 Regulation of ADH, specifically with the pituitary.

insufficiency, or SIADH. Therefore, the next steps in work-up are typically confusing, and a patient is commonly labeled as having SIADH because the clinician has difficulty interpreting the numbers. Fortunately, however, the standard of care is to make changes to normalize the effective arterial volume (by giving crystalloids, colloids, blood, or diuresis) and checking for and treating hypothyroidism or adrenal insufficiency when it is clinically suspected. Consequently, most hospitalized patients with incidental hyponatremia are effectively treated without much of a work-up. They all tend to have a near normal sodium concentration by the time they leave the hospital. If not, then SIADH is seriously considered at that time. However, the full work-up should be done because sometimes it is very fruitful and can improve patient care. This is especially the case when the patient has one cause of hyponatremia, and then work-up is quick and makes a lot of sense clinically.

The most valuable test you can order next is a urine sodium concentration. This gives you a key into understanding what the kidneys themselves are experiencing and what is going on physiologically with the patient. When there is a low EAV state, then there is low kidney perfusion. Consequently, the renin-angiotensin system is activated, and sodium is retained by the kidneys. This low EAV/high renin state (and pretty much only this state) can dramatically lower the urine sodium concentration. Therefore, a low urine sodium concentration is very useful because it confirms that a patient is experiencing a low EAV state.

If the urine sodium concentration is low and the low EAV state is confirmed, then the next step is to figure out why there is a low effective arterial volume. That is where the physical exam and assessing the volume status of the patient are of utmost importance. If a patient is hypovolemic, then the hyponatremia is due to extra-renal losses such as dehydration or hemorrhage. If the patient is euvolemic, then the hyponatremia is likely due to sepsis or another state of systemic arterial vasodilation. If the patient is hypervolemic, then the patient has venous congestion from CHF or third spacing from cirrhosis or nephrotic syndrome. However, this interpretation can only happen when the patient is not on a diuretic or in renal failure as these situations cause an increase in urine sodium concentration, which confuses the interpretation as previously discussed (see Fig. 12.3).

Alternatively, if the urine sodium is high then it is difficult to tell exactly what is happening with the patient. However, the physical exam is also very useful in this situation. If the patient is hypovolemic, then the hyponatremia is due to a diuretic or mineralocorticoid deficiency (which is effectively a potassium sparing diuretic). If the patient is euvolemic, then the hyponatremia is due to hypothyroidism, adrenal insufficiency, or SIADH (thyroid stimulating hormone, free T4, and morning cortisol should be tested at that point to investigate further). If the patient is hypervolemic, then the hyponatremia is likely due to renal failure (see Fig. 12.3).

The patient's lab values are shown below:

	Our Patient	Normal Values
Serum osmolality	260 mmol/kg	275-295 mmol/kg
Urine osmolality	600 mOsm/kg	300-900 mOsm/kg
Urine sodium	65 mEq/L	20 mEq/L

You then send for a urine sodium and it comes back at 65 mEq/L, which is above normal. You look back at your original physical exam and note that the patient is euvolemic. Since the patient is not on a diuretic and is not in renal failure, you correctly suspect hypothyroidism, adrenal insufficiency, or SIADH at this time. You then order a thyroid stimulating hormone, free T4, and morning cortisol. In the meantime, you free water restrict him because he is euvolemic. The next day these tests all come back normal. You are now highly suspicious that your patient has SIADH. You remember his history of smoking, weight loss, and clubbing on physical exam and decide to start a work-up for lung cancer, so you order a chest radiograph (CXR). The patient's CXR (see Fig. 12.4) reveals a mass in the left hilum measuring 5 cm × 8 cm, suspicious for malignancy. The patient undergoes a computed tomography (CT) of the chest and then bronchoscopy with biopsy the next day. Unfortunately, the findings reveal poorly differentiated small cell cancer of the lung, and you consult oncology.

Diagnosis: SIADH due to primary lung carcinoma

What are the principles of treating hyponatremia?
Treatment of hyponatremia consists of the following principles:
1. If the patient is acutely altered or confused due to hyponatremia, it does not matter what the cause of their hyponatremia is. You should immediately begin to infuse hypertonic 3% normal saline and check electrolytes frequently as to avoid overcorrection.
2. For the edematous *(hypervolemic)* patient from CHF, cirrhosis, or chronic renal failure use water restriction, diuretics, and occasionally IV albumin (for cirrhosis). Remember, although the sodium concentration is low in these patients, the total body sodium is very high, hence the pitting edema. Do not give sodium unless they have symptoms of hyponatremia as discussed in principle one.

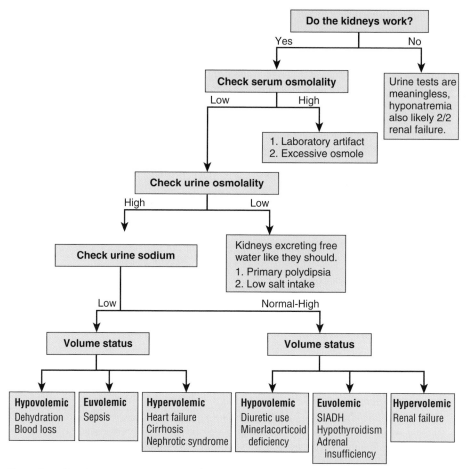

Figure 12.3 Algorithm for evaluation of hyponatemia. This figure is a graphic representation of the algorithm that was explained in the text regarding how to work up hyponatremia. Classically, most algorithms start the decision tree based on volume status, because it helps to group causes of hyponatremia based on their treatment. However, this alternative algorithm instead ends the decision tree with volume status. Doing this groups the causes of hyponatremia together based on their similar pathologic mechanisms. This should help with understanding the causes of hyponatremia, not just knowing how to treat them.

3. For the volume-depleted *(hypovolemic)* patient from gastrointestinal or other losses, use isotonic saline or oral salt replacement. The sodium in the saline (concentration is 154 mEq/L) will offer more osmoles to the serum and increase volume, thus correcting the hypovolemia. Then, ADH will decrease and excess water will be excreted. You can also consider stopping a diuretic if the hyponatremia is severe.

4. In the setting of primary polydipsia (excessive water intake) *(euvolemic)* and SIADH, it is best to treat with water restriction. Water restriction is usually to less than 2 L of free water or other liquids in 24 hours. Hypertonic saline can also be given if there are severe symptoms of hyponatremia. Long-term treatment is correcting the underlying condition as well.

5. Hypothyroidism and cortisol deficiency are treated by correcting the underlying condition. Replacing the deficient hormones will correct the metabolic derangements.

6. Medication side effect is treated by stopping the offending medication.

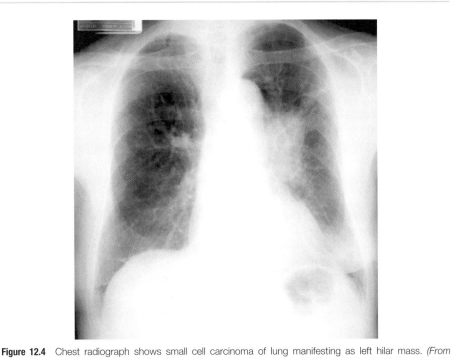

Figure 12.4 Chest radiograph shows small cell carcinoma of lung manifesting as left hilar mass. *(From Weinberger SE, Cockrill BA, Mandel J. Lung cancer: clinical aspects. In: Weinberger SE, Cockrill BA, Mandel J, eds.* Principles of Pulmonary Medicine. *6th ed. Philadelphia: W.B. Saunders; 2014:266-279.)*

CLINICAL PEARL   **STEP 3**

A 60-kg female will have a higher rise in serum sodium than a 70-kg male due to the male's higher volume of distribution.

What are the pharmacologic therapies for SIADH?

Vasopressin receptor antagonists emerged on the market for treating SIADH and "reset osmo-stats." The vasopressin antagonists selectively bind to the V2 receptors and block the effect of ADH on the collecting ducts, thus causing aquaresis. Tolvaptan, mozavaptan, satavaptan, and lixivaptan are all oral agents. The intravenous agent is conivaptan. These drugs are costly and have variable effects.

Oral salt tablets operate on the same principles as hypertonic saline.

Oral salt tablets plus a loop diuretic can be effective, especially in mixed causes of hyponatremia (SIADH and volume overload states).

Oral urea can be used in ambulatory patients and is well tolerated. It operates by increasing solutes in the serum. However, its use is limited by lack of availability in U.S. pharmacies.

How would you summarize the evaluation of hyponatremia in this case?

Hyponatremia is caused by a number of different clinical pathologies, and it is typical that a patient has more than one cause of hyponatremia. The work-up includes checking the kidney function, a serum osmolality, a urine osmolality, a urine sodium, and then examining the volume status of the patient. At that point, use your history to guide you further and other specific tests as necessary as illustrated in Figure 12.3. Once you know the cause of the hyponatremia, then you will be able to appropriately treat it. In this patient's case, he was found to have SIADH from lung cancer and should be treated with free water restriction.

BEYOND THE PEARLS

- 1 L of normal saline contains 154 mEq of Na and Cl = 308 mOsm.
- Vasopressin antagonists such as tolvaptan selectively bind to the V2 receptors and block the effect of ADH on the collecting ducts, thus causing aquaresis.
- The sodium deficit equation is: sodium deficit = volume of distribution × sodium deficit per liter.

References

Braun MM, Barstow CH, Pyzocha NJ. Diagnosis and management of sodium disorders: hyponatremia and hypernatremia. *Am Fam Physician*. 2015;91(5):299-307.

Rose BD. *Renal Pathophysiology: The Essentials*. Baltimore: Williams & Wilkins; 1994.

Sterns RH. Treatment of hyponatremia: syndrome of inappropriate antidiuretic hormone secretion (SIADH) and reset osmostat. UpToDate. 2014. Available at <www.uptodate.com/home/index.html>. Accessed 09.12.15.

Sterns RH. Overview of the treatment of hyponatremia in adults. UpToDate. 2014. Available at <www.uptodate.com/home/index.html>. Accessed 09.12.15.

John Khoury ■ Carla LoPinto-Khoury

A 65-Year-Old Male With Dysphagia

A 65-year-old male who is a pack-a-day smoker presents to your outpatient office complaining of weakness and choking. He says he noticed these symptoms gradually over the last 6 months.

What is your differential diagnosis for dysphagia?

Dysphagia can be either neurological or mechanical. Mechanical dysphagia is more likely to present with problems swallowing solid foods whereas neurological dysphagia is more noticeable with liquids than with solids. Examples of nonneurological causes of dysphagia include obstruction from esophageal carcinoma or oropharyngeal muscle involvement in patients with inflammatory myositis. Neurological causes of dysphagia may include a brainstem lesion or neuromuscular disorders.

CLINICAL PEARL   **STEP 2/3**

Neurological dysphagia is more prominent with liquids than with solids, and the reverse is true for mechanical dysphagia.

The patient reports that his dysphagia is worse with liquids. He describes the weakness as being unable to lift objects over his head, which waxes and wanes to the point that sometimes he tires from combing his hair.

On exam, he has normal pupils, mild ptosis of the right eye, and normal-appearing extraocular muscles; however, he does report diplopia in all directions. He states that this was noticeable over the last few months and has been meaning to get new glasses. Also noted while testing cranial nerves is that there are no tongue fasciculations.

His motor exam is significant for 4/5 strength in the bilateral deltoids, biceps, and triceps but a normal grip strength. His lower extremity strength is normal and reflexes are mildly decreased at the ankles but otherwise normal. He has 1+ reflexes at the ankles.

What is the significance of the absence of tongue fasciculations?

Although the absence of tongue fasciculations does not rule out a diagnosis of amyotrophic lateral sclerosis (ALS), the presence of tongue fasciculations, especially on a board exam question, is highly specific for ALS. ALS is a motor neuron disease that often presents with dysphagia, weakness, a combination of upper and lower motor neuron signs including brisk reflexes and atrophy, including the tongue.

With the previous exam, what could the proximal muscle weakness indicate?
Proximal muscle weakness as opposed to distal weakness is typically seen with disorders of muscle or the neuromuscular junction. For instance, myopathies, myositis, and muscular dystrophies all may present with proximal muscle weakness, and some disorders are associated with ocular involvement as well such as diplopia and ptosis. However, the pattern of waxing and waning would point to a myasthenic syndrome—most commonly myasthenia gravis (MG) or the rarer Lambert-Eaton myasthenic syndrome (LEMS).

CLINICAL PEARL	STEP 2/3

Myasthenia gravis patients typically have fatigable weakness that worsens with exercise, whereas Lambert-Eaton patients improve with exercise.

What other conditions can you consider with a unilateral ptosis?
The most common cause of ptosis is disinsertion of the levator palpebrae superioris tendon from the tarsal plate, which is more common in older patients. It is a benign nonneurological condition unless it interferes with vision, in which case surgery can be performed. Ptosis can be a sign of dysfunction of the third cranial (oculomotor) nerve, which innervates the levator palpebrae; third nerve dysfunction can also cause pupillary dilatation (mydriasis) as well as a "down and out" eye as the actions of the VI and IV cranial nerves are unopposed. A diabetic third nerve palsy will result in ptosis as well as diplopia but should spare the pupil.

Unilateral partial ptosis in association with the inability to properly constrict the pupil (meiosis, best seen in a dark room) and decreased sweating on one side of the face are seen with Horner's syndrome. The ptosis is partial because it affects the tiny Mueller's muscle, which is innervated by the sympathetic nerves. The sympathetic pathway to the Mueller's muscle includes the hypothalamus, cervical spine, superior cervical ganglion, the adventitia of the internal carotid artery, and then the ophthalmic artery.

CLINICAL PEARL	STEP 2/3

Classic conditions that result in a Horner's syndrome of ptosis, meiosis, and anhydrosis are a Pancoast tumor or a carotid dissection. If a patient presents with head/neck trauma and Horner's syndrome, order a computed tomography angiogram (CTA) of the neck to evaluate for a dissection. If a patient presents with cough and history of smoking, order a chest radiograph or chest computed tomography (CT) scan.

In this patient's case, the ptosis is unaccompanied by pupillary abnormalities, and the diplopia seen in all directions is not consistent with a third nerve palsy. Therefore, the possibility of a neuromuscular junction disorder is more likely, especially when seen in combination with limb weakness and dysphagia.

What is the next step in diagnosis?
At this point the patient's differential diagnosis includes myasthenia gravis, LEMS, ALS myopathies, or upper cervical cord or brainstem lesions. Blood testing for acetylcholine-receptor antibodies would be appropriate as would myopathy labs including thyroid-stimulating hormone (TSH) and creatine kinase (CPK).

CLINICAL PEARL STEP 2/3

Patients with decreased reflexes may have peripheral neuropathies or myopathies, whereas increased reflexes indicate upper motor neuron involvement, as in cervical cord central lesions or ALS, which is a mixed upper and lower motor neuron degenerative disease.

What neurodiagnostic test would be appropriate?

Electromyography/nerve conduction studies (EMG/NCS) are appropriate because they may rule in a diagnosis of ALS or myopathy. In addition, a type of EMG know as repetitive nerve stimulation (RNS) can confirm the presence of myasthenia gravis and distinguish it from LEMS. Single-fiber EMG might also be performed. If this patient were much younger and myasthenia gravis was confirmed, a CT scan of the chest to look for a thymoma would be important.

CLINICAL PEARL STEP 2/3

Young women with myasthenia gravis have a higher incidence of thymomas, and a thymectomy can reverse their disease or be curative.

Acetylcholine-receptor antibodies are checked, which return positive.

Diagnosis: Myasthenia gravis (generalized)

Based on the history and exam and the lab work, the patient has antibody-positive myasthenia gravis. A single-fiber EMG may be performed to confirm the diagnosis, which is not part of a routine EMG/NCS. The single-fiber EMG can be especially helpful for patients who are seronegative myasthenia gravis to aid in diagnosis.

What are treatment options for myasthenia gravis?

For mild to moderate disease, pyridostigmine is an acetylcholinesterase inhibitor and appropriate first-line therapy. Treatment for the condition often includes immunosuppression with steroids as primary prevention for relapses. Other treatment options include azathioprine, mycophenolate mofetil, cyclosporine, cyclophosphamide, and rituximab for maintenance. For exacerbations, intravenous immunoglobulin and plasma exchange are beneficial.

CLINICAL PEARL STEP 2/3

3-4 Diaminopyridine is the agent used to treat symptoms of LEMS, but because it is a paraneoplastic disorder, definitive treatment is aimed at an underlying tumor that might not be known at the time of the diagnosis of LEMS.

CLINICAL PEARL STEP 2/3

Although antibodies to the postsynaptic acetylcholine receptor are present in most cases of myasthenia gravis, antibodies to muscle-specific tyrosine kinase (MuSK) may also be positive and should be checked in patients who have weakness limited to the ocular muscles.

BEYOND THE PEARLS

- Thymomas are more likely to be present when acetylcholine-receptor antibodies are present.
- Patients who have thymomas should get thymectomies for myasthenia gravis, as this has been shown to be curative. What may be less obvious to clinicians is that for patients who do not have a thymoma, a thymectomy may still be considered an option to improve the chance of treatment remission (this is an American Academy of Neurology practice parameter).
- Although the tensilon test is rarely used in clinical practice, it can be useful when antibodies and EMG are nondiagnostic. Incremental doses of edrophonium chloride are given, and the patient is watched for improvement over 1 minute. It is especially prominent when patients have ptosis or diplopia. It can, however, cause bradyarrhythmias, and thus atropine should be available. Patients with MuSK antibodies may have a paradoxical reaction to this test and get weakness or fasciculations.
- In 1993, superoxide dismutase *(SOD-1)* was the first gene discovered for ALS. This gene accounts for 20% of familial ALS cases. As of 2014, two thirds of familial ALS and 10% of sporadic ALS can be linked to a specific genetic cause.
- Primary lateral sclerosis (PLS) is an upper motor neuron disease similar to ALS, but it spares the anterior horn cells of the spine; thus, the lower motor neuron findings (such as atrophy, hypotonia, and fasciculations) are not present in PLS.
- Certain commonly prescribed drugs, including aminoglycosides, fluoroquinolones, and antiarrhythmic drugs, may in fact worsen or exacerbate myasthenia. However, there are many more medications that may worsen the disease as well. Before prescribing a new medication to a myasthenia gravis patient, check to make sure the medication is not contraindicated on www.myasthenia.org.

References

Deady JP. Recognizing aponeurotic ptosis. *J Neurol Neurosurg Psychiatry.* 1989;52:996-998.
Gronseth GS, Barohn RJ. Practice parameter: thymectomy for autoimmune myasthenia gravis (an evidence based review): report of the Quality Standards Subcommittee of the American Academy of Neurology. *Neurology.* 2000;55(1):7-15.
Myasthenia Gravis Foundation of America, Inc. Available at <www.myasthenia.org>. Accessed 10.12.15.
Pascuzzi RM. The edrophonium test. *Semin Neurol.* 2003;23(1):83-84.
Sanders DB, Guptill JT. Myasthenia gravis and Lambert-Eaton myasthenic syndrome. *Continuum (Minneap Minn).* 2014;20(5 Peripheral Nervous System Disorders):1413-1425.

Arzhang Cyrus Javan ▪ Andrea Censullo

A 60-Year-Old Male With Acute Headache and Fever

A 60-year-old male presents to the emergency department with the acute onset of a severe headache associated with subjective fever. He also reports a stiff neck.

What medical emergency must you consider in this patient based solely on these initial symptoms?

You must consider the diagnosis of acute bacterial meningitis. Patients with acute bacterial meningitis usually present with some combination of headache, fever, nuchal rigidity, and altered mental status. Nuchal rigidity (i.e., stiff neck) is the hallmark sign of irritated meninges and can be demonstrated when the neck resists passive flexion.

CLINICAL PEARL   **STEP 2/3**

The classic triad of fever, nuchal rigidity, and altered mental status is present in approximately 21 to 66% of patients with acute meningitis, but the absence of all three findings nearly rules out acute meningitis.

This patient is presenting with three of the four aforementioned signs and symptoms, therefore favoring a diagnosis of acute meningitis. Nausea, vomiting, and photophobia are other common components of the presentation. Keep in mind that a higher level of suspicion is required to diagnose bacterial meningitis in elderly and immunocompromised patients. These patients can have an atypical presentation, with lethargy and confusion serving as the main clinical manifestations.

What factors should be considered when evaluating the cause of a patient's suspected meningitis?

The list of organisms that can cause meningitis is long and can be daunting, but conducting a thorough history can sometimes help narrow the differential diagnosis.

Assessing the patient's immune status is paramount, as certain immunodeficiencies can predispose patients to distinct opportunistic pathogens. For example, the elderly (considered age 50 or older), diabetics, alcoholics, pregnant patients, patients on immunosuppressive medications, and those with impaired cell-mediated immunity are more susceptible to *Listeria monocytogenes* meningitis. Patients with human immunodeficiency virus (HIV) have a significantly increased risk of *Cryptococcus neoformans* meningitis.

111

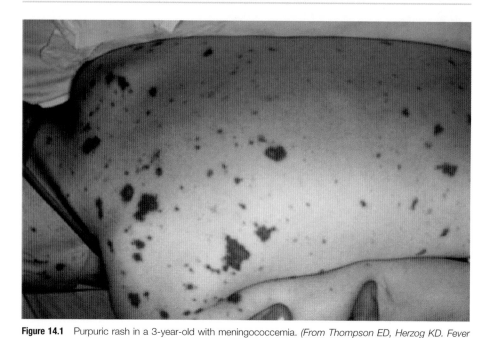

Figure 14.1　Purpuric rash in a 3-year-old with meningococcemia. *(From Thompson ED, Herzog KD. Fever and rash, In: Zaoutis LB, Chiang VW, eds.* Comprehensive Pediatric Hospital Medicine. *Philadelphia: Mosby; 2007:329-339.)*

CLINICAL PEARL   **STEP 2/3**

Patients without a functional spleen are at increased risk of infection with encapsulated bacteria such as *Streptococcus pneumoniae, Neisseria meningitidis,* and *Haemophilus influenzae.*

Patients with deficiencies in terminal complement are predisposed to recurrent *N. meningitidis* bacteremia (i.e., meningococcemia) and, rarely, meningitis.

CLINICAL PEARL   **STEP 2/3**

A rash occurs in about 50% of patients with meningococcemia, independent of the presence or absence of meningitis, beginning as a diffuse macular rash that rapidly evolves into petechiae and purpura. Lesions can occur on the trunk, lower extremities, mucous membranes, and occasionally on the palms and soles (see Fig. 14.1).

The presence of other risk factors, independent of the patient's immune status, can also assist with the evaluation. For example, patients with recent head trauma or neurosurgical procedures are at greater risk for infection with *Staphylococcal* spp., *H. influenzae,* and nosocomial gram-negative rods.

Certain elements from the history of present illness or the past medical history can also help elucidate the cause. A clinical picture of recent or active pneumonia, otitis media, or sinusitis can point towards a diagnosis of *S. pneumoniae.* A history of herpes may place herpes simplex virus (HSV) meningitis or encephalitis higher on the differential. Recent constitutional symptoms suggesting upper respiratory tract infection (URI) or a viral gastroenteritis should prompt one to think of other, more common causes of viral meningitis such as enteroviruses.

Certain elements of the social history can be very helpful. High-risk sexual behavior should prompt one to consider syphilis or acute HIV infection in the differential diagnosis. Recent tick exposure should alert one to the possibility of Lyme disease, human granulocytic anaplasmosis (HGA), ehrlichiosis, or Rocky Mountain spotted fever (RMSF). Recent mosquito bites can be a clue for meningitis or encephalitis from arboviruses such as West Nile virus. Recent contact with sick children makes enterovirus meningitis a real possibility. Coccidioidal meningitis should be considered in patients with recent travel to certain regions of the southwestern United States with high endemicity for this soil-dwelling fungus. There have been outbreaks of *N. meningitidis* in crowded living conditions such as college dormitories and military barracks.

Further history is obtained. The patient denies similar headaches in the past and has not been recently ill. He does have a past medical history of well-controlled hypertension, and his surgical history is significant for splenectomy due to a ruptured spleen from a motor vehicle accident 30 years prior.

On review of systems he denies nausea or vomiting, chest pain, cough, shortness of breath, or any other significant complaints.

On physical exam, temperature is 39 °C (102.4 °F), pulse rate is 110/min, blood pressure is 120/88 mm Hg, respiration rate is 18/min, and oxygen saturation is 95% on room air.

He is awake but appears fatigued and in mild distress. Cardiac exam is notable for tachycardia. His lungs are clear and abdominal exam is unremarkable. He resists passive flexion of his neck and has mild photophobia. He has no rash, no papilledema, and the neurologic exam shows no focal deficits. Kernig's and Brudzinski's signs are negative.

What are Kernig's and Brudzinski's signs, and how reassuring is it that they are normal in this patient?
Kernig's and Brudzinski's signs are used to test for meningeal irritation. To elicit Kernig's sign, while the patient is supine, the practitioner passively flexes the patient's hip 90 degrees and passively extends the knee from a 90-degree flexed position. The test is considered positive when the patient resists the straightening of the knee due to pain. Brudzinski's sign involves flexing the neck of a patient who is supine. The test is considered positive if the patient reflexively flexes the hips and/or knees due to pain.

A positive Kernig's or Brudzinski's sign can help point toward meningitis, but a negative test does not rule it out, as the sensitivity of these maneuvers is only roughly 5%.

What is your differential diagnosis at this point?
The clinical presentation of acute onset of headache, fever, and symptoms of meningeal irritation, along with neck stiffness and photophobia, is most concerning for meningitis. When considering meningitis, it is helpful to break it down further into two categories: acute bacterial meningitis and aseptic meningitis. Viral encephalitis is also on the differential but less likely.

Other diseases to consider, though less likely in this patient with no focal neurologic findings, are a focal infection of the central nervous system such as a brain abscess, epidural empyema, or subdural empyema. One critical noninfectious diagnosis to keep in mind is subarachnoid hemorrhage.

As described previously, acute bacterial meningitis is a medical emergency with an overall mortality around 25%. The mortality rate is even higher in patients with pneumococcal meningitis.

TABLE 14.1 ■ Common Bacterial Pathogens in Meningitis and Recommended Empiric Antibiotic Therapy Based on Age and Risk Factors

Predisposing Factor	Common Bacterial Pathogens	Empiric Antimicrobial Therapy
Age 16-50 years old	S. pneumoniae, N. meningitidis	Vancomycin + third-generation cephalosporin
Age >50 years old or alcoholism	S. pneumoniae, N. meningitides, L. monocytogenes, aerobic gram-negative bacilli	Vancomycin + third-generation cephalosporin + ampicillin
Immunocompromised (i.e., HIV, immunosuppressive medication)	S. pneumoniae, N. meningitides, L. monocytogenes, aerobic gram-negative bacilli (including pseudomonas)	Vancomycin + ampicillin + cefepime or meropenem
Basilar skull fracture	S. pneumoniae, H. influenzae, Group A strep	Vancomycin + third-generation cephalosporin
Postneurosurgery, cerebrospinal shunt, or penetrating head trauma	S. aureus, coagulase negative staph, aerobic gram-negative bacilli including Pseudomonas spp., Propionibacterium acnes	Vancomycin + cefepime or ceftazidime or meropenem

(Adapted from Tables 89-5 and 89-12 from Tunke AR, van de Beek D, Scheld WM. Acute meningitis. In: Bennett JE, Dolin R, and Blaser MJ. *Principles and Practice of Infectious Diseases.* 8th ed. Philadelphia; Elsevier; 2015:1097-1137.)

The most common bacterial causes of meningitis in this patient's age group (>50 years old) include *S. pneumoniae,* which is the most common cause of meningitis in adults overall, followed by *N. meningitidis* and *L. monocytogenes. H. influenzae* has become an exceedingly rare cause of meningitis in adults because of the widespread use of the *H. influenzae* type B vaccine, although it can still be seen in adults with predisposing factors such as cerebrospinal fluid (CSF) leak, recent neurosurgery, trauma, or mastoiditis. Common bacteria that cause meningitis in specific age groups and populations are displayed in Table 14.1.

BASIC SCIENCE PEARL   **STEP 1**

Once bacteria enter the subarachnoid space, they are able to rapidly multiply because of decreased host defenses in the CSF, specifically a decreased level of complement and immunoglobulins. This prevents effective opsonization of encapsulated bacteria, which is the first necessary step in phagocytosis.

Aseptic meningitis is a term used to categorize any meningitis that has a negative CSF bacterial Gram stain and culture. The differential diagnosis is comprised of a broad range of both infectious and noninfectious etiologies, many of which can lead to an acute clinical picture that very closely resembles acute bacterial meningitis. Table 14.2 reviews many of the etiologies of aseptic meningitis.

Viruses are the most common cause of aseptic meningitis. Coxsackieviruses, echoviruses, and human enteroviruses 68-71, all of which are members of the *Enterovirus* group of viruses, are the

TABLE 14.2 ■ Differential Diagnosis of Aseptic Meningitis

Viral Meningitis

- Enterovirus (e.g., coxsackievirus, echovirus, poliovirus)
- Herpes simplex virus (HSV)
- Human immunodeficiency virus (HIV)
- West Nile virus (WNV)
- Varicella-zoster virus (VZV)
- Lymphocytic choriomeningitis virus (LCM)

Other Pathogens

- *Mycobacterium tuberculosis*
- *Treponema pallidum* (syphilis)
- *Borrelia burgdorferi* (Lyme disease)
- *Rickettsia rickettsii* (Rocky Mountain spotted fever)
- Agents of ehrlichiosis
- *Cryptococcus neoformans*
- *Coccidioides immitis*

Neoplasms

- Large cell lymphoma
- Acute leukemia
- Certain solid tumors (breast cancer, lung cancer, melanoma, gastrointestinal cancers)

Drug-Induced Meningitis

- Nonsteroidal antiinflammatory drugs (NSAIDs)
- Trimethoprim-sulfamethoxazole (TMP/SMX)

Systemic Illness

- Systemic lupus erythematosus (SLE)
- Sarcoidosis
- Behçet's disease

Para Meningeal Focus of Infection

- Brain or epidural abscess

(Adapted from Singh A, Promes SB. Meningitis, encephalitis, and brain abscess in emergency medicine. In: Adams JG, ed. *Emergency Medicine*. Philadelphia: Elsevier; 2013:1443-1453.)

most frequent causes of viral meningitis. The other, less common causes of viral meningitis are HIV, HSV type 1 and 2 (type 2 more often than type 1), varicella-zoster virus (VZV), mumps, adenovirus, lymphocytic choriomeningitis virus, cytomegalovirus (CMV), and Epstein-Barr virus (EBV).

CLINICAL PEARL	STEP 2/3

Enteroviruses are the leading recognizable cause of aseptic meningitis in both adults and children. Enterovirus infections occur worldwide, more frequently in the summer and fall, but can occur year round in tropical areas.

Among the bacterial causes of aseptic meningitis are spirochetes such as *Treponema pallidum* (syphilis) and *Borrelia burgdorferi* (Lyme disease), rickettsial organisms including *Rickettsia rickettsii* (RMSF), and *Mycobacterium tuberculosis*.

TABLE 14.3 ■ **Indications for Brain Imaging Prior to Lumbar Puncture**

History of immunocompromised state
History of central nervous system disease (e.g., mass lesion, stroke, focal infection)
New-onset seizure (or new-onset seizure within 1 week of presentation)
Papilledema on funduscopic exam (or elevated optic nerve sheath diameter on ultrasound)
Abnormal neurologic exam
Altered mental status
Altered level of consciousness

(Adapted from Singh A, Promes SB. Meningitis, Encephalitis, and brain abscess in emergency medicine. In: Adams JG, ed. *Emergency Medicine*. Philadelphia: Elsevier; 2013:1443-1453.)

Can you clinically distinguish meningitis from encephalitis, and is this distinction important?

Meningitis refers to inflammation of the leptomeninges, which surround the brain and spinal cord, whereas encephalitis is inflammation of the brain parenchyma itself. Although there is considerable overlap in the clinical presentation, patients with encephalitis more often have altered mental status as the primary feature early in the disease course, with personality changes, speech deficits, or other focal neurologic findings often noted. In bacterial meningitis, headache and signs of meningeal irritation tend to predominate early, but as the disease progresses, a decreased level of consciousness occurs in greater than 75% of patients and can vary from lethargy to coma. Seizures and focal neurological deficits are also possible findings in a patient with bacterial meningitis but would be atypical of viral meningitis, which again is the most common cause of aseptic meningitis. Many patients with encephalitis also have evidence of meningitis. This entity is known as meningoencephalitis.

Although there can be significant overlap in the clinical presentation of the above entities, reminding yourself that these disease processes are two separate entities remains paramount during both evaluation and management of these patients, as the list of pathogens that have a predilection to cause meningitis differs from the list that causes encephalitis.

What is the most critical diagnostic test that should be performed as soon as possible?

Unless contraindicated, every patient with suspected meningitis should have a lumbar puncture (LP) performed as soon as possible.

What CSF studies should you perform?

The CSF should be sent for Gram stain, culture, cell count with differential, glucose, and protein. The opening pressure should also be recorded. If a viral etiology is suspected, especially based on the results of the initial CSF profile, polymerase chain reaction (PCR), and antibody testing should be performed on the CSF. Additional studies should be performed based on the clinical picture.

Should brain imaging always be performed prior to an LP?

In certain patients, brain imaging with either computed tomography (CT) scan (usually more readily available) or magnetic resonance imaging (MRI) should be performed before an LP to rule out mass effect (brain shift) caused by a space-occupying lesion or brain edema. This is recommended because the presence of mass effect increases the risk of herniation from an LP. (Table 14.3 lists indications for head imaging prior to LP.)

CLINICAL PEARL STEP 2/3

Brain imaging should be performed before LP in the following situations: new-onset seizure, immunocompromised state (HIV, immunosuppressive medications), history of space-occupying CNS lesion, focal neurologic deficits or papilledema, severely impaired consciousness, or age older than 60.

CLINICAL PEARL STEP 2/3

Over 90% of patients with bacterial meningitis have some degree of elevated intracranial pressure (ICP), which can lead to the dreaded complication of herniation. Significantly increased ICP can potentially lead to a reduced level of consciousness, papilledema, dilated poorly reactive pupils, sixth nerve palsies, decerebrate posturing, and the Cushing reflex (bradycardia, hypertension, and irregular breathing).

Should you start empiric antibiotics? If so, which antibiotics would be most appropriate?

When bacterial meningitis is suspected, empiric antibiotics should be administered as soon as possible after two sets of blood cultures are drawn and the LP is performed. Bacterial meningitis has a high mortality rate, and timely administration of antibiotics improves outcomes.

If an LP must be delayed while awaiting brain imaging, antibiotics should be administered before the patient undergoes the diagnostic exams. Administering antibiotics a few hours prior to LP should not have a significant impact on the CSF white blood cell (WBC), glucose concentration, or Gram stain results.

The choice of empiric antibiotics while awaiting LP results depends on the patient's clinical picture and risk factors for certain pathogens.

BASIC SCIENCE PEARL STEP 1

Many antibiotics poorly penetrate the CNS of a patient with an intact blood–brain barrier. Bacterial meningitis increases the blood–brain barrier permeability and therefore allows for higher CSF concentrations of antibiotics. Despite this, high doses of antibiotics are still required in order to achieve adequate therapeutic CSF antibiotic concentrations.

This patient is at risk for the two most common causes of community acquired bacterial meningitis: *S. pneumoniae* and *N. meningitidis*. Because he is over 55 years old, he is also at risk for *L. monocytogenes*. Therefore, he should be empirically started on a third-generation cephalosporin (cefotaxime or ceftriaxone), plus vancomycin and ampicillin. The third-generation cephalosporin will treat *N. meningitidis* and cephalosporin-susceptible *S. pneumoniae*. Penicillin is highly active against penicillin-susceptible strains of *S. pneumoniae* but should never be used as empiric therapy because there is more penicillin resistance in *S. pneumoniae* in the community than cephalosporin resistance. Because of the increasing prevalence of cephalosporin-resistant *S. pneumoniae*, vancomycin is added while awaiting culture and susceptibility data. Ampicillin is added to cover for the possibility of *Listeria*.

When the patient's clinical picture suggests a possible encephalitis component, empiric intravenous (IV) acyclovir along with good hydration and IV fluid (to prevent IV acyclovir-induced renal crystal buildup and resultant acute kidney injury) should also be initiated.

A patient with acute meningitis will typically be hospitalized for treatment. However, if certain criteria are met and adequate monitoring can be ensured, a trial of outpatient management is appropriate. In order to consider outpatient treatment, the patient must be immunocompetent,

TABLE 14.4 ■ Initial Results From Patient's CSF
Testing (With Normal Values in Parenthesis)

Opening pressure	260 mm H$_2$0 (60-200 mm H$_2$0)
Glucose	20 mg/dL (40-80 mg/dL or CSF/ serum ratio >0.6)
Protein	80 mg/L (15-50 mg/L)
White blood cell count	1500 cells/μL (98% neutrophils, 2% lymphocytes) (0-5 cells/μL)
Red blood cell count	3 cells/μL (0-5 cells/μL)

have a normal level of consciousness, have received no prior antibiotic treatment, and have CSF studies consistent with viral meningitis. If there is failure to improve within 48 hours, the patient must be promptly reevaluated by a physician and have repeat imaging and laboratory studies, and often a repeat LP.

Should you add glucocorticoids?
Absolutely.

CLINICAL PEARL   **STEP 2/3**

Glucocorticoids have been shown to improve survival and neurologic outcomes in *S. pneumoniae* meningitis, so dexamethasone should be started in every adult patient with suspected acute bacterial meningitis.

The timing of glucocorticoid administration is critical; glucocorticoids must be given prior to, or in conjunction with, the first dose of antibiotics. Glucocorticoids can be discontinued later if a diagnosis of *S. pneumoniae* meningitis is not established.

Laboratory testing reveals a peripheral WBC of $18 \times 103/\mu L$ (normal 4 to $11 \times 103/\mu L$), with neutrophilic predominance. Results of other basic laboratory testing are within normal limits. Two sets of blood cultures are drawn. An LP is performed, and the patient is started on empiric vancomycin, ceftriaxone, and ampicillin along with IV dexamethasone.
   Results of CSF analysis are provided in Table 14.4.

Does this CSF profile help further narrow your differential?
Yes, this CSF profile is consistent with a diagnosis of bacterial meningitis. The classic CSF profile in bacterial meningitis includes an elevated opening pressure (>200 mm H$_2$O in 90% of cases), elevated WBC (pleocytosis) with neutrophilic predominance, low glucose, and high protein. The fluid is often found to be cloudy. No single CSF finding can definitively distinguish between bacterial and aseptic meningitis, but the evaluation of the CSF findings in conjunction with the clinical picture should lead to the diagnosis. Keep in mind, however, that in a patient with partially treated bacterial meningitis, the CSF profile will likely lead to a diagnosis of aseptic meningitis.
   Table 14.5 outlines the classic CSF findings in the various types of meningitis.

TABLE 14.5 ■ Classic CSF Profiles in Various Types of Meningitis

Parameter (Normal)	Bacterial Meningitis	Viral Meningitis	Fungal Meningitis	Tuberculosis Meningitis	Neoplastic Meningitis
Opening pressure (6-20 cm H₂O)	>20 cm H_2O	Normal to mildly elevated	>20 cm H_2O	>20 cm H_2O	>20 cm H_2O
CSF WBC (<5 cells/mL)	>1000 cells/mL	<1000 cells/mL	<500 cells/mL	<500 cells/mL	<500 cells/mL
PMNs (<80%) Lymphocytes (<10%)	>80%	<50% >50%	<50% >80%	<50%	<50%
CSF glucose (>40 mg/dL)	<40 mg/dL	>40 mg/dL	<40 mg/dL	<40 mg/dL	<40 mg/dL
CSF protein (<50 mg/dL)	>150 mg/dL	<100 mg/dL	>100 mg/dL	>100 mg/dL	>100 mg/dL

PMN, Polymorphonuclear leukocytes; WBC, white blood cell count.
(Adapted from Singh A, Promes SB. Meningitis, encephalitis, and brain abscess in emergency medicine. In: Adams JG, ed. *Emergency Medicine*. Philadelphia: Elsevier; 2013:1443-1453.)

CSF Gram stain shows gram-positive cocci in pairs.

What is your presumptive diagnosis, and how will you confirm the diagnosis?
The presumptive diagnosis is *S. pneumoniae* meningitis, which can be confirmed by culture. CSF bacterial cultures are positive in 80 to 90% of patients with bacterial meningitis, and CSF Gram stain reveals the organism in 60 to 90% of cases.

CLINICAL PEARL   **STEP 2/3**

If the CSF Gram stain identifies organisms, the empiric antibiotics should be modified accordingly. *S. pneumoniae* are gram-positive diplococci, *N. meningitidis* are gram-negative diplococci, and *H. influenzae* are small pleomorphic gram-negative coccobacilli. Gram stain for *L. monocytogenes* will reveal gram-positive rods.

CSF Gram stain and culture remains the gold standard in the evaluation of acute bacterial meningitis, but it is important to be aware that newer testing modalities do exist. Although studies evaluating the use of CSF bacterial antigen tests (latex agglutination) have shown that they do not appear to significantly change management, studies evaluating the use of PCR testing for bacteria have been promising and they may play a more prominent role in the future. CSF viral PCR testing is already an important testing modality used in clinical practice today.

CSF culture shows penicillin (PCN) and cephalosporin-susceptible *S. pneumoniae*. The patient's antibiotics are subsequently narrowed to IV PCN G. His symptoms gradually improve, and he is discharged with a 2-week total course of IV antibiotics.

Diagnosis: Acute bacterial meningitis caused by *Streptococcus pneumoniae*

Is there any role for a repeat LP?

In a patient with *S. pneumoniae* meningitis treated with dexamethasone who is not improving as expected, or if the pneumococcal isolate has a minimum inhibitory concentration (MIC) >2 for cefotaxime, the LP should be repeated 36 to 48 hours after initiation of therapy to ensure the CSF is sterilized.

Because this patient's pneumococcal isolate was a sensitive organism and he improved with treatment, repeat LP is not indicated.

> Upon completing his course of antibiotics, he returns to your clinic with his wife. He reports full resolution of his symptoms, but his wife is now concerned about getting meningitis.

Should you provide, or should you have provided, chemoprophylaxis for his close contacts?

Prophylaxis is not routinely indicated for the close contacts of patients with *S. pneumoniae* meningitis. However, chemoprophylaxis is recommended for the close contacts of patients with meningitis caused by either *N. meningitidis* or *H. influenzae*.

N. meningitidis and *H. influenzae* are spread by droplets of oropharyngeal secretions; close contacts are defined as household or daycare members who sleep or eat in the same dwelling as the index patient and therefore may have had contact with the secretions. Health care workers generally do not require chemoprophylaxis unless they had close contact with the patient's oropharyngeal secretions such as during mouth-to-mouth resuscitation or oropharyngeal intubation.

Close contacts of patients with *N. meningitidis* should receive chemoprophylaxis with a 2-day regimen of rifampin. Note that pregnant women should not take rifampin. Alternate regimens are a single dose of ciprofloxacin (also not to be used during pregnancy) or one intramuscular dose of ceftriaxone. In areas with high prevalence of ciprofloxacin-resistant *N. meningitidis*, azithromycin is another option.

Chemoprophylaxis of adult close contacts of patients with *H. influenzae* meningitis should be done only if the contact shares a household with an unvaccinated or immunocompromised child. Because there are no good alternatives for prevention of meningitis caused by *H. influenzae*, consultation with an infectious disease specialist is recommended when rifampin is contraindicated.

CLINICAL PEARL   STEP 2/3

Colonization of the nasopharynx is the requisite first step in the pathogenesis of meningitis caused by the two most common causes of community-acquired bacterial meningitis: *S. pneumoniae* and *N. meningitidis*. Once in the bloodstream, the presence of a polysaccharide capsule helps these bacteria avoid phagocytosis and complement-mediated killing.

BEYOND THE PEARLS

- Bacterial meningitis is a medical emergency and LP with initiation of empiric antibiotics should be performed as soon as possible.
- Brain imaging prior to LP is only indicated in certain clinical situations. If indicated, empiric antibiotics should be given while awaiting the studies.
- In adults, the meningococcal conjugate vaccine should be given to adolescents 16 to 18 years old and in those with asplenia or complement deficiency. Certain local health

BEYOND THE PEARLS—cont'd

departments also recommend the vaccine for those with HIV and for men who have sex with men as a result of recent outbreaks of meningococcal meningitis in New York City and Los Angeles.

- Eosinophilic meningitis is a syndrome characterized by >10 eosinophils/mm^3 in the CSF, or eosinophils >10% of the CSF lymphocytes. The differential diagnosis of eosinophilic meningitis includes parasitic diseases (e.g., *Angiostrongylus,* cysticercosis, schistosomiasis, and *Baylisascaris*), nonparasitic infections (e.g., Coccidioidomycosis, Cryptococcosis), and noninfectious causes (e.g., NSAIDs, antibiotics, ventriculoperitoneal shunts, CNS leukemia/lymphoma).
- Although not widely used at this time, PCR assays for the diagnoses of bacterial meningitis have shown good sensitivity and specificity (>98% for both), and further studies may prove this to be a useful test in the future. PCR assays have also been shown to aid in the diagnosis of meningitis caused by *Mycoplasma pneumoniae,* which can mimic viral meningitis and encephalitis.
- Petechiae, if identified in a patient with suspected infection with *N. meningitidis,* should be biopsied in order to evaluate for the presence of the organisms. Meningococcemia may lead to a rash as a result of dermal seeding of organisms with resultant damage to the vascular endothelium.
- In patients with systemic hyperglycemia, the CSF/serum glucose ratio, rather than the absolute value of CSF glucose, should be used. A CSF/serum glucose ratio <0.6 is considered low, and a ratio <0.4 is highly suspicious for bacterial meningitis, although it can be seen in other disorders such as fungal, TB, sarcoid, and carcinomatous meningitis.
- Administering bactericidal antibiotics in meningitis leads to the release of bacterial cell-wall components that then activate macrophages and microglia to secrete tumor necrosis factor (TNF)-alpha. The rationale for giving glucocorticoids prior to antibiotics in bacterial meningitis is that glucocorticoids inhibit the synthesis of TNF-alpha by these cells, but only if administered before the cells are activated by endotoxin.
- If either penicillin, ampicillin, or chloramphenicol are used to treat a patient with *N. meningitidis* or *H. influenzae* meningitis, then chemoprophylaxis should also be administered to the patient to completely eradicate nasopharyngeal colonization; these antibiotics are not reliable at doing so.
- Many of the complications of bacterial meningitis are the result of the host immune response to the pathogen rather than by direct injury from the organism. As a result, CNS damage can continue even after antibiotics have sterilized the CSF.
- CSF findings of lymphocytic pleocytosis with low glucose should prompt consideration of fungal or tuberculous meningitis, *Listeria* meningoencephalitis, or noninfectious disorders (sarcoid, malignancy).
- Up to 40% of patients with VZV meningitis do not present with a rash.
- The CSF HSV PCR may be negative in the first 72 hours, so if there still is a high suspicion, the LP should be repeated and retested for HSV PCR.
- CSF lactate may be helpful in differentiating between bacterial and viral meningitis. In those who have not received antibiotics, elevated CSF lactate is seen in bacterial meningitis and may have better accuracy than CSF WBC, glucose, or protein in making this distinction.

References

Bamberger D. Diagnosis, initial management, and prevention of meningitis. *Am Fam Physician.* 2010;82(12):1491-1498.

Tunkel A. Approach to the patient with central nervous system infection. In: Bennett J, Dolin R, Blaser M, eds. *Mandell, Douglas, and Bennett's Principles and Practice of Infectious Diseases.* 8th ed. Philadelphia: Elsevier; 2015:1091-1096.

Tunkel A, van de Beek D, Scheld M. Acute meningitis. In: Bennett J, Dolin R, Blaser M, eds. *Mandell, Douglas, and Bennett's Principles and Practice of Infectious Diseases*. 8th ed. Philadelphia: Elsevier; 2015:1097-1137.

Tunkel A, Hartman B, Kaplan S, et al. Practice guidelines for the management of bacterial meningitis. *Clin Infect Dis*. 2004;39(9):1267-1284.

Roos K, Tyler K. Meningitis, encephalitis, brain abscess, and empyema. In: Fauci A, Braunwald E, Kasper D, et al., eds. *Harrison's Principles of Internal Medicine*. 17th ed. New York: McGraw-Hill; 2008:2621-2641.

Roos K, Tyler K. Meningitis, encephalitis, brain abscess and empyema. In: Kasper D, Fauci A, eds. *Harrison's Infectious Diseases*. 2nd ed. New York: McGraw-Hill; 2013:330-350.

van de Beek D, Gans J, Tunkel A, et al. community-acquired bacterial meningitis in adults. *N Engl J Med*. 2006;54(1):44-53.

Andrew Morado ■ Raj Dasgupta ■ Ahmet Baydur

A 66-Year-Old Male With Progressive Dyspnea on Exertion

A 66-year-old male presents for outpatient evaluation of progressive shortness of breath on exertion for the past 6 months. He becomes short of breath after ambulating two blocks and has noted a productive cough during this time. With rest, his shortness of breath resolves.

With shortness of breath, what organ systems should be considered as a potential cause?

Anytime shortness of breath or dyspnea are encountered, it is best to keep the differential broad to help organize a diagnostic approach. The three main categories are the lungs, heart, and anemia. In an older male such as this, the most likely causes are cardiac or pulmonary in nature, though you can never exclude less common causes on history alone. There is no immediate history of coronary artery disease, chest pain, or orthopnea that might suggest congestive heart failure (CHF) as a potential etiology. Additionally, a productive cough could support a primary pulmonary pathology as a cause of his symptoms, though CHF and other cardiac etiologies such as arrhythmias and a dilated left atrium can be other potential culprits. Anemia, regardless of the cause, can manifest as dyspnea on exertion because of decreased oxygen delivery to tissues.

He denies shortness of breath while recumbent, uses one pillow to sleep at night, and denies lower extremity edema. He describes his sputum as thick and moderate in consistency and yellowish in color. He denies fevers or chills. Further review of systems is negative.

What clues in the history might point toward CHF?

Heart failure can be due to a low ejection fraction (systolic dysfunction), most commonly caused by myocardial infarction, or with preserved ejection fraction (diastolic dysfunction), which is strongly associated with long-standing, poorly controlled hypertension. Regardless of the type, the common complaints typically are dyspnea with exertion, orthopnea reported as need to remain upright while sleeping, and peripheral edema. With the absence of orthopnea and lower extremity edema, CHF becomes lower on the differential while pulmonary causes remain high.

He reports well-controlled hypertension and no other past medical conditions. He had an uneventful cholecystectomy 20 years prior. He has no contributing family conditions. He reports occasional alcohol use, no illicit drug use, and smoking 40 cigarettes per day for the past 30 years. He has taken lisinopril for his hypertension for the past 10 years and denies allergies.

CLINICAL PEARL   **STEP 2/3**

Pharmacology and adverse effects are commonly tested on all board exams, and it is worthwhile to know the effects of the more common drugs. Angiotensin-converting enzyme (ACE) inhibitors have several well-known side effects and can be remembered by the acronym CAPTOPRIL: cough, angioedema, palpitations, taste, orthostatic hypotension, potassium elevation, renal impairment, impotence, and leukocytosis. The dilation of the efferent arteriole at the level of the glomerulus is responsible for the decrease in glomerular filtration rate, while inhibition of ACE inhibitor results in potassium retention. Cough and angioedema occur from the effect on bradykinin. The cough itself can be confused clinically as a marker for worsening pulmonary disease when in fact it is an adverse effect. Additionally, make note of medications that can exacerbate chronic disease such as beta blockers in obstructive airway disease.

He reveals a 60 pack-year smoking history and no other pertinent findings. Given his presenting symptoms and his smoking, chronic obstructive pulmonary disease (COPD) rises to the top of the differential.

CLINICAL PEARL   **STEP 2/3**

To calculate pack-years, multiply the number of cigarettes × years smoked and divide by 20. Risk of developing COPD substantially increases in those with more than 10 pack-years; however, only about 15% of all smokers will develop this disease.

On exam, he is a thin male in no distress. The temperature is 37.9 °C (100.3 °F), blood pressure is 118/70 mm Hg, pulse rate is 110/min, respiration rate is 28/min, and oxygen saturation is 86% on room air. Heart sounds are distant. He exhibits an increased anterior/posterior diameter of his chest wall. Breath sounds are faint with end expiratory wheezes diffusely. There is no clubbing or lower extremity edema present.

His faint heart and breath sounds suggest increased lung volumes, as does his chest wall diameter (barrel chest; see Fig. 15.1). His small stature is typical of patients with COPD while the absence of peripheral edema further refutes CHF. Clubbing is almost never seen with emphysema or chronic bronchitis (unlike in cystic fibrosis, bronchiectasis, or congenital heart disease).

What is your differential diagnosis?

This is a 66-year-old male with progressive dyspnea on exertion, productive cough, and a 60 pack-year smoking history. Physical exam demonstrates evidence of hyperinflation and obstructive airway disease. COPD remains number one on the differential. We gave consideration earlier to left heart failure as it can cause dyspnea as well as wheezing if significant pulmonary edema is present. However, the absence of other classic history and exam findings such as elevated jugular venous pressure (JVP), S3 gallop, or orthopnea makes it less likely. Other considerations are other causes of obstructive airway disease. Chronic asthmatics could present in such a way, though he denies having a history of asthma as a younger male or child. He is too old to be newly diagnosed with cystic fibrosis. Alpha-1 antitrypsin (A1AT) deficiency is a definite consideration but is still less likely than COPD as a cause of this patient's symptoms. (A1AT deficiency typically presents at a young age, especially if patients are homozygous for the mutation. Other clues to the diagnosis are necrotizing panniculitis, a rare skin lesion, and abnormalities in liver enzymes.)

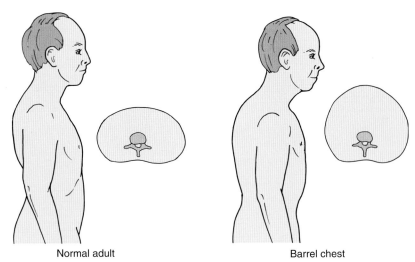

Normal adult   Barrel chest

Figure 15.1   Normal chest wall compared to barrel chest, a sign suggestive of hyperinflation. *(From Lippincott Williams & Wilkins Instructor's Resource CD-ROM to Accompany* Fundamentals of Nursing: The Art and Science of Nursing Care. *5th ed. Philadelphia: Lippincott Williams & Wilkins; 2005.)*

CLINICAL PEARL   **STEP 2/3**

A1AT deficiency is a codominant genetic disorder resulting in increased neutrophil elastase within the lung parenchyma. The effect of elastase is a panacinar emphysema that can eventually lead to COPD. Patients can present as early as their 30s without significant smoking history but demonstrating clinical and objective signs of COPD. Computed tomography (CT) imaging usually reveals predominantly lower lobe emphysema. Serum enzyme levels confirm the diagnosis, whereas genetic testing for the mutation determines disease severity. A1AT is less commonly associated with cystic fibrosis and bronchiectasis.

BASIC SCIENCE PEARL   **STEP 1**

Emphysema or destruction of lung parenchyma can have varying patterns depending on the etiology of disease. For example, A1AT tends to present with panacinar emphysema, whereas smoking typically causes centrilobular emphysema. The difference pathologically is how the secondary pulmonary lobule is affected. In Figure 15.2, the functional unit of the lung otherwise known as the secondary pulmonary lobule is shown and typically houses 3 to 12 acini. Centrilobular emphysema involves loss of the proximal respiratory bronchiole within the acinus but sparing of distal alveolitis. This sparing of lung parenchyma produces the effect of normal- and abnormal-appearing lung that can be discerned by the naked eye and typically involves the upper lobes. In contrast, panacinar emphysema results in destruction of the entire acinus and mainly affects the lower lobes.

What labs would you order and why?

Basic labs including a complete blood count (CBC) and basic metabolic panel (BMP) should be ordered, as they can reveal erythrocytosis suggesting chronic hypoxemia, though anemia is the most common blood abnormality, while an elevated bicarbonate suggests carbon dioxide retention. A1AT enzyme levels should be ordered to rule out this diagnosis.

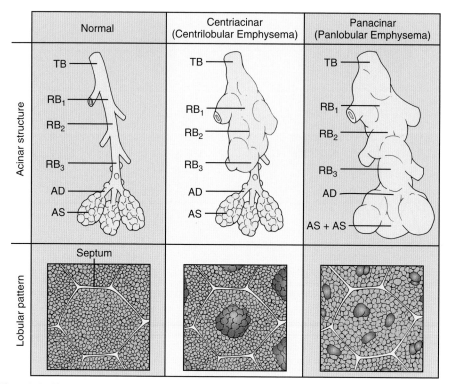

Figure 15.2 The secondary pulmonary lobule and types of emphysema based on location of anatomical changes. *(From WEBMD Inc. 2004.)*

Labs including a CBC and BMP are unremarkable. A1AT enzyme level is normal. An echocardiogram reveals normal ejection fraction and right-sided pressures.

How should you proceed with his workup?

The hallmarks of COPD are entrenched in the chest radiograph (CXR) and pulmonary function tests. Examine the CXR in Figure 15.3. Notice the hyperinflated lungs (more than 10 posterior rib shadows), air under the heart, widened intercostal spaces, and scalloping of the diaphragms. These findings are consistent with air trapping, but this should be confirmed by pulmonary function testing. There is also evidence of emphysematous changes, predominantly in the upper lobes, consistent with the physiology of emphysema. This results in the apices being overventilated relative to the perfusion at the apex of the lung compared to the bases.

How would you diagnose COPD?

The diagnosis is cinched by the pulmonary function tests, which also give information regarding disease severity and management options. Obstructive airway disease is defined as a forced expiratory volume in 1 second/forced vital capacity (FEV_1/FVC) ratio <70% while reduction in FEV_1 classifies disease severity. The FEV_1/FVC is simply the amount of the forced vital capacity expired in 1 second and defines airflow limitation if the ratio is less than 0.7 after maximal inspiration. The FEV_1 is an index of pulmonary reserve. Mild disease is FEV_1 >80%, moderate disease is FEV_1 50 to 80%, severe disease is FEV_1 30 to 50%, and very severe disease is <30%.

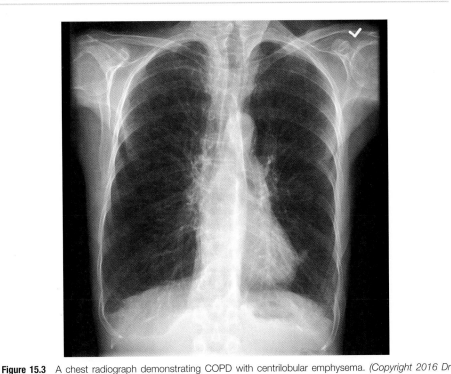

Figure 15.3 A chest radiograph demonstrating COPD with centrilobular emphysema. *(Copyright 2016 Dr Frank Gaillard. Image courtesy of Dr Frank Gaillard and* Radiopaedia.org. *Used under license.)*

CLINICAL PEARL	STEP 2/3

Remember your flow volume loops as they pertain to the patient because they will help determine the type of airway disease. For COPD, look for the classic scalloped expiratory phase with a normal inspiratory limb (shown in Fig. 15.4). This is typical of obstructive airway disease.

Diagnosis: Acute COPD exacerbation

What is the difference between emphysema and chronic bronchitis?

Remember pink puffers and blue bloaters? COPD has been classified as two main forms for the past 50 years: emphysema, which we have previously discussed as destruction of lung parenchyma, and chronic bronchitis. So what about chronic bronchitis? Chronic bronchitis is a clinical diagnosis defined as a chronic productive cough for at least 3 months of the year for 2 consecutive years in a smoker. Patients suffering from chronic bronchitis have problems stemming from airway inflammation and increased mucous production. The increased mucous production is the stimulus for the chronic cough, and over time mucous impaction can lead to recurrent pulmonary infections. The mucous impaction results in early air trapping and hyperinflation (bloater), while the severe ventilation/perfusion (V/Q) mismatch leads to hypoxemia (blue). In contrast, emphysema results in simultaneous destruction of alveolar spaces and capillary beds resulting in a near-normal alveolar/oxygen difference. Over the last 15 years, gene studies have proposed a reclassification of COPD into exacerbators with emphysema or chronic bronchitis, and patients with asthma-COPD overlap, or those with none of these features.

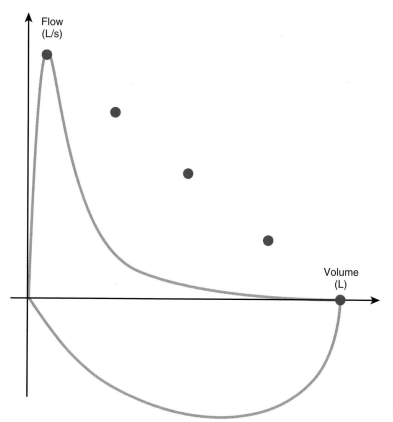

Figure 15.4 A flow-volume loop demonstrating marked obstructive airway disease with a normal flow volume depicted by the black dots. *(From Han MK, Lazarus SC.* Murray and Nadel's Textbook of Respiratory Medicine. *6th ed. Philadelphia: Elsevier; 2016:767-785.e7, Figure 44-3.)*

Why is emphysema a disease of expiratory flow limitation?

To answer this question, we need to understand the normal physiology of the lung. In the non-intubated patient, respiration is via negative pressure. The diaphragm contracts and expands the intrathoracic volume, thereby decreasing intrathoracic pressure, allowing for a pressure gradient for air to flow into the lungs. This is an active process needing the muscles of respiration to be accomplished. Exhalation, however, is passive and is accomplished by the natural tendency of the alveolar air spaces to collapse on themselves. What prevents the alveolar air spaces from being persistently collapsed? The lung parenchyma that surrounds the respiratory bronchioles and alveoli contains connective tissue that applies an outward force, known as radial traction, to keep the airways open. This allows for full expiration to occur without the airway collapsing, preventing air trapping and hyperinflation. In COPD, substantial destruction of the lung parenchyma leads to loss of radial traction of airways. Full expiration cannot occur before the terminal airway collapse, leading to dynamic hyperinflation of the lung. This phenomenon also contributes to the generation of intrinsic positive end-expiratory pressure (PEEP), a major contributing factor to dyspnea.

BASIC SCIENCE PEARL	STEP 1

As daunting as it may seem, histology representing pathophysiology is fair game for the exam. Note in Figure 15.5 the appearance of emphysematous lung on the left compared to the normal appearing lung on the right.

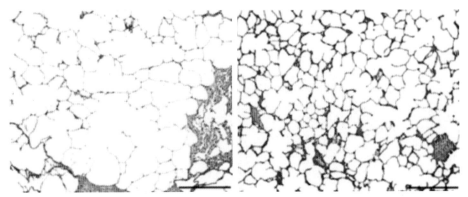

Figure 15.5 Pathology cuts of the lung demonstrating emphysema (left) versus normal lung (right). *(From Bruun CS, Jørgensen CB, Bay L, et al. Phenotypic and genetic characterization of a novel phenotype in pigs characterized by juvenile hairlessness and age dependent emphysema. BMC Genomics. 2008;9:283.)*

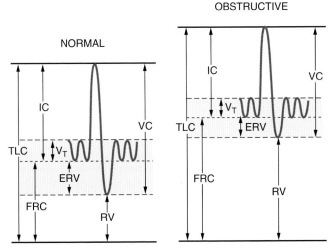

Figure 15.6 The effect of dynamic hyperinflation on respiratory physiology. *(From Al-Ruzzeh S, Kurup V. Respiratory diseases. In: Hines RL, Marschall KE. Stoelting's Anesthesia and Co-Existing Disease. Saunders: Elsevier; 2012:181-217.)*

How does the physiology of the lung change in someone with COPD?

Total lung capacity (TLC) is divided into inspiratory capacity (IC) and functional residual capacity (FRC). Inspiratory capacity comprises tidal volume (TV), essentially normal breathing, and inspiratory reserve volume (IRV; forced inspiration). The FRC is expiratory reserve volume (ERV) plus residual volume (RV). In COPD, FRC increases due to air trapping at the IC. As shown in Figure 15.6, increasing FRC effectively decreases IRV, and TV must be maintained at a higher than normal end-expiratory volume. Therefore, when these patients try to exert themselves, they have less volume available to increase minute ventilation, which then contributes to dyspnea on exertion. Additionally, increasing FRC flattens the diaphragm and makes the work of breathing difficult. This occurs because of a decrease in the diaphragm's area of apposition with respect to the chest wall and increase in its Laplace radius, resulting in decreased force generation.

How should you institute management for this patient?

Management of COPD is divided into acute and chronic management. As this patient is visiting your clinic, the question focuses more on chronic management of COPD and thus the focus is

GOLD Therapy at Each Stage of COPD

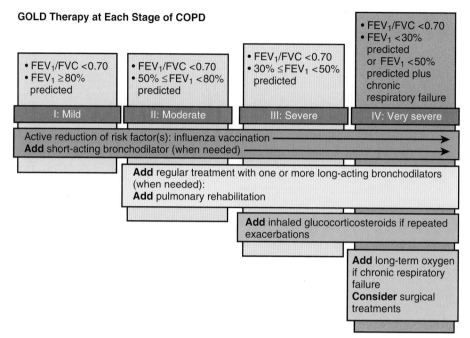

Figure 15.7   The GOLD guidelines for the management of COPD. *(From the Global Strategy for Diagnosis, Management and Prevention of COPD 2015, © Global Initiative for Chronic Obstructive Lung Disease [GOLD], all rights reserved. Available from* http://www.goldcopd.org.*)*

on decreasing long-term mortality. The only proven therapies to decrease mortality are smoking cessation, supplemental oxygen, and lung transplant. For this purpose, the Global Initiative for Chronic Obstructive Lung Disease (GOLD) guidelines are helpful in formulating a therapeutic strategy. Regardless of GOLD staging (shown in Fig. 15.7), all patients should receive pneumonia and influenza vaccinations as well as short-acting bronchodilators and smoking cessation guidance. As FEV_1 declines to moderate severity, patients should be referred for pulmonary rehabilitation to improve physical stamina and quality of life, and long-acting bronchodilators should be initiated. As disease progresses, inhaled glucocorticoids should be added. Although evidence of inhaled glucocorticoids is not strong, they have been shown to reduce the number of exacerbations. Once very severe disease is present, patients should be evaluated for home oxygen therapy and surgical interventions.

To meet criteria for home oxygen therapy, patients should demonstrate hypoxia less than 88% with activity or at rest or partial pressure of oxygen (PO_2) on arterial blood gas less than 55 mm Hg. These criteria are liberalized to hypoxemia <90% or PO_2 less than 60 mm Hg in the presence of polycythemia or right heart failure.

What are therapeutic strategies for smoking cessation?
Twenty percent of the U.S. population continues to smoke, which stresses the importance of effective smoking cessation guidance. Smoking cessation requires a multipronged approach consisting of both cognitive behavioral therapy and pharmacological intervention. Each has been proven to work well on its own; however, combined therapy is superior. All patients that smoke should be assessed for readiness to quit at every clinic visit. The pharmacologic approach chosen is patient preference and includes nicotine replacement therapy (patch, gum) or centrally acting

agents like varenicline, cytisine, or bupropion. E-cigarettes have not been granted FDA approval for this specific purpose.

CLINICAL PEARL	STEP 2/3

Varenicline (Chantix) has been recently approved for smoking cessation and is at least as effective as nicotine replacement therapy if not more in inducing cessation. A recent study revealed cessation rates using cytisine comparable to nicotine replacement therapy. Varenicline can exacerbate underlying psychiatric conditions and should be avoided in this population. Similarly, bupropion is known to decrease the seizure threshold and thus is not recommended for patients with epilepsy.

What are some nonmedical interventions for COPD?

Surgical interventions include lung volume reduction surgery, but patients must meet specific guidelines to receive maximum benefit from this option and to avoid potential adverse events. These criteria include FEV_1 of 30 to 50%, diffusing capacity of the lungs for carbon monoxide (DLCO) >30%, and predominantly upper lobe emphysema. To help understand these selection criteria, remember that FEV_1 is a marker of pulmonary reserve, and thus patients with disease that has progressed to <30% will not be able to tolerate any further loss of lung that is inherent with this procedure. Similarly, DLCO cannot be low enough to where normal gas exchange cannot occur following removal of lung. Lastly, emphysema confined to the upper lobes makes surgical removal far easier and allows for preservation of normal lung.

What about acute management of COPD exacerbations?

To round up our discussion of COPD, consider this same patient who is seen in the emergency department for worsening shortness of breath over several days with increased cough and sputum production. These findings are suggestive of a COPD exacerbation. Exacerbations are most commonly triggered by pulmonary infections, even as simple as common colds, or medication noncompliance resulting in increased airflow limitation due to airway inflammation. The treatment then depends largely upon improving expiratory airflow, reducing airway inflammation, and treating any infectious causes that may be present.

Supplemental oxygen is recommended for achieving an arterial oxygen saturation of 88 to 92%. The lower limit is set to allow adequate oxygen delivery for tissue perfusion, while the upper limit is set to avoid worsening of hypercapnia. If COPD has progressed far enough to impair gas exchange, some patients may be prone to carbon dioxide retention that can be evaluated by measuring an arterial blood gas. In patients with relatively high levels of PO_2, delivering high fractions of inspired oxygen (FiO_2) can worsen this hypercapnia and push patients into carbon dioxide narcosis exhibited by profound altered mental status. However, prevention of hypercapnia should not take precedence over patients with severe hypoxemia.

Improving airflow is best accomplished with short-acting beta agonists like albuterol. Short-acting anticholinergic agents like ipratropium, although not having as good of evidence for efficacy, are used in combination with a beta agonist. Typical administration is via a nebulizer. Airway inflammation is treated with administration of glucocorticoids. Parenteral glucocorticoids are given initially and then can be transitioned to oral agents depending on clinical improvement. Typical treatment courses are full dose for 5 days followed by a gradual taper over the next 2 weeks.

There is no recommended antibiotic regimen for COPD exacerbations. It is recommended that an appropriate antibiotic be given for all patients admitted to the hospital for an exacerbation when infection is suspected.

BEYOND THE PEARLS

- Long-standing hypoxia can lead to class 3 pulmonary hypertension.
- If pulmonary hypertension persists, patients can exhibit signs of right ventricular failure including lower extremity edema, right axis deviation, and dilated right atrial/right ventricle.
- Roflumilast is a new phosphodiesterase 4 (PDE-4) inhibitor that has been shown to decrease exacerbations and improve FEV1, though the effect is modest.
- The BODE index (BMI, FEV1, Dyspnea, Exercise Capacity) is an effective tool to predict mortality in patients with COPD.
- Once the BODE index becomes >7, patients should be evaluated for lung transplant if contraindications do not exist.
- Lung transplantation for COPD has been shown to improve quality of life and improve survival.
- Lung volume reduction surgery (LVRS) improves survival only for patients with upper lobe emphysema and a diminished exercise capacity.
- Noninvasive positive pressure ventilation has been shown to be beneficial for patients with COPD exacerbation as long as contraindications do not exist.
- Opiates are the most effective medication for relieving dyspnea in hospice patients.

References

Calverley PMA, Anderson JA, Celli B, et al. Salmeterol and fluticasone propionate and survival in chronic obstructive pulmonary disease. *N Engl J Med.* 2007;356:775-789.

D'Angelo ED, Agostoni E. Statics of the chest wall. In: Roussos C, Macklem PT, eds. *The Thorax.* 2nd ed. New York: Dekker; 1995:457-493.

McDonough JE, Yuan R, Suzuki M, et al. Small-airway obstruction and emphysema in chronic obstructive pulmonary disease. *N Engl J Med.* 2011;365:1567.

Rennard S, Thomashow B, Crapo J, et al. Introducing the COPD Foundation Guide for Diagnosis and Management of COPD, recommendations of the COPD Foundation. *COPD.* 2013;10:378.

Vestbo J, Hurd SS, Aqusti AG, et al. Global strategy for the diagnosis, management, and prevention of chronic obstructive pulmonary disease: GOLD executive summary. *Am J Respir Crit Care Med.* 2013;15;187(4):347-365.

Walker N, Howe C, Glover M, et al. Cytisine versus nicotine for smoking cessation. *N Engl J Med.* 2014;371:2353-2362.

R. Michelle Koolaee

A 26-Year-Old Female With Joint Pain

A 26-year-old female is evaluated in the emergency department for diffuse joint pain and malaise, along with a 2-week history of shortness of breath and pleuritic chest pain. She reports no fevers, weight loss, or cough. She has a history of iron deficiency anemia, which she has attributed to a history of heavy menses (a Pap smear performed recently was normal). Her medications include ferrous sulfate and a multivitamin.

What are critical questions to ask in anyone with a history of joint pain?
The most important question to ask is the duration of symptoms, as the differential diagnosis can be vastly different for acute (<6 weeks) versus chronic (>6 weeks) joint pain. Secondly, questions such as the presence/duration of morning stiffness and presence of joint swelling help to determine whether the joint pain is due to an inflammatory (versus noninflammatory) arthritis. Morning stiffness greater than 1 hour along with joint swelling is more typical of an inflammatory arthritis. Last, the distribution and number of joints involved should always be elicited, as this may also help determine the etiology of joint pain. *Monoarticular* refers to one joint, *oligoarticular* refers to fewer than five joints, and *polyarticular* refers to five or more joints.

BASIC SCIENCE/CLINICAL PEARL   **STEP 1/2/3**

Identifying the cause of joint pain can be difficult because of the extensive differential diagnosis. A thorough history and complete physical exam are essential, and their value should not be overlooked (especially given the myriad diagnostic and imaging tools available). In rheumatology, a history and physical exam often help just as much as (if not more than) diagnostic tools to determine the diagnosis.

Common considerations for someone with acute arthritis include infectious etiologies as well as crystalline arthritis (i.e., gout and pseudogout). Causes of acute viral polyarthritis include parvovirus B19, hepatitis B virus (HBV), hepatitis C virus (HCV), and rubella. Other infectious etiologies include septic arthritis (usually monoarticular), Lyme arthritis (a late manifestation of Lyme disease characterized usually by a monoarticular or oligoarticular arthritis), poststreptococcal reactive arthritis (arthritis following throat infection with β-hemolytic group A streptococcus), and reactive arthritis (arthritis in the setting of a recent urethritis or enteric infection).

Causes of chronic arthritis are vast but would usually exclude common infectious causes or crystalline arthritis. As broad categories, connective tissue disease and paraneoplastic processes would be higher considerations in someone with chronic symptoms and less likely in someone with acute symptoms.

On further questioning, the patient tells you that the joint pain initially began 6 months ago and is worse in her bilateral knees and bilateral hands, wrists, and knees. The pain is associated with joint swelling and more than 2 hours of morning stiffness. The pain initially improved with nonsteroidal antiinflammatory drugs (NSAIDs) but is now progressively worse despite oral analgesics.

How does this information help you to form a differential diagnosis?

The patient has chronic polyarticular joint pain, which likely represents an inflammatory arthritis. The duration of her symptoms (in conjunction with her other clinical manifestations) make an infectious or crystalline arthritis less likely (furthermore, a crystalline arthritis would not explain her systemic manifestations). She is young and has no constitutional symptoms, so malignancy-associated arthritis is less likely at this point. Her shortness of breath and pleuritic chest pains are suspicious for serositis. Serositis can be a manifestation of many connective tissue diseases, although most commonly associated with systemic lupus erythematosus (SLE) and rheumatoid arthritis (RA). Thus, overall, the suspicion is highest at this time for a connective tissue disease–associated illness.

On physical exam, temperature is 37.2 °C (99 °F), blood pressure is 115/80 mm Hg, pulse rate is 90/min, and respiration rate is 22/min. Cardiac exam is normal. Pulmonary exam reveals a left pleural friction rub. There is synovial thickening of the wrists and metacarpophalangeal (MCP) and proximal interphalangeal (PIP) joints bilaterally as well as small bilateral knee effusions. Several diffuse areas of petechiae are noted over the forearms bilaterally.

What is synovial thickening and how do you test for it? What does it mean?

The term *synovial thickening* is often used interchangeably with *synovitis*. The synovial membrane is a structure that resides in between the joint capsule and the joint cavity (see Fig. 16.1) and is responsible for producing synovial fluid. This membrane can become inflamed in any type of inflammatory arthritis, which may include infectious, autoimmune, crystalline, or neoplastic etiologies. Physical findings of synovial thickening are usually characterized by a "boggy" sensation to the joint, which is typically associated with tenderness and swelling. Effusions are also a feature of synovial thickening.

Initial laboratory and radiographic tests are provided in Table 16.1.

What is your differential diagnosis at this point?

This is a young female who presents with a chronic polyarticular inflammatory arthritis, serositis (pleural effusions), and fatigue, with laboratory evidence of leukopenia, anemia, and marked thrombocytopenia.

    Connective tissue disease is highest on the differential at this time, particularly given the chronicity of the inflammatory arthritis in conjunction with evidence of other systemic organ involvement. The combined arthritic, pleuritic, and hematologic manifestations are very characteristic features of SLE, which would carry the strongest likelihood of all the connective tissues illnesses. RA is also a possibility, given the chronic polyarticular inflammatory arthritis and serositis; however, it usually does not present with severe pancytopenia. Patients with Sjögren's

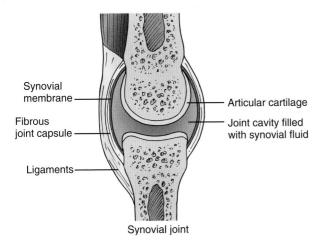

Synovial membrane

Fibrous joint capsule

Ligaments

Articular cartilage

Joint cavity filled with synovial fluid

Synovial joint

Figure 16.1 Synovial joint. *(From http://commons.wikimedia.org/ wiki/File:Illu_synovial_joint.jpg)*

TABLE 16.1 ▓ **Initial Laboratory Tests**

Leukocyte count	3000/μL (3.0 × 10⁹/L)
Hemoglobin	9.8 g/dL (98 g/L)
Platelet count	8000/μL (8 × 10⁹/L)
Leukocyte differential	Normal
Erythrocyte sedimentation rate	86 mm/h
Serum creatinine	0.6 mg/dL
Urinalysis	1+ protein; 0-2 erythrocytes/ HPF; 5-10 leukocytes/HPF
Chest radiograph	Blunted costophrenic angles bilaterally without infiltrate

HPF, High power field.

syndrome may present with extraglandular manifestations and occasionally do lack overt symptoms of oral or ocular dryness. However, this would be much lower on the differential. Pancytopenia and serositis are not usual manifestation of the seronegative spondyloarthritis (SpA) and would be very unlikely as well. Systemic vasculitis should always be considered in anyone with multisystem organ involvement; however, this would not be a consideration at this time given the much higher likelihood of SLE.

BASIC SCIENCE PEARL	**STEP 1**

You should form two or three diagnoses that are highest on your differential, along with the diagnoses that could result in significant morbidity if missed. The other diagnoses should be considered individually and only eliminated after careful assessment. (This is especially important in patients with complex, multisystem organ involvement, where many disease features can mimic other illnesses.)

Infectious etiologies would be less likely given the constellation of symptoms and because the arthritis has been chronic in duration. Paraneoplastic processes can sometimes mimic connective

TABLE 16.2   Follow-Up Laboratory Tests

Antinuclear antibody	1 : 1280 dilution
Anti-double-stranded DNA antibody	Positive
Anti-smith antibody	Positive
Anti-SS-A/Anti-SS-B antibodies	Negative
Complement C3	Low
Complement C4	Low
Rheumatoid factor	Negative
Anticyclic citrullinated peptide antibodies	Negative

tissue disease, but there are no constitutional symptoms such as fever or weight loss, so this is less likely at this time. If a workup for connective tissue disease is unrevealing, it would not be unreasonable to consider a neoplastic process (particularly given the patient's pancytopenia).

BASIC SCIENCE/CLINICAL PEARL   **STEP 1/2/3**

In patients with multisystem illness, it may be easier to compartmentalize the differential diagnosis into three broad categories: infection, malignancy, and autoimmune (and elaborate on diagnoses within each broad category). There are many disease mimics of rheumatic illness, and establishing the proper diagnosis starts with organizing your thoughts.

Follow-up laboratory tests are provided in Table 16.2.

Diagnosis: Systemic lupus erythematosus

How did the autoantibody profile help establish this diagnosis?

A diagnosis of SLE requires most importantly a careful history and physical exam. There is not one single laboratory test that establishes a diagnosis. Autoantibody testing should not be used as a sole means of establishing a diagnosis but should rather be used in conjunction with the history, physical exam, and initial laboratory tests to confirm or refute the diagnosis.

The antinuclear antibody (ANA) test is positive in virtually all patients with SLE but can also be present in patients without an autoimmune illness. Anti-double-stranded DNA (anti-dsDNA) and anti-smith (anti-Sm) antibodies are highly specific for SLE but lack sensitivity for disease. Anti-dsDNA antibodies may be particularly high in patients with renal disease in SLE. Anti-Ro/SSA and anti-La/SSB antibodies may be present in patients with SLE; however, they are more frequently associated with Sjögren's syndrome.

What are the classification criteria for SLE and how are they helpful in this case?

Classification criteria for SLE were derived as a uniform way to categorize patients for study purposes. Although they lack the sensitivity and specificity to be used as diagnostic criteria, they can be of help to clinicians in order to systematically organize and document key features.

In 2012, a group of experts from the Systemic Lupus International Collaborating Clinics (SLICC) proposed revised classification criteria for SLE (the previous criteria were from 1997);

this includes both clinical and immunologic criteria. Clinical criteria include detailed descriptions of mucocutaneous, arthritic, pleuritic (i.e., pleural or pericardial effusions), renal, neurologic, and hematologic manifestations. For instance, hematologic criteria include hemolytic anemia, leukopenia ($<4{,}000/mm^3$), lymphopenia ($<1{,}000/mm^3$), and/or thrombocytopenia ($<100{,}000/mm^3$) in the absence of other known causes. A diagnosis of SLE requires 4 or more of the 11 criteria present, with at least one clinical criterion and one laboratory criterion being met. A patient with biopsy-proven SLE nephritis may also be classified, provided that the patient has either a positive ANA or anti-dsDNA antibodies.

This patient meets classification criteria based on the presence of serositis (pleural effusions), inflammatory arthritis, leukopenia, and thrombocytopenia in the setting of low serum complement levels, and positive ANA, anti-dsDNA, and anti-Sm antibodies.

BASIC SCIENCE PEARL   **STEP 1**

B-cell activating factor (BAFF, also known as B-lymphocyte stimulator or BLyS) is a protein that acts as a potent B-cell activator; it has also been shown to play a role in the proliferation and differentiation of B cells. Increased BAFF (BLyS) serum levels have been implicated in autoimmunity and are elevated in many patients with SLE. Belimumab is a human monoclonal antibody that inhibits BLyS, and it is the newest available medication for the treatment of SLE.

How would you approach treatment acutely?

Treatment for anyone with SLE is very individualized and depends not only on the extent of organ involvement but also on the severity of disease. Often, therapy is further adjusted and fine-tuned depending on clinical responses to therapy. This patient has both moderate (arthritis, serositis, leukopenia) and severe lupus involvement (severe thrombocytopenia). In cases of severe or life-threatening manifestations, patients are treated for a short period of time with high doses of systemic glucocorticoids (i.e., 1 to 2 mg/kg/day of prednisone or equivalent or intermittent intravenous (IV) "pulses" of methylprednisolone). Generally, "pulses" of methylprednisolone are reserved for life-threatening manifestations (i.e., renal and central nervous system involvement), none of which this patient has. Therefore, a dose of prednisone 1 mg/kg/day would be a reasonable acute therapy.

CLINICAL PEARL   **STEP 2/3**

The arthritis in SLE is rarely erosive. In contrast to RA, hand deformities in SLE are easily reducible and are thought to be due to laxity in the tendons and ligaments, leading to joint instability (i.e., Jaccoud's arthropathy).

Patients with low to moderate lupus involvement (i.e., disease that is significant but is not organ-threatening) usually respond to short-term therapy with prednisone (or equivalent) 5 to 15 mg daily along with hydroxychloroquine. Given the long-term side effects of glucocorticoids, every effort should be made to limit their exposure.

How do you approach treatment chronically in this patient?

The approach to therapy is highly variable and is generally guided by the predominant disease manifestations. As a general rule, glucocorticoids (at variable doses) are started for acute manifestations and are tapered off as soon as possible. It is not unusual, however, for some patients to remain on low doses of glucocorticoids given the challenges of tapering the drug.

All patients with SLE with any degree of disease activity should be treated indefinitely with hydroxychloroquine or chloroquine, unless contraindicated. There is a high level of evidence that antimalarials play a role in preventing SLE flares and increasing long-term survival; there is moderate evidence of protection against thrombosis, bone loss, and irreversible organ damage. Sun protection with agents that have a sun protection factor (SPF) ≥55 should also be emphasized to patients, as ultraviolet (UV) light may induce or flare many of the systemic manifestations of SLE.

CLINICAL PEARL   **STEP 2/3**

Advise SLE patients to choose a broad-spectrum sunscreen, which will protect against both UV-A and UV-B light (both rays can exacerbate SLE; some sunscreens contain only UV-B protection, which is the ray that causes sunburns).

Pleural disease in SLE may be treated initially with NSAIDs and a short course of moderate-to-high-dose glucocorticoids if there is no response within a few days. Glucocorticoids often raise the platelet counts within a few weeks in patients with severe immune thrombocytopenia (ITP). If this is not effective, then therapy with IV rituximab is considered. Rituximab would have benefits for this patient's inflammatory arthritis as well as the pleural disease. Methotrexate is an option for persistent inflammatory arthritis.

BASIC SCIENCE PEARL   **STEP 1**

There are several proposed mechanisms of action of methotrexate. One hypothesis is that it increases serum adenosine release (adenosine has potent antiinflammatory properties), which contributes to decreases in leukocyte migration to tissues, thereby decreasing systemic inflammation.

What is the patient's prognosis?

Patients with SLE have mortality rates two to five times higher than that of the general population, despite the fact that the 5-year survival rate has dramatically increased over the last several decades to greater than 90%. The major causes of death include active disease (i.e., central nervous system [CNS] and renal disease), active infection, treatment complications, and cardiovascular disease.

CLINICAL PEARL   **STEP 2/3**

Maintain a high index of suspicion for coronary heart disease in SLE patients. Remember that these patients may present with atypical, nonspecific, or absent symptoms despite the presence of significant coronary artery disease (similar to the presentation for diabetics).

The patient is doing well 9 months after her initial hospital visit, and her disease is well-controlled on methotrexate and hydroxychloroquine. She was tapered off of prednisone 6 months prior. She reports no further joint pain, chest pain, or shortness of breath. Her complete blood count is normal. She is recently married and expresses to you that she would like to become pregnant.

How do you approach therapy now? What changes should be made?

It is recommended that disease activity be very low for at least 6 months prior to pregnancy (particularly in patients with renal disease). Her disease activity is low at this time; however, the methotrexate should be discontinued, and this may affect disease activity. Methotrexate is teratogenic and should not be administered during conception or pregnancy.

CLINICAL PEARL   **STEP 2/3**

SLE patients are considered as fertile as women in the general population, unless they have received medications that are known to decrease fertility (i.e., cyclophosphamide).

NSAIDs and low-dose aspirin may be continued until the beginning of the third trimester (after which there is a risk of premature closure of the ductus arteriosus). NSAIDs may be used during lactation but have an increased risk of causing jaundice and kernicterus. Both hydroxychloroquine and sulfasalazine are safe to continue during both pregnancy and lactation. Glucocorticoid therapy is not contraindicated during pregnancy but may increase the risk of premature rupture of the membranes (PROM) and intrauterine growth restriction. Their dose should be limited as much as possible. It is excreted into breast milk, so breastfeeding should occur 4 hours after the last dosing. In moderate to severe disease, azathioprine, cyclosporine, tacrolimus, and IV immunoglobulin may be used. Data are limited to support the use of tumor necrosis factor (TNF) inhibitors or rituximab during pregnancy; their use should take into account patient preference (after discussion of risks versus benefits).

BEYOND THE PEARLS

- Avascular necrosis (AVN) of the hips and knees is recognized frequently in SLE patients, who often have increases in total glucocorticoid exposure. Patients present with subacute or chronic joint pain. Magnetic resonance imaging (MRI) is a more sensitive tool to detect AVN than plain films.
- Platelet counts in patients with SLE-related idiopathic thrombocytopenic purpura (ITP) can be labile, so be mindful of how rapidly glucocorticoids are tapered in these patients and monitor platelet counts very closely.
- In trials of efficacy, patients with musculoskeletal or mucocutaneous manifestations responded best to belimumab, which is the newest agent available for the treatment of SLE.
- The direct Coombs test is valuable to order in SLE patients with anemia; there is a subset of patients that can have a positive Coombs test (indicating the presence of autoantibodies against red blood cells) without clinical signs of hemolysis. This is part of the 2012 SLICC classification criteria for SLE.
- Osteoporosis is a significant problem in patients with SLE, especially given their increased exposure to glucocorticoids. A rapid decline in bone mineral density (BMD) begins within the first 3 months of glucocorticoid use, so it is recommended that patients on doses of prednisone as low as 5 to 7.5 mg daily for ≥3 months be started on bisphosphonate therapy.
- Always ask the duration the patient has had symptoms of inflammatory arthritis; chronicity of symptoms (>6 to 8 weeks) generally decreases the likelihood of infectious etiologies of arthritis.
- Autoantibody testing should not be used as a sole means of establishing a diagnosis of SLE but should rather be used in conjunction with the history, physical exam, and initial laboratory tests to confirm or refute the diagnosis.

References

Borchers AT, Keen CL, Shoenfeld Y, et al. Surviving the butterfly and the wolf: mortality trends in systemic lupus erythematosus. *Autoimmun Rev.* 2004;3(6):423-453.

Mies Richie A, Francis ML. Diagnostic approach to polyarticular joint pain. *Am Fam Physician.* 2003;68(6):1151-1160.

Petri M, Orbai AM, Alarcón GS, et al. Derivation and validation of the Systemic Lupus International Collaborating Clinics classification criteria for systemic lupus erythematosus. *Arthritis Rheum.* 2012;64(8):2677-2686.

Ruiz-Irastorza G, Ramos-Casals M, Brito-Zeron P, et al. Clinical efficacy and side effects of antimalarials in systemic lupus erythematosus: a systematic review. *Ann Rheum Dis.* 2010;69(1):20-28.

Temprano KK, Bandlamudi R, Moore TL. Antirheumatic drugs in pregnancy and lactation. *Semin Arthritis Rheum.* 2005;35(2):112-121.

Steven M. Naids ■ Brian K. Do

A 57-Year-Old Male With Blurred Vision

A 57-year-old male with a past medical history of type 2 diabetes mellitus diagnosed 10 years prior to presentation presents for evaluation of 2 months of blurred vision in both eyes. The right eye is more bothersome than the left. He has been unable to drive for the last 2 months due to his vision. He was fitted for a new pair of glasses less than a month ago, but they have not improved his vision. There has been no associated eye pain or redness.

Why is it important to ask about eye pain and redness in association with vision loss?
It is important to ask about eye pain and redness when evaluating the etiology of vision loss because painless vision loss is most commonly associated with a process involving the more posterior portion of the eye (i.e., the retina, vitreous, choroid, and in some cases the optic nerve). Painful vision loss with redness on exam should alert you that the front of the eye (i.e., the cornea, conjunctiva, anterior sclera, iris, or ciliary body) is involved. A red eye can provide helpful information on the acuity of the inciting event and may or may not be associated with vision loss.

He denies headache, dizziness, nausea, and vomiting. He complains of a persistent mild burning sensation on the plantar surfaces of both feet for the past year. His other review of systems is negative.

BASIC SCIENCE PEARL   **STEP 1**

Sometimes, an ophthalmologist may be the first doctor that a diabetic patient presents to. Even though the focus of this case is the eye, it is important to take a complete history, including review of systems in diabetic patients. This can provide you with important clues as to the duration and control of the patient's disease. In this case, the patient has stocking-glove neuropathy, indicating poor control or long duration of the disease. This is associated with more advanced eye disease.

The patient's other past medical history is significant for a known 15-year history of hypertension, for which he takes lisinopril. He has been taking metformin since diagnosis and has never used insulin. He has never had surgery, including eye surgery. His family history is significant for hypertension in both parents and for myocardial infarction suffered by his father at age 65. He has a 30-pack/year history of cigarette smoking. He works long hours as a construction site supervisor and admits that his job has prevented him from following up regularly with his primary care physician.

BASIC SCIENCE PEARL   **STEP 1**

Obtaining a good social history is important in these patients. Although control of blood sugar over the duration of the disease is important, other cardiovascular risk factors such as hypertension and hyperlipidemia must be addressed. Ask patients about their diet, exercise, smoking, and alcohol habits, as modifying these can help better achieve treatment goals.

When should a diabetic patient be initially screened for diabetic retinopathy?

It is currently estimated that as of 2014, only about 60% of diabetics have a yearly screening for diabetic retinopathy. Currently, screening is recommended for type 1 diabetics 5 years after the onset of their disease. Type 2 diabetics should be screened at diagnosis and yearly thereafter.

The duration of diabetes is a major risk factor in the development of diabetic retinopathy. After 5 years, approximately 25% of type 1 patients have retinopathy. After 10 years, 60% develop retinopathy, and after 15 years, 80% will be affected.

Of type 2 patients over the age of 30 who have had diabetes for less than 5 years, 40% of those taking insulin and 24% of those not taking insulin have retinopathy. The percentages increase to 84% and 53%, respectively, when the duration has been documented for up to 19 years.

Currently, the gold standard imaging for the diagnosis and classification of diabetic retinopathy is stereoscopic color photographs using seven standard fields. However, this is very labor intensive. There is evidence that single-field fundus photographs in the hands of trained readers can serve as an effective screening tool.

The Snellen best-corrected distance visual acuity is 20/150 in the right eye and 20/50 in the left eye as measured with his glasses. A refraction done in the office does not improve his vision. His pupils are equally round and reactive to light. There is no relative afferent pupillary defect in either eye. Extraocular movements are full. The intraocular pressures are 14 and 17 in the right and left eye, respectively.

On slit lamp exam of his eyes, there are no eyelid or adnexal abnormalities. His conjunctiva and sclera are noninjected and both corneas are clear. The anterior chambers are deep without evidence of cell, flare, or blood. He has lightly pigmented, hazel irises. On careful inspection, there are no abnormal blood vessels present on either iris.

CLINICAL PEARL   **STEP 2/3**

Iris neovascularization, or rubeosis iridis, is a sign of ocular ischemia and has a variety of etiologies, including diabetic retinopathy. It is most commonly seen at the border of the pupil. It is clinically significant because it may be an indicator of neovascularization of the anatomic angle of the eye. The drainage outflow for aqueous humor is found in the angle, and these vessels may contract to seal it off, resulting in a secondary angle-closure attack.

For dilation, one drop of tropicamide 1% and one drop of phenylephrine 2.5% are instilled into both eyes. The lenses both have cataract changes, including central posterior subcapsular cataracts.

BASIC SCIENCE/CLINICAL PEARL   **STEP 1/2/3**

To dilate the eye for exam purposes, most ophthalmologists use phenylephrine 2.5% to stimulate the alpha-1 receptors of the iris dilator muscle. Tropicamide 1% is an anticholinergic that induces dilation, or mydriasis, by inhibiting acetylcholine (ACh) at the level of the pupillary sphincter muscle. Anticholinergics also inhibit accommodation.

What are the three primary types of age-related cataracts?
As the lens ages, it increases in mass and thickness. This results in changes in the refractive index of the lens, causing light to scatter and transparency to decrease.

The first cataract type is the nuclear sclerotic cataract, which results in yellowing/browning of the nucleus of the lens. This type tends to progress slowly and causes a greater impairment of distance vision.

Cortical cataracts are associated with local disruption of the structure of the mature lens fiber cell, leading to protein oxidation and precipitation. A common complaint of patients with cortical cataracts is glare, particularly from intense light sources such as car headlights.

Posterior subcapsular cataracts are often seen in younger patients compared with people who have nuclear or cortical cataracts. However, they can also occur in diabetics as a result of trauma, in patients taking systemic or topical glucocorticoids, and in uveitis patients. These patients complain of glare and poor vision in bright light because the small pupil prevents light from entering more peripheral parts of the lens. Near vision tends to be reduced more than distance vision for the same reason (decreased accommodation/near reflex).

The dilated funduscopic exam in both eyes is significant for dot and blot hemorrhages and microaneurysms within the macula. There is hard exudate involving the fovea, which appears elevated. Intraretinal hemorrhages are scattered outside of the macula. There is no neovascularization of either optic nerve or neovascularization seen elsewhere (Fig. 17.1).

BASIC SCIENCE/CLINICAL PEARL   **STEP 1/2/3**

There are many descriptive terms for retinal findings in diabetic retinopathy. Some of these may overlap with other retinal diseases as well. For example, "dot and blot" and "flame" hemorrhages are used to describe blood found within the retina, which takes a different shape depending on in which retinal layer it is found. Dot and blot hemorrhages are located deeper in the retina, where the cells have a more vertical orientation. Flame hemorrhages are more superficial, where they become more linear with the horizontal orientation of the nerve fibers. "Cotton-wool spots" are localized areas of nerve fiber layer infarction with axoplasmic stasis.

How would you classify this patient's disease on the spectrum of diabetic retinopathy?
There are two primary classifications of diabetic retinopathy: nonproliferative and proliferative. When retinopathy is confined to the retina and does not cross the barrier into the vitreous, it is classified as nonproliferative.

This male has moderate nonproliferative diabetic retinopathy in both of his eyes.

What is diabetic macular edema?
Diabetic patients may lose vision due to macular edema. Retinal blood vessels become abnormally permeable, which allows intravascular fluid to accumulate within the layers of the retina. Patients usually become symptomatic when the thickening and edema involves the center of the macula, known as the fovea. The leakage can either be focal, from a leaking microaneurysm (areas of dilated retinal vessels with a tendency to leak), or diffuse from widespread capillary leakage and blood–retina barrier breakdown.

Resorption of the fluid component occurs at a faster rate than the plasma lipids. This leaves behind yellow-white deposits, or so-called "hard exudates" within the retina.

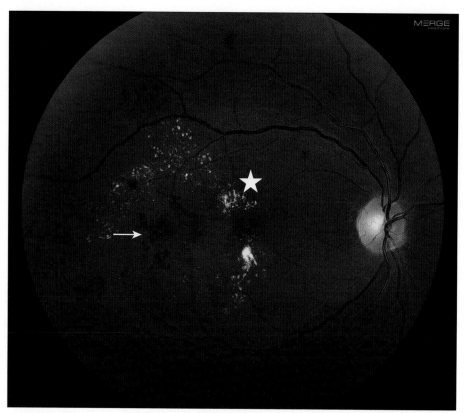

Figure 17.1 Color fundus photograph of the patient's right eye. Note the hard exudate involving the fovea (*) and the intraretinal macular hemorrhages *(arrow)*.

What types of retinal imaging should you obtain on this patient?

Fluorescein angiography (FA) and optical coherence tomography (OCT) are important ancillary tests to determine the presence and etiology of macular edema.

 FA allows the study of the circulation of the retina and choroid. After intravenous injection of sodium fluorescein, blue light is used to excite the molecule, which then emits a yellow-green light that is captured by the camera. Eighty percent of fluorescein is bound to albumin in the intravascular space. The remaining 20%, and any molecules that have leaked out of vessels in diseases like diabetes, fluoresce. An FA can show a potential area that is leaking or demonstrate that the leakage is widespread (Fig. 17.2). This has important treatment implications. It can also, perhaps more importantly, delineate areas of poor retinal perfusion as well as retinal and optic nerve neovascularization, which may help guide treatment.

 OCT is a noninvasive imaging modality that produces micrometer-resolution, cross-sectional images of ocular tissue. This technique is based on imaging reflected light (Fig. 17.3). It is important in diabetics to determine the presence and anatomical location of macular edema. Also, follow-up studies are useful in monitoring the response to treatment.

FA and OCT are obtained. In both eyes, there is foveal-involving macular edema on OCT and widespread leakage. Hemoglobin A1C is 10.9%.

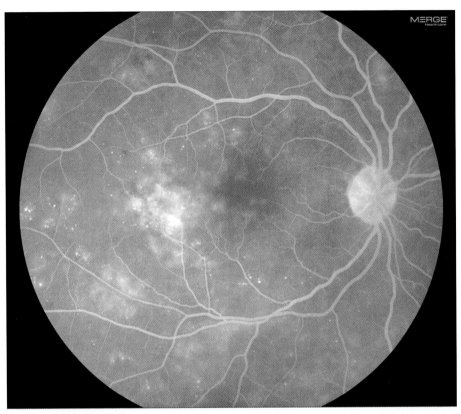

Figure 17.2   FA of the right eye at 7 minutes after injection. Areas of leakage appear white with indistinct borders and can be seen within the macula and fovea.

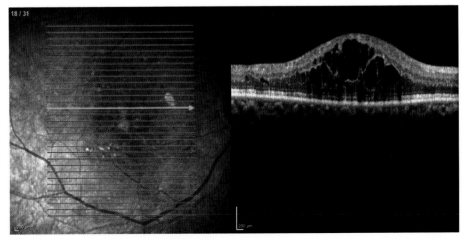

Figure 17.3   An OCT of the patient's right eye. This section is from the foveal center, showing cystic spaces of fluid within the retina (cystoid macular edema).

Diagnosis: Moderate nonproliferative diabetic retinopathy with diabetic macular edema in both eyes

What is the next step in the management of this patient?

Diabetic retinopathy is one manifestation of a systemic disease. Ophthalmologists must work in partnership with the patient's primary care physician to make sure that all potential risk factors (blood sugar, blood pressure, cholesterol, smoking, etc.) are addressed. In this patient's case, the hemoglobin A1C is quite high. His treatment, including the possible addition of insulin, should be tailored to a specific hemoglobin A1C goal (usually less than 7%). The retinopathy will not improve, and may worsen, if the systemic disease is not optimized.

What are the options for treatment of this patient's macular edema?

Diabetic macular edema is treated with intraocular pharmacologic agents, laser photocoagulation, or a combination of both.

The target for the majority of drugs is vascular endothelial growth factor (VEGF). Currently used anti-VEGF medications include bevacizumab, ranibizumab, and aflibercept. These are administered by injection into the vitreous cavity through the pars plana. For patients with edema refractory to these medications, intraocular or periocular glucocorticoids may be considered. Patients receiving anti-VEGF therapy are initially seen and treated monthly. Therapeutic response is followed by clinical exam and OCT.

Laser may be used to focally coagulate areas of leakage or to treat areas of ischemia. Laser is avoided in the fovea, as it can cause a permanent scotoma, or blind spot, although more recent technological developments may not preclude the use of focal retinal laser photocoagulation in the treatment of foveal edema.

BEYOND THE PEARLS

- Clinically significant macular edema (CSME) is a clinical diagnosis (i.e., without the help of imaging) based on retinal thickening and hard exudate. It is, therefore, possible for a patient to have very minimal diabetic retinopathy but still have CSME.
- One of the landmark diabetic retinopathy studies, the ETDRS, found that aspirin at doses of 650 mg a day does not slow the progression of diabetic retinopathy.
- There are two components of the blood–retinal barrier: the vascular endothelium of the retinal vessels and the retinal pigment epithelium.
- It is important to identify patients meeting the severe nonproliferative diabetic retinopathy criteria. This can be done by remembering the 4:2:1 rule: 4 quadrants of intraretinal hemorrhage, 2 quadrants of venous beading, intraretinal microvascular abnormalities (IRMAs) in 1 quadrant.
- Patients with severe nonproliferative diabetic retinopathy have a 15% chance of progression to high-risk proliferative diabetic retinopathy within 1 year.
- Intraocular surgery (i.e., cataract surgery) can be a cause of macular edema. It can also worsen preexisting diabetic macular edema. It is generally accepted that diabetic macular edema be maximally treated before a patient has surgery.
- A recent study demonstrated that aflibercept was more effective at improving vision when the initial acuity was worse than 20/40 as compared to ranibizumab or bevacizumab.

References

American Academy of Ophthalmology. Diabetic Retinopathy Summary Benchmarks for Preferred Practice Pattern Guidelines. October 2014, San Francisco.

American Academy of Ophthalmology. Information Statement: Screening for Diabetic Retinopathy. November 2006, Update October 2014, San Francisco.

Bobrow, et al. Basic and Clinical Science Course: Section 11 Lens and Cataract. American Academy of Ophthalmology. 2013-2014. pp. 39-46, San Francisco.

Schubert, et al. Basic and Clinical Science Course: Section 12 Retina. American Academy of Ophthalmology. 2013-2014. pp. 95-99, San Francisco.

Schubert, et al. Basic and Clinical Science Course: Section 12 Retina. American Academy of Ophthalmology. 2013-2014. pp 20-21, San Francisco.

Schubert, et al. Basic and Clinical Science Course: Section 12 Retina. American Academy of Ophthalmology. 2013-2014. pp 26-27, San Francisco.

Diabetic Retinopathy Clinical Research Network. Aflibercept, bevacizumab, or ranibizumab for diabetic macular edema. *N Engl J Med*. 2015;372(13):1193-1203.

Albert Huang

A 52-Year-Old Male With Radiating Leg Pain

A 52-year-old male presents with low back pain. His symptoms began 2 days ago while lifting a boat to go fishing. The pain is severe and is rated a 10/10. He has been unable to move from his couch since it started 2 days ago. It is associated with another radiating pain that extends down his right leg. His has suffered low back pain in the past but never of this severity. His past medical history includes dyslipidemia.

What symptoms associated with acute low back pain could potentially warrant emergent management?

When presented with acute low back pain, one of the chief concerns is neurologic involvement. It is important to ask questions related to leg strength and bowel/bladder function to assess for damage of the spinal cord or the cauda equina. Patients may note leg weakness or difficulty walking. Damage to the sacral segments can lead to saddle paresthesia, urinary retention, or bowel/bladder incontinence. Diagnostic imaging, ideally with magnetic resonance imaging (MRI), can help identify the cause and determine whether urgent neurosurgical consultation is necessary for immediate interventional management. An acute spinal cord injury or cauda equina syndrome may be the result of severe spinal stenosis, severe herniated vertebral disc, cyst, abscess, or neoplasm. In the event one of these other causes is identified, appropriate management should be initiated.

BASIC SCIENCE/CLINICAL PEARL   **STEP 1/2/3**

In the embryonic stage, the spinal cord and vertebrae form from the neural tube and are even in length. As they grow, the vertebral column and its elements grow at a faster rate as compared to the spinal cord. At birth, the tip of the spinal cord ends around the L3 vertebral body and eventually L1 as an adult. If the tip is any lower, there is suspicion for a tethered cord, which may have been previously undiagnosed early on and can also present with symptoms of low back pain, radiating leg pain, bowel/bladder dysfunction, leg weakness, and sensory loss.

What other red flags should be elicited on the history?

After a cauda equina syndrome has been excluded, acute low back pain can be divided into three groups: nonspecific low back pain, back pain related to radiculopathy or spinal stenosis, and an alternative cause. The third group may present with a pattern of symptoms consistent with a specific diagnosis, which are commonly referred to as red flags because the pathology can be particularly concerning. Possibilities include an infectious, neoplastic, or inflammatory cause. Questions regarding the presence of fevers, history of infection with human immunodeficiency virus (HIV), use of immunosuppressant medications, or intravenous (IV) drug abuse suggest the possibility of an infection. Recent unintentional changes in weight, increased fatigue, and pain worse at night can be suggestive of a spinal tumor. A younger individual with increased pain and stiffness in the morning that improves through the day could be presenting with a spondyloar-thropathy. Recent trauma or fall, especially in an older individual with a history of osteoporosis, can result in a new vertebral fracture, associated back pain, and possible neurologic damage. Because no single symptom can definitively confirm the presence of a diagnosis, it is important to perform a thorough history and exam to form a complete picture of the possible diagnosis.

> On further questioning, the patient describes the pain in his low back as dull and achy. He has experienced it in the past, but it always resolved within a few days and was never this severe. The pain that runs down his leg is new, sharper, and described as a burning sensation. It runs down along the outside of his right leg, past the knee, and ends along the outside of his right foot. He denies any numbness or weakness. The review of systems is negative for significant weight loss, fatigue, fever, chills, or recent illness.

What specific symptom description can help differentiate between a referred pain and radiculopathy?

Pain that occurs outside of the original location is considered referred pain. Although it typically emanates from the original source, it can also occur as a new discomfort in a separate location that begins about the same time. A common example is a myocardial infarction with pain that extends into the left shoulder, down the left arm, or into the back. When evaluating low back pain with associated symptoms, it can be difficult separating referred pain from a radiculopathy, which is a separate injury caused by damage to a nerve root as it exits the vertebral column.

One way to delineate the two is by asking questions regarding the specific course of the radia-tion. Pain that travels past the knee and into the foot is typically associated with a radiculopathy. If it extends down into the medial aspect of the lower leg, there is suspicion for L4 nerve root involvement. Pain that goes down the lateral aspect of the thigh and leg and ends along the outside of the foot suggests L5 involvement. If the pain runs along the posterior thigh and extends down to the heel, it may be due to an S1 nerve root.

However, pain that does not extend beyond the knee does not automatically rule out a radicu-lopathy. Damage to the L2, L3, and L4 nerve roots can cause pain to radiate from the low back anteriorly into the groin, anterior thigh, or knee. Involvement of the S2, S3, and S4 roots may remain proximal by extending into the sacral or gluteal regions and potentially end in the perineal area.

BASIC SCIENCE/CLINICAL PEARL   **STEP 1/2/3**

Sciatica is commonly used by patients to describe a pain that extends from the low back and down the posterior thigh. It refers to the sciatic nerve, which is made up of the tibial and common fibular nerves. Although the term was originally coined in reference to a radiculopathy, it should not be considered synonymous because there are many other conditions that can be associated with posterior leg pain such as peripheral injury to the sciatic nerve. Examples include piriformis syndrome or pregnancy when the weight of the growing fetus in the pelvis puts increased pressure on the sciatic nerve. Furthermore, the pain being described by patients as sciatica could also be a referred pain unrelated to the sciatic nerve, such as referred low back pain or a hamstring injury.

On exam, the patient's oral temperature is 36.4 °C (97.5 °F), pulse rate is 80/min, blood pressure is 122/78 mm Hg, and respiration rate is 16/min. Inspection is negative for rashes or signs of trauma along his back and legs. Palpation of his abdomen is soft and negative for tenderness or masses. Palpation along the lumbar vertebral spine, around the hip girdle, and over the greater trochanter are negative for tenderness. Patellar reflex is 2+ bilaterally and symmetrical. Ankle reflex is 2+ on the left and absent on the right. Sensation to light touch is intact throughout the lower extremities, except over the right lateral foot. Muscle strength is 5/5 throughout the left limb and 4/5 on the right limited by pain.

How can sensation and muscle function contribute to the diagnosis?

Dermatomes and myotomes refer to associations between a specific area of skin or muscle groups innervated by a single nerve root or set of nerve roots. Numerous maps have been created, though due to variations in development from one person to the next there are variations between different versions. Although not always an exact representation of nerve root involvement, deficits in sensation and muscle strength elicited on a physical exam can yield clues to the involved nerve root of a suspected radiculopathy. Decreased sensation over the medial knee can suggest involvement of the L4 nerve root, the lateral malleolus with L5, and the heel with S1.

Common myotomes of the lower limbs are L2 with hip flexion, L3 with knee extension, L4 with ankle dorsiflexion, L5 with extension of the great toe, and S1 with ankle plantar flexion. Despite these generalities, each action is typically the result of multiple muscles. For example, hip flexion can occur via contraction of the iliopsoas or rectus femoris portion of the quadriceps and both are innervated by L2, L3, and L4. The tensor fascia latae (TFL) also contributes to hip flexion and is innervated by levels L4, L5, and S1. Weakness in hip flexion can be a result of any one or multitude of levels. Damage to one level may not cause detectable weakness on exam because the remaining muscles can make up for the loss. Thus, weakness in an action can prompt suspicion of nerve injury, but intact strength does not necessarily rule it out.

What special exam maneuvers are good for diagnosing acute radiculopathy?

When suspecting the presence of an acute radiculopathy, there are several special exam maneuvers that aid in diagnosis. The straight leg raise (SLR or Lasègue's sign) is most common. To perform it, the patient lies supine and the examiner passively raises the affected leg while the knee remains fully extended. When the pain is first reproduced, the angle of the leg compared to the horizontal is noted. Although the angle range is debatable, a positive finding is generally between 30 and 70 degrees. Outside of this range, the pain can be attributed to another cause such as hamstring or gluteal muscle tightness. This maneuver can be repeated on the unaffected leg, which is referred to as the contralateral SLR. If it causes pain in the affected side, the test is considered positive. Unlike most exam findings that have little associated research or low reliability, studies have resulted in general acceptance of the SLR and contralateral SLR. A Cochrane review found the former to have 90% sensitivity and the latter 90% specificity when diagnosing a radiculopathy.

BASIC SCIENCE/CLINICAL PEARL	STEP 1/2/3

Specificity and sensitivity are commonly differentiated by the mnemonic SPIN and SNOUT. Namely, high SPecificity can rule IN a diagnosis and high SeNsitivity can rule it OUT. As applied to the crossed SLR and SLR discussed in the text, if the physical exam reveals a positive crossed SLR that has a high specificity, then a radiculopathy is likely present. If the supine SLR on the affected side that has a high sensitivity is negative, then there is low probability for a radiculopathy.

The purpose of these tests is to cause increased tension or stretch on the damaged nerve and reproduction of the symptom. Other tests have been developed with similar intent, and any positive findings have been collectively referred to as neural root tension signs. Examples include the sitting SLR where the knee is extended while the patient is sitting at the edge of an exam table. Dorsiflexion of the ankle while the leg is extended during the SLR adds further tension. The slump sign is the observation of a patient slumping forward during a sitting SLR in an attempt to decrease tension on the nerve root. The flip test is when the patient changes posture from a forward leaning position to a rearward position when the leg is raised during a sitting SLR. Unlike the supine SLR and contralateral SLR, these and other tests like them have little evidence to support their reliability. Thus, an isolated positive sign may not strongly indicate the cause of the symptoms, whereas a collection of positive signs that correlate with this patient's chief complaint can help narrow down diagnosis.

Additional exam includes a supine SLR that is positive on the right at 50 degrees. Crossed SLR on the left side is positive for reproduced pain on the right when the left leg is raised to 60 degrees. Seated SLR bilaterally does not produce any pain, although there is a notable flip sign associated on the right. Passive dorsiflexion of the right ankle during the seated SLR on that side reproduces the symptoms. Slump sign is negative bilaterally.

What is the differential diagnosis?
The differential for low back pain and associated radiating pain can be broad but easily narrowed down to one of the three groups mentioned above: nonspecific low back and referred pain, radiculopathy, or another cause. Even after ruling out red flags and diagnoses that necessitate urgent attention, many other possibilities exist. It may be a peripheral neuropathy caused by nerve damage outside the vertebral column, such as mechanical compression by the piriformis muscle (piriformis syndrome). Considering the high prevalence of low back pain in the general population (up to 60% in general and over 80% over the course of a year), there is the possibility of an acute low back injury occurring simultaneously with an unrelated leg pain. Examples include greater trochanteric bursitis, stress or insufficiency fractures, osteonecrosis, osteoarthritis, and shingles. Additional history and exam can help narrow down the differential. Greater trochanteric bursitis is typically associated with palpable tenderness over the greater trochanter of the femur, chronic glucocorticoid use can suggest the presence of related osteonecrosis, and a rash associated with pain distributed along a specific dermatome will clue in the possibility of shingles.

In this case, there is no rash or pain with light touch to suggest the presence of a herpes zoster infection. The patient denies any recent trauma, and there is little (such as history of osteoporosis or chronic glucocorticoid use) to suggest the presence of a vertebral fracture and subsequent narrowing of the transforaminal space. Palpation along the hip is also negative for pain, which could suggest the presence of a greater trochanteric bursitis.

Based on the history and exam, a radiculopathy involving the L5 nerve root is highly suspected. Supporting evidence include the description of a burning pain that extends beyond the knee to the right lateral ankle, decreased sensation and muscle weakness consistent with the L5 nerve root, and positive nerve root tension signs, particularly the contralateral SLR, which has a high specificity. However, imaging is necessary to confirm the diagnosis and more importantly the etiology. The most common cause of radiculopathy is a disc herniation that compresses the nerve root and/or a ruptured disc with material from the nucleus pulposus causing an inflammatory response. A tumor, metastatic or primary, can also cause transforaminal narrowing and radicular symptoms. However, without a history, symptoms, or exam findings concerning for a neoplasm, this possibility is lower on the differential. The lack of fever or other signs of infection also make the presence of an epidural abscess less likely. Because the patient denies presence of any impairments that would be concerning for cauda equina syndrome or spinal stenosis with spinal cord compression, an urgent MRI or neurosurgical evaluation is not needed.

What is the natural history of acute low back pain and associated radiculopathy?

Low back pain is very common, with a lifetime prevalence of at least 60 to 80% and the annual incidence of 10 to 12%. However, only a quarter of those affected seek out formal care. The low percentage of adults who seek care is due to a favorable natural course of acute low back pain, which is often self-limiting and does not require extensive evaluation and management. Approximately 30 to 60% will recovery within a week, 60 to 90% in 6 weeks, and 95% within 12 weeks.

Similarly, an acute lumbar radiculopathy also has a favorable natural course. Although large studies are lacking, it is generally accepted that the majority of disc herniations with lumbosacral radiculopathy will resolve with conservative management alone, which includes medication management and physical therapy. In one study of 208 patients, 70% of patients reported significant improvement in pain after 4 weeks with improved function and 60% were able to return to work.

CLINICAL PEARL   **STEP 2/3**

Studies examining the natural course of a disc herniation and associated radiculopathy show spontaneous resolution is possible and most significant with larger protrusions as compared to smaller bulges.

Is a definitive diagnosis or further testing necessary before beginning management?

Not necessarily. As discussed above, the history and physical are consistent with a lumbar radiculopathy, but the diagnosis is not certain without diagnostic imaging to better identify the involved nerve root(s) and cause. As long as the history and physical lack evidence of severe underlying pathology, further diagnostic imaging is not necessary for management of an acute musculoskeletal injury. Guidelines generally do not recommend early imaging for care of nonspecific low back pain or lumbar radiculopathy. Diagnostic imaging prior to treatment is recommended if red flags are identified or in anticipation of an interventional procedure with a transforaminal epidural steroid injection (TFESI) or lumbar surgery. In this case, the patient presents with low back and leg pain, but without any symptoms or signs concerning for infection, inflammation, or tumors. Considering the early presentation, it is reasonable to start with a conservative approach.

How can conservative management be approached initially?

When treating acute nonspecific low back pain with and without radicular symptoms, the first step is to emphasize their natural course because the majority of cases will resolve spontaneously. It is also important to emphasis early mobilization. Studies have shown bed rest is ineffective for low back pain and may delay recovery, whereas early mobilization and return to daily activities can improve both recovery time and decrease chronic disability. Due to the severe nature of pain associated with the low back and radiculopathy, it is reasonable to expect reluctance by the patient, which is why early education about the natural course of both conditions is essential.

To assist the patient with early mobilization, pharmaceutical treatment is often considered. Treatment should be tailored toward the patient's particular symptoms and can minimize symptoms with the aim of improving activity and participation in formal therapy if necessary.

For analgesic treatment of mild to moderate cases, acetaminophen and nonsteroidal antiin-flammatory drugs (NSAIDs) are first line and preferred for their nonabuse potential. The latter should be used cautiously in individuals with cardiovascular, renal, and gastrointestinal concerns. Muscle relaxants such as cyclobenzaprine and tizanidine are helpful for spasms and difficulty sleeping due to their central mechanism of action, which can cause sedation, a common side effect. Opiates are often utilized when the symptoms are severe. However, their potential for dependence and lack of evidence demonstrating shorter improvement times or decreased dis-ability warrants judicious use. Their purpose is mainly as a temporary measure to allow for increased activity and participation in therapy. If the patient demonstrates concurrent depressive symptoms or if psychiatric illness is suspected, a selective serotonin reuptake inhibitor (SSRI) or serotonin-norepinephrine reuptake inhibitor (SNRI) can also be trialed.

Nerve membrane stabilizers can be started for treatment of a radiculopathy. Gabapentin and its derivative pregabalin are commonly utilized. There is evidence to show the former can lead to improved function and rest pain. High daily dosages of gabapentin may be necessary for effectiveness. Like the centrally acting muscle relaxants, gabapentin and pregabalin can also cause increased drowsiness at both lower and higher dosages. A course of oral glucocorticoids can also be considered if a chemical radiculitis is suspected, although their mechanism is unclear and there is little evidence regarding their use (as opposed to epidural corticosteroid injections). A short, tapered course over 1 to 2 weeks is reasonable.

CLINICAL PEARL   **STEP 2/3**

The evidence for using opioids in managing both acute nonspecific low back pain and radiculopathy was initially derived from other pain conditions. Although effective in the short term, there is limited evidence to show its efficacy for chronic back pain. Considering the risk for depression, addiction, overdose-related mortality, and risk of falls in the elderly, long-term use must be administered cautiously.

Because low back pain and radiculopathy are often self-limited, it is acceptable to begin with education and medication. Physical therapy (PT) can also be included with the treatment regimen initially or later if symptoms fail to show adequate improvement after several weeks. There are numerous approaches when it comes to PT and developing a home exercise program. Common techniques include stretching the muscles of the pelvic girdle and hamstrings and strengthening the core musculature. More specific programs exist for management of radiculopathy, though little evidence shows one is superior over another. The paradigm behind mechanical diagnosis and therapy (MDT or McKenzie program) is to assess for movements that aggravate or benefit radicular symptoms and coaching on exercises based on the patient's directional preference. PT programs can utilize other techniques such as neural mobilization, spinal manipulation, and lumbar traction. Yoga can also be helpful because it emphasizes flexibility and core stability and its meditative component can help address psychological issues if present.

Considering the lack of any suspicious symptoms or signs concerning for malignancy, infection, or inflammation along with a history and physical exam consistent with a radiculopathy, the patient is initially treated conservatively. He is instructed to limit bed rest, begin ambulating when possible, and resume daily activities as soon as tolerated. Over-the-counter NSAIDs such as ibuprofen are also recommended for treating pain as needed. For the radicular symptoms, he is started on a low dosage of gabapentin twice a day. He is instructed to note sedentary symptoms and, if tolerated, the gabapentin will be increased until the radiating pain improves.

Continued

Four weeks later, he returns with minimal improvement of his symptoms. Although he is able to walk slowly and manage simple tasks such as dressing and toileting, advanced daily activities are considerably more difficult and he has not been able to return to work. In light of the persistent pain, an MRI scan without contrast of the lumbar and sacral spine is scheduled in anticipation of a transforaminal epidural glucocorticoid injection. For further management of pain, he is started on a short and scheduled course of the antiinflammatory meloxicam, twice a day for approximately 2 weeks. A glucocorticoid taper is also prescribed over the course of 2 weeks. The patient is referred to PT with specific instructions for stretching the hamstrings and pelvic girdle and gradual transition to core stabilization exercises and a home exercise regimen as he is able to tolerate increased activity.

Diagnosis: Low back pain with right-sided radiculopathy due to right L5-S1 disc protrusion with impingement on the L5 nerve root

---

What other studies can be used in the event MRI is contraindicated?

MRI is the imaging modality of choice when evaluating low back pain with suspected radiculopathy and neurologic damage. It provides excellent visualization of soft tissue structures such as the vertebral discs and neural roots and can provide information regarding impingements. When reviewing diagnostic imaging, it is important to match the suspected nerve root involved on history and physical with pathology seen on the MRI. A left disc protrusion at the L2-L3 interval has little clinical significance if the patient is complaining of radiating pain extending down his or her right leg.

Aside from identifying a herniated disc that can cause nerve root damage, other causes that can be identified on MRI such as a cyst, abscess, and tumor can be better visualized with the addition of IV gadolinium contrast. Despite its utility in diagnosing radiculopathies, it is not recommended when managing nonspecific low back pain.

When an MRI is contraindicated, such as with the presence of a pacemaker, the next modality of choice is a computed tomography (CT) scan with myelography. CT alone, even with IV contrast, is unable to provide adequate definition of vertebral discs and the nerve roots as they exit the neuroforaminal space. Myelography is the introduction of contract material into the epidural space for improved definition and identification of any neuroforaminal narrowing or nerve root impingement consistent with the suspected radiculopathy.

CLINICAL PEARL   **STEP 2/3**

Not all implanted devices are a contraindication to an MRI. Recent joint replacements are commonly composed of the nonferrous metal titanium, which is not affected by a magnet and labeled as MRI compatible. However, the implant itself can cause significant artifact and render certain images difficult to interpret. Although a titanium hip or knee replacement are not contraindications to an MRI, the hip replacement may make images near the pelvis difficult to visualize, whereas the knee replacement will have little effect at that level.

Electrodiagnostic testing can also be performed when the affected level is unclear based on the history, exam, and imaging modalities. It is not recommended as a sole diagnostic study for identification of an affected nerve root but can help narrow down the possibilities if the diagnosis is unclear based on the history, exam, and imaging.

BASIC SCIENCE/CLINICAL PEARL   **STEP 1/2/3**

Peripheral nerve damage can be categorized as neuropraxia (damage of the myelin sheath with an intact axon), axonotomesis (damage of the axon with an intact myelin sheath), and neurotomesis (damage to both the myelin sheath and axon). For nerve regeneration to occur, the neural cell body must be intact. After Wallerian degeneration of the distal nerve segment, the proximal end can grow at an average rate of 1 mm per day.

What interventional and surgical options are available for treatment of radiculopathy?

After conservative measures have been attempted, symptoms may persist and require more invasive management. Once the specific root level is identified as the cause, a TFESI can be considered. This procedure is performed under fluoroscopic guidance and involves injecting an anesthetic and glucocorticoid preparation at the site of inflammation near the neuroforamen. There is reasonable evidence that TFESIs are effective for acute radiculopathies, although there is little evidence for long-term use.

The presence of acute and worsening neurologic impairments, such as cauda equina syndrome, are a clear indication for an urgent neurosurgical consultation and possible intervention. Surgery can also be considered following a conservative course of treatment and TFESI without significant improvement, although optimal timing of surgery for radiculopathy has not been well established. Surgical options for radiculopathy include the minimally invasive microdiscectomy, which is a percutaneous procedure to remove a section of the vertebral disc that may be protruding into the involved area. Open surgery can also be performed by removing the lamina and a portion of the disc for decompression of the affected level. It can be performed via a hemilaminectomy where the lamina is removed entirely at a particular level or a hemilaminotomy, which involves removal of a section of the lamina. If the surgery involves only one level unilaterally, fusion is not typically necessary. Recommendations on which procedure is ideal have also not been well established. The presence of a worker's compensation claim or psychological distress has been identified as a poor prognostic indicator for success following surgery of a disc herniation to manage radiculopathy.

The MRI reveals a right posterolateral disc protrusion at the L5-S1 disc level with significant impingement on the L5 nerve root. The patient undergoes a TFESI at the right L5-S1 level with significant improvement of the radicular pain. He is started on the mild opiate analgesic tramadol due to continued low back pain and to aid with daily activity and to tolerate PT, which is continued. Eight weeks later, the symptoms are significantly improved. He completes his course of formal PT and continues with a home exercise regimen. Tramadol is discontinued and the gabapentin decreased as tolerated. He eventually returns to work without further issues.

BEYOND THE PEARLS

- It is important to avoid leading questions during the physical in additional to the historical exam when evaluating pain and keeping questions open ended when possible. For instance, performing an SLR and asking what the patient feels is different from asking whether they experience a shooting sensation that goes to their foot. In their desire to provide the examiner with positive symptoms, they may respond positively to the latter question when in fact they may only have pain down the posterior thigh, possibly related to tight hamstring musculature and not a true radiculopathy.

Continued

BEYOND THE PEARLS—cont'd

- Disc bulges and protrusions are distinctly different from a disc extrusion, prolapse, or sequestration. The disc material in the former is still contained within the outer layers of the annulus fibrosis.
- When proinflammatory substances from the nucleus pulposus escape the confines of the annulus fibrosis, they may cause chemical irritation with or without mechanical compression of a nerve root. The substances from the nucleus pulposus that may cause an inflammatory response include tumor necrosis factor-alpha (TNF-α), interleukin-1 (IL-1), IL-6, prostaglandin E2, and nitric oxide.
- Although epidural injections are commonly performed as a minimally invasive procedure for low back pain and radiculopathy, the available evidence only supports the use of TFESI for short-term relief of acute radicular symptoms. There is little evidence supporting relief of radiculopathy related to a disc herniation beyond 12 months.
- Several prospective trials have been attempted to determine the efficacy of surgery in radiculopathy and disc herniation. Results show improved recovery time of the radiculopathy, although it is difficult to determine whether surgery is better than conservative management alone in the long term beyond 1 year. A common difficulty with such trials is high crossover between conservative and interventional arms, as noted even in the most recent multicenter study labeled Spine Patient Outcomes Research Trial (SPORT).
- Guidelines agree that conservative management with medications and therapy is the first line of care for nonspecific low back pain and radiculopathies, yet there is little guidance regarding a specific program or intensity of nonoperative services. The literature suggests there are patients who can benefit from conservative management without adequate nonsurgical options. A Danish study demonstrated a reduction in lumbar disc surgery for patients with sciatica after the implementation of nonsurgical spine clinics.

References

Benny B, Azari P. The efficacy of lumbosacral transforaminal epidural glucocorticoid injections: a comprehensive literature review. *J Back Musculoskelet Rehabil.* 2011;24:67-76.

Casey E. Natural history of radiculopathy. *Phys Med Rehabil Clin N Am.* 2011;22:1-5.

Chou R, Qaseem A, Snow V, et al. Diagnosis and treatment of low back pain: a joint clinical practice guideline from the American College of Physicians and the American Pain Society. *Ann Intern Med.* 2007;147:478-491.

Deyo RA, Mirza SK, Martin BI. Back pain prevalence and visit rates: estimates from U.S. national surveys, 2002. *Spine.* 2006;31:2724-2727.

Deyo RA, Von Korff M, Duhrkoop D. Opioids for low back pain. *BMJ.* 2015;350:g6380.

Donelson R. Mechanical diagnosis and therapy for radiculopathy. *Phys Med Rehabil Clin N Am.* 2014;25:75-89.

Efstathiou MA, Stefanakis M, Savva C, Giakas G. Effectiveness of neural mobilization in patients with spinal radiculopathy: a critical review. *J Bodyw Mov Ther.* 2015;19:205-212.

Fox J, Haig AJ, Todey B, Challa S. The effect of required physiatrist consultation on surgery rates for back pain. *Spine.* 2013;38:E178-E184.

Grimm BD, Blessinger BJ, Darden BV, et al. Mimickers of lumbar radiculopathy. *J Am Acad Orthop Surg.* 2015;23:7-17.

Hoy D, Brooks P, Blyth F, Buchbinder R. The Epidemiology of low back pain. *Best Pract Res Clin Rheumatol.* 2010;24:769-781.

Kinkade S. Evaluation and treatment of acute low back pain. *Am Fam Physician.* 2007;75:1181-1188.

Kreiner DS, Hwang SW, Easa JE, et al. An evidence-based clinical guideline for the diagnosis and treatment of lumbar disc herniation with radiculopathy. *Spine.* 2014;14:180-191.

Krisner M, Van Tulder M. Low back pain (non-specific). *Best Prac Res Clin Rheumatol.* 2007;12:77-91.

Longa DL. Sciatica. *N Engl J Med*. 2015;372:1240-1248.

Quraishi NA. Transforaminal injection of corticosteroids for lumbar radiculopathy: systematic review and meta-analysis. *Eur Spine J*. 2012;21:214-219.

Rasmussen C, Nielsen GL, Hansen VK, Jensen OK, Schioettz-Christensen B. Rates of lumbar disc surgery before and after implementation of multidisciplinary nonsurgical spine clinics. *Spine*. 2005;30:2469-2473.

Rubinstein SM, Van Tulder M. A best-evidence review of diagnostic procedures for neck and low-back pain. *Best Prac Res Clin Rheumatol*. 2008;22:471-482.

Saal JA, Saal JS, Herzog RJ. The natural history of lumbar intervertebral disc extrusions treated nonoperatively. *Spine*. 1990;15:683-686.

Spijker-Huiges A, Vermeulen K, Winters JC, Wijhe MV, Van Der Meer K. Epidural steroids for lumbosacral radicular syndrome compared to usual care: quality of life and cost utility in general practice. *Arch Phys Med Rehabil*. 2015;96:381-387.

Van der Windt DA, Simons E, Riphagen II, et al. Physical examination for lumbar radiculopathy due to disc herniation in patient with low-back pain. *Cochrane Database Syst Rev*. 2010;(2):CD007431.

Visco CJ, Cheng DS, Kennedy DJ. Pharmaceutical therapy for radiculopathy. *Phys Med Rehabil Clin N Am*. 2011;22:127-137.

Waddell G, Feder G, Lewis M. Systematic reviews of bed rest and advice to stay active for acute low back pain. *Br J Gen Pract*. 1997;47:647-652.

Gina Rossetti ■ Nida Hamiduzzaman ■ Eric Hsieh

A 78-Year-Old Male With Palpitations and Lightheadedness

A 78-year-old male with a long-standing history of both type 2 diabetes mellitus and hypertension presents to your clinic with 3 days of intermittent palpitations and lightheadedness. His blood pressure is 140/80 mm Hg and his pulse rate is 134/min. His oxygen saturation is 96% on room air. His heart beat is irregularly irregular on cardiac exam. An electrocardiogram (ECG) is obtained in the clinic (Fig. 19.1).

How would you interpret this ECG?
This ECG shows atrial fibrillation with a rapid ventricular response. This is characterized by an irregularly irregular ventricular rhythm, the absence of discrete P waves, and a narrow QRS complex. Atrial fibrillation can present with a rapid ventricular response characterized by a ventricular rate greater than 100 beats/minute. The ventricular rate generally ranges from 120 to 160 but can sometimes be greater than 200 beats/minute.

Diagnosis: Atrial fibrillation

What are the common presenting signs and symptoms of atrial fibrillation?
Approximately 5% of all adults older than 70 years old will experience atrial fibrillation. Many patients are asymptomatic and the arrhythmia is found incidentally during medical evaluation. Patients can present with palpitations, dizziness, fatigue, and poor exercise tolerance. They can also have chest pain due to cardiac demand ischemia caused by the increased ventricular rate. This usually occurs in patients who have underlying coronary artery disease (CAD). Patients may present with signs of fluid overload such as an elevated jugular venous pulsation, crackles on lung exam, and peripheral pitting edema. Fluid overload can be due to decreased cardiac output caused by poor contraction of the ventricle or underlying structural heart disease. Hypotension due to reduced cardiac output can occur and may progress to cardiogenic shock.

CLINICAL PEARL	**STEP 2/3**

Signs of fluid overload, murmurs, or extra heart sounds on physical exam may indicate underlying congestive heart failure or valvular disorders.

How do you classify the types of atrial fibrillation?
Atrial fibrillation is classified into three types. Lone atrial fibrillation occurs in patients with no structural heart disease and no identifiable precipitants. Despite no identifiable cause, the arrhythmia tends to recur and then becomes permanent. Paroxysmal atrial fibrillation occurs when the episodes of the arrhythmia are intermittent. The patient will often have episodes of atrial fibrillation that can last minutes to days and then will convert back to normal sinus rhythm

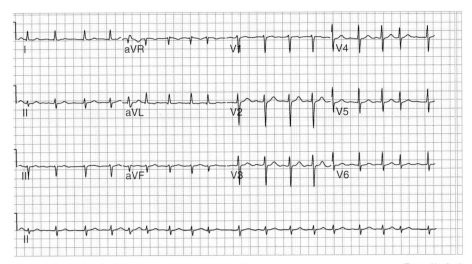

Figure 19.1   Resting ECG that demonstrated atrial fibrillation with fast ventricular response. *(From Alsaileek A, Alharthi M, Almallah, M. Coronary computed tomography angiography in a patient with atrial fibrillation, case report.* J Saudi Heart Assoc. *2011;23(4):245-247.)*

spontaneously. Persistent atrial fibrillation indicates that the arrhythmia will not convert to normal sinus rhythm and thus will need medical therapy. Permanent atrial fibrillation indicates that the arrhythmia will not respond to therapy and normal sinus rhythm cannot be achieved.

What is the pathophysiology of atrial fibrillation?

In a normal heart, the sinoatrial node in the right atrium will send an electric impulse to the atrioventricular (AV) node, which will generate a ventricular heartbeat at a rate of 50 to 80 beats/minute. This coordinated electrical impulse allows for effective contraction of the myocardium and thus normal cardiac output. In atrial fibrillation, electric impulses are produced by multiple ectopic foci, usually next to the origin of the pulmonary veins. This causes the atria to fibrillate, or contract in a disordered manner. The resulting disordered conduction through the AV node to the ventricles causes rapid, inefficient ventricular contraction and decreased cardiac output.

What are some underlying etiologies of atrial fibrillation?

The most common etiology is underlying structural heart disease in patients older than 65. Common causes of heart disease include long-standing hypertension, CAD, congestive heart failure (CHF), and valvular disease. If there is underlying heart pathology, atrial fibrillation is more likely to become persistent or permanent. In addition, there are identifiable triggers that are reversible. The most common are alcohol, hyperthyroidism, electrolyte abnormalities, stimulants, and pulmonary disease. Atrial fibrillation also occurs in the postoperative setting, specifically after cardiopulmonary operations in elderly patients and often abates on its own over 1 to 2 days. A portion of atrial fibrillation cases will have no identifiable cause and be deemed idiopathic.

BASIC SCIENCE PEARL   **STEP 1**

Many substances and medications can induce atrial fibrillation. Examples include caffeine, theophylline, pseudoephedrine, and albuterol. When evaluating a patient with atrial fibrillation, it is important to obtain a thorough medication history, especially in the elderly population due to polypharmacy. Treatment includes withdrawal of the offending drug.

What are the criteria for hospitalization for atrial fibrillation?
Patients are admitted if they show evidence of hypotension or fluid overload or if they have an associated medical condition that justifies admission. Examples include hypertensive emergency, cardiac ischemia, infection, or hyperthyroidism.

What medications could you use to control the pulse rate?
Patients with significant tachycardia or complications such as hypotension or fluid overload should be given a short-acting AV nodal blocking agent for immediate control of their pulse rate. The two main classes of medications are beta blockers and calcium channel blockers. The cardioselective beta blockers such as atenolol or metoprolol are used. The nondihydropyridine calcium channel blockers such as verapamil or diltiazem are used. These medications have more effect on the AV node and less effect on the peripheral vasculature. Alternative medications include amiodarone and digoxin. Amiodarone has both rate- and rhythm-control properties. Digoxin should be added if rate control cannot be achieved with the above medications alone.

CLINICAL PEARL   **STEP 2/3**

Verapamil and diltiazem are contraindicated in patients with systolic heart failure. Therefore, beta blockers or amiodarone should be used to control pulse rate.

CLINICAL PEARL   **STEP 2/3**

Long-term use of amiodarone can lead to many side effects. These include thyroid disease, pulmonary fibrosis, liver toxicity, corneal deposits, optic neuropathy, and blue discoloration of the skin.

The patient is treated with intravenous (IV) metoprolol. His palpitations and lightheadedness subside. His pulse rate is now 85/min. He continues to have an irregularly irregular rhythm on cardiac exam.

What lab and imaging studies do you want to send at this point?
The initial laboratory evaluation should include serum electrolytes, a complete blood count (CBC), a thyroid-stimulating hormone (TSH), and a urinary toxicology. Additionally, a lipid panel and hemoglobin A1C are frequently sent. A chest radiograph (CXR) is obtained to evaluate for pulmonary edema. A transthoracic echocardiograph is obtained to evaluate for underlying structural heart disease.

The patient's electrolytes, CBC, TSH, and urine toxicology are normal. A CXR shows bilateral pulmonary edema. A transthoracic ECG shows mild diastolic dysfunction with a normal ejection fraction and normal chamber sizes.

Should this patient be offered rhythm control as treatment for his arrhythmia?
Rhythm control is an option for both acute and chronic treatment of atrial fibrillation. It involves delivering therapies that will terminate the electrical impulses from the ectopic foci and attempt to maintain normal sinus rhythm. This can be achieved with either pharmacologic therapies or electrocardioversion. This is in contrast to maintaining rate control with oral AV nodal blocking

agents. Though there are some theoretical benefits to maintaining a patient in normal sinus rhythm, many trials have assessed morbidity and mortality outcomes in rhythm versus rate control. The Atrial Fibrillation Follow-up Investigation of Rhythm Management (AFFIRM) trial showed that there was no difference in overall mortality, risk of ischemic stroke, or adverse events between the two groups. In addition, a recent meta-analysis of 10 randomized controlled trials showed that there is no difference in stroke, cardiac mortality, and all-cause mortality. Because of this, the physician will often decide on a case-by-case basis; however, the majority of patients are given rate control. This is because antiarrhythmia medications have many side effects and are sometimes not effective.

CLINICAL PEARL   **STEP 2/3**

Amiodarone is the preferred antiarrhythmia medication because it is safe for systolic heart failure patients and has a low potential to precipitate ventricular arrhythmias. It also has some AV nodal blocking properties and can be used for rate control.

CLINICAL PEARL   **STEP 2/3**

Cardioselective beta blockers are often the preferred agent for rate control in patients with systolic CHF. Beta blockers have been shown to reduce all-cause mortality in patients with systolic heart failure.

CLINICAL PEARL   **STEP 2/3**

The goal pulse rate in patients on rate-control therapy is less than 90/min at rest and less than 110/min with exertion.

When would you choose electric and/or pharmacologic cardioversion over rate control?

Rate control should be avoided in patients with a preexcitation syndrome such as Wolff-Parkinson-White syndrome. Patients who cannot achieve effective rate control with multiple medications should be considered for rhythm control. Also, emergent electrocardioversion is indicated if the patient has signs of hemodynamic instability, such as hypotension, severe fluid overload, or cardiogenic shock.

The physician on call elects to continue rate control therapy. The patient is transitioned to oral metoprolol, and his resting pulse rate is 85/min. His fluid overload resolves, and the furosemide is discontinued.

Should this patient be referred for elective electrocardioversion?

Patients with no underlying cardiac disease who are having their first documented episode of atrial fibrillation are often referred for elective electrocardioversion.

If electric cardioversion is successful, how would you manage the patient after sinus rhythm is restored?

After sinus rhythm is restored, the atria are stunned and may not resume normal functioning for several weeks. Stasis in the atria may form a thrombus, and the risk of thromboembolism in the

TABLE 19.1 ▓ The CHA$_2$DS$_2$-VASc Scoring System

C	Congestive heart failure	1 point
H	Hypertension	1 point
A	Age >75 years old	2 points
D	Diabetes mellitus	1 point
S	History of stroke or transient ischemic attack (TIA)	2 points
VA	Vascular disease	1 point
Sc	Sex or gender	1 point for female

first month postcardioversion is 5%. This includes pharmacologic cardioversion. Therefore, every patient must be placed on anticoagulation for 1 month postcardioversion.

What are some other treatment options for atrial fibrillation if rate or rhythm control is not successful?

Patients can be referred to a cardiologist for catheter ablation of the AV node with pacemaker insertion. A second option is ablation of the pulmonary veins, which carries a risk of cardiac perforation and subsequent cardiac tamponade. A cardiothoracic surgeon can perform a maze procedure in some cases, although it is usually performed in patients undergoing valvular replacement surgery.

Do patients with atrial fibrillation need lifelong anticoagulation for stroke prevention?

The average patient with atrial fibrillation has a 4% risk of stroke annually. The risk of stroke is significantly higher if certain risk factors are present. The CHA$_2$DS$_2$-VASc scoring system is used to assess the risk of stroke in atrial fibrillation patients (Table 19.1).

A score of zero (0) is considered low risk, and the patient may receive aspirin therapy alone. A score of 1 is considered moderate risk, and the patient may receive aspirin or warfarin. This is left to the discretion of the physician. A score of ≥2 is high risk, and warfarin is recommended. Bleeding risk and fall risk must always be considered when making the decision to prescribe anticoagulation.

The patient reports that he has no history of stroke or transient ischemic attack. He has a CHA$_2$DS$_2$-VASc of 3 given his hypertension, diabetes, and age older than 75. He is discharged on warfarin for anticoagulation and oral metoprolol for rate control.

BEYOND THE PEARLS

- Atrial fibrillation can be associated with Wolff-Parkinson-White syndrome or a preexcitation pathway. On ECG, you will see an irregularly irregular rhythm with a wide QRS complex. This is due to the delta wave associated with preexcitation pathways. AV nodal blockers are contraindicated for rate control of the rapid ventricular response. Beta blockers may exacerbate the syndrome by blocking the AV nodal pathway, thus allowing further conduction through the preexcitation pathway. This can lead to life-threatening ventricular arrhythmias.

BEYOND THE PEARLS—cont'd

- If paroxysmal atrial fibrillation is suspected and you have been unable to diagnose an episode on a 12-lead ECG, you can send the patient home with a Holter monitor. This portable device records the heart rhythm 24 hours a day. The patient usually wears the device for 1 to 2 days; however, some monitors can record for up to 1 week. Dronedarone is a new drug approved for the treatment of atrial fibrillation. It is in the same class as amiodarone but has fewer side effects.
- A subanalysis of patients with CHF in the AFFIRM trial showed no difference in mortality in the rate control versus rhythm control groups.
- There are three electrocardioversion scenarios that physicians will encounter in clinical practice. First, if the atrial fibrillation has been present for more than 48 hours, oral anticoagulation must be given for 3 weeks prior to the procedure to treat a possible thrombus and avoid embolization. If the atrial fibrillation has been present for less than 48 hours, parenteral short-acting anticoagulation can be given immediately prior to the procedure. Physicians can also consider transesophageal echocardiogram cardioversion if the proper equipment and personnel are present. This procedure involves placing an ultrasound probe in the esophagus and visualizing the cardiac chambers. If no thrombus is present, cardioversion is performed.

References

Al-Khatib SM, LaPointe NM, Chatterjee R, et al. Rate and rhythm control therapies in patients with atrial fibrillation: a systematic review. *Ann Intern Med.* 2014;160:760-773.

van der Hooft CS, Heeringa J, van Herpen G, et al. Drug-induced atrial fibrillation. *J Am Coll Cardiol.* 2004;44(11):2117-2124.

Hart R, Pearce L, Aguilar M. Meta-analysis: anti-thrombotic therapy to prevent stroke in patients who have non-valvular atrial fibrillation. *Ann Intern Med.* 2007;146:857-867.

Packer M, Fowler MB, Roecker EB, et al. Effect of carvedilol on the morbidity of patients with severe chronic heart failure: results of the carvedilol prospective randomized cumulative survival (COPERNICUS) study. *Circulation.* 2002;106(17):2194-2199.

The Atrial Fibrillation Follow-up Investigation of Rhythm Management (AFFIRM) Investigators. A comparison of rate control and rhythm control in patients with atrial fibrillation. *N Engl J Med.* 2002;347:1825-1833.

Arzhang Cyrus Javan   ■   Andrea Censullo

A 56-Year-Old Male With Acute Cough and Fever

A 56-year-old male is evaluated in an outpatient clinic during the month of May for a 2-day history of productive cough and fever. His past medical history is significant for well-controlled hypertension and osteoarthritis of the knees.

What are some important initial questions to ask in a patient who presents with a cough?
Cough is very commonly encountered in medical practice and has a broad differential diagnosis. To help narrow the differential, first determine the duration of cough. This patient has an acute cough (defined as <3 weeks), which is most often caused by a viral upper respiratory tract infection (URI) but can also be a presenting symptom in patients with pneumonia (infection of the lung parenchyma, i.e., the lower respiratory tract), chronic obstructive pulmonary disease (COPD) exacerbation, pulmonary malignancy, pulmonary embolism, or congestive heart failure (CHF)-related pulmonary edema. A subacute cough (3 to 8 weeks) is most commonly postinfectious in origin, whereas a chronic cough (>8 weeks) is most commonly caused by postnasal drip, asthma, or gastroesophageal reflux disease (GERD). Keep in mind that this is by no means an exhaustive list as the differential for cough is quite broad.

Next, ask about symptoms associated with pneumonia. It is important to distinguish this relatively common and serious entity from the less common or less serious causes of cough. The classic symptoms of bacterial pneumonia are acute-onset cough, sputum production, dyspnea, chest pain (often pleuritic), and fever. Patients with pneumonia may also report nonpulmonary symptoms such as fatigue, sweats, headache, nausea, myalgias, and occasionally abdominal pain and diarrhea. Remember that the elderly often present with fewer of the classic symptoms just described.

Asking about the presence and quality of sputum can help when formulating a strong differential. Purulent sputum (containing pus) can suggest pneumonia but is nonspecific and can also point toward COPD, bronchiectasis, lung abscess, and even a viral URI. Hemoptysis (bloody sputum) is commonly caused by viral bronchitis but should raise suspicion for cancer or tuberculosis in those with risk factors.

Finally, ask about medication use because some patients develop a dry cough while taking angiotensin-converting enzyme (ACE) inhibitors.

On further questioning, the cough is productive of thick, yellow sputum and is associated with dyspnea and pleuritic chest pain. He also reports fatigue and nasal congestion. He denies myalgias, weight loss, night sweats, or hemoptysis.

His medications include hydrochlorothiazide 25 mg orally once daily and acetaminophen 650 mg every 6 hours as needed for pain.

TABLE 20.1 ▇ **Noninfectious Conditions That Should Be Considered in the Differential for CAP**

- Congestive heart failure-associated pulmonary edema
- Lung cancer
- Pulmonary embolism with infarction
- Cryptogenic organizing pneumonia (COP)
- Collagen vascular disease
- Drug toxicity
- Radiation pneumonitis

What is at the top of your differential?

This 56-year-old male is presenting with an acute cough productive of purulent sputum, fevers, dyspnea, and pleuritic chest pain. These collective signs and symptoms point toward an infection and should place pneumonia at the top of your differential. There may be a considerable amount of overlap in the signs and symptoms of pneumonia and the other causes of acute cough, so important clues already gathered from the history must be used to help sort through the differential.

CLINICAL PEARL   **STEP 2/3**

Pneumonia occurs by one of the following mechanisms: aspiration of upper airway colonizing microbiota (most common), inhalation of aerosolized material, or less likely, hematogenous seeding of the lung.

He has no known history of COPD or CHF, so a COPD or CHF exacerbation would be highly unlikely. He lacks the chronic constitutional symptoms that would suggest an underlying malignancy. Pulmonary embolism (PE) is still on the differential as it too often manifests with dyspnea and pleuritic chest pain (Table 20.1). Although patients with PE can occasionally have fevers, the purulent sputum in this case makes this a less likely diagnosis. Viral URI is still on the differential but somewhat less likely because of the presence of dyspnea.

Further history reveals that the patient lives in Ohio with his wife and works as an accountant. He denies smoking, alcohol use, or illicit drug use. He has a pet dog but denies recent travel or significant outdoor exposures. He denies recent exposure to sick contacts.

How does the information gathered from taking a thorough social history influence your initial evaluation and management of patients with suspected pneumonia?

By taking a thorough social history, you can determine a patient's risk factors for unusual pathogens that may not be covered by a standard empiric antibiotic regimen. Any disorder that increases the risk of aspiration, including alcoholism, increases the risk for pneumonia caused by oral anaerobes and gram-negative enteric pathogens including *Klebsiella pneumoniae*.

CLINICAL PEARL   **STEP 2/3**

Aspiration can cause a chemical pneumonitis shortly thereafter, whereas aspiration pneumonia occurs more insidiously, several days after the initial aspiration event.

CLINICAL PEARL   **STEP 2/3**

An elderly, alcoholic male presenting with "currant-jelly" sputum is the classic clinical picture used to describe pneumonia caused by *K. pneumoniae*.

Tobacco smokers and those with COPD have an increased risk for pneumonia with *Streptococcus pneumoniae, Haemophilus influenzae, Moraxella catarrhalis, Legionella* species including *L. pneumophila* and, less commonly, *Pseudomonas* species.

CLINICAL PEARL   **STEP 2/3**

The influenza (flu) viruses can cause a primary pneumonia and can also predispose the patient to a secondary bacterial pneumonia with *Staphylococcus aureus* or other pathogens.

A travel history is important because some infections are geographically limited. Exposure to bat or bird droppings in the Mississippi and Ohio River valleys raises the possibility of pneumonia caused by *Histoplasma capsulatum,* whereas infection with *Coccidioides immitis,* another endemic fungi, occurs mainly in the southwest United States. Ask about a recent hotel or cruise ship stay that can increase the chance of an infection with *Legionella.* Emerging infectious diseases are also initially geographically limited, such as Middle East respiratory syndrome coronavirus (MERS-CoV) (Arabian peninsula) and avian influenza (Asia). Tuberculosis (TB) is more likely in those who have lived in or traveled to an endemic region for TB and also in those who are homeless.

Although rare, certain zoonotic organisms can cause pneumonia in humans. This list of pathogens includes *Chlamydophila psittaci* (bird exposures), *Coxiella burnetti,* the agent of Q fever (farm animals), and *Francisella tularensis* (rabbits). This is why it is always important to ask about animal exposures.

CLINICAL PEARL   **STEP 2/3**

When pneumonia is caused by a suspected bioterrorism agent, infection with *Bacillus anthracis* (anthrax), *Yersinia pestis* (plague), and *Francisella tularensis* (tularemia) should be considered.

If the history reveals risk factors for human immunodeficiency virus (HIV), opportunistic pathogens such as *Pneumocystis jiroveci* (which causes *Pneumocystis* pneumonia, also known as PCP) in addition to *Mycobacterium tuberculosis* should be added to your differential. With that said, *S. pneumoniae* is still the leading cause of pneumonia in those with HIV/acquired immunodeficiency syndrome (AIDS).

Unfortunately, no cause is found in approximately half of the patients diagnosed with pneumonia in the United States.

On physical exam, temperature is 38.5 °C (101.3 °F), blood pressure is 120/80 mm Hg, pulse rate is 110/min, respiration rate is 22/min, and oxygen saturation is 95% on room air. He is alert and oriented but in slight distress from mild tachypnea. He is not using any accessory muscles of respiration. Cardiac exam reveals a rapid pulse rate with regular rhythm and no jugular venous distension.

Pulmonary exam reveals dullness to percussion, rales, and bronchial breath sounds at the right lung base without wheezing. He has no peripheral edema.

What diagnostic test should you perform next?

There are signs of lung consolidation on physical exam, which further supports a diagnosis of pneumonia. All patients with suspected pneumonia should have a chest radiograph (CXR), ideally a posterior-anterior (PA) and lateral view.

> Due to logistical concerns, a single view, portable CXR is performed rather than a PA and lateral CXR (Fig. 20.1).

Does this CXR help narrow your differential?

This patient has a consolidation in the right lower lobe, thus solidifying the diagnosis of pneumonia. Although no one pattern on CXR is specific for any one pathogen, the general radiographic appearance can sometimes provide the clinician with important clues as to the cause of the pneumonia. Lobar consolidation, as seen in this patient, points toward (but does not equal) infection with a "typical" bacterial pathogen. In contrast, an interstitial pattern on chest radiograph is more often associated with "atypical" pathogens.

What are the typical and atypical pathogens? Why does it matter to distinguish them?

The typical bacterial pathogens are *S. pneumoniae, H. influenzae,* and, in certain patient populations, the gram-negative bacilli and *S. aureus. Mycoplasma, Chlamydophila, Legionella,* as well as the respiratory viruses comprise the atypical category. The atypical organisms are distinguished from the typical by the fact that they generally cannot be visualized on Gram stain or cultured via standard media. The history cannot be used to definitively differentiate between the typical and atypical pathogens. With that said, the typical pathogens generally cause a more acute presentation, whereas the atypicals, excluding *Legionella,* generally present with a more indolent course, often in younger patients.

This distinction has treatment implications because the atypical bacteria are resistant to all beta lactams (which encompass the penicillin, cephalosporin, carbapenem, and monobactam families of antibiotics). Macrolides, fluoroquinolones, or tetracyclines are the antibiotics of choice for these pathogens.

> Upon further questioning, the patient denies recent hospitalization or antibiotic use within the last year.

Why is it important to ask about recent contact with the health-care system, including recent antibiotic use, in a patient diagnosed with pneumonia?

In addition to the typical versus atypical pneumonia syndromes, pneumonia can be further classified into four broad categories: community-acquired pneumonia (CAP), hospital-acquired pneumonia (HAP), health care-associated pneumonia (HCAP), and ventilator-associated pneumonia (VAP). The goal of these distinctions is to predict the most likely pathogens, including the risk for multidrug-resistant pathogens, because this will have implications when choosing an empiric antibiotic regimen. HAP occurs 48 hours or more after admission, whereas VAP is defined as pneumonia that occurs 48 hours after intubation. HCAP is the most heterogeneous group and occurs in patients who have either been hospitalized for 2 or more days within the previous 90 days or who have at least one of the following risk factors: resided in a nursing home within the last 30 days; visited a hemodialysis center; or received intravenous (IV) antibiotic therapy, chemotherapy, or wound care. By definition, patients classified as having CAP have none of these risk factors.

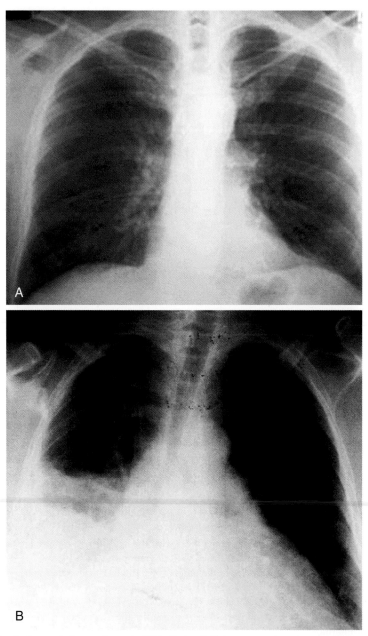

Figure 20.1　**A,** A normal chest radiograph (CXR); **B,** the CXR from our patient demonstrating a right lower lobe infiltrate that obscures the diaphragm. *(Adapted from* https://commons.wikimedia.org/wiki/Pneumonia#/media/File:Pneumonia_x-ray.jpg.*)*

> **Diagnosis:** Community-acquired pneumonia (CAP)

CLINICAL PEARL   **STEP 2/3**

The use of any antibiotics within the previous 3 to 6 months increases the probability of infection with a penicillin- or macrolide-resistant strain of *S. pneumoniae;* because of this, these agents are not recommended as initial empiric monotherapy for pneumonia in these cases. It should also be noted that the antibiotics chosen should be from a different class than used previously.

Should laboratory testing be performed in this patient?

While CXR is recommended in all patients with suspected pneumonia, the decision to perform blood or sputum cultures is more complex. The 2007 Infectious Disease Society of America/American Thoracic Society (IDSA/ATS) guidelines for CAP state that further testing after CXR in an outpatient diagnosed with CAP is optional and should be done when a specific pathogen is suspected that would change the empiric management. In this patient, no unusual pathogen is strongly suggested by history, so no laboratory testing needs to be performed. However, you could consider urine antigen testing for *Histoplasma capsulatum* because he resides in an endemic area (Ohio). Pneumonia caused by *H. capsulatum* in those with an intact immune system is usually self-limited and does not require any specific antifungal treatment.

In contrast, for cases of HAP, HCAP, and VAP, or when CAP is severe enough to warrant hospitalization, further laboratory testing should be performed. At a minimum, blood and sputum should be sent for Gram stain and culture (ideally before antibiotic administration to increase yield), and critically ill patients with CAP should also have *Legionella* and *S. pneumoniae* urine antigen testing performed.

CLINICAL PEARL   **STEP 2/3**

Only sputum samples of good quality should be analyzed; this includes those with >25 neutrophils and ≤10 epithelial cells. Inducing sputum with nebulized hypertonic saline can increase chances of obtaining a good-quality specimen rather than saliva.

It is especially important to attempt to make a microbiologic diagnosis in immunocompromised patients, and early bronchoscopy should be considered to aid in this effort.

What is the most likely pathogen in this patient?

S. pneumoniae is by far the most likely cause, followed by *H. influenzae* because he is a smoker. Historically, *S. pneumoniae* has caused the vast majority of cases of pneumonia (about 95% of cases). Although it is still the most commonly identified cause of CAP, its frequency has declined, likely because of widespread pneumococcal immunization and antismoking campaigns.

The most common causes of CAP treated in the outpatient setting are *S. pneumoniae, M. pneumoniae, H. influenzae, C. pneumoniae,* and respiratory viruses including influenza (Table 20.2). Because we have opted to not perform further testing, it is unlikely that we will ever establish a microbiologic diagnosis. This is of little clinical consequence because the recommended empiric antibiotic regimen should appropriately treat the most likely bacterial pathogens involved. If this patient were ill enough to warrant hospitalization, *S. pneumoniae* would still be the most likely cause. However, other bacteria such as *S. aureus, Legionella* spp., and the gram-negative bacilli would also need to be considered.

TABLE 20.2 ■ Common Etiologies of Community-
Acquired Pneumonia (CAP)

Clinical Scenario	Microorganism
Outpatient	S. pneumoniae M. pneumoniae H. influenzae C. pneumoniae Respiratory viruses including influenza A and B
Inpatient (non-ICU)	S. pneumoniae M. pneumoniae C. pneumoniae H. influenzae Legionella species Respiratory viruses
Inpatient (ICU)	S. pneumoniae S. aureus Legionella spp. Gram-negative bacilli H. influenzae

(Adapted from Mandell L, Wunderink R, Anzueto A, et al.
Infectious Diseases Society of America/American Thoracic
Society consensus guidelines on the management of
community-acquired pneumonia in adults. *Clin Infect Dis.*
2007;44[suppl 2]:S27-S72.)

CLINICAL PEARL   **STEP 2/3**

Community-associated methicillin-resistant *S. aureus* (CA-MRSA) can cause a severe,
rapidly progressive bilateral pneumonia in previously healthy young patients. The Panton-
Valentine leukocidin toxin is associated with increased virulence and is often present in
these strains of *S. aureus* found in the community.

In contrast, HAP, HCAP, and VAP are most frequently caused by aerobic gram-negative bacilli
(50 to 60% of the time) including *Pseudomonas,* followed by *S. aureus* (especially MRSA). Polymicrobial pneumonias comprised of anaerobes and aerobes can also occur in these patients. *S. pneumoniae* and *H. influenzae* are rare in VAP, HAP, and HCAP and comprise only 5 to 15% of cases.
Legionella as a cause of HAP, HCAP, and VAP can occur in the context of a *Legionella* outbreak.

**Should this patient be hospitalized or treated as an outpatient? Are there any tools to guide
us in our decision?**
Ultimately, whether to hospitalize a patient with CAP is left to the discretion of the treating
clinician, but there are several validated prediction scores to assess mortality risk in those with
pneumonia, which in turn can help inform this decision. These scoring systems include the
PORT score, Pneumonia Severity Index (PSI), CURB-65, and CRB-65 (Table 20.3).
    The CRB-65 does not require laboratory testing (blood urea nitrogen [BUN] is omitted), so
it may be a good option for an otherwise healthy outpatient, although studies have suggested
that the CURB-65 and CRB-65 may be less accurate in predicting mortality than the other
scoring systems mentioned.

TABLE 20.3 ■ CURB-65 Scoring System

A patient with 2 or more points should be hospitalized (non-ICU), whereas a patient with 3 or more points should be hospitalized in an ICU.

Clinical Criteria	Points Awarded
Confusion	1
BUN >20	1
Respiratory rate ≥30	1
Blood pressure (systolic) <90	1
Age >65	1

ICU, Intensive care unit.

This patient has received a score of 0 on the CRB-65. Therefore, assuming he has a safe home environment and the ability to be closely followed by his health care provider, he can be safely treated as an outpatient.

What should be the initial empiric antibiotic therapy? How long should he be treated for?
CAP patients treated in an outpatient setting with no significant comorbidities and no recent antibiotic use should be treated with a macrolide (if <25% of pneumococcal isolates in the community have macrolide resistance) or alternatively with doxycycline.

In patients with recent antibiotic use or with risk factors for poor outcomes secondary to significant comorbidities, fluoroquinolone monotherapy (levofloxacin or moxifloxacin) or combination therapy comprised of a macrolide plus a beta lactam are recommended, given the concern for resistant *S. pneumoniae*. The macrolide is added to the beta lactam to cover for the possible atypical bacteria (*Mycoplasma, Chlamydophila,* and *Legionella*). Fluoroquinolones themselves have excellent atypical coverage and also are effective against more drug-resistant *S. pneumoniae,* hence their use as monotherapy in CAP. Doxycycline also has atypical bacterial coverage but is not the preferred agent for *Legionella.*

Patients with CAP should be treated for a minimum of 5 days and must be afebrile for 48 to 72 hours before stopping therapy (Table 20.4). If a specific pathogen is identified on sputum Gram stain, culture, or through other testing, therapy should be narrowed appropriately. See Table 20.5 for recommended empiric antibiotic regimens for CAP in various clinical settings.

CLINICAL PEARL   **STEP 2/3**

CAP patients treated as inpatients can be safely transitioned to oral antibiotics and discharged home once signs of clinical instability (fever, tachycardia, tachypnea, hypotension, desaturation, altered mental status, or inability for oral intake) are absent.

The patient is sent home with a prescription for 5 days of azithromycin and instructed to call the office or go to the emergency room if his condition worsens or fails to improve.

What potential factors may lead to treatment failure?
A patient that either worsens of fails to improve after 72 hours of antibiotic therapy should be reevaluated. Some possible explanations for failure to respond to antibiotics include infection

TABLE 20.4 ■ Recommended Empiric Antibiotic Regimens for Community Acquired Pneumonia (CAP)

Clinical Scenario	Treatment Option 1	Treatment Option 2	Penicillin Allergic
Outpatient			
Previously healthy and no antibiotics in prior 3 months	Macrolide	Doxycycline	n/a
Presence of comorbidities (e.g., diabetes; heart, lung, liver disease; immunosuppressed)*	Respiratory fluoroquinolone (moxifloxacin, gemifloxacin, or levofloxacin)	Beta lactam† plus macrolide	n/a
Inpatient			
Non-ICU	Respiratory fluoroquinolone	Beta lactam plus macrolide	n/a
ICU	Beta lactam plus macrolide	Beta lactam plus respiratory fluoroquinolone	Respiratory fluoroquinolone plus aztreonam
Special Considerations			
Concern for pseudomonas	Antipseudomonal beta lactam‡ plus ciprofloxacin or levofloxacin	Antipseudomonal beta lactam plus aminoglycoside and azithromycin or antipseudomonal fluoroquinolone§	Substitute aztreonam for beta lactam
If MRSA is consideration	Add vancomycin to selected regimen	Add linezolid to selected regimen	n/a

*In regions with high rates (>25%) of macrolide resistant *S. pneumoniae,* consider using these regimens even in those without comorbidities.
†Preferred beta lactam options: amoxicillin, amoxicillin-clavulanate, cefpodoxime or cefuroxime. IV beta lactam options: cefotaxime, ceftriaxone, or ampicillin.
‡Antipseudomonal beta lactams are piperacillin-tazobactam, cefepime, imipenem, meropenem
§Antipseudomonal fluoroquinolone: ciprofloxacin or levofloxacin
MRSA, Methicillin-resistant *Staphylococcus aureus.*
(Adapted from Mandell L, Wunderink R, Anzueto A, et al. Infectious Diseases Society of America/American Thoracic Society consensus guidelines on the management of community-acquired pneumonia in adults. *Clin Infect Dis.* 2007;44[suppl 2]:S45.)

with a resistant organism, infection with an unaccounted-for organism such as an endemic fungus, the presence of a parapneumonic effusion or empyema, the presence of a postobstructive pneumonia caused by a mass such as cancer, or misdiagnosis.

What are some strategies for preventing pneumonia-related morbidity and mortality in adults?
Pneumonia is the most common cause of infection-related mortality in the United States, so many efforts have been appropriately focused on prevention. There are currently two vaccines available for prevention of invasive *S. pneumoniae* disease: the pneumococcal polysaccharide vaccine (PPSV23) and the pneumococcal conjugate vaccine (PCV13). In addition to preventing

TABLE 20.5 ■ **Antibiotic Recommendations for HAP/VAP/HCAP**

Clinical Scenario	Empiric Antibiotic Regimen
Early onset (<5 days) and no risk factors risk for multidrug-resistant organisms (MDRO)	Ceftriaxone *or* Levofloxacin, moxifloxacin, or ciprofloxacin *or* Ampicillin-sulbactam *or* Ertapenem
Late onset (>5 days) or at risk for MDRO	Antipseudomonal beta lactam *plus* Antipseudomonal fluoroquinolone (levofloxacin or ciprofloxacin) or aminoglycoside (amikacin, gentamicin, or tobramycin) *plus* Linezolid or vancomycin

(Adapted from American Thoracic Society and Infectious Disease Society of America. Guidelines for the management of adults with hospital-acquired, ventilator-associated, and healthcare-associated pneumonia. *Am J Respir Crit Care Med.* 2005;171:388-416.)

invasive pneumococcal disease, the PCV13 vaccine also has been shown to prevent pneumococcal pneumonia. Specific indications for these vaccines are beyond the scope of this text.

Another strategy to reduce pneumonia in adults is to recommend yearly influenza vaccination according to the CDC guidelines; currently, influenza vaccination is recommended for all patients 6 months of age or older without contraindications.

Finally, in patients who smoke cigarettes, strongly recommend they quit and offer assistance when possible.

BASIC SCIENCE PEARL   **STEP 1**

Cigarette smoke disrupts mucociliary transport and alters macrophage B- and T-lymphocyte functionality, which can predispose patients to pneumonia.

BEYOND THE PEARLS

- The *Legionella* urine antigen detects only the L1 serotype, which accounts for 90% of community-acquired *Legionella* infections in the United States.
- *Mycoplasma* and *Chlamydophila* are two agents of atypical pneumonia and generally present indolently in younger patients with an interstitial pattern on CXR; *Legionella* also is considered an atypical pathogen but usually presents more acutely in older patients.
- *Legionella* can be associated with severe gastrointestinal and neurologic symptoms, elevated liver enzymes, increased creatinine levels, and abnormalities of other organ systems simultaneously.
- While evaluating patients with CAP, it is imperative to evaluate immune status and recent exposure to health care and/or antibiotics before choosing an empiric regimen.
- If high rates of *S. pneumoniae* resistance are prevalent or if the patient is at risk for poor outcomes, macrolides, doxycycline, or beta lactams should not be used empirically as monotherapy.

Continued

BEYOND THE PEARLS—cont'd

- Parapneumonic effusions are pleural effusions that occur as a result of contiguous extension of a bacterial pneumonia. They are common and usually resolve with antibiotic therapy.
- Parapneumonic effusions should be sampled (i.e., diagnostic thoracentesis) if they are sizeable or appear loculated radiographically. Complicated parapneumonic effusions that have a pH <7.2, a glucose <60, a positive Gram stain or culture, and empyemas (frank pus) usually require further drainage to achieve full resolution.
- Radiographic abnormalities often resolve weeks after the patient has successfully completed the antibiotic course. A follow-up CXR should be considered 4 to 6 weeks after completion of therapy to ensure disease resolution and to help rule out the possibility of an underlying neoplasm.
- Between 10 and 15% of CAP are polymicrobial in nature.
- Anaerobic bacterial pathogens should be considered in patients who present with CAP days to weeks after an aspiration event. These pneumonias often lead to abscess formation, parapneumonic effusions, or empyemas. Patients with significant dental disease in the setting of an unprotected airway (as can be seen in drug overdose, alcohol abuse, or seizure disorders) are at greatest risk.
- *Pseudomonas aeruginosa* can be a significant pathogen in patients with cystic fibrosis, severe COPD, bronchiectasis, and other structural lung diseases.
- Pneumonia in a patient with recent travel to southeast Asia should raise suspicion for melioidosis, which is caused by the gram-negative bacteria *Burkholderia pseudomallei*.

References

American Thoracic Society and Infectious Disease Society of America. Guidelines for the management of adults with hospital-acquired, ventilator-associated, and healthcare-associated pneumonia. *Am J Respir Crit Care Med.* 2005;171:388-416.

Ellison R, Donowitz G. Acute pneumonia. In: Bennett JE, Dolin R, Blaser MJ, eds. *Mandell, Douglas, and Bennett's Principles and Practice of Infectious Diseases.* 8th ed. Philadelphia: Elsevier; 2015:823-846.

Mandell L, Wunderink R. Pneumonia. In: Kasper DL, Fauci AS, eds. *Harrison's Infectious Disease.* 2nd ed. New York: McGraw-Hill; 2013:207-221.

Mandell L, Wunderink R, Anzueto A, et al. Infectious Diseases Society of America/American Thoracic Society consensus guidelines on the management of community-acquired pneumonia in adults. *Clin Infect Dis.* 2007;44(suppl 2):S27-S72.

Musher D, Thorner A. Community-acquired pneumonia. *N Engl J Med.* 2014;371(17):1619-1628.

Weinberger S, Lipson D. Cough and hemoptysis. In: Fauci AS, Braunwald E, Kasper DL, et al., eds. *Harrison's Principles of Internal Medicine.* 17th ed. New York: McGraw-Hill; 2008:225-228.

Andrew Morado ▦ Raj Dasgupta ▦ Ahmet Baydur

A 34-Year-Old Female With Left Lower Extremity Edema

A 34-year-old female presents for outpatient evaluation of acute onset left lower extremity edema over the past 2 days. She reports tenderness to the leg especially with palpation over the calf muscle. Associated erythema of the left leg has been present for the past day.

What are common causes of peripheral edema and the mechanism?
Edema is accounted for by capillary permeability and the balance between hydrostatic and oncotic pressure (Fig. 21.1). Diffuse edema typically is a result of heart, kidney, or liver dysfunction. Systolic heart failure causes peripheral edema from increased hydrostatic pressure as a result of poor forward flow as left ventricular function deteriorates. Chronic kidney disease (CKD) causing oliguria or anuria arises from destruction of glomeruli resulting in decreased glomerular filtration rate and fluid retention. Alternatively, any of the many causes of nephrotic syndrome causing excessive loss of plasma proteins, especially albumin, can cause peripheral edema from loss of serum oncotic pressure within the vasculature. Finally, liver disease can cause edema via the underfill theory stating that vasodilation of the splanchnic circulation results in decreased blood flow to the kidneys. This stimulates the renin-angiotensin-aldosterone system and results in sodium retention, and water naturally follows. Hypoalbuminemia from impaired synthetic function also contributes to edema.

What are causes of unilateral peripheral edema?
When edema is confined to a single extremity, then systemic causes become less likely. Instead, consider local processes at the limb involved that may be the culprit. Cellulitis can cause edema because of local inflammation resulting in increased capillary permeability. Patients with history of trauma or surgery can suffer damage of the lymphatics causing retention of fluid. Additionally, deep vein thrombosis (DVT) is a common cause of unilateral edema, usually caused by vascular obstruction of venous return from the affected limb.

The patient denies trauma to the left leg and subjective fevers or chills. She has no prior medical or surgical history. Her family history is noncontributory. She has smoked 10 cigarettes per day for the past 4 years, drinks alcohol on the weekends, and uses marijuana occasionally. She takes an oral contraceptive pill daily and denies allergies. Exam reveals 2+ nonpitting edema with associated erythema. Peripheral pulses are palpable.

What are risk factors for development of DVT?
Given the lack of trauma or surgery to the affected leg and no systemic signs of infection, DVT becomes our likely diagnosis. Risk factors for DVT are described by Virchow's triad:

175

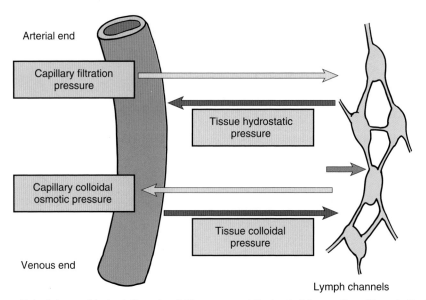

Arterial end

Capillary filtration pressure

Tissue hydrostatic pressure

Capillary colloidal osmotic pressure

Tissue colloidal pressure

Venous end

Lymph channels

Figure 21.1   Balance of hydrostatic and colloid pressures at the level of the capillary. *(From Aukland K, Reed RK. Interstitial-lymphatic mechanisms in the control of extracellular fluid volume. Physiol Rev. 1993;73:1-78.)*

hypercoagulability, injury to the vascular endothelium, and variation in blood flow. Any condition that affects these three parameters will predispose to development of a DVT. This includes pregnancy, malignancy, inherent disorders of coagulation, birth control, smoking, surgery, immobilization, and nephrotic syndrome.

CLINICAL PEARL   **STEP 2/3**

Occult malignancy should always be considered in patients with recurrent idiopathic DVT. 1.8% of patients with this finding are diagnosed with malignancy within 2 years of the initial clot. Given this finding, age-appropriate malignancy evaluation should be done in these patients.

How would you proceed with her care to make a diagnosis?

D-dimer levels in the serum and compression ultrasonography are primary modalities for diagnosing DVT. However, knowing the pretest probability of your presumed diagnosis is important as it determines the usefulness of your tests. The Wells score for DVT (see Table 21.1) helps stratify patients into low, moderate, or high risk based on clinical findings in the history or exam. For low-risk patients, a D-dimer is sufficient to exclude DVT, but for higher-risk patients, compression ultrasound becomes the diagnostic test of choice.

BASIC SCIENCE PEARL   **STEP 1**

Pretest probability is the likelihood of a patient having a positive test and is dependent upon the prevalence of the disease and associated risk factors. For example, the pretest probability of a positive cardiac stress test is high in men over age 65 with history of chest pain, hypertension, and diabetes.

TABLE 21.1 ■ The Wells Probability Score for Predicting Deep Vein Thrombosis

Clinical Characteristic	Score
Active cancer (treatment within past 6 months or palliative)	1
Calf swelling ≥3 cm compared to asymptomatic calf (measured 10 cm below tibial tuberosity)	1
Collateral superficial veins (nonvaricose)	1
Pitting edema (confined to symptomatic leg)	1
Swelling of entire leg	1
Localized tenderness along distribution of deep venous system	1
Paralysis, paresis, or recent cast immobilization of lower extremities	1
Recently bedridden ≥3 days or major surgery requiring regional or general anesthetic in the previous 12 weeks	1
Previously documented deep vein thrombosis	1
Alternative diagnosis at least as likely as deep vein thrombosis	−2

Note: A score of ≥2 indicates that probability of deep vein thrombosis is likely; a score of <2 indicates that a probability of deep vein thrombosis is unlikely.
(From Wells PS, Anderson DR, Bormanis J, et al. Value of assessment of pretest probability of deep-vein thrombosis in clinical management. *Lancet.* 1997;350[9094]:1795-1798.)

What inherited coagulopathies should be considered for recurrent DVT?
Numerous inherited defects of coagulation have been identified and include factor V Leiden (most common), protein C/S deficiency, antithrombin 3 deficiency, antiphospholipid antibodies, and hyperhomocysteinemia. Testing for each can be time consuming and expensive with relatively low yield. Thus, exhaustive workup should be reserved for those with thrombi occurring at a young age, family history of clots, recurrent thrombosis, or atypical locations, especially arterial thrombi in the absence of predisposing risks.

CLINICAL PEARL   **STEP 2/3**

Factor V Leiden is the most common inherited disorder of coagulation and affects 8% of the population. Risk of clot formation is substantially increased with homozygous inheritance. Antiphospholipid antibodies include the lupus anticoagulant, beta-2 glycoprotein, and anticardiolipin antibodies. Arterial thrombosis is more common in this disorder as well as hyperhomocysteinemia.

D-dimer is elevated >10,000 mcg/mL. Compression ultrasonography is ordered of the bilateral lower extremities and reveals extensive thrombosis of the left popliteal vein extending to the left femoral vein.

How should therapy be instituted for this patient?
Traditionally, warfarin had been the standard of care for treatment of DVT, but with the advent of newer drugs including low molecular weight heparin, factor 10a inhibitors, and direct thrombin inhibitors, our arsenal is far more varied. Because we all love the coagulation cascade, Figure 21.2 shows how each class of drug exerts its effect on clot formation to prevent further propagation

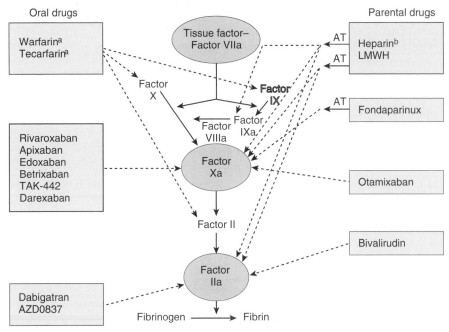

Figure 21.2 Coagulation cascade with current sites of potential pharmacologic action. *(From Davis EM, Packard KA, Knezevich JT, Campbell JA. New and emerging anticoagulant therapy for atrial fibrillation and acute coronary syndrome. Pharmacotherapy. 2011;31[10]:975-1016.)*

of any thrombi, thereby allowing for natural fibrinolysis and resolution of the remaining clot. For patients who cannot undergo chemical anticoagulation or have failed other therapies and have lower extremity DVT, inferior vena cava filters are a viable option to prevent propagation of large pulmonary emboli. They do not prevent recurrence of clots and are in fact a risk for clot formation themselves.

CLINICAL PEARL   **STEP 2/3**

With the new oral anticoagulants becoming more popular, be prepared for questions to begin appearing on exams. Remember that these agents are approved for treatment of DVT and nonvalvular atrial fibrillation. They are exorbitantly expensive compared to warfarin but do not need to be followed for levels in clinic. They are contraindicated in chronic kidney disease because of primarily renal clearance. Additionally, there are no approved antidotes for patients taking these agents and presenting with severe bleeding.

Confusion is common in determining the length of anticoagulation. Try to remember that long-term anticoagulation always will be favored in those with recurrent DVT or who have significant irreversible risk factors for developing further clots. Additionally, never anticoagulate patients with absolute contraindications (see Table 21.2). To summarize, patients with a first DVT and a known reversible cause should be treated for 3 months. Unprovoked DVT occurring for the first time can be treated for 3 months followed by a D-dimer assay. If positive, continued anticoagulation is preferred. Patients with DVT and malignancy should be treated with low molecular weight heparin indefinitely or until the cancer resolves because of its mortality benefit

TABLE 21.2 ▓ **Absolute and Relative Contraindications for Chronic Anticoagulation**

Absolute	Propensity to bleed
	Active bleeding processes
	Severe, uncontrollable hypertension
	Hemorrhagic retinopathy
	Intracranial aneurysm or neoplasm
	History of intracranial hemorrhage or severe liver or kidney disease
Relative	Chronic liver disease
	Nonbleeding active gastroduodenal ulcer
	Hiatal hernia
	Steatorrhea
	Chronic alcoholism
	Pregnancy
	Low cognitive status
	Pericarditis with effusion
	Mental disorder

(Perez IM, Garcia, JM, Castroseiros EF, et al. Use of anticoagulation at the time of discharge in patients with heart failure and atrial fibrillation. *Rev Esp Cardiol.* 2003;56:880-887.)

over warfarin. Recent studies suggest that direct thrombin inhibitors, as opposed to indirect inhibitors (such as heparin and warfarin) or factor Xa inhibitors, are associated with increased risk for coronary thrombosis.

BASIC SCIENCE/CLINICAL PEARL   **STEP 1/2/3**

Immediate initiation of anticoagulation for patients with DVT is crucial. Studies have shown improved mortality for treated patients because of lower incidence of recurrent DVT and pulmonary embolism. Remember to bridge warfarin with a heparin agent until the international normalized ratio (INR) is therapeutic due to the paradoxical hypercoagulation that occurs with vitamin K antagonists as protein C and S levels tend to drop prior to other factors.

The patient's DVT is attributed to combined oral contraceptive pill use and smoking. You counsel her on the risks of further DVT and she elects to stop oral contraceptive pill use and quit smoking. She receives a 3-month course of warfarin with resolution.

Two years later, you are paged to the emergency room to evaluate a new patient for acute onset shortness of breath and chest pain. To your surprise, it is the same patient. She reports edema of the left lower extremity, similar to her prior occurrence, and had been planning to make a visit to her primary care physician when she developed onset of shortness of breath and chest pain. Her chest pain is aggravated with deep inspiration and vital signs reveal tachycardia and tachypnea.

What is your differential diagnosis for chest pain?
A common presenting complaint to any clinic, emergency room, or hospitalized patient is chest pain, so it is crucial to have a broad differential to guide your workup. Some advocate a "what is

the worst thing this could be?" and "what is the most likely thing this could be?" approach to chest pain. Our "worst things" are myocardial infarction, dissecting aortic aneurysm, and pulmonary embolism as each carries high mortality. Less emergent causes are gastroesophageal reflux disease and musculoskeletal disorders. If we ask ourselves what is most likely for this patient with prior history of DVT, current complaints of recurrent DVT, pleuritic pain and tachycardia, then pulmonary embolism becomes our number one concern.

How should you proceed with her care to make a diagnosis?

We have numerous tools that can help confirm our diagnosis, though some are more helpful than others. An arterial blood gas can be done with typical findings in patients suffering from pulmonary embolism being a respiratory alkalosis (due to tachypnea) and an increased alveolar-arterial gradient (due to ventilation/perfusion [V/Q] mismatch). However, this finding is not specific for pulmonary embolism. Electrocardiogram (ECG) findings most commonly show tachycardia, but with larger pulmonary embolism it is possible to see right axis deviation as a possible consequence of right ventricular strain. Classically reported is the S1/Q3/T3 or a deep S wave in lead 1, Q wave in lead 3, and an inverted T wave in lead 3 (see Fig. 21.3).

Chest radiograph (CXR) most commonly is normal but helps exclude other diagnoses. Keep in mind the classic findings on CXR for patients with pulmonary emboli. These are Hampton's hump, Westermark's sign, atelectasis, and pleural effusions. Examples of Hampton's hump and Westermark's sign are shown in Figure 21.4 and Figure 21.5.

What imaging modalities can be used to diagnose pulmonary embolism?

Pulmonary angiogram is the gold standard for diagnosis but is invasive and requires contrast exposure. Ventilation-perfusion scans were the most commonly used modality prior to computed tomography pulmonary angiograms (CTPA) but are still useful for ruling out pulmonary embolism in the presence of a normal CXR, those that cannot receive intravenous (IV) contrast, or if chronic pulmonary embolism is a concern. The current preferred test is the CTPA because of its ease of use and high sensitivity and specificity.

BASIC SCIENCE PEARL   **STEP 1**

Statistics in some form or shape will be represented on exams, and questions can be as simple as knowing the definition of statistical terms. These are the "gimme" points and cannot be missed. Remember, sensitivity is the proportion of people with a disease who test positive for it, whereas specificity is the proportion of people without a disease who test negative for it. Sensitive tests are good for screening because they have low false-negative rates. Specific tests are good for confirmatory testing.

A CTPA is ordered and reveals a left middle segmental pulmonary embolism. The patient is still tachycardic and tachypneic but otherwise is hemodynamically stable.

Diagnosis: Pulmonary embolism

What therapy should be instituted for this patient and how would it change if she were hypotensive and hypoxemic?

Her pulmonary embolism should be treated similarly to her DVT that she had 2 years prior. Unfractionated or low molecular weight heparin should be started immediately and then a decision made regarding choice of a long-term anticoagulant. Assuming she stopped smoking and is no longer on oral contraceptive pills, she now falls under the category of recurrent DVT and

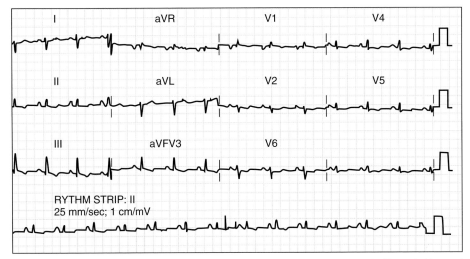

Figure 21.3 ECG with S1/Q3/T3 findings. *(From Davis EM, Packard KA, Knezevich JT, et al. New and emerging anticoagulant therapy for atrial fibrillation and acute coronary syndrome. Pharmacotherapy. 2011;31[10]:975-1016.)*

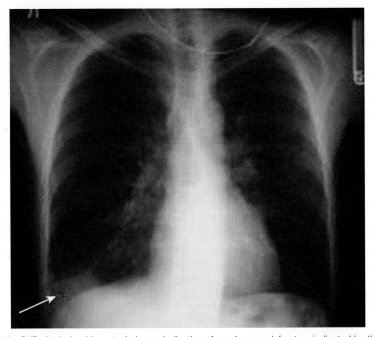

Figure 21.4 CXR displaying Hampton's hump indicative of a pulmonary infarct as indicated by the arrow.

should be treated lifelong. Strong consideration should be given to looking for an underlying thrombophilic condition.

In the event this patient was admitted with severe hypotension or hypoxemia in the presence of a pulmonary embolism, tissue plasminogen activator (tPA) should be given as long as no absolute contraindications are present. The risk of intracranial bleed following tPA is about 3%. For patients who are not candidates, mechanical thrombectomy can be attempted in experienced

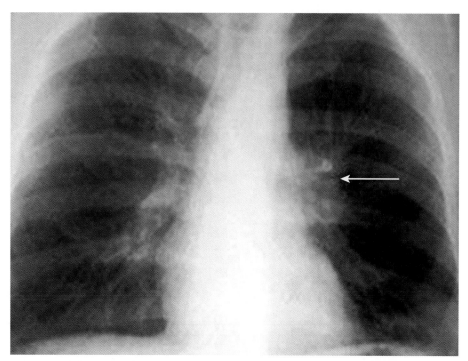

Figure 21.5 CXR displaying Westermark's sign indicating loss of vascular markings distal to embolus as indicated by the arrow.

centers though mortality is high. Table 21.3 lists absolute and relative contraindications for tPA administration.

When can patients be treated as outpatients for pulmonary embolism?

After diagnosis of pulmonary embolism, decisions should be made regarding the aggressiveness of therapy. As detailed above, tPA is indicated for patients who demonstrate clinical instability. The pulmonary embolism severity index stratifies 30-day mortality for patients with pulmonary embolism. Those with very low risk (0 to 1.6%) can be treated as outpatients.

BEYOND THE PEARLS

- Both pneumatic compression devices and prophylactic chemical anticoagulation have been shown to reduce risk of DVT formation in hospitalized patients.
- Low molecular weight heparin has a mortality benefit for patients with DVT and malignancy that goes beyond simply the anticoagulative effect. It is believed that low molecular weight heparin also provides additional benefit by suppressing the vascular growth factors that are released by malignant tumors.
- ECGs are fast, safe bedside exams that can be done to evaluate for signs of right ventricular strain best described as paradoxical bowing of the intraventricular septum to the left during systole.
- Patients with evidence of right heart strain on ECG or biochemical markers (brain natriuretic peptide, troponin) are defined as having submassive pulmonary embolism (PE).
- Patients with submassive PE can be considered for tPA to prevent development of pulmonary hypertension, though there is no mortality benefit.

TABLE 21.3 ■ **Absolute and Relative Contraindications for tPA Administration**

Absolute contraindications	History of hemorrhagic stroke
	Known intracranial neoplasia (primary or metastatic)
	Known intracranial vascular malformation (fistula or aneurism)
	Nonhemorrhagic stroke in the previous 3 months
	Suspicion of aortic dissection
	Active bleeding or known hemorrhagic diathesis (excluding menses)
	Significant cranial or facial surgery or trauma in previous 3 months
Relative contraindications (individual assessment of risk/benefit ratio)	Uncontrolled hypertension on admission (>180/110 mm Hg)*
	History of chronic, severe, or poorly controlled HTN
	History of previous CVA or other intracerebral disease not included in absolute contraindications
	Prolonged or traumatic CPR (>10 min) or major surgery in the previous 3 weeks
	Recent internal bleeding (previous 2 to 4 weeks)
	Noncompressible vascular punctures
	Pregnancy
	Chronic anticoagulant use (INR >2-3)
	Active peptic ulcer

*In patients with low-risk AMI, this would be an absolute contraindication.
AMI, Acute myocardial infarction; *CPR,* cardiopulmonary resuscitation; *CVA,* cerebrovascular accident; *HTN,* hypertension; *INR,* international normalized ratio.
(Khatri P, Wechsler LR, Broderick, JP. Intracranial hemorrhage associated with revascularization therapies. *Stroke.* 2007;38:431-440.)

References

Aukland K, Reed RK. Interstitial-lymphatic mechanisms in the control of extracellular fluid volume. *Physiol Rev.* 1993;73:1-78.

Davidson BL. The association of direct thrombin inhibitor anticoagulants with cardiac thromboses. *Chest.* 2015;147(1):21-24.

Davis EM, Packard KA, Knezevich JT, Campbell JA. New and emerging anticoagulant therapy for atrial fibrillation and acute coronary syndrome. *Pharmacotherapy.* 2011;31(10):975-1016.

Kearon C, Akl EA, Comerote AJ, et al. Antithrombotic therapy for VTE disease: antithrombotic therapy and prevention of thrombosis, 9th ed: American College of Chest Physicians evidence-based clinical practice guidelines. *Chest.* 2012;141:e419s-e494s.

Khatri P, Wechsler LR, Broderick JP. Intracranial hemorrhage associated with revascularization therapies. *Stroke.* 2007;38:431-440.

Konstantinides SV, Torbicki A, Agnelli G, et al. 2014 ESC guidelines on the diagnosis and management of acute pulmonary embolism. *Eur Heart J.* 2014;35(43):3033-3069.

PIOPED Investigators. Value of the ventilation/perfusion scan in acute pulmonary embolism. Results of the prospective investigation of pulmonary embolism diagnosis. *JAMA.* 1990;263(20):2753-2759.

Segal JB, Streiff MB, Hofmann LV, Thornton K, Bass EB. Management of venous thromboembolism: a systematic review for a practice guideline. *Ann Intern Med.* 2007;146(3):211-222.

Carla LoPinto-Khoury ■ John Khoury

A 25-Year-Old Male With Seizures

A 25-year-old male is brought to the emergency room by ambulance after having a witnessed seizure while at a football game. In the emergency room, he is lethargic and unable to provide a coherent history. No family members are currently available, but a friend who was at the game is at his bedside.

What questions are important to ask witnesses about the convulsion to determine what caused his seizure?

Was he was sitting or standing at the time of the seizure? What prodromal symptoms did he exhibit and for how long (i.e., did he complain of any headache, lightheadedness, or nausea, or did he stare blankly or behave oddly, like smack his lips or pick absently at his clothes)? What sort of movements did he make during the seizure itself (i.e., were his eyes opened or closed, did he forcibly turn his head or body during the seizure, did he twitch his face or one side of his body first, did his limbs stiffen first then shake or just stiffen or shake or neither)? Was he responsive during the seizure or did he vocalize or cry out? Did he fall? How long did the seizure itself last if it could be timed?

The semiology of a seizure is important to determine its type and cause. *Semiology* refers to the pattern of behavior. The prodrome is a nonspecific set of preceding symptoms that may last for hours before a seizure, like feeling fatigued or having headaches; however, an *aura* is typically a very specific set of psychosensory symptoms that precedes a seizure by a minute or less (classically deja-vu, a rising epigastric sensation like nausea, a foul taste or smell). Physiologically, an aura is the beginning of a focal epileptic seizure before it has spread enough to cause obvious motor or behavioral symptoms. Seizure semiology can vary considerably depending on the type, location, and spread of a seizure.

CLINICAL PEARL	STEP 2/3

Not all seizures have auras—only *focal* or *partial-onset* seizures should have auras, and not every focal seizure has an identifiable aura.

What are some different types of seizures?

Epileptic seizures can either be generalized, meaning starting in both hemispheres at once, or focal/partial in onset, meaning starting within one hemisphere then spreading. Typical motor seizure types are *tonic-clonic*, in which the limbs first stiffen then shake, and *clonic*, in which one or both sides of the body shake. *Absence seizures* are a very specific subtype of childhood-onset generalized seizures in which a patient stares briefly. However, focal or partial-onset seizures may also involve staring and unresponsiveness with or without automatisms like lip smacking or absent picking at clothes and little or no motor activity (these are termed *complex partial or focal seizures* and should not be called *absence*). The terms *grand mal* and *petit mal* seizures are old terms that can be misused and should be clarified when taking a history.

BASIC SCIENCE PEARL **STEP 1**

Ethosuximide is the classic treatment option for childhood absence epilepsy. It is not indicated for complex partial seizures, which may resemble absence seizures as they both may involve staring spells.

How do you correctly distinguish epileptic seizures from other types of events?

Certain features of the history will lead one to consider a diagnosis other than an epileptic seizure. Syncope is often positional, preceded by nonspecific symptoms including lightheadedness or chest pain, and seen in the context of illness, dehydration, or to a strong emotional stimulus causing a vagal response. Eye closure can be seen with syncope or with psychogenic, nonepileptic seizures (PNES, often termed *pseudoseizures*). Brief, bilateral convulsions may be seen with syncope as well (termed *convulsive syncope*), but this can be confusing because some seizures, namely myoclonic seizures, might look similar. A typical seizure lasts for 2 to 3 minutes, so seizure durations of longer than 5 minutes either indicate status epilepticus or a nonepileptic event. A patient returning to baseline quickly (within a few seconds) without a period of postictal confusion or lethargy after a prolonged, convulsive event is less likely to have had a true epileptic seizure. Responsiveness during an event of bilateral clonic activity is also less likely to be an epileptic seizure, as involvement of the bilateral motor regions is unlikely to be seen in isolation without diffuse bilateral cerebral dysfunction causing altered state of awareness.

On the other hand, patients may vocalize incoherently during partial-onset seizures, and odd, complex, and almost psychotic-appearing behavior is common with frontal lobe seizures. An ictal cry is a disturbing sound made during tonic contraction of the diaphragm usually during a generalized tonic-clonic seizure. Lateral tongue bites, urinary or bowel incontinence, and injuries such as fractures or dislocations are also strongly suggestive of epileptic seizures. Cataplexy seen in narcolepsy may be another seizure mimic, but cataplexy is a sudden loss of muscle tone often at the knees that is triggered by an emotional response and has preserved consciousness.

The patient's friend reports that they were walking together to the concession stand when the patient suddenly stopped, was not answering questions, and instead stared straight ahead. For a second or two his mouth twitched, then he suddenly fell down, his body stiffened then shook "all over"; the friend thinks the patient's eyes were open and "rolled back" and he was "foaming" at the mouth. He thinks the seizure lasted less than 5 minutes altogether. He thinks his friend wet himself and bit his tongue because blood was coming out of his mouth.

On exam, the patient is afebrile, blood pressure is 125/80 mm Hg, pulse rate is 90/min, respiration rate is 14/min, and oxygen saturation is 100% on room air, and he is currently arousable but disoriented to time and place. His general exam reveals abrasions on his scalp and elbows and a left lateral tongue laceration. His pupils are 4 mm and equally reactive to light, and on his motor exam his left arm and leg drift downward slightly when raised. His reflexes are 2+ and symmetric and there is no Babinski sign.

Does it seem that the patient had an epileptic seizure? What type of seizure does it sound like, and why does it seem that he had it? What are the next steps for the evaluation of this patient?

The history provided by the witness is fairly convincing for a true epileptic seizure, likely a tonic-clonic seizure. The brief period of staring and unresponsiveness, twitching of the face, and a postictal Todd's paralysis of the left side of the body might suggest a focal or partial-onset seizure arising from the right hemisphere, but a generalized seizure is entirely possible even with these features. At this point, we do not know whether he has had similar seizures in his history, in which case perhaps he has epilepsy. He may have had a provoked seizure, such as from intoxication (i.e., from cocaine, phencyclidine [PCP]), alcohol or benzodiazepine withdrawal, diabetic ketoacidosis or hypoglycemia, or infection (meningitis—although at this time he is afebrile) or to an acute structural lesion in the brain like a brain hemorrhage, neoplasm, abscess, or even an infarction.

How is epilepsy defined?

Epilepsy is defined as the presence of two or more unprovoked seizures occurring greater than 24 hours apart, or a single seizure with a risk of recurrence greater than 60% in the next 10 years. The risk of recurrence after a single unprovoked seizure varies in the literature but is about 30% or less in absence of an abnormal electroencephalogram (EEG), family history of epilepsy, seizure from waking (nocturnal seizures carry a higher recurrence rate), abnormal perinatal or developmental history, a history of febrile convulsions, a history of central nervous system (CNS) infections or trauma, or known structural lesions.

CLINICAL PEARL   **STEP 2/3**

Brain trauma if recent (within 1 week) may be considered a provoking factor for an isolated seizure.

The patient undergoes head computed tomography (CT), which is normal, and lab work reveals a normal urine drug screen, elevated white blood cell count of 14,000/µL, normal electrolytes, and a serum glucose of 85 mg/dL. A phenytoin level is measured at 8 mg/dL, which is subtherapeutic (normal range is 10 to 20 mg/dL). At this time, his father arrives and explains that the patient has a history of epilepsy since he was a teenager and was taking phenytoin for years. The patient is still not completely awake and alert, and has a milder left-sided hemiparesis. The emergency room orders a fosphenytoin load of 10 mg/kg and he is admitted to the medicine service after having a seizure without returning to baseline mental status.

What is the reason to admit to the hospital for this patient?

The patient is being admitted to evaluate for concerns of status epilepticus. Status epilepticus is defined as a single seizure lasting more than 5 minutes or two or more seizures without a return to baseline mental status in between. This may simply be a case of a prolonged postictal state, but he might have ongoing subclinical or nonconvulsive seizures and might be at risk of having further convulsive seizures.

An EEG is ordered by the medicine resident on the advice of a phone consultation with the neurologist to rule out nonconvulsive status epilepticus. However, as the technician arrives to the patient's room on the medical floor, the patient begins to have tonic-clonic activity lasting 3 minutes. Intravenous (IV) lorazepam 2 mg is ordered immediately and administered. The shaking ceases but the patient is still lethargic, he is tachycardic to 120/min, respiration rate is 18/min, and his oxygen saturation is 95% on room air.

What is the next step in treating this patient?
The patient is now in clinical status epilepticus. He appears to not be in danger of respiratory failure, thus intubation at this time is not necessary; however, admission to an intensive care unit would be appropriate. If his seizures recur without return to baseline, then repeated boluses of IV lorazepam 2 mg up to 8 mg total or IV diazepam 10 mg can be given with careful consideration of the need for intubation. Phenytoin (best given as a bolus of fosphenytoin through a peripheral IV to avoid peripheral necrosis or "purple glove" syndrome) is also on the standard algorithm to treat status epilepticus but has already been given to this patient. Another phenytoin level may be drawn, but in the meantime, a second antiepileptic medication can be considered. Valproate or levetiracetam is commonly used next in the algorithm.

The patient has yet another 2-minute seizure after 15 minutes and a second dose of lorazepam is administered. Pulse oximetry remains above 95%, but oxygen is now administered via nasal cannula. His outpatient pharmacy is contacted, and he is actively prescribed two antiepileptic medications: phenytoin and levetiracetam. Levetiracetam is then administered intravenously. No further seizures are reported overnight. The next morning, he is back to his baseline mental status, his repeat phenytoin level is 18 mg/dL, and he is discharged on his home medications (phenytoin 200 mg orally twice daily and levetiracetam 1000 mg orally twice daily) with follow up with the office in one week as an outpatient.

Why did this patient likely have this admission for status epilepticus? What should be considered in the follow up of this patient and need for specialist care?
In this patient with epilepsy on chronic antiepileptic medication, nonadherence to the medication regimen is a probable trigger for status epilepticus. Adverse reactions to medications can cause patients not to adhere to their medication regimens. Other triggers for seizures in patients with epilepsy include underlying infections, substance use, and sleep deprivation. In approximately one third of patients with epilepsy, their seizures can be refractory to medical management alone and surgical options such as resective surgery (often of the temporal lobe) or neurostimulation (i.e., vagus nerve stimulator placement) might be considered.

CLINICAL PEARL   **STEP 2/3**

If you are presented a case of a compliant patient who has failed multiple medications, referral to an epilepsy specialist is highly recommended. The specialist will reconfirm the epilepsy diagnosis, usually through epilepsy monitoring, and consider surgical approaches to treatment.

The patient arrived at his one-week appointment complaining of sluggishness and imbalance. He is mildly ataxic on exam. His father is with him and reports that his son is moody and irritable. A phenytoin level drawn the day before is 24 mg/dL. He reports compliance with both medications but says that last night he woke up with his tongue bitten again and the bed sheets wet.

What is the reason for the patient's symptoms? What is the next best step in this patient's treatment and evaluation?
The patient is experiencing ataxia and sedation due to slight phenytoin toxicity, and his irritability is probably an adverse effect of levetiracetam. Decreasing his dose of phenytoin to 300 mg daily

will reduce his toxicity symptoms, but the patient is still having seizures despite taking his medications. A referral to a neurologist is required, who will likely request an EEG if not already done, and a brain magnetic resonance imaging (MRI) scan.

Diagnosis: Medically refractory epilepsy and status epilepticus

The patient returns for a follow-up visit 1 year later asking for medical clearance for a temporal lobectomy. The neurologist's note states that he had an MRI demonstrating right-sided mesial temporal sclerosis, and his EEGs demonstrated right temporal sharp waves. He is currently taking lamotrigine and oxcarbazepine as his antiepileptic medications. He reports a much better mood and lower side effects, but he still has occasional seizures and wishes to proceed with surgery. His exam is normal, but his lab work demonstrates a sodium level of 131 mmol/L (the normal threshold is 134 mmol/L).

CLINICAL PEARL   STEP 2/3

In women who are already taking lamotrigine, oral contraceptive pills will lower serum drug levels, as will pregnancy. Fortunately, the patient in this discussion is not affected by this problem.

What is the underlying reason for the hyponatremia?

Hyponatremia is a common side effect of medications including oxcarbazepine, carbamazepine, and phenytoin. Mild decreases in sodium can be monitored, but more severe decreases should be addressed with the neurologist for a possible therapy change as hyponatremia may provoke seizures.

The patient successfully undergoes a right anterior temporal lobectomy and comes back to your office 1 year later telling you that he is seizure free and is in the process of getting his driver's license back.

BEYOND THE PEARLS

- Over a dozen antiepileptic medications are available. Few head-to-head comparison studies are available for efficacy. However, some medications are indicated for partial-onset seizures rather than for generalized seizures: oxcarbazepine and carbamazepine are two of these. These two may even worsen generalized epilepsy such as juvenile myoclonic epilepsy. For primary generalized epilepsy, valproate or divalproex is considered to be most efficacious, although several safety concerns, especially teratogenicity for women of childbearing age, limit its use in many patients.
- "Newer" generation antiepileptic drugs, such as levetiracetam, lamotrigine, topiramate, zonisamide, oxcarbazepine, and lacosamide, are becoming more commonly prescribed because they have minimal to no effect on the hepatic enzymes responsible for drug metabolism. This reduces their drug–drug interactions compared to phenytoin, phenobarbital, primidone, and carbamazepine, which induce hepatic enzymes, and divalproex, which inhibits hepatic enzymes. Antibiotics, oral contraceptive pills,

BEYOND THE PEARLS—cont'd

chemotherapeutic agents, and cardiac medications are among those that utilize the hepatic enzyme system, and therefore patients with multiple comorbidities may have difficulty with using older-generation antiepileptic medications.

- When choosing an antiepileptic drug for a patient, it is often useful to consider his or her other comorbidities. For example, if a patient has both epilepsy and migraine, topiramate or divalproex may be useful to help treat both disorders. Patients who have a history of bipolar disorder may have both conditions managed with medications such as lamotrigine, divalproex, carbamazepine, or oxcarbazepine.

- Driving laws vary by state in the United States. In some states, a physician is required to report a patient who had a seizure or any loss of consciousness to the State Department of Motor Vehicles.

- A specialized epilepsy surgery center will have various options for surgical treatment of epilepsy for patients who do not have good control or seizure freedom with medication alone. For patients with severe refractory generalized epilepsy with falls, a corpus callosotomy can reduce falls and morbidity but does not cure seizures. Vagus nerve stimulation can reduce the frequency of seizures. Temporal lobectomy, however, can bring about complete seizure freedom in up to 70% of patients. Other types of surgeries, such as frontal lobectomy and multiple subpial transections, can bring about seizure freedom at lower rates. Responsive neurostimulation is a newer technology designed for patients who cannot have respective surgery because of the location of their seizure onset zone.

References

Kwan P, Brodie M. Early identification of refractory epilepsy. *N Engl J Med*. 2000;342:314-319.

Sperling MR, O'Connor MJ, Saykin AJ, Plummer C. Temporal lobectomy for refractory epilepsy. *JAMA*. 1996;276(6):470-475.

Wyllie E, ed. *Wyllie's Treatment of Epilepsy*. 6th ed. Philadelphia: Wolters Kluwer; 2015.

R. Michelle Koolaee

A 58-Year-Old Female With Dyspnea on Exertion and Renal Failure

A 58-year-old female presents for evaluation for 5 months of progressive dyspnea on exertion associated with a dry cough. She has a history of diffuse scleroderma (SSc) diagnosed 2 years prior, and her manifestations include sclerodactyly, Raynaud's phenomenon (RP), and gastro-esophageal reflux disease (GERD). She denies any fevers or recent travel history. Her medications include omeprazole twice daily and amlodipine.

CLINICAL PEARL   **STEP 2/3**

Despite the lack of specific randomized trials, experts believe that proton pump inhibitors (PPIs) should be used both for the treatment and prevention of SSc-related GERD. GERD symptoms in SSc patients can be subtle and can result in silent aspiration if not recognized and treated.

What are helpful ways to elicit a history of RP?

RP is an exaggerated response of the digits to cold temperatures and is characterized by distinct color changes of the skin of the digits. It is thought to be due to an abnormal vascular response, causing vasoconstriction of the digital arteries and cutaneous arterioles. An attack of RP classi-cally manifests as a triphasic color change, white to blue to red. RP is considered primary if not associated with an underlying disease (i.e., many young, thin females who are long-distance runners have primary RP; this is usually benign) and secondary RP if it is associated with a connective tissue disease.

BASIC SCIENCE PEARL   **STEP 1**

The white phase is due to excessive vasoconstriction and interruption of local blood flow. This phase is followed by a cyanotic phase, as the residual blood in the finger desaturates. The red phase is due to hyperemia as the attack subsides and blood flow is restored.

There is no standardized way to elicit a history of true RP. The author prefers these screening questions:

- Do your fingers change colors in the cold? If so, what colors? (The author prefers not to disclose the specific color changes, in order to allow the patient to describe what exactly occurs during an attack.)

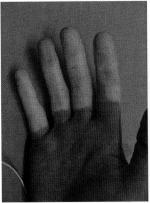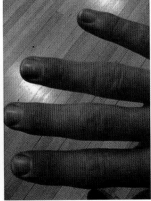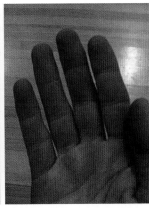

Figure 23.1   Raynaud's phenomenon involving the digits of the hand. *(Courtesy of* http://commons.wikimedia. org/wiki/File:Raynaud_phenomenon.jpg#filelinks*)*

TABLE 23.1 ▓ **Limited Versus Diffuse Systemic Scleroderma**

Features	Limited Scleroderma	Diffuse Scleroderma
Sclerodactyly	Distal to the wrists; spares the face and neck	Proximal to the wrists and knees; also affects the face, neck, and trunk
Raynaud's phenomenon	May be evident years before other features of limited SSc	RP and skin changes often occur closely together in time
Morbidity	PAH is more common in limited disease; the severity of PAH is correlated with the risk of premature death	Greater risks for renal (SRC), lung (ILD), and cardiac disease (pericardial/myocardial disease)
Other	Prominent vascular manifestations; may be classified as having the CREST syndrome (**C**alcinosis cutis, **R**aynaud phenomenon, **E**sophageal dysmotility, **S**clerodactyly, and **T**elangiectasia)	May also have vascular manifestations

ILD, Interstitial lung disease; *PAH,* pulmonary arterial hypertension; *RP,* Raynaud's phenomenon; *SRC,* scleroderma renal crisis; *SSc,* scleroderma.

• Are your fingers unusually sensitive in places such as the frozen food section of the grocery store?

What can be very helpful for the clinician is for the patient to take photographs of the digits during an episode of RP and show this to you during the visit (see Fig. 23.1).

How is diffuse SSc distinguished from limited SSc?

Table 23.1 describes clinical differences between diffuse and limited SSc.

On physical exam, the patient's blood pressure is 130/80 mm Hg, pulse rate is 70/min, respiration rate is 28/min, and oxygen saturation is 91% on room air. There are fine inspiratory rales at the lung bases. Cardiac exam reveals regular rhythm without murmurs. Dilated nailfold capillaries are present. Cutaneous exam reveals sclerodactyly of both hands as well as skin induration of the forearms and anterior chest. There are no digital ulcers.

TABLE 23.2 ■ Cutaneous Manifestations of Scleroderma

Skin Finding	Description
Sclerodactyly	Usually begins in the fingers, hands, and face; variable in extent and severity
Nail-bed abnormalities	Dilated and tortuous nail-fold capillaries alternating with capillary dropout; cuticular overgrowth
Skin pigment changes	"Salt and pepper" appearance of the affected skin due to areas of hypopigmentation alternating with areas of hyperpigmentation
Digital ulceration	As a result of severe skin thickening (resulting in skin breakdown) and/or poor peripheral circulation
Telangiectasias	Small dilated blood vessels near the surface of the skin; more frequently a feature of limited scleroderma
Calcinosis cutis	Soft tissue calcifications; more frequently a feature of limited scleroderma
Edema of the hands	Edematous swelling and erythema may precede skin induration; this may be associated with pruritus of the skin

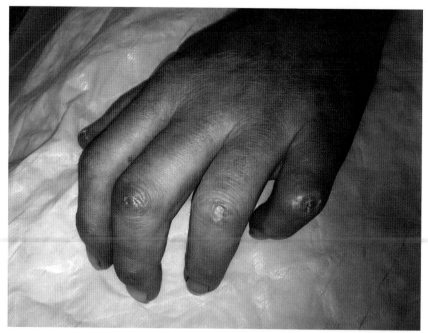

Figure 23.2 Sclerodactyly and resolving skin ulcerations, most prominent at the third and fifth proximal interphalangeal joints. (Courtesy of Dr. Chris Derk.)

What skin changes are seen in patients with SSc?

Table 23.2 describes the cutaneous manifestations of SSc. Figure 23.2 demonstrates a patient with sclerodactlyly and resolving skin ulcerations, most prominent at the third and fifth proximal interphalangeal joints. Figure 23.3 demonstrates classic "salt and pepper" skin changes seen in SSc.

What are possible causes of this patient's dyspnea?

Dyspnea in a patient with SSc should always prompt evaluation. Pulmonary involvement is seen in more than 70% of patients with SSc; the most common pulmonary manifestations include

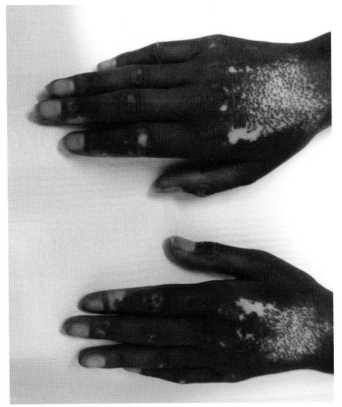

Figure 23.3 "Salt and pepper" skin changes apparent in the dorsal hand of a patient with diffuse SSc.

interstitial lung disease (ILD) and pulmonary vascular disease, leading to pulmonary arterial hypertension (PAH). PAH is amenable to medical management; this should be assessed for initially with a transthoracic echocardiogram (TTE). However, echocardiograms give both false-negative and false-positive results; right heart catheterization is essential to confirm the diagnosis and exclude other disease processes. Often severe and progressive, PAH can lead to cor pulmonale and right-sided heart failure.

CLINICAL PEARL   **STEP 2/3**

Typical features of ILD include progressive dyspnea, dry cough, and bibasilar "Velcro" crackles on auscultation. Most but not all patients will have crackles on auscultation. The breath sounds may be diminished or absent in patients with ILD. Thus, pulmonary function tests and chest radiograph should be ordered in anyone with SSc who complains of dyspnea.

BASIC SCIENCE/CLINICAL PEARL   **STEP 1/2/3**

A significant cause of morbidity and mortality in SSc arises from PAH, particularly in diffuse SSc. A TTE should be ordered annually as a screening tool in patients with SSc; right heart catheterization is the gold standard for diagnosis of PAH.

TABLE 23.3 ■ Initial Laboratory Tests

Complete blood count	Normal
Blood urea nitrogen	40 mg/dL
Serum creatinine	3.2 mg/dL
Urinalysis	2+ protein; 10-15 erythrocytes/HPF; 0-5 leukocytes/HPF; erythrocyte casts present
Antinuclear antibody	1 : 1280 dilution
Peripheral blood smear	No schistocytes
Anti-topoisomerase I (anti–Scl-70) antibodies	Positive

HPF, High power field.

Dyspnea may also be due to cardiac involvement. Patients with systemic cardiac involvement in SSc have a poor prognosis, with 5-year mortality rates greater than 60%. Often, cardiac involvement is a result of pulmonary hypertension, but primary cardiac involvement has been recognized. Primary cardiovascular manifestations of SSc include pericardial disease (i.e., symptomatic pericarditis, pericardial effusions), myocardial disease, conduction abnormalities, and cardiac arrhythmias. Myocardial fibrosis in SSc can lead to systolic or diastolic ventricular dysfunction. Furthermore, patients with SSc have an increased risk of acute myocardial infarction, even after adjusting for age, sex, and comorbidities.

Initial laboratory tests are provided in Table 23.3.

What is your differential diagnosis?

This is a 58-year-old female with diffuse SSc who presents with progressive dyspnea on exertion, acute renal failure, and microscopic hematuria associated with erythrocyte casts.

Erythrocyte casts characterize a nephritic urine sediment and indicate the presence of glomerulonephritis. Glomerulonephritis in the setting of a severely reduced estimated glomerular filtration rate raises suspicion for disorders that include mixed cryoglobulinemia, antineutrophil cytoplasmic antibody (ANCA)-associated vasculitides (i.e, granulomatosis with polyangiitis [GPA], microscopic polyangiitis [MPA], eosinophilic granulomatosis with polyangiitis [EGPA; formerly known as Churg-Strauss syndrome]), IgA nephropathy, Goodpasture's disease, and postinfectious glomerulonephritis. This patient does not have any symptoms of pulmonary hemorrhage; however, it is worth noting the diseases that are characterized by pulmonary hemorrhage and renal failure (also called pulmonary-renal syndrome); these include GPA, MPA, and Goodpasture's disease. Renal biopsy is essential to confirm diagnosis; certain autoantibody testing (i.e., ANCA testing) can also guide diagnosis. It is important to note that glomerulonephritis is not a common finding in patients with SSc.

CLINICAL PEARL	STEP 2/3

Diffuse alveolar hemorrhage (DAH) from all causes is confirmed via bronchoalveolar lavage. During the procedure, lavage aliquots are progressively more hemorrhagic, confirming the diagnosis. Hemosiderin-laden macrophages are also found in bronchoalveolar lavage fluid from DAH.

It is critical to consider scleroderma renal crisis (SRC) in anyone with SSc (particularly diffuse disease) who presents with renal failure. SRC is a potentially life-threatening complication and should be recognized and managed immediately. Patients with SRC typically present with the following findings:

- Abrupt onset of marked hypertension (although normotensive renal crisis occurs in approximately 10% of patients).

BASIC SCIENCE PEARL   **STEP 1**

The histopathologic changes in SRC occur in the glomeruli and the small arcuate and interlobular arteries. Findings include intimal proliferation with concentric "onion-skin" hypertrophy, leading to significant vessel narrowing; these findings are nonspecific and can be found in other causes of thrombotic microangiopathy (i.e., antiphospholipid syndrome, thrombocytopenic purpura/hemolytic uremic syndrome).

- The urine sediment is usually bland, with few cells or casts. The presence of glomerulonephritis (as in this patient) would not be characteristic for SRC and would suggest another etiology.
- Acute onset of renal failure.
- Additional findings may include headaches, blurred vision, hypertensive encephalopathy, pulmonary edema, thrombocytopenia, and characteristic findings on renal biopsy.
- Peripheral smear may reveal schistocytes (a sign of microangiopathic hemolytic anemia).

What is the role of autoantibody testing at this point in the patient's presentation?
This patient's diagnosis of diffuse SSc has already been established, so there is no role for autoantibody testing to diagnose SSc. Anti-topoisomerase I (anti–Scl-70) antibodies are associated with diffuse SSc as well as a higher incidence of ILD. There is no role for checking anticentromere antibodies (ACA), as these are more characteristic of limited SSc. Anti-RNA polymerase III antibodies are worthwhile to order for patients with diffuse SSc; these autoantibodies are associated with rapidly progressive skin disease, increased risk for SRC, as well as a possible increased risk for cancer. All three of these antibodies are specific for SSc but only moderately sensitive. Several other SSc-associated antibodies have more prognostic implications but are not readily available in all laboratories. In instances where there is concern for overlap with other systemic rheumatic diseases, other antibodies (i.e., rheumatoid factor, antibodies to citrullinated peptides, lupus-associated antibodies) could be useful; however, not in this particular case.

BASIC SCIENCE PEARL   **STEP 1**

Over 95% of patients with SSc will have a positive ANA; consider alternate causes of fibrosing skin diseases if the ANA is negative (i.e., scleredema, nephrogenic systemic fibrosis). A significant proportion will also have a history of Raynaud's phenomenon.

BASIC SCIENCE PEARL   **STEP 1**

Be mindful of health care costs when ordering tests and understand that there is no role for repeating the ANA test serially, or following titers of the ANA test to follow disease activity.

Testing for ANCA antibodies plays more of a role for diagnosis of the ANCA-associated vasculitides (AAVs) and would be helpful in this patient with acute renal failure with glomerulonephritis. There are two types of ANCA assays currently used:

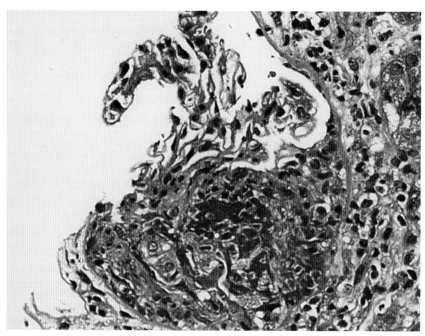

Figure 23.4 Trichrome stain reveals areas of fibrinoid necrosis (seen in red), also a feature of the ANCA-vasculitides.

- Indirect immunofluorescence assay (where there is a subjective component to interpretation; this describes either a cytoplasmic [c-ANCA] or perinuclear [p-ANCA] pattern).
- Enzyme-linked immunosorbent (ELISA) assay (which is a confirmatory test that targets vasculitis-specific antigens; in vasculitis, the two relevant target antigens are proteinase 3 [PR3] and myeloperoxidase [MPO]).

Of these two techniques, the immunofluorescence assay is more sensitive and the ELISA is more specific. There are pitfalls to reliance upon immunofluorescence alone, and so a positive c-ANCA or p-ANCA test should always be confirmed by antigen-specific ELISA testing (i.e., MPO-ANCA or PR3-ANCA). Furthermore, a positive ANCA test does not necessarily obviate the need for a renal biopsy, as in this case. Antiglomerular basement membrane (GBM) antibodies are associated with Goodpasture's disease and would also not be unreasonable to order.

Additional serologic testing reveals a positive p-ANCA/myeloperoxidase antibody (MPO-ANCA). A renal biopsy is performed and demonstrates a pauci-immune necrotizing crescentic glomerulonephritis (see Fig. 23.4). Computed tomography (CT) of the chest reveals patchy bilateral groundglass opacities with extensive honeycombing at the lung bases and periphery. A TTE is normal.

Diagnosis: ANCA-associated vasculitis associated with SSc; SSc-associated ILD

Is concurrent vasculitis a common finding with SSc?
AAV is an uncommon complication of SSc, and to date has been described only in case reports. In a review of 37 cases of SSc and AAV, the characteristics of patients include a mean age of

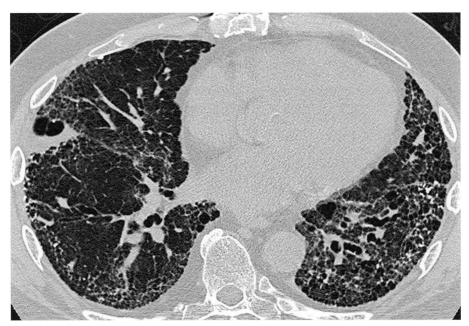

Figure 23.5   Multiple cystic air spaces are noted at the lung periphery, characteristic of honeycombing. Additionally noted are interstitial thickening, architectural distortion, and bronchiectasis. *(Courtesy of* http:// commons.wikimedia.org/wiki/File:UIP_[Usual_interstitial_pneumonia]-CT_scan_[4744513424].jpg*)*

57 ± 12 (19 to 82) years, 57% of whom have diffuse SSc, 97% with MPO-ANCA positivity, and 83% who present with rapidly progressive glomerulonephritis (RPGN). In terms of outcome, 51% had improvement, 14% progressed to end-stage renal disease (ESRD), and 34% died.

What is the significance of "honeycombing"?
Honeycombing is a feature of end-stage ILD and is characterized by clustered, multilayered, or multitiered cystic air spaces with well-defined walls, located mostly in the lung bases and periphery on CT imaging (see Fig. 23.5). Not all patients with ILD will have honeycombing, but when it is noted on imaging, it relays a poor prognosis.

How would you treat the renal disease in this patient?
Patients with AAV associated with severe end organ damage are treated aggressively with immunosuppressive therapy. This would include a "pulse" dose of methylprednisolone 1000 mg daily for 3 days, followed by prednisone or equivalent 1 mg/kg/day. Glucocorticoids are tapered over several months (and sometimes more); the rate of taper depends on clinical response. Patients with moderate to severe disease (as in this case) also receive either cyclophosphamide (oral or intravenous) or rituximab.

CLINICAL PEARL   **STEP 2/3**

Glucocorticoid use (particularly in doses ≥15 mg daily) is associated with a markedly increased risk of SRC; as a general rule, avoid glucocorticoids in SSc patients whenever possible. This patient has life-threatening organ damage, however, and without glucocorticoids has a high risk of morbidity and mortality.

How would you treat ILD in this patient?

There are currently no curative measures for SSc-associated ILD; advanced ILD carries a grim prognosis. In patients with severe SSc-associated ILD, cyclophosphamide is an option and has shown modest benefit; however, those benefits are lost after 24 months of follow-up. Mycophenolate mofetil (MMF) has shown stabilization or improvement in lung function and could be an option in the future. Targeting B cells with rituximab in patients with SSc-associated ILD resulted in significant improvements in forced vital capacity (FVC) and carbon monoxide diffusion capacity (DLCO) in a small study. Glucocorticoids are widely used to treat SSc-associated ILD with variable benefit; glucocorticoids as a general rule carry an increased risk for SRC so should be carefully used, if at all. In this case, however, the most acutely life-threatening feature is renal vasculitis; this does require glucocorticoid therapy. Selection of immunosuppressive agents should be focused first on the patient's renal vasculitis.

The patient receives a "pulse" dose of methylprednisolone 1000 mg daily for 3 days, followed by prednisone 1 mg/kg daily. She is also started on intravenous (IV) rituximab; the first dose of 1000 mg is administered inpatient and the second is given 2 weeks later. Within a week, her serum creatinine improves to 1.4 mg/dL and microscopic hematuria resolves. She is discharged with home oxygen therapy.

BEYOND THE PEARLS

- Autologous hematopoietic stem cell transplantation has shown efficacy in early diffuse SSc (particularly in those with ILD) but is associated with increased treatment-related mortality in the first year after treatment.
- Pirfenidone is a new antifibrotic agent (approved October 15, 2014, by the U.S. Food and Drug Administration [FDA]) that has shown efficacy in slowing ILD related to idiopathic pulmonary fibrosis (IPF). Its role in connective tissue disease–related ILD has not yet been defined but will likely be pursued in the near future.
- There is a strong association with SSc and primary biliary cirrhosis (PBC), a cholestatic liver disease characterized by inflammatory infiltrates and fibrosis within the portal tracts. Unexplained itching, right-upper-quadrant pain, elevated serum alkaline phosphatase, and/or presence of antimitochondrial antibodies are suggestive of PBC.
- Pregnancy is an absolute contraindication for women with PAH; the necessary increase in cardiac output cannot be achieved by these patients, resulting in right heart failure with significant morbidity and mortality.
- Very severe Raynaud's phenomenon can lead to digital ulcers and even necrosis, requiring surgical amputation. Aggressive vasodilator therapy is implemented in these patients. This includes an IV prostacyclin analog drip (i.e., alprostadil, epoprostenol) for 3 to 5 days; this may not necessarily heal the existing skin lesions but can potentially prevent involvement of other digits.
- SSc sine scleroderma is a rare form of disease characterized by visceral organ involvement and typical vascular features, without sclerodactyly.

References

Arad U, Balbir-Gurman A, Doenyas-Barak K, et al. Anti-neutrophil antibody associated vasculitis in systemic sclerosis. *Semin Arthritis Rheum.* 2011;41(2):223-229.

Chu SY, Chen YJ, Liu CJ, et al. Increased risk of acute myocardial infarction in systemic sclerosis: a nationwide population-based study. *Am J Med.* 2013;126(11):982.

Cooke JP, Marshall JM. Mechanisms of Raynaud's disease. *Vasc Med.* 2005;10(4):293-307.

Daoussis D, Liossis SN, Tsamandas AC, et al. Experience with rituximab in scleroderma: results from a 1-year, proof-of-principle study. *Rheumatology (Oxford)*. 2010;49:271-280.

Herzog EL, Mathur A, Tager AM, et al. Review: interstitial lung disease associated with systemic sclerosis and idiopathic pulmonary fibrosis: how similar and distinct? *Arthritis Rheumatol*. 2014;66(8):1967-1978.

Janosik DL, Osborn TG, Moore TL, et al. Heart disease in systemic sclerosis. *Semin Arthritis Rheum*. 1989;19(3):191.

Mukerjee D, St George D, Coleiro B, et al. Prevalence and outcome in systemic sclerosis associated pulmonary arterial hypertension: application of a registry approach. *Ann Rheum Dis*. 2003;62(11):1088.

Tashkin DP, Elashoff R, Clements PJ, et al. Effects of 1-year treatment with cyclophosphamide on outcomes at 2 years in scleroderma lung disease. *Am J Respir Crit Care Med*. 2007;176:1026-1034.

Brandon A. Miller

A 46-Year-Old Male Referred for Hyperglycemia

A 46-year-old male is referred to your primary care clinic after he was found to have a random blood sugar of 296 mg/dL at a health screening fair. He hasn't seen a primary care physician in over 20 years due to lack of insurance. As a result, he has no *known* past medical or surgical history and takes no medications. His family history is positive for heart disease in his father and type 2 diabetes in his mother. He currently works in construction and does not smoke, drink, or use illicit substances. His diet consists largely of prepackaged and fast foods, sports drinks, and sodas. Review of systems is positive for fatigue, urinary frequency, and thirst for the past several weeks that he attributes to working outside in the heat. He has noticed that his vision is blurry over the past several days. His blood pressure at the visit is 144/98 mm Hg, pulse rate is 82/min, and body mass index (BMI) is 30 kg/m² (he states that he used to weigh more, but lost 10 pounds recently, which he again attributes to work). The physical exam reveals a middle-aged male with central obesity in no distress. The skin exam discloses a hyperpigmented velvety-appearing rash (Fig. 24.1) on the back of his neck, but the remainder of the exam is otherwise unremarkable. He states that he was told to make an appointment with a primary care doctor because his elevated blood sugar could mean that he has diabetes.

Does your patient have diabetes?

Type 2 diabetes is a chronic disease with numerous adverse effects on health, but unfortunately many people are asymptomatic with it for years. As such, screening tests are recommended to diagnose the condition early so that lifestyle modifications and treatments can begin to prevent long-term complications. Several professional organizations, including the American Diabetes Association (ADA) and the U.S. Preventive Services Task Force (USPSTF), have guidelines for screening asymptomatic patients for diabetes. In general, patients over 45 years old or those with risk factors for developing diabetes such as obesity (BMI >25 kg/m²), hypertension, hypercholesterolemia, vascular disease, a sedentary lifestyle, or a family history of diabetes should be screened. Screening is accomplished using either a fasting plasma glucose (FPG) test (patients are asked not to have anything to eat or drink for 8 hours prior to having their blood drawn), hemoglobin A1C (HbA1C; a measure of the amount of glucose that attaches to proteins on red blood cells over time) or an oral glucose tolerance test (OGTT; a test rarely used in clinical practice in which a patient is given an oral glucose load and the blood sugar level is measured 2 hours later). A diagnosis of diabetes is made when either the:

- FPG is ≥126 mg/dL,
- HbA1C is ≥6.5% or
- Plasma glucose ≥200 mg/dL 2 hours after an oral glucose load.

A fourth way to diagnose diabetes is by a random (without regard for time since last meal) plasma glucose level that is ≥200 mg/dL with accompanying signs and symptoms of hyperglycemia like fatigue, weight loss, polydipsia, and polyuria. This patient has all of the symptoms of hyperglycemia and a random plasma glucose of 296 mg/dL; therefore, he does have type 2 diabetes.

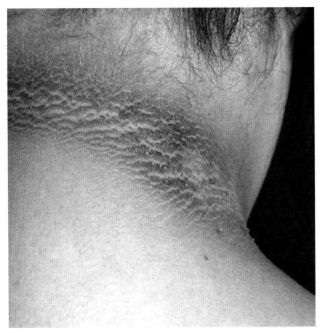

Figure 24.1   Acanthosis nigricans.

Diagnosis: Type 2 diabetes mellitus

What elements of the physical exam are important for you to focus on in an outpatient with type 2 diabetes?

Elevated blood sugar damages the walls of blood vessels (from capillaries to arteries) and nerves. The physical exam in patients with type 2 diabetes should focus on uncovering findings that suggest that microvascular/macrovascular or neurologic complications have occurred. Microvascular damage can be apparent in the capillaries in the retina (retinopathy), glomeruli (nephropathy), and nerves (both sensory and autonomic; neuropathy). Fundoscopy should be attempted, though this is best accomplished with a dilated exam by an eye-care professional. Although nephropathy is difficult to assess on exam, lower extremity edema suggesting low oncotic pressure from glomerular protein loss can be a clue. Neuropathy should be assessed annually by performing a detailed exam of the foot. Vibration sense should be tested using a 128 Hz tuning fork on the big toe. A monofilament should be pressed against multiple areas on the plantar surface of the foot until it bends to test pressure sensation. A safety pin or broken tongue depressor should be used to test two-point discriminant sensation. Finally, ankle and patellar reflexes should be tested. Visual inspection of the feet should be performed to assess for areas of ulceration that a patient with decreased sensation may not feel. Open ulcers are a major risk factor for the development of infections in diabetics such as cellulitis and osteomyelitis. The toenails should be inspected for onychomycosis (as evidenced by yellow discoloration and hypertrophied nail matrix) and the interdigital areas assessed for tinea pedis (which can manifest as dry, cracked skin). Both conditions can create portals of entry for bacteria that can lead to cellulitis. Dorsalis pedis and posterior tibialis pulses should be assessed for strength and symmetry as diminished pulses are a macrovascular manifestation of diabetes.

The patient is curious to know how he got diabetes. You explain to him that in type 2 diabetes, environmental (obesity, sedentary lifestyle) and genetic factors converge to cause the disease. Being an excellent clinician, you don't want to miss any other potential causes of hyperglycemia and insulin resistance.

What are some secondary causes of diabetes and how can the physical exam be helpful in diagnosing them?

Type 2 diabetes is responsible for approximately 90% of the cases of diabetes. The remaining 10% of cases are type 1 diabetes (mostly patients who are teenagers or younger) and secondary forms. The disease process in type 2 diabetes starts with tissue resistance to insulin (the hormone responsible for allowing cells to uptake and metabolize glucose) due to dietary and genetic factors. As a result of less glucose available inside the cells to utilize, pancreatic beta cells continue to increase the production of insulin and the liver continues to produce glucose (via gluconeogenesis). If diabetes goes untreated for long enough, the pancreatic beta cells can "burn out" and lose their synthetic ability altogether.

Insulin resistance and the ensuing elevated circulating levels of both glucose and insulin are responsible for a number of historical and physical findings. Insulin resistance and the decreased uptake of glucose into cells for use in cellular metabolism is responsible for the patient's fatigue and weight loss. Elevated levels of insulin are responsible for acanthosis nigricans, the hyperpigmented velvety rash your patient has on his neck. Elevated levels of blood glucose are responsible for increasing the osmolality of his blood leading to increased urination (osmotic diuresis), increased thirst, and dehydration and can also result in blurry vision due to swelling of the lens.

Though the etiology is different, secondary forms of diabetes can present in a similar fashion. Patients with recurrent pancreatitis can develop diabetes owing to beta cell destruction and pancreatic fibrosis. These patients have recurrent bouts of epigastric abdominal pain associated with nausea and vomiting, but sometimes patients can develop chronic, painless pancreatitis. The most common causes of pancreatitis include frequent alcohol use, medications, and elevated triglyceride levels. Therefore, a thorough review of the patient's social habits and medications is warranted. Hemochromatosis is an inherited disorder of increased iron absorption leading to iron deposition in the liver, pancreas, heart, joints, and skin. It can also be acquired via frequent blood transfusions. A patient presenting with darkened skin (due to iron deposition), joint pain, and new onset diabetes should prompt one to think of this disease, also known as "bronze diabetes."

Several endocrine conditions can cause secondary diabetes as well. Diabetes can be the first sign of acromegaly (caused by a growth hormone–secreting pituitary tumor) in approximately 5% of cases. However, the disease usually presents in adults with frontal bossing; enlargement of the tongue, lips, and nose; and occasionally carpal tunnel syndrome. Cushing's syndrome (in which excess cortisol stimulates the production of glucose leading to hyperinsulinemia) presents with a number of physical exam findings including proximal muscle weakness, central adiposity, a "buffalo hump," and purple striae on the abdomen that appear as stretch marks. Cushing's syndrome is caused by an adrenocorticotropic hormone (ACTH)–secreting tumor or exogenous glucocorticoids, so again, a thorough review of medications is always warranted. Lastly, pheochromocytoma is a rare tumor that secretes dopamine, epinephrine, and norepinephrine (all of which can stimulate glucose production) and presents with severe episodic hypertension, palpitations, sweating, flushing, and sometimes arrhythmia.

Finally, medications such as thiazide diuretics and beta blockers have been associated with the development of diabetes, though these medications are sometimes necessary to control blood pressure and other conditions frequently encountered in diabetics. Pentamidine, an antiparasitic medication used as prophylaxis or treatment for pneumocystis pneumonia in patients with acquired immune deficiency syndrome (AIDS), has been associated with insulin-dependent diabetes after its use. The atypical antipsychotics are also strongly correlated with the development of the metabolic syndrome and type 2 diabetes mellitus.

Your clinic is a busy one and you have only 20 minutes to spend with your patient today. He is overwhelmed with the new diagnosis and has so many questions he doesn't even know what to ask.

In the short period of time you have to spend with him today, what is important for you to accomplish?

Many patients are asymptomatic when they are diagnosed with diabetes and can be surprised to hear they have it. In a time-restricted setting such as a busy clinic, it is not often feasible to explain everything patients need to know about the etiology, complications, treatment, and monitoring of diabetes. Comprehensive care of the diabetic is best achieved in an integrated and collaborative fashion with a team of medical professionals that can include other physicians, nurses, nurse practitioners, dietitians, pharmacists, and mental health providers, and a referral should be made to a diabetes education/management program when available. Patients should be made aware that diabetes is a chronic, most often lifelong disease with potentially serious complications that can be prevented by controlling hyperglycemia, an obtainable goal that requires active participation on their part.

Initial treatment options should be discussed and initiated. Lifestyle modifications with weight loss and exercise are indicated in all patients with type 2 diabetes at the first and all subsequent visits and are aimed at improving tissue insulin sensitivity. (Remember, insulin resistance plays a fundamental role in the development of diabetes.) Because eating habits are deeply and culturally ingrained, a great place to start at the first visit is by educating patients that bread, pasta, candy, juice, and soda contain large amounts of processed carbohydrates that break down in the body to form glucose and are a major cause of high blood sugar. A goal should be set to cut down on these types of foods and drinks before the next visit. Patients should be told that the U.S. Department of Health and Human Services recommends 150 minutes/week of moderate-intensity aerobic exercise or 75 minutes/week of vigorous aerobic exercise, and *reasonable* goals should be set to increase aerobic activity before the next visit.

Medications designed to decrease circulating blood sugar levels should be discussed and initiated. The initial treatment for type 2 diabetes is metformin and sometimes insulin as well (depending on the severity of the patient's hyperglycemia and comfort with giving self-injections and closely monitoring blood sugar levels). Metformin, an oral medication of the biguanide class, decreases hepatic gluconeogenesis. (A neat way to remember this is "notformin," as in "not formin' glucose"). If there are no changes in the patient's diet, metformin alone can achieve a 1 to 1.5% decrease in HbA1C. The most common adverse effects are on the gastrointestinal tract and include upset stomach, nausea, vomiting, and diarrhea. It should not cause hypoglycemia. The most feared adverse effect is lactic acidosis, which can occur in the setting of renal insufficiency. (Do not start this medication if your patient has a creatinine ≥1.5 mg/dL.)

Patients should be sent for a number of labs at the first visit (including liver function tests, lipid panel, urine for microalbumin to creatinine ratio, and creatinine and thyroid hormone testing in some) to establish a baseline, assess for evidence of complications, and determine whether additional medications need to be prescribed. An HbA1C should be ordered if not done within the past 3 months. The HbA1C correlates with average blood sugar over a 3-month time period, or roughly the lifespan of a healthy red blood cell.

Finally, patients should be referred to an eye-care professional (either an optometrist or ophthalmologist) for a dilated eye exam to look for changes in the eye consistent with diabetic retinopathy. Whereas patients with type 1 diabetes (diagnosed at a younger age, oftentimes by diabetic ketoacidosis) are referred 5 years after the initial diagnosis, patients with type 2 diabetes are referred at the initial visit as it is often not known when their diabetes developed.

CLINICAL PEARL   **STEP 2/3**

Consider starting insulin at the first visit in patients with symptoms of hyperglycemia: fasting blood sugars >250 mg/dL, random blood sugars >300 mg/dL, or an HbA1C >10%.

The patient agrees to start metformin but is not comfortable at this time with insulin injections. He agrees to go to the lab after his initial visit and is provided with referrals to a diabetes education class and a local ophthalmologist. He sets a goal to cut down to only one soda per day and plans on purchasing a bicycle because he has knee pain with running. He returns to your office several weeks later and is feeling better. His blurry vision has resolved, he is less thirsty, and his energy level is improved. His blood pressure at today's visit is 156/96 mm Hg. His HbA1C after the first visit was 12.5%. He still does not want to start taking insulin.

What is the patient's goal hemoglobin A1C? What other oral medication options are available to help achieve it?

It is not unusual for patients to be apprehensive about starting insulin, so it is useful to explore these trepidations. The target HbA1C is the same in patients taking insulin and those on oral hypoglycemics. In most patients, the goal HbA1C is less than 7.0%. A more stringent goal of less than 6.5% is appropriate in certain patients if there is a long life expectancy and can be achieved without significant risk of hypoglycemia. A higher goal of 8.0% can be set for the elderly, those with short life expectancies, or those with multiple episodes of hypoglycemia.

When metformin (at maximum tolerated dosages) and lifestyle modifications fail to achieve target HbA1C values after 3 months, a second oral agent should be added. Choosing a second agent should be patient-centered, and considerations should include cost, effect on weight, and side-effect profile. Options include medications from the sulfonylurea class, thiazolidinedione (glitazones) class, dipeptidyl peptidase (DPP)-4 inhibitor class (gliptins), and alpha-glucosidase inhibitors. In general, each of these classes of medications can further decrease the HbA1C by 0.5 to 1%.

Sulfonylureas were the first oral hypoglycemics and are the most inexpensive. They work by altering pancreatic adenosine triphosphate (ATP) pumps leading to increased insulin secretion. Whereas metformin is *not* known to cause hypoglycemia and can lead to weight loss, sulfonylureas *can cause significant hypoglycemia* and lead to weight gain.

Thiazolidinediones (glitazones) act on receptors in adipose tissue and alter adipose metabolism, ultimately leading to increased tissue insulin sensitivity. Unlike metformin, thiazolidinediones can be used in patients with diminished renal function and have less gastrointestinal side effects. They do not cause hypoglycemia unless combined with another medication that does, and they can also cause weight gain and peripheral edema. The most feared adverse effect is heart failure, and they should be avoided in patients with a history of heart disease.

DPP-4 (dipeptidyl peptidase) inhibitors (gliptins) work by inhibiting an enzyme (DPP-4) that degrades glucagon-like peptide-1 (GLP-1) in small intestinal cells. These medications are newer and therefore more expensive. They are not known to cause hypoglycemia, have no major known side effects, and do not cause weight gain or loss.

Finally, alpha-glucosidase inhibitors block GI enzymes from converting polysaccharides into monosaccharides and slow the intestinal absorption of glucose. Their main side effect is excessive flatulence.

BASIC SCIENCE PEARL   **STEP 1**

GLP-1 is an incretin hormone that acts in response to a meal to stimulate insulin release from the pancreas and inhibits inappropriate postmeal glucagon release.

The patient wants to know the results of the other labs that were drawn prior to the visit. His serum creatinine is 0.85 mg/dL (glomerular filtration rate [GFR], 110 mL/min), urine microalbumin to creatinine ratio is 35 mcg/mg, total cholesterol is 210 mg/dL, triglycerides are 154 mg/dL, high-density lipoprotein (HDL) is 41 mg/dL, and low-density lipoprotein (LDL) is 120 mg/dL. His liver function tests are normal.

What additional medications are indicated for the patient?

In addition to medications aimed at lowering blood glucose, patients with diabetes should be managed with other medications intended to prevent cardiovascular complications. (Cardiovascular disease is the number one cause of morbidity and mortality in patients with diabetes.)

The blood pressure goal for a patient with diabetes is less than 140/90 mm Hg (as recommended by the Joint National Committee [JNC] 8 Guidelines). Several classes of medications can be used to achieve this goal, including beta blockers, diuretics, calcium channel blockers, and angiotensin-converting enzyme (ACE) inhibitors/angiotensin receptor blockers (ARBs). The first choice in diabetics is usually an ACE inhibitor or ARB as they confer additional renal protection by decreasing the amount of microalbuminuria/proteinuria, which helps to preserve the GFR. Your patient should be started on an ACE inhibitor given his elevated microalbumin to creatinine ratio coupled with his blood pressure that is not currently at goal.

In 2013 the American College of Cardiology/American Heart Association (ACC/AHA) released new guidelines for the primary prevention of cardiovascular disease in type 2 diabetics. The guidelines recommend statin therapy for patients with diabetes aged 40 to 75 years with an LDL between 70 and 189 mg/dL. The type of statin (moderate or high intensity) is based on the 10-year atherosclerotic cardiovascular disease risk percentage, which is calculated using the patient's age, race, total cholesterol, HDL, systolic blood pressure, and smoking history. Calculators are easily found online and there's even a free app for smartphones released by ACC/AHA. Your patient's 10-year atherosclerotic cardiovascular disease risk is 6.6%, which warrants treatment with a moderate intensity statin. Patients with a 10-year atherosclerotic cardiovascular disease risk greater than 7.5% should be started on a high-intensity statin, according to guidelines.

Finally, aspirin should be considered in type 2 diabetics for primary prevention of myocardial infarction and stroke in high-risk patients. This includes those with a 10-year atherosclerotic cardiovascular disease risk greater than 10% and men older than 50 years old/women older than 60 years old with multiple risk factors for coronary disease (i.e., a family history of cardiovascular disease, hypertension, hypercholesterolemia, smoking). Aspirin should not be recommended for those with atherosclerotic cardiovascular disease risk less than 5% and men younger than 50 years old/women younger than 60 years old with no additional coronary artery disease risk factors. Clinical judgment should be used for those with atherosclerotic cardiovascular disease risk between 5 and 10% in the above age groups. Given your patient's age and his 10-year atherosclerotic cardiovascular disease risk, aspirin would not be warranted now and should be considered in the future.

Finally, patients with diabetes are considered to be immunocompromised (due to reduced neutrophil and T-cell activity resulting from hyperglycemia), and a number of immunizations are important. Patients should receive the influenza vaccine on a yearly basis, the 23-valent pneumococcal vaccine (which should be repeated at age 65 or 5 years after the initial immunization), and the hepatitis B vaccine if they have not been previously vaccinated.

CLINICAL PEARL   **STEP 3**

If a patient's urine dipsticks and urinalysis frequently reveal any degree of proteinuria, he or she is already past the stage of microalbuminuria 30 to 300 mg/day. The dipstick/urinalysis detects only albumin excretion greater than 300 mg/day, which is considered overt proteinuria.

The patient is started on an ACE inhibitor for his blood pressure and microalbuminuria, and a moderate intensity statin for primary prevention of cardiovascular disease. He does not want to start another medicine for his diabetes as he is now on three medications, including metformin. He promises to follow up with a dietitian, improve his diet, and exercise more. He returns to your office 3 months later and reports that he has not been able to change his diet or exercise due to constraints at work. His repeat HbA1C is 11.0%. After you reinforce the potential complications of poorly controlled diabetes and again encourage a better diet, weight loss, and exercise, he reluctantly agrees to start taking a sulfonylurea in addition to his metformin. He does not show up for his next scheduled appointment. Approximately a year later, he returns to your office for a posthospital follow-up visit. He was recently hospitalized for cellulitis and told by the hospital doctor that his HbA1C was 10.1%. His blood sugars were managed in the hospital with basal and meal insulin (his metformin and sulfonylurea were held), and he was surprised how painless the injections were and how well his blood sugars responded. He did not want to start insulin at that point without talking to you first and was restarted on his metformin and sulfonylurea at discharge.

How will you treat your patient's persistent hyperglycemia at this point?
Patients should be reminded regularly that diabetes is a progressive disease, and most patients who have it for long enough eventually require insulin. They should be reassured that starting insulin is not a failure on their part and can provide the excellent blood sugar control that will get them to meet their HbA1C goals. At this point, after the patient has experienced about a year of poorly controlled blood sugar on two medications, you should strongly recommend that he start insulin. Your patient already has some familiarity with it from his recent hospitalization.

Insulin is injected subcutaneously and comes in several preparations with differences in regard to their duration of cost and action (short-acting for use premeal and sometimes "sliding scale," and long-acting for basal use). Starting insulin should be based on a patient's comfort with self-administration and with the blood sugar monitoring (with a glucometer) that it requires.

In general, a long-acting insulin (either Neutral Protamine Hagedorn [NPH] or glargine) is started once at bedtime, and the initial dose is based on weight (0.2 units/kg), though many clinicians will start with a lower dose as a trial (10 units of NPH or glargine) to prevent hypoglycemia. The goal is to target a before breakfast (or "fasting") blood sugar of 90 to 130 mg/dL. Patients who are savvy can up-titrate their bedtime insulin by 1 to 2 units every three nights until they reach this goal. In patients that you feel may have difficulty with this, it is prudent to have frequent in-office or telephone visits to help titrate dose adjustments. When it is not possible to see a patient frequently or discuss changes in regimens over the phone, a diabetes management program (as discussed earlier) can be of great help.

In addition to checking a fasting blood sugar in the morning, checking premeal (also known as preprandial) and bedtime blood sugars are helpful in further titrating insulin doses.

The patient prefers to take glargine insulin because of its convenient once-daily administration. He should be instructed to continue to take his metformin to suppress hepatic gluconeogenesis (remember, this medication is rarely associated with hypoglycemia) and should be taken off the sulfonylurea (as the combination of insulin and sulfonylurea will greatly increase the risk of hypoglycemia).

CLINICAL PEARL   **STEP 3**

Always inform patients of the risks of hypoglycemia with the medications they are taking. Make sure they know the signs and symptoms of hypoglycemia (i.e., sweating, palpitations, anxiety, confusion) and what to do if they develop any (check their blood sugar and administer glucose if necessary). Pharmacies sell over-the-counter glucose tablets, which are cheap and portable and can come in handy if a patient is not around food (for example, in the car) when symptoms arise.

The patient is started on 10 units at bedtime of glargine insulin. His fasting blood sugars for the first 3 days are 191 mg/dL, 212 mg/dL, and 186 mg/dL. He self-titrates his glargine until his morning blood sugars are consistently around 100 mg/dL. He does not report any episodes in which the fasting blood sugar is below 70 mg/dL and denies feeling any symptoms of hypoglycemia (sweating, confusion, palpitations, anxiety). He states that he is only able to check his blood sugar once in the morning due to his job. He returns to your office 3 months later on 24 units of glargine at bedtime. His repeat HbA1C is improved but still not at goal. On today's visit it is 8.5%.

If his fasting blood sugars are now at goal, why is his HbA1C still elevated? What needs to be done to fix this?

Your patient is almost there. He has successfully titrated his basal insulin, and his fasting blood sugars are well controlled, but there's more to controlling just the hyperglycemia that occurs while fasting. Insulin is secreted naturally in the body in a basal state and as a bolus in response to meals. Your patient most likely has hyperglycemia throughout the day as the basal insulin doesn't cover the spikes in blood sugar that occur with meals. He needs insulin to cover what he eats during the day and should be instructed to do a fingerstick before lunch, before dinner, and at bedtime. In your patient, these numbers are probably higher than the fasting number from the morning.

Mealtime, or prandial, insulin comes in several forms that also vary based on their onset, peak, and duration of action. They should be injected between 15 and 45 minutes before a meal depending on the type of insulin prescribed. Usually 4 units per meal is the starting dose and can be titrated upward in a similar fashion to the basal insulin: 2 units every 3 days until the blood sugar is in the recommended range (between 90 and 130 mg/dL) before the next meal. The prandial insulin injected before breakfast affects the blood sugar level before lunch and so on with all daily meals. Patients who do not eat consistent meals during the day may need adjustments in their prandial doses. If the HbA1C is still not controlled after seeing goal blood sugars in the morning and before meals, instruct the patient to check his blood sugar after a meal. The goal is less than 180 mg/dL 2 hours after a meal.

CLINICAL PEARL	STEP 3

Do not let the different types of insulin overwhelm you. It is important to remember a few intermediate/long-acting and prandial insulin types. Glargine (a long-acting insulin) is typically paired with a very rapid-acting insulin such as lispro. Glargine starts to work after 4 to 6 hours and has no peak. Lispro starts to work after less than 15 minutes and peaks at 0.5 to 3 hours; it lasts 3 to 5 hours. NPH (an intermediate/long-acting insulin) is typically paired with a short-acting insulin such as Regular insulin. NPH starts working after 2 to 4 hours, peaks at 4 to 10 hours, and lasts 10 to 18 hours. Regular insulin starts working at 0.5 to 1 hour, peaks at 2 to 4 hours, and lasts 4 to 8 hours.

The patient is started on prandial insulin. Although it is difficult to check his fingerstick at work, he is committed to trying to control his diabetes. He has an appointment with an ophthalmologist right after his appointment with you. He asks why you cannot just perform the eye exam and why he needs to see an eye doctor if he has no problems with his vision.

What should you tell him?

Diabetic retinopathy is the leading cause of blindness in the United States, and patients with diabetes are 25 times more likely to go blind than patients without it. Blindness is the result of macular edema and microvascular changes in the retina. The best treatment for diabetic retinopathy is early detection and prevention. Detection is accomplished by a dilated exam (allowing for more complete visualization of the retina) done once a year by an eye-care professional. Prevention is achieved by you and the patient working together to control his or her hyperglycemia.

Diabetic retinopathy occurs in two stages: nonproliferative and proliferative. The first stage, nonproliferative, can occur within the first decade of having poorly controlled diabetes and is characterized by microvascular retinal damage that leads to retinal ischemia. Nonproliferative diabetic retinopathy (NPDR) is characterized by microvascular aneurysms and hemorrhages ("blot hemorrhages") and "cotton wool spots" that appear as white patches and represent damaged nerves.

Proliferative diabetic retinopathy (PDR) can be seen after just 5 years of poorly controlled NPDR. Neovascularization, or the formation of new blood vessels in response to prolonged retinal ischemia/hypoxia, is seen at the optic disc and leads to further hemorrhages and retinal fibrosis.

Both NPDR and PDR are treated with laser photocoagulation, which is focal in the case of macular edema and NPDR and panretinal in the case of PDR.

The patient is scheduled for a phone visit 3 months later to review his ophthalmology visit and HbA1C. He has no evidence of NPDR or PDR and his HbA1C is 6.9%. He did it! Congratulate him on his efforts and be satisfied that you are playing a significant role in keeping him healthy for years to come.

BEYOND THE PEARLS

- Adults who are thin and fit and who present with new-onset diabetes in their 20s or 30s may actually have type 1 diabetes. Check an antiglutamic acid decarboxylase antibody, which will be positive in type 1 diabetics.

BEYOND THE PEARLS—cont'd

- Be careful when checking the HbA1C in the hospital if a patient recently received a blood transfusion, as the transfused red blood cells will not be as glycosylated as the patient's own, and the HbA1C will therefore be falsely low. Consequently, the HbA1C may be falsely elevated in low red blood cell turnover states such as iron deficiency anemia.
- Acanthosis nigricans is seen in conditions other than insulin resistance. It can also be seen in paraneoplastic fashion, so consider internal malignancy in patients without a history of diabetes who develop this condition suddenly.
- Although not an oral medication, GLP-1 agonists (incretin mimetics) are a noninsulin subcutaneous injectable medication for controlling hyperglycemia in type 2 diabetics. They work in a similar fashion to DPP-4 inhibitors and are considered a second- or third-line addition for hyperglycemia not controlled with metformin or the combination of metformin and another oral hypoglycemic.
- There are two types of lactic acidosis. Type A lactic acidosis is associated with tissue hypoperfusion leading to a low oxygen state and a switch to anaerobic metabolism. It is seen in states that cause shock, such as sepsis or hemorrhage. Type B lactic acidosis, the type caused by metformin, occurs via drug-induced impairment of cellular metabolism. Patients with renal insufficiency and those receiving intravenous (IV) contrast are at highest risk of type B lactic acidosis. Hold metformin on hospitalized patients and those who are receiving IV contrast for outpatient CT scans. Type B lactic acidosis can also be seen in human immunodeficiency virus infection, lymphoma, and drugs other than metformin.
- Vascular endothelial growth factor (VEGF) inhibitors are a newer treatment for proliferative diabetic retinopathy that are injected directly into the eye to halt the progression of proliferative diabetic retinopathy.
- Diabetics who are allergic to aspirin should be started on clopidogrel as primary prevention for cardiovascular disease if they are considered high risk.
- Insulin is a liquid that comes in a bottle in two forms for injection: U-100 (100 units/mL) and U-500 (500 units/mL). U-100 is the standard form that almost all type 1 and type 2 diabetic patients are on. For patients who require very high doses of insulin to control their diabetes, refer to endocrinology for the highly concentrated U-500 form of insulin. Patients inject less fluid subcutaneously, which helps with absorption.
- Short- and long-acting insulin can be mixed in the same syringe. There are also premixed versions of insulin, like 70/30, that contain 70% NPH and 30% Regular insulin. The downside to this preparation is that you cannot titrate the long-acting insulin independent of the short-acting insulin. Consider prescribing this to patients who need long- and short-acting insulin but who are not reliable enough or unwilling to titrate their doses.
- Insulin is cleared via the kidneys. Be careful about increasing insulin doses in patients with chronic kidney disease as the decreased clearance can lead to hypoglycemia.

References

American Diabetes Association. Standards of medical care in diabetes—2014. *Diabetes Care*. 2014;3(1): S14-S80.

Ganda O. Prevalence and incidence of secondary and other types of diabetes. In: *Diabetes in America*. 2nd ed. National Diabetes Information Clearinghouse; 1995:69-84.

Henske JA, Griffith ML, Fowler MJ. Initiating and titrating insulin in patients with type 2 diabetes. *Clin Diabetes*. 2009;27(2):72-76.

Koliaki C, Doupis J. Incretin-based therapy: a powerful and promising weapon in the treatment of type 2 diabetes mellitus. *Diabetes Ther*. 2011;2:101-121.

Powers AC. Diabetes mellitus. In: Longo D, Fauci A, Kasper D, et al., eds. *Harrison's Principles of Internal Medicine*. 18th ed. New York: McGraw-Hill; 2012:2968-3003.

Stumvoll M, Goldstein BJ, van Haeftan TW. Type 2 diabetes: principles of pathogenesis and therapy. *Lancet*. 2005;365:1333-1346.

Walia A, Molitch ME. Insulin therapy for type 2 diabetes mellitus. *JAMA*. 2014;311(22):2315-2325.

Nirav Patel ■ Arzhang Cyrus Javan

A 23-Year-Old Female With Dysuria

A 23-year-old female presents to your clinic with complaints of dysuria, urinary frequency, and urinary urgency. The symptoms have progressed over the past 2 days. She denies fevers, chills, nausea, vomiting, or abdominal pain. She is currently sexually active with a male partner and has had three prior partners. She takes oral contraceptive medication though denies using barrier protective devices during sexual activity.

What is the differential diagnosis of a patient presenting with dysuria?

Dysuria (a burning pain during urination) is a frequent complaint associated with a number of infectious and noninfectious etiologies. Dysuria is a common clinical manifestation of urinary tract infection (UTI), though its presence may vary based on the anatomic location of the infection along the urinary tract. Cystitis, which is a UTI localized to the bladder epithelium, classically presents with dysuria but may also present with concomitant urinary urgency, urinary frequency, change in urine color, malodorous urine, and/or suprapubic pain. Dysuria may also be caused by cervicitis (inflammation/infection of the cervix), urethritis (inflammation/infection of the urethra), vaginitis (inflammation/infection of the vaginal tract), interstitial cystitis (a chronic condition), as well as noninfectious vaginal or vulvar irritation. Frequent causes of cervicitis and urethritis include sexually transmitted infections such as *Chlamydia trachomatis*, *Neisseria gonorrhoeae*, and occasionally herpes simplex virus. Vaginitis may be infectious, such as with *Trichomonas vaginalis*, or associated with organism overgrowth, such as with *Candida albicans* or *Gardnerella vaginalis*.

CLINICAL PEARL   **STEP 2/3**

There is considerable overlap between the symptoms of UTI and sexually transmitted infection. Many patients are reluctant to discuss infections of a sexually transmitted nature and instead only complain of urinary symptoms. Directed questions and a nonjudgmental approach are necessary to best treat the patient.

Cystitis was mentioned as a type of UTI. What are the other types of UTIs?

UTIs can be classified based on anatomic parameters or clinical parameters. Lower UTIs involve the urethra (urethritis) or the bladder (cystitis). Upper UTIs involve the kidney (pyelonephritis) and include perinephric abscesses and renal abscesses. In men, prostatitis can also be considered an "upper" UTI.

UTIs can also be classified based on clinical parameters as either uncomplicated or complicated UTI. Uncomplicated UTI encompasses cystitis or pyelonephritis in nonpregnant women without any other structural or functional abnormalities of the urinary tract. In general, uncomplicated UTIs have a high likelihood of responding to empiric therapy. A complicated UTI includes essentially all other types of infections, both lower and upper tract, including those that occur in males, are associated with stones, involve urinary catheters, are associated with anatomic or functional abnormalities, or that occur after procedures or surgery.

CLINICAL PEARL   **STEP 2/3**

Distinguishing between upper and lower UTI does not necessarily indicate disease severity or risk of progression. For example, uncomplicated pyelonephritis can be managed on an outpatient basis using oral antibiotics.

What clinical clues help differentiate between the different types of UTIs?

There is considerable overlap in symptoms among the various types of UTIs; however, some historical elements can be distinguishing. As discussed earlier, cystitis typically presents with dysuria, urgency, and frequency but can also be associated with a change in urinary color, malodorous urine, and suprapubic pain. Fever is frequently absent, and finding fever usually suggests an upper UTI. Urethritis frequently is associated with discharge. In males, prostatitis is associated with symptoms of urinary obstruction, such as dribbling, hesitancy, a weak urinary stream, and incomplete voiding. Tenderness of the prostate or perineal pain may also be unique features.

Patients with pyelonephritis are frequently more toxic, with more systemic signs and symptoms, such as fevers, chills, back or flank pain, nausea, and vomiting. Symptoms of cystitis may or may not be present with pyelonephritis. Typically perinephric and renal abscesses have symptoms similar to pyelonephritis; however, they can be poorly responsive to antibiotic therapy alone.

The physical exam is notable for blood pressure of 116/70 mm Hg, pulse rate of 70/min, and temperature of 37.1 °C (98.8 °F). She is in no acute distress and is nontoxic in appearance. The exam is unremarkable overall. She has a benign abdomen, no costovertebral angle tenderness, and a normal genitourinary exam.

Does the physical exam help narrow the differential diagnosis?

A thorough physical exam can help establish a diagnosis as the various causes of dysuria often manifest with characteristic findings. Cystitis most frequently presents with no specific findings, though suprapubic tenderness can be present. The presence of fever would suggest pyelonephritis, renal abscess, or perinephric abscess, all of which can be associated with costovertebral angle tenderness. The presence of genitourinary discharge would make cervicitis, urethritis, or vaginitis more likely. This patient has a benign physical exam and does not display any systemic signs of infection, suggesting a diagnosis of cystitis rather than an upper UTI or one of the other previously described causes of dysuria.

CLINICAL PEARL   **STEP 2/3**

Dysuria from *Neisseria gonorrhoeae* can be extremely severe and is often accompanied by significant discharge. On the other hand, *Chlamydia trachomatis* is associated with much less pain and scant discharge and may occasionally be asymptomatic, especially in men. If treating empirically for one, always treat for the other.

What additional testing is appropriate at this time?

Urinary testing would be reasonable because UTI, specifically cystitis, is high on the differential diagnosis. Some clinicians may treat a clear-cut case of uncomplicated UTI based on symptoms alone; however, a urine dipstick test is warranted and provides point-of-care information if the diagnosis of UTI is still in question after a thorough history and physical exam.

It should be noted that a negative urine dipstick test does not rule out UTI. This is why further testing via microscopic exam of the urine and urine culture are recommended when urine dipstick testing is negative. Urine should be collected as a clean-catch, midstream sample in order to avoid contamination with the microbial flora of the urogenital tract.

As our patient is otherwise healthy, without coexistent medical problems and without systemic signs of illness, no further blood testing is necessary. However, testing for pregnancy and screening for sexually transmitted infections is warranted as the patient is sexually active and does not use barrier protective devices. This may include testing for *C. trachomatis, N. gonorrhoeae,* and human immunodeficiency virus (HIV).

CLINICAL PEARL   **STEP 2/3**

Always remember to evaluate whether a patient at reproductive age is pregnant, as some antimicrobials are teratogenic.

How does one interpret a urine dipstick test for infection?

A urine dipstick provides a number of useful diagnostic tests on one panel. To assist with the diagnosis of infection, two tests are included on the panel: nitrite reduction and detection of leukocyte esterase. Only organisms within the family Enterobacteriaceae convert nitrate to nitrite, thus the test may miss detection of certain other organisms. Additionally, the concentration must be high enough to reach the level of detection, which may not occur if a patient is consuming a significant amount of fluid, resulting in dilute urine, and/or urinating frequently.

Leukocyte esterase is an enzyme found in polymorphonuclear cells and is a reflection of the host's response to infection. Many clinicians consider it a surrogate of pyuria (white blood cells seen on microscopic analysis of the urine); however, the leukocyte esterase test may be positive with intact or lysed polymorphonuclear cells.

A positive test (detection of either nitrite or leukocyte esterase) in the presence of typical symptoms of cystitis is highly suggestive of UTI and warrants the initiation of empiric antibiotics. Again, a negative urine dipstick should prompt additional testing via urine microscopic analysis and culture and an evaluation for alternative causes of symptoms.

How does one interpret a microscopic exam of the urine?

Urine microscopy allows for the visualization of intact white blood cells in the urine, as well as other types of cells (red blood cells), bacteria, or yeast. The findings must be evaluated carefully, as sample contamination frequently occurs. Nonetheless, the advantage is the direct detection of pyuria, which is present in the vast majority of cases of cystitis.

How does one interpret a urine culture?

The gold standard diagnostic study for UTI is the detection of organisms on urine culture. Although most patients diagnosed with cystitis have $\geq 10^5$ colony forming units/mL (CFU/mL) of bacterial growth, the guidelines utilize a positive cutoff of $\geq 10^2$ CFU/mL in women. Different thresholds have been used for men and for patients with indwelling urinary catheters.

Obtaining a clean urinary tract sample is of vital importance, as specimens can become easily contaminated by the normal flora of the urogenital tract. Thus, a definitive diagnosis of UTI requires a patient to have all of the following: symptoms consistent with a UTI, significant pyuria, and a urine culture positive for an organism that has a predilection to cause UTIs.

The urine dipstick shows 3+ leukocyte esterase and is positive for nitrites. Rapid HIV testing is negative. Nucleic acid amplification testing of the urine for gonorrhea and chlamydia are also negative.

Diagnosis: Acute, uncomplicated cystitis

What are the typical organisms that cause UTI?

Most cases of uncomplicated cystitis are caused by enteric organisms, primarily aerobic gram-negative bacilli, of which *Escherichia coli* is by far the most common. *Klebsiella* spp., *Citrobacter* spp., and *Proteus* spp. (often associated with stone formation) are other frequent pathogens. *Staphylococcus saprophyticus* is another organism that can be commonly found in uncomplicated infection, particularly in young, sexually active females. *Enterococcus* spp., which are gram-positive cocci, are also occasional agents of uncomplicated cystitis. Although *E. coli* remains the primary cause of complicated UTI, other commonly isolated gram-negative pathogens include *Pseudomonas aeruginosa*, *Morganella* spp., and *Acinetobacter* spp., as well as the above-mentioned gram-negative bacilli that are typical culprits of uncomplicated cystitis. *Enterococcus* spp. and *Candida* spp. also play a prominent role in complicated UTI.

How would you treat this patient?

In general, uncomplicated cystitis should be treated with oral antibiotics. According to the 2010 Infectious Diseases Society of America guidelines, one of the following empiric regimens is recommended: nitrofurantoin 100 mg orally twice daily for 5 days, trimethoprim-sulfamethoxazole double strength 1 tablet orally twice daily for 3 days, fosfomycin 3 g orally for one dose, or pivmecillinam 400 mg orally twice daily for 5 days; not available in the United States. The choice of one of these agents (typically either of the first two) is based on allergy, tolerability, and community-resistance patterns. When a culture has been obtained, the antibiotics should be tailored to the isolated organism's *in vitro* susceptibility.

Fluoroquinolones (specifically, ofloxacin, ciprofloxacin, and levofloxacin) are noted to have excellent, experimentally proven efficacy. However, given concerns about resistance and selection of more resistant pathogens, they are recommended as alternatives. Other beta-lactam agents are noted to be inferior and are therefore also considered alternatives. These include penicillins (only beta-lactam/beta-lactamase inhibitor combinations, such as amoxicillin/clavulanate, should be considered in the empiric treatment of UTI) or cephalosporins such as cefpodoxime or cefdinir.

In this patient, a treatment course with nitrofurantoin 100 mg orally twice daily for 5 days would be a reasonable option.

How does the treatment of complicated UTI differ?

Generally, the empiric regimen chosen for complicated UTI should have broader antimicrobial coverage than that used to treat uncomplicated UTI. Oral fluoroquinolones are appropriate for stable patients; however, those who have a more severe presentation, are postsurgery, or have been exposed to prior antibiotics will need more extensive antimicrobial coverage until the causative organism is identified. Depending on the clinical situation, this can include broad-spectrum beta-lactam/beta-lactamase inhibitor combinations, such as piperacillin/tazobactam, a third- or fourth-generation cephalosporin, or a carbapenem. Again, therapy should be tailored toward the culture results and *in vitro* susceptibility testing.

Longer treatment durations are generally appropriate for complicated UTI. The exact treatment duration varies based on the individual patient's clinical situation and response to therapy.

CLINICAL PEARL   STEP 2/3

An obstructing stone can frequently lead to an infection proximal to it. Thus, sampling urine distal to the obstruction may not reflect the true nature of the infection. Obstructed and infected urine can act as a functional abscess and needs to be drained in order to achieve source control. This may require a urologic procedure.

BEYOND THE PEARLS

- Dysuria is a common complaint in patients presenting with UTI, but symptoms may also include urinary urgency, frequency, change in urine color, malodorous urine, and/or suprapubic pain.
- UTIs can be anatomically categorized into lower urinary tract infections, involving the urethra or bladder, or upper urinary tract infections, involving the kidney or the prostate. UTIs can also be categorized based on clinical parameters as uncomplicated UTIs, which involve nonpregnant women without structural or functional abnormalities of the urinary tract, or complicated UTIs, which include all other types of infection.
- The most frequent cause of UTI is *E. coli,* though other enteric gram-negative bacilli are common causative agents as well. *S. saprophyticus,* a gram-positive organism, is commonly identified in uncomplicated cystitis in young, sexually active females.
- Empiric treatment of uncomplicated cystitis is typically with nitrofurantoin 100 mg orally twice daily for 5 days or trimethoprim-sulfamethoxazole double strength 1 tablet orally twice daily for 3 days.
- Fosfomycin and nitrofurantoin are only appropriate for treatment of cystitis as they do not reach adequate tissue drug levels and are therefore not effective in pyelonephritis or prostatitis.
- Most UTIs arise from an ascending route (i.e., they ascend the urethra into the urinary tract). Occasionally, certain organisms can hematogenously spread to the kidney and then leak into the urine. *Salmonella* spp. and *Staphylococcus aureus* isolated from a urine culture should prompt an evaluation for bacteremia (though *S. aureus* UTI can also occur posturologic procedure or in association with an indwelling urinary catheter).
- Candiduria frequently occurs in association with urinary catheters. In a patient without a catheter, it may also reflect disseminated infection.
- In complicated UTI occurring in elderly patients, especially those with dementia, the classical symptoms may be difficult to elucidate. Frequently, these patients present with alteration in mental status, lethargy, falls, metabolic derangements, renal failure, and/or sepsis syndrome. Despite the severity of illness, they frequently respond rapidly to aggressive therapies.
- Patients will occasionally present with typical UTI symptoms and with pyuria on urine microscopic exam; however, cultures will be negative. This is considered "sterile pyuria" and has a unique differential diagnosis. Although urethritis is the most common etiology, other causes can include concurrent antibiotic use, pelvic inflammatory disease, urinary stones/foreign bodies, bladder tumor, interstitial cystitis, or more unusual infections, such as tuberculosis, schistosomiasis, blastomycosis, coccidioidomycosis, histoplasmosis, cryptococcosis, or other fungal etiologies.
- Asymptomatic bacteriuria does not warrant antibiotic therapy unless the patient is pregnant or is about to undergo a urologic procedure. Neutropenic patients and recipients of renal transplants can also be considered for therapy.

References

Dellinger RP, Levy MM, Rhodes A, et al. Surviving sepsis campaign: international guidelines for management of severe sepsis and septic shock: 2012. *Crit Care Med.* 2013;41(2):580-637.

Drekonja DM, Rector TS, Cutting A, Johnson JR. Urinary tract infection in male veterans: treatment patterns and outcomes. *JAMA Intern Med.* 2013;173(1):62-68.

Foxman B. Urinary tract infection syndromes: occurrence, recurrence, bacteriology, risk factors, and disease burden. *Infect Dis Clin North Am.* 2014;28(1):1-13.

Grigoryan L, Trautner BW, Gupta K. Diagnosis and management of urinary tract infections in the outpatient setting: a review. *JAMA.* 2014;312(16):1677-1684.

Gupta K, Hooton TM, Naber KG, et al. International clinical practice guidelines for the treatment of acute uncomplicated cystitis and pyelonephritis in women: a 2010 update by the Infectious Diseases Society of America and the European Society for Microbiology and Infectious Diseases. *Clin Infect Dis.* 2011; 52(5):e103-e120.

Gupta K, Trautner BW. Urinary tract infections, pyelonephritis, and prostatitis. In: Kasper D, Fauci A, eds. *Harrison's Infectious Diseases.* 2nd ed. New York: McGraw-Hill; 2013.

Hooton TM. Clinical practice. Uncomplicated urinary tract infection. *N Engl J Med.* 2012;366(11): 1028-1037.

Hooton TM, Bradley SF, Cardenas DD, et al. Diagnosis, prevention, and treatment of catheter-associated urinary tract infection in adults: 2009 international clinical practice guidelines from the Infectious Diseases Society of America. *Clin Infect Dis.* 2010;50(5):625-663.

Takhar SS, Moran GJ. Diagnosis and management of urinary tract infection in the emergency department and outpatient settings. *Infect Dis Clin North Am.* 2014;28(1):33-48.

John Khoury ■ Carla LoPinto-Khoury

A 40-Year-Old Female With Headaches

A 40-year-old right-handed obese female presents to your office complaining of headaches as far back as she can remember but worse over the past year. She reports that her headaches originally started as unilateral pressure-type feelings that would radiate to the back of the head and start to throb. These headaches would last about 8 hours and would be associated with a sensitivity to smell and light. She often gets nausea with her headaches and rarely vomits. Headaches are worse with movement and better if she lies down in a dark room. She denies ever having warnings to her headaches.

Why is it important to ask the patient for a description of the headache?

With most headache disorders, a proper history must be obtained as physical exam rarely leads to a diagnosis. Factors including age of onset, location, duration, radiating locations, quality, associated symptoms, exacerbating factors, and ameliorating factors are all important to determine the diagnosis to aid in treatment. In the history provided, the patient's diagnosis is consistent with migraine and the correct medications can be administered appropriately.

CLINICAL PEARL	STEP 2/3

Although photophobia and phonophobia are often features of migraine headache, the presence of osmophobia (smell sensitivity) is one of the most specific features of migraine headache.

You inquire about medications she has used for treatment. She occasionally takes ibuprofen, and this usually helps but not always. If that does not work she will use sumatriptan to help abort her headache.

CLINICAL PEARL	STEP 2/3

Triptan medications are FDA (U.S. Food and Drug Administration) approved for the treatment of acute migraine headache. To date there are seven triptans available in the United States: sumatriptan (Imitrex), rizatriptan (Maxalt), naratriptan (Amerge), frovatriptan (Frova), zolmatriptan (Zomig), almotriptan (Axert), and eletriptan (Relpax). If a patient does not respond to a single triptan medication, the physician should try a different one. Failure of one triptan medication does not mean the patient will fail all.

What are contraindications to the use of triptans for migraine?

Because triptans bind to $5HT_{1B}$ and $5HT_{1D}$ serotonin receptors, they can cause vasoconstriction and are contraindicated in patients with a history of heart attack, coronary artery disease, stroke, transient ischemic attach (TIA), familial hemiplegic migraine, and uncontrolled hypertension. Although category C, triptans are not used during pregnancy in clinical practice.

CLINICAL PEARL   **STEP 2/3**

The use of preventative agents is recommended when patients have disabling or frequent migraine headaches. Preventive agents include beta blockers such as propranolol, antiepileptic medications such as topiramate, or antidepressant medications such as nortriptyline.

CLINICAL PEARL   **STEP 2/3**

The mnemonic SNOOPS is often used to evaluate for secondary causes of headache:

Systemic symptoms (fever, weight loss)
Neurologic signs or symptoms (confusion, impaired consciousness, focal weakness)
Onset (sudden, abrupt, thunderclap)
Older age of onset (age >50 increases risk for giant cell arteritis)
Prior headache history (first headache or change in pattern)
Secondary risk factors (human immunodeficiency virus, cancer)

The patient indicates that over the past year, her headaches have worsened and seem to occur nearly daily. Even on days when she does not have a severe headache, she often feels a milder, dull bifrontal headache that does not go away with medication. You confirm that she is not overusing over-the-counter analgesics and has not been prescribed narcotics.

CLINICAL PEARL   **STEP 2/3**

It is important to determine the presence of medication overuse headache in patients who have a history of previously stable migraine headache as medication overuse is a common cause of refractory headache.

The patient informs you that over the past year when her headaches get severe she starts to hear a pulsating ringing in her ears during the headache. Her headaches get slightly worse when she coughs. She also reports headaches are now associated with blurry vision, which is a new symptom.

What would you do next to aid in the diagnosis of this patient's headache?

The presence of pulsatile tinnitus and headaches that are worsening with valsalva may be indicative of a mass lesion causing an increase in intracranial pressure. Fundoscopic exam is very important, as the presence of papilledema confirms suspicion of increased intracranial pressure. Although malignant hypertension can also present with bilateral papilledema, this cause can easily be ruled out by taking the patient's blood pressure.

On physical exam, you determine that the patient's blood pressure is 130/82 mm Hg. On cranial nerve exam you note that she complains of horizontal diplopia on far left gaze, which is resolved when she looks right. Diplopia is absent when one eye is closed.

Which extraocular muscle is involved?

This patient has binocular diplopia secondary to a left 6th nerve palsy, which controls the lateral rectus muscle. Only a 6th nerve lesion can cause pure horizontal diplopia in this manner. A 3rd nerve lesion would cause diagonal diplopia and a 4th nerve palsy often causes vertical diplopia, although patients may complain of diagonal diplopia instead.

CLINICAL PEARL	STEP 2/3

A 6th nerve palsy alone has poor localizing value. Downward displacement of the brain due to either high or low cerebrospinal fluid (CSF) pressures stretch the 6th nerve as it exits the pons through Dorello's canal. Thus, in isolation the lesion may have nothing to do with the orbit or the brainstem.

On fundoscopic exam you note bilateral papilledema.

What tests should you order next?

Although it is tempting to perform a spinal tap to relieve pressure, a magnetic resonance image (MRI) with and without contrast should be ordered to evaluate for mass lesions. Tumors of the 4th ventricle may cause hydrocephalus, and a spinal tap may cause entrapment of the tumor and collapse of the spinal column due to drainage of CSF. Magnetic resonance venography (MRV) would also be appropriate and can be ordered with the MRI to evaluate for venous sinus thrombosis, which is another cause of increased intracranial pressure.

MRI is negative for a mass lesion and MRV is negative for a venous sinus thrombosis.

What other findings would you look for if you still suspect an increase in intracranial pressure?

Patients with idiopathic intracranial hypertension (IIH, also known as pseudotumor cerebri) have some classic MRI findings, including an empty (or partially empty) sella turcica, slitlike ventricles, dilated perioptic CSF spaces, tortuous bilateral optic nerves, or posterior globe flattening. MRV may show narrowing without thrombosis of a transverse sinus.

A spinal tap is performed on the patient while the patient is in the lateral decubitus position. The opening pressure is 32 cm of H_2O. You remove 25 mL of CSF, and the patient notes immediate relief of her headache.

BASIC SCIENCE PEARL	STEP 1

The amount of CSF in the brain and spinal system is about 150 mL. CSF is made by the choroid plexus and is removed via arachnoid granulations. CSF is produced at a rate of 400 to 700 mL per day. In healthy individuals, the rate of CSF absorption is equal to the rate of production, but in persons with IIH, the rate of absorption is lower than the rate of production, and a spinal tap is not a long-term or maintenance treatment. Because CSF production is so fast, oral medications are needed to help maintain a lower CSF pressure, which will not only reduce headaches but will prevent permanent visual loss due to chronic optic nerve edema.

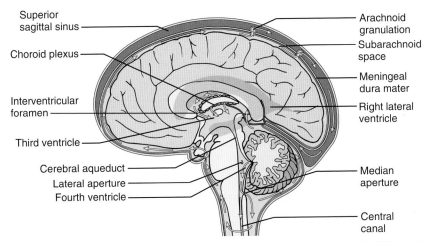

Figure 26.1 The choroid plexus in the four ventricles produce cerebrospinal fluid (CSF), which is circulated through the ventricular system and then enters the subarachnoid space through the median and lateral apertures. The CSF is then reabsorbed into the blood at the arachnoid granulations, where the arachnoid membrane emerges into the dural sinuses. *(From* http://cnx.org/contents/14fb4ad7-39a1-4eee-ab6e-3ef2482e3e22@6.27:89/Circulation-and-the-Central-Ne.*)*

What is the pathway of CSF production and excretion?

CSF is produced in the choroid plexus, which is located in each of the four ventricles (Fig. 26.1). The choroid plexus is *not* located in the cerebral aqueduct. (This pertinent negative point is a common point of testing.) The choroid plexus is made up of tufts of capillaries with fenestrated endothelial cells. They appear bright on computed tomography (CT) scans because of calcifications that form with aging.

Starting at the lateral ventricles where CSF is produced most superiorly, CSF travels through the interventricular foramen of Monro into the 3rd ventricle. From the 3rd ventricle, CSF then travels through the cerebral aqueduct of Sylvius into the 4th ventricle. CSF then leaves the 4th ventricle into the subarachnoid space via the lateral aperture (foramen of Luschka) and through the median aperture (foramen of Magendie). In the subarachnoid space, CSF lines the brain and spinal cord. CSF is finally absorbed into venous sinuses via arachnoid granulations.

> **Diagnosis:** Idiopathic intracranial hypertension (also known as pseudotumor cerebri)

What are some treatment options for this patient with idiopathic intracranial hypertension?

The most important intervention is patient education as to the prognosis of the disease. If left untreated, blindness may occur. Treatment adherence is paramount. Low-salt diet may reduce intracranial pressures. Medication treatment options include acetazolamide, topiramate, and furosemide. These agents have been shown to decrease CSF pressures, but acetazolamide has been shown to also improve vision. Studies are lacking regarding vision specifically and topiramate and furosemide. Weight loss has also been shown to reduce CSF pressures, and even as little as a 5% weight loss may be enough to control the disease. Given the difficulty in weight loss it should generally be used in conjunction with medications initially. Both acetazolamide and topiramate have weight loss properties; however, patients improve even if they remain weight neutral. Regular dilated fundoscopic evaluations are recommended to check for resolution of papilledema.

CLINICAL PEARL STEP 2/3

What are some secondary causes of intracranial hypertension? Venous sinus thrombosis, meningitis, hypoparathyroidism, vitamin A intoxication, renal disease or side effects of: tetracyclines, tretinoins, human growth hormone, and steroid withdrawal.

BEYOND THE PEARLS

- Although the overwhelming majority of cases of IIH have papilledema on presentation, there are some IIH patients who have headaches without papilledema.
- Optic nerve sheath fenestration has been shown to reverse visual losses due to IIH.
- Repeated lumbar punctures are not recommended as treatment when patients complain of worsening headache with IIH. The rapid rate of CSF production makes relief transitory and not worth the risk of serial lumbar punctures because alternative treatments are available.
- In some cases, optic nerve fenestrations or ventriculoperitoneal shunts are necessary to control IIH when medications fail or cannot be used.
- Botox was recently FDA approved for treatment of migraine headaches.

References

Corbett JJ. Problems with the diagnosis and treatment of pseudotumor cerebri. The 1982 Silverides Lecture. *Can J Neurol Sci.* 1982;10:221-229.

Silberstein SD, Lipton RB, Dodick DW. *Wolff's Headache and Other Head Pain.* 8th ed. New York, NY: Oxford University Press; 2007.

Wall M, McDermott MP, Kieburtz KD, et al. Effect of acetazolamide on visual function in patients with idiopathic intracranial hypertension and mild visual loss: the idiopathic intracranial hypertension treatment trial. *JAMA.* 2014;311(16):1641-1651.

Monisha Bhanote   ▨   Wen Chen   ▨   Daniel Martinez

A 35-Year-Old Male With Substernal Chest Pain

A 35-year-old male presents for an annual health exam for work. He has a past medical history of asthma and seasonal allergies, which are well controlled. However, he reports a 3- to 4-year history of burning, substernal, nonradiating chest pain that can last up to 2 to 3 hours, is associated with large meals, and is worse at night when he lays down to go to bed. Upon questioning, he denies any feelings of chest pressure or heaviness or a tearing/ripping feeling in his back. The patient also notes an occasional acidic taste in his mouth. He had not sought medical attention because the pain quickly resolved with antacids, but now the pain seems to be more severe and frequent, and antacids no longer provide relief. He denies nausea, vomiting, hematemesis, melena, hematochezia, diarrhea, or constipation.

On exam, blood pressure is 132/75 mm Hg in his right arm and 130/70 mm Hg in his left arm, pulse rate is 74/min, respiration rate is 14/min, and oxygen saturation is 100% on room air. He is well developed and comfortable appearing. There are equal pulses bilaterally, proximally, and distally. There is no jugular venous distension or carotid bruits. The chest pain is not reproducible upon palpation. The heart and lung sounds are unremarkable, and his abdomen is soft, nontender, and nondistended. There is no peripheral edema, nail clubbing, or nail telangiectasias.

How should you approach chest pain?

Chest pain is one of those red-flag symptoms that require a clinician to at least consider several life-threatening pathologies, including acute coronary syndrome, aortic dissection, pneumothorax, and pulmonary embolism. Because the tests to rule out these conditions are costly, time consuming, and include radiation exposure, a detailed history and physical exam is the most important first step in evaluation. It is important to know all the risk factors for these conditions, ask questions relating to them, and evaluate them specifically on physical exam with each patient presenting with chest pain. Given that the patient is comfortable appearing, not tachycardic, not tachypneic, and this has been a chronic problem for many years, these acute life-threatening etiologies are very unlikely.

What is most likely in this patient?

The patient describes a substernal chest pain associated with acidic regurgitation, precipitated by large meals and lying flat, and initially relieved by over-the-counter antacids. Given this history, the most likely diagnosis is gastroesophageal reflux disease (GERD). When a relatively young patient without risk factors for other conditions has this classic set of symptoms, it is appropriate to start empiric treatment for GERD with close follow up to ensure resolution of symptoms. However, you should first evaluate whether the patient has any risk factors for other conditions on the differential diagnosis or any alarm symptoms (see Table 27.1 and Table 27.2).

TABLE 27.1 ■ Differential Diagnosis of
Gastroesophageal Reflux Disease

- Infectious esophagitis
- Pill esophagitis
- Ingestion of corrosive agents (lye)
- Chemotherapy
- Collagen vascular diseases
- Graft versus host disease
- Trauma

TABLE 27.2 ■ Alarm Features in Someone Presenting
With Gastroesophageal Reflux Disease

- Dysphagia
- Odynophagia
- Hematochezia
- Melena
- Hematemesis
- Recurrent vomiting
- Weight loss
- Anemia

CLINICAL PEARL   **STEP 2/3**

The classic symptoms of GERD include substernal burning discomfort and acidic
regurgitation. Atypical symptoms include chest pain, asthma, hoarseness, chronic cough,
and laryngitis.

What other conditions should be considered?

Other gastrointestinal causes of his chest pain include other types of esophagitis such as infectious, eosinophilic, and pill esophagitis.

Infectious esophagitis typically presents in immunocompromised individuals and can be caused by viruses, fungi, and bacteria. The most common pathogens include *Herpes simplex*, *Cytomegalovirus*, and *Candida* species. These patients typically present with chest pain, odynophagia, and endoscopic findings of ulcerations.

Eosinophilic esophagitis also typically presents with odynophagia, and patients may report that they have a sensation that food is getting stuck in their throat. Patients with eosinophilic esophagitis do not respond to antireflux therapy and tend to have normal pH monitoring.

Pill esophagitis can be caused by long-standing use of medications. This has a similar presentation as other forms of esophagitis with odynophagia, dysphagia, and retrosternal pain and is typically seen in patients who are taking medications such as nonsteroidal antiinflammatory drug (NSAIDs), bisphosphonates, and antibiotics (Table 27.3).

Diagnosis: Gastroesophageal reflux disease (GERD)

How do you manage a patient who presents with GERD?

The initial management consists of an empiric trial of acid-reducing agents as well as lifestyle and dietary modifications. These can include eating smaller meals, avoiding late-night meals or snacks 2 to 3 hours before bed, avoiding the common precipitating foods, stopping smoking, losing weight, and elevating the head of the bed for sleeping.

TABLE 27.3 ■ **Medications Associated With Pill Esophagitis**

NSAIDs	Bisphosphonates	Antibiotics	Other Medications
Aspirin	Alendronate	Clindamycin	Ferrous sulfate
Ibuprofen	Risedronate	Doxycycline	Potassium chloride
Naproxen		Tetracycline	

NSAIDs, Nonsteroidal antiinflammatory drugs.

You explain to the patient that his clinical presentation is most consistent with a diagnosis of GERD and that you recommend initiating treatment. He is counseled about weight loss, lifestyle modifications, and trigger foods to avoid. He is also prescribed a proton pump inhibitor (PPI) and scheduled for a follow-up visit in 1 month.

What is the mechanism of reflux in GERD?

Physiologically, the gastroesophageal junction (GEJ) is a barrier formed by the lower esophageal sphincter (LES) and the diaphragm that prevents the acidic contents of the stomach from flowing back into the esophagus (Fig. 27.1). In the act of swallowing, the GEJ relaxes momentarily to allow food to pass from the esophagus into the stomach before closing to reestablish the barrier between the esophagus and the stomach.

GERD is caused by the abnormal reflux of acidic gastric contents back into the esophagus and can be precipitated by physical abnormalities within the GEJ such as a hiatal hernia or abnormal GEJ tone as can be seen in scleroderma. Other contributing factors include a defective LES, delayed gastric emptying, and increased gastric acid production.

CLINICAL PEARL   STEP 2/3

Patients with scleroderma often have gastrointestinal complaints, including dysphagia and reflux symptoms. Scleroderma can cause the lower esophageal sphincter to be abnormally loose. Patients with scleroderma will typically present with other signs of scleroderma such as skin changes, Raynaud's phenomenon, calcinosis cutis, and telangiectasias and may complain of dysphagia as well.

What are some risk factors and/or precipitating factors for GERD?

Risk factors include abnormalities in the GEJ such as a hiatal hernia, obesity, pregnancy, and abnormal GEJ tone.

Obesity is thought to increase intragastric pressure as well as increase the frequency of transient lower esophageal sphincter relaxations.

Pregnancy is thought to increase GERD through the effects of high serum levels of estradiol and progesterone, which can relax the smooth muscles of the GEJ.

Factors that may cause reflux include gastric distension, satiety (mediated through the effect of cholecystokinin, a hormone released from satiety), smoking, specific foods, and various medications (Table 27.4).

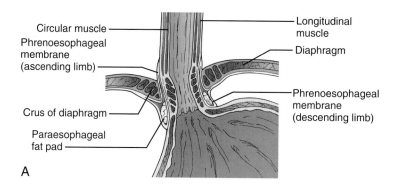

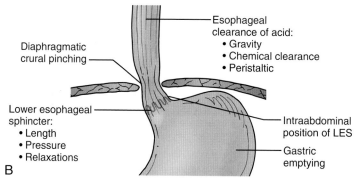

Figure 27.1 A, Anatomy of a normal gastroesophageal junction. **B,** In a hiatal hernia, the diaphragm cannot effectively participate in maintaining lower esophageal sphincter (LES) tone. *(From Fischer J. Fischer's Mastery of Surgery. 6th ed. Philadelphia: Wolters Kluwer Health/Lippincott Williams & Wilkins; 2012.)*

TABLE 27.4 ▓ Common Foods and Medications That Can Precipitate Gastroesophageal Reflux Disease

Foods	Medications
Chocolate	Antidepressants (amitriptyline, imipramine)
Peppermint	Anticholinergics (prochlorperazine, promethazine)
Caffeinated beverages	Beta-2 agonists
Alcohol	Theophylline
Tomatoes	Sedatives (diazepam, temazepam)
Spicy foods	Estrogen containing medications (oral contraceptives)
High-fat meals	

A month later, the patient returns, stating that his symptoms have improved somewhat but he is still having bothersome symptoms despite being adherent to his medication. He is worried that something else might be going on and would like a definitive diagnosis.

What are some indications to refer a patient for endoscopy?

Indications for referral for endoscopy include alarm features, failure of an empiric trial of twice-daily PPI therapy, or male gender greater than 50 years of age with a history of symptoms greater than 5 years to screen for Barrett's esophagus. The purpose of endoscopy is to rule out alternative diagnoses, assess the severity of mucosal damage, and to screen for long-term complications of GERD such as intestinal metaplasia, which is sine qua non for the diagnosis of Barrett's esophagus and the development of dysplasia (Fig. 27.2).

CLINICAL PEARL   **STEP 2/3**

Indications for endoscopy:
- Alarm symptoms
- Failure of twice-daily PPI therapy
- Long-standing GERD in a male >50 years of age (in order to evaluate for Barrett's esophagus)

You explain that further diagnostic testing is still premature at this time and that conservative measures should be taken first. You recommend that the patient instead increase his PPI therapy to twice a day to see whether this will relieve his symptoms. The patient is agreeable and is scheduled for a follow up of his symptoms. After a month of therapy, the patient returns for further evaluation. He reports that he still has persistent symptoms despite adherence to twice-daily PPI and all the recommended lifestyle modification. His persistence of symptoms is unusual for a patient simply with GERD, so you refer the patient to a gastroenterologist for an upper endoscopy.

Besides endoscopy, what are some other tests that can be used in someone presenting with GERD, and what are their indications?

A manometry and 24-hour gastric pH monitor may be indicated in patients with persistent GERD. Esophageal manometry is a study typically performed in the endoscopy suite during which pressures along the entire length of the esophagus are monitored at rest and during a swallow. It can be used to diagnose esophageal motility disorders such as achalasia, diffuse esophageal spasm, or esophageal hypomotility as can be seen in scleroderma. Manometry is a mandatory procedure prior to surgical intervention with Nissen fundoplication.

A 24-hour gastric pH monitor can be inserted immediately following an esophageal manometry study. During this study, a pH probe is inserted intranasally with its tip ending in the stomach. The probe continually measures the pH in the stomach and along its length up the esophagus over the next 24 hours. Patients may also keep a log of reflux events so that the symptoms of GERD can be correlated with pH readings suggestive of reflux.

Both of these studies are used to rule out alternative diagnoses and to rule in gastric reflux as the cause of the patient's symptoms.

The patient arrives as his gastroenterologist and describes what has happened over the past few months. The gastroenterologist agrees that an endoscopy is the next best step in the workup. The patient then has an endoscopy showing mucosal inflammation in the distal esophagus consistent with Los Angeles grade A esophagitis and a small hiatal hernia. Biopsies taken from the affected area are consistent with GERD-induced esophagitis. The patient also receives an esophageal manometry study showing a mildly reduced lower esophageal sphincter tone, and a 24-hour pH monitor study shows acidic reflux that correlates with the patient's symptoms of reflux.

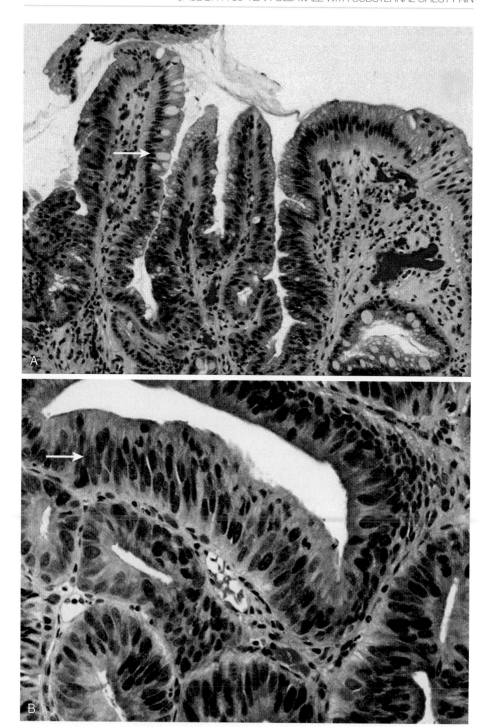

Figure 27.2 A, Histology of intestinal metaplasia at the gastroesophageal junction *(arrow)*, consistent with Barrett's esophagus. **B,** Histology of low-grade dysplasia as indicated by the arrow in patient with Barrett's esophagus.

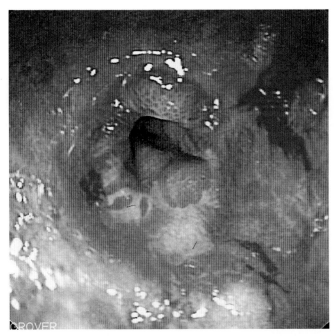

Figure 27.3 Endoscopic image of peptic stricture showing narrowing of the esophagus near the junction with the stomach due to chronic gastroesophageal reflux in the setting of scleroderma. *(From* http:// commons.wikimedia.org/wiki/File%3APeptic_stricture.png.*)*

What types of changes can be seen on endoscopy in a person with GERD?
Long-standing GERD can cause esophagitis, typically linear or irregular ulcerations seen in the distal esophagus (Fig. 27.3). The severity of the esophagitis is graded using the Los Angeles classification, which is based on the endoscopic appearance of the lesions (Fig. 27.4). Endoscopy may also show abnormalities such as an esophageal hernia.

CLINICAL PEARL   **STEP 2/3**

Reflux esophagitis is an endoscopic diagnosis characterized by distal esophageal erythema or ulcerations. The severity of reflux esophagitis can be graded using the Los Angeles classification, with grade D esophagitis being the most severe.

In a patient presenting with reflux symptoms, an upper endoscopy may also show mucosal changes that may point to other diagnoses such as eosinophilic esophagitis, infectious esophagitis, or pill-induced esophagitis.

During the endoscopy, biopsies are also typically taken of normal- and abnormal-appearing mucosa in order to establish a diagnosis and to rule out alternative diagnoses like eosinophilic esophagitis and infectious esophagitis.

What are some histologic changes associated with GERD-induced esophagitis, and how do these compare with the histology seen in other causes of esophagitis?
It is recommended that all symptomatic patients undergo biopsy because of the discordance between endoscopy and histologic findings. Biopsies should be taken at least 2 cm above the levels of the GEJ. Common features seen in reflux esophagitis include basal cell hyperplasia,

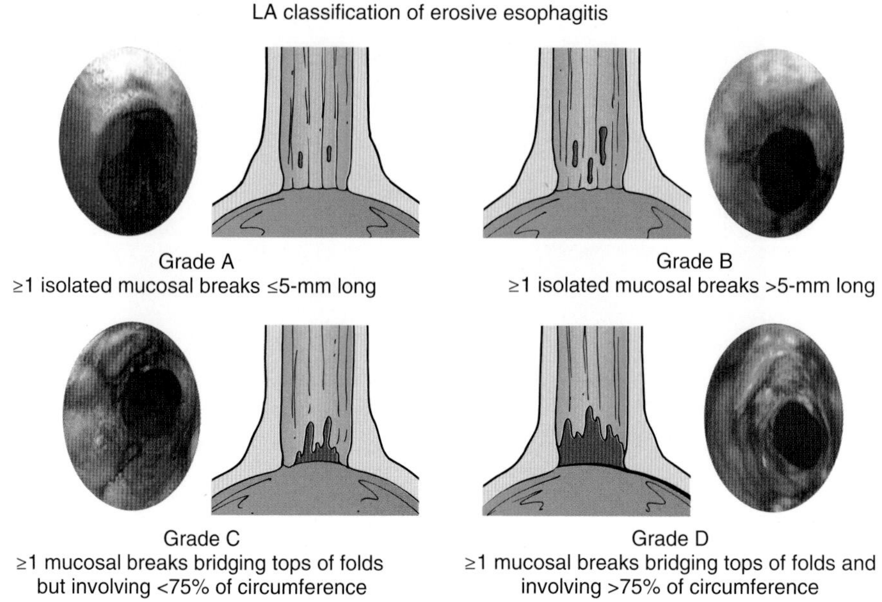

LA classification of erosive esophagitis

Grade A
≥1 isolated mucosal breaks ≤5-mm long

Grade B
≥1 isolated mucosal breaks >5-mm long

Grade C
≥1 mucosal breaks bridging tops of folds
but involving <75% of circumference

Grade D
≥1 mucosal breaks bridging tops of folds and
involving >75% of circumference

Figure 27.4 Comparison of endoscopic findings of Los Angeles grade A, B, C, and D esophagitis. *(Source: Richter JE. The many manifestations of gastroesophageal reflux disease: presentation, evaluation, and treatment,* Gastroenterol Clin North Am. *2007;36[3]:577-599.)*

elongation and congestion of the lamina propria papillae, intraepithelial inflammation (eosinophils, neutrophils, and lymphocytes), acantholysis, and ulcerations (Fig. 27.5).

The presence of organisms is typically seen in infectious esophagitis. In esophagitis caused by the *Herpes* virus, the histology typically shows multinucleated giant cells with nuclear molding and ground glass nuclei (Fig. 27.6). In esophagitis caused by the *Cytomegalovirus*, the histology typically shows large intranuclear inclusions. In esophagitis caused by *Candida*, the histology typically shows fungal hyphae and yeast forms, which can be confirmed with additional stains.

Pill esophagitis typically has nonspecific findings. However, crystalline material may be present.

Eosinophilic esophagitis is distinguished by a greater number of intraepithelial eosinophils, generally greater than 15 per high power field, and microabscesses. Involvement of the proximal and distal esophagus is more common in eosinophilic esophagitis, whereas the involvement of just the distal esophagus is commonly seen in reflux esophagitis (Fig. 27.7).

What are some long-term consequences of GERD?
The long-term consequences of GERD can be divided into two categories: esophageal and extraesophageal.

Esophageal consequences include esophageal stricture and intestinal metaplasia (Barrett's esophagus). These consequences are a direct result of the healing and adaptation to mucosal injury induced by long-standing acid reflux.

Esophageal stricture is typically treated with endoscopic esophageal dilation.

Barrett's esophagus is managed with surveillance endoscopy to assess for dysplasia and malignant transformation as well as treatment of the underlying GERD (Table 27.5). If dysplasia is discovered on surveillance endoscopy, endoscopic ablative procedures, endoscopic mucosal resection, or surgical resection can be used to treat the dysplasia depending on its grade and extent.

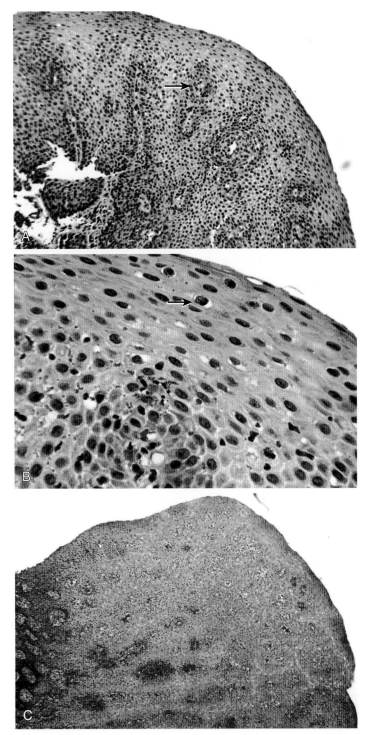

Figure 27.5 Histology of reflux esophagitis showing squamous mucosa with increased eosinophils as indicated by the arrows (**A,** high and **B,** low power) and **(C)** congestion of the lamina propria papillae.

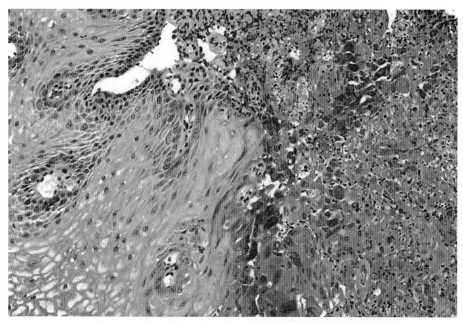

Figure 27.6 Histology of Herpes esophagitis demonstrating the three Ms: nuclear molding, margination, and multinucleation. *(From* https://commons.wikimedia.org/wiki/File:Herpes_esophagitis_-_high_mag.jpg#/media/File:Herpes_esophagitis_-_high_mag.jpg.*)*

TABLE 27.5 ■ **American Gastroenterological Association Screening Guidelines for Barrett's Esophagus**

- If no dysplasia is found on upper endoscopy and biopsy: repeat upper endoscopy (also called a esophagogastroduodenoscopy [EGD]) in 3 to 5 years
- If low-grade dysplasia is found: repeat EGD in 6 to 12 months
- If high-grade dysplasia is found in the absence of eradication therapy: repeat EGD in 3 months

---

CLINICAL PEARL	STEP 2/3

Barrett's patients with high-grade dysplasia can now be treated with radiofrequency ablation and endoscopic mucosal resection, avoiding the need for esophagectomy, which has a high mortality rate.

Extraesophageal complications of GERD include chronic cough, asthma, laryngitis, and laryngeal cancer.

CLINICAL PEARL	STEP 2/3

Esophageal complications of GERD include esophageal stricture, Barrett's esophagus, dysplasia, and carcinoma. Extraesophageal complications of GERD include chronic cough, asthma, laryngitis, and laryngeal cancer.

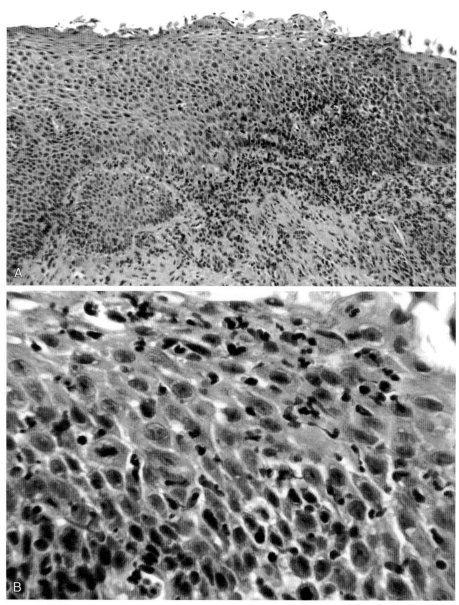

Figure 27.7 Proximal esophagus biopsies at **(A)** low and **(B)** high power show reactive squamous hyperplasia and numerous intraepithelial eosinophils, consistent with eosinophilic esophagitis.

What are some therapy options for patients with GERD refractory to twice-daily PPI?

If a patient still has symptoms after a trial of lifestyle modification and twice-daily PPI, other medical therapies that can be tried include a histamine 2 (H2) blocker for a patient who has breakthrough symptoms at night or less commonly used baclofen to reduce the frequency of transient lower esophageal sphincter pressure.

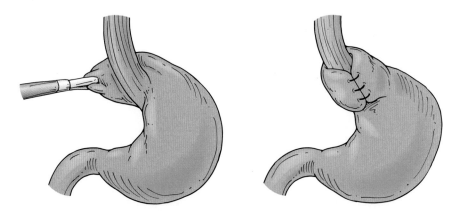

Figure 27.8 Anatomy of Nissen fundoplication. In fundoplication, the upper part of the stomach (known as the fundus), is wrapped around the lower part of the esophagus. *(From Nissen fundoplication. [2015, March 13]. In* Wikipedia, The Free Encyclopedia. *Retrieved 05:04, April 1, 2015, from* http://en.wikipedia.org/w/index.php?title=Nissen_fundoplication&oldid=651157350.*)*

CLINICAL PEARL	STEP 2/3

Adjunctive therapies for patients with refractory GERD who may not be good surgical candidates or who do not want to proceed yet with surgery include the addition of histamine 2 (H2) blockers at night such as famotidine as well as the addition of less commonly used baclofen, which is not risk-free, especially in patients with renal insufficiency, and can cause seizures if withdrawn suddenly.

After a patient has failed optimal medical management and lifestyle modification, surgery is the next step, especially in severe symptomatic GERD or if there are signs of intestinal metaplasia (Barrett's esophagus) on endoscopy. The most widely used surgical procedure for the treatment of GERD is the Nissen fundoplication (Fig. 27.8) in which the fundus of the stomach is wrapped around the distal esophagus to increase the pressure across the lower esophageal sphincter.

CLINICAL PEARL	STEP 2/3

The Nissen fundoplication improves the symptoms of GERD in 85 to 90% of cases; however, it does not address the presence of Barrett's esophagus.

You explain to the patient that the tests have confirmed the diagnosis of GERD as a cause for his symptoms. However, it seems that he has failed medical therapy and lifestyle modifications. He is counseled about the risks and benefits of surgeries and a laparoscopic Nissen fundoplication as an option. Because his symptoms are very bothersome and affect his daily life, he decides to proceed with a Nissen fundoplication. Fortunately, the procedure goes well without complications and the patient's symptoms are finally under control.

What are some long-term adverse consequences that can be seen after a Nissen fundoplication?

The most common adverse consequence of a fundoplication is dysphagia. Most patients have a period of dysphagia postoperatively that may last months and may require a modified diet during that period of time. However, patients with dysphagia greater than 3 months postoperatively should be evaluated with a barium swallow. These patients may require either esophageal dilation or a fundoplication revision in order to relieve their dysphagia.

CLINICAL PEARL	STEP 2/3

Common complications from a Nissen fundoplication include dysphagia and gas-bloat syndrome.

BEYOND THE PEARLS

- Asthma can worsen GERD by two mechanisms: increased negative intrathoracic pressure on inhalation and the use of short- and/or long-acting beta-2 agonists, which both can lead to lower esophageal sphincter relaxation.
- In young college-age females presenting with acne and symptoms of esophagitis, remember to review their medication list as doxycycline is a frequently used therapy for refractory acne and can cause pill esophagitis.
- Acid perfusion test, also known as the Bernstein test, is a test done to reproduce the pain when the lower esophagus is irrigated with a 0.1 molar hydrogen chloride (HCl) solution attempting to reproduce the patient's GERD symptoms. This test is obsolete and replaced by 24-hour pH monitoring, which is the gold standard diagnosis for GERD.
- PPIs are weak bases that are concentrated in the acidic environment of the parietal cell. They require the acidic environment of the parietal cell in order to be activated to irreversibly bind the H-K-ATPase pump, which occurs when parietal cells are stimulated by the act of eating.
- Patients should take omeprazole 30 to 60 minutes before their meal to ensure that there is enough circulating drug in the bloodstream ready to inhibit the enzyme. If patients take the medication too early, the medication will be cleared before the parietal cells achieve their acidic environment, allowing the medication to be concentrated and bind to its target.
- About 66% of Caucasians are fast metabolizers of PPIs and 5% are slow metabolizers. Fast metabolizers may have breakthrough symptoms at night and slow metabolizers may experience more drug–drug interactions.
- Cimetidine (a histamine receptor antagonist) is an inhibitor of many of the hepatic p450 enzymes. Because of this inhibition, it has many interactions with other medications and substances that require those enzymes for their metabolism (examples include warfarin, theophylline, phenytoin, propranolol, metronidazole, and alcohol). Thus, famotidine (another histamine receptor antagonist) is preferred as it has very little effect on p450 system.
- Gas-bloat syndrome is a common adverse consequence of a Nissen fundoplication in which the patient has the sensation of needing to but being unable to belch. This sensation usually decreases in severity over time but can be treated symptomatically with gas-reducing agents such as simethicone and, in extreme cases, may be treated with surgical procedures such as a pyloric stent.

References

Fass R. *Approach to refractory gastroesophageal reflux disease in adults.* In: Post TW, ed. *UpToDate.* Waltham, MA. Updated Feb. 18, 2015. Available at <www.uptodate.com>. Accessed 10.02.16.

Gelhot SM. Gastroesophageal reflux disease: diagnosis and management. *Am Fam Physician.* 1999;59(5): 1161-1169, 1199.

Kahrilas PJ. *Clinical manifestations and diagnosis of gastroesophageal reflux in adults.* In: Post TW, ed. *UpToDate.* Waltham, MA. Updated Mar. 11, 2015. Available at <www.uptodate.com>. Accessed 10.02.16.

Kahrilas PJ. Gastroesophageal reflux disease. *N Engl J Med.* 2008;359:1700-1707.

Kahrilas PJ. *Medical management of gastroesophageal reflux disease in adults.* In: Post TW, ed. *UpToDate.* Waltham, MA. Updated Apr. 27, 2015. Available at <www.uptodate.com>. Accessed 10.02.16.

Odze RD, Goldblum JR. *Surgical Pathology of the GI Tract, Liver, Biliary Tract, and Pancreas.* 3rd ed. Philadelphia: Saunders; 2014.

Nida Hamiduzzaman ▓ Seth Politano

A 62-Year-Old Male With Dyspnea at Rest and Lower Extremity Edema

A 62-year-old male with a history of type 2 diabetes mellitus, hypertension, and dyslipidemia presents with orthopnea, dyspnea at rest, and lower extremity edema. He reports two pillow orthopnea for the past week. Prior to a week ago, he was able to walk two blocks without any dyspnea. He also reports an 8-pound weight gain over the past few days. His medications include metformin, lisinopril, aspirin, and atorvastatin. He has a 30 pack-year history of smoking cigarettes but quit 2 years ago.

What is the differential diagnosis for dyspnea at rest?
Differential diagnosis for dyspnea at rest can be caused by heart disease, renal disease, lung disease, or hematologic abnormalities. One must consider acute ischemia or heart disease as a cause of such. Fluid retention from chronic kidney disease, interstitial lung disease, chronic obstructive pulmonary disease, anemia, or bone marrow suppression due to malignancy or chronic infection should be considered as well.

On physical exam, the patient's temperature is 37°C (98.6°F), blood pressure is 102/80 mm Hg, pulse rate is 98/min, and oxygen saturation is 88% on room air. Jugular venous distention is present; the lung exam reveals bilateral crackles in lower lobes; the cardiac exam reveals a regular rhythm and an S3 heart sound; and lower extremity edema is present with bilateral pitting to the knees.

Laboratory testing reveals a hemoglobin of 11.0 g/dL, creatinine of 1.3 mg/dL, sodium of 133 mEq/L, and troponin of 0.1 ng/mL. The patient's electrocardiogram (ECG) is shown in Figure 28.1. His chest radiograph is shown in Figure 28.2

What additional laboratory test would you order at this point?
You should order a B-type natriuretic peptide (BNP).

Laboratory results show a BNP of 782 pg/mL.

What is the role of BNP?
Serum levels of BNP and N-terminal-pro B-type natriuretic peptide (NTproBNP) increases in response to an increase in ventricular volume and pressure overload. NTproBNP has a longer half-life in the serum than BNP. The plasma half-life of BNP is estimated to be about 20 minutes. Both BNP and NTproBNP are used to help distinguish acute dyspnea caused by heart failure from other non-heart failure causes. Most patients with heart failure have values above 400 pg/mL.

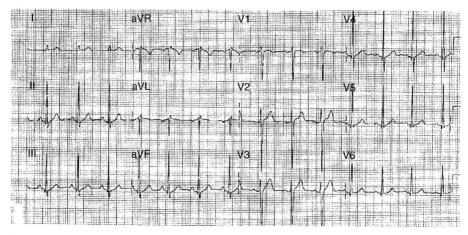

Figure 28.1   12-lead ECG with left ventricular hypertrophy pattern. Note absence of ST segment and T wave changes. *(From Brady WJ, Lentz B, Barlotta K, Harrigan RA, Chan T. ECG patterns confounding the ECG diagnosis of acute coronary syndrome: left bundle branch block, right ventricular paced rhythms, and left ventricular hypertrophy.* Emerg Med Clin North Am. *2005;23[4]:999-1025.)*

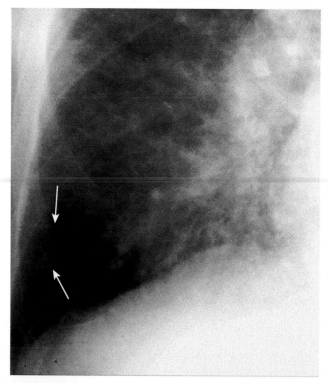

Figure 28.2   Chest radiograph detail showing Kerley B lines *(arrows). (From Milne D. Chest radiography. In: Sidebotham D, Mckee A, Gilham M, Levy JH, eds.* Cardiothoracic Critical Care. *Philadelphia: Butterworth Heinemann Elsevier; 2007:87-104.)*

CLINICAL PEARL	**STEP 2/3**

BNP levels can be elevated in women, older patients, persons with renal disease, obese patients, and acute MI.

Transthoracic echocardiography reveals a left ventricular ejection fraction of 30%, mild to moderate mitral regurgitation, and left ventricular enlargement.

Diagnosis: Acute congestive heart failure exacerbation

What diagnostic tests are needed for evaluation of heart failure?

- ECG is indicated in all patients with acute heart failure or risk factors for heart disease. Look for ventricular hypertrophy, active ischemia, or arrhythmias.
- Echocardiography can show ventricular size and function, wall function abnormalities, and reveal valvular function.
- Stress testing is used to determine functional capacity, exercise-induced arrhythmias, and ventricular function.
- Coronary angiography is indicated if ischemic heart disease is suspected as a cause of heart failure.

What are risk factors for heart failure in this patient?

Risk factors for heart failure in this case include hypertension, diabetes, dyslipidemia, and history of smoking cigarettes. Other risk factors for heart failure are use of cardiotoxic substances, such as alcohol and cocaine, thyroid disorders, tachycardia, valvular disease, and coronary artery disease (CAD). In obese patients, sleep apnea should be ruled out as it can cause hypertension, which can lead to heart failure. Treatment for risk factors reduces the risk for heart failure.

What is the functional difference between systolic and diastolic heart failure?

The difference between the two is based on preserved left ventricular function. Systolic heart failure is when the heart is dilated and ejection fraction is less than 50%. Common causes of systolic heart failure are CAD, smoking, diabetes, and hypertension. Diastolic heart failure is when there is less dilatation of the heart and ejection fraction is preserved. The most common cause of diastolic heart failure is hypertension. Both types of heart failure present with the same symptoms.

BASIC SCIENCE PEARL	**STEP 1**

Cardiac dilation in heart failure is caused by greater ventricular end diastolic volume.

How do you assess functional capacity in heart failure patients?

Functional capacity is assessed by using the New York Heart Association (NYHA) classification system. It is important to track changes in the NYHA class to help identify patients with worsening heart failure as well as to tailor medical therapy based on the NYHA classification (Table 28.1).

TABLE 28.1 ■ **New York Heart Association (NYHA) Classification System**

NYHA Class I	Patient has asymptomatic left ventricular dysfunction. Normal physical activity does not cause fatigue, palpitation, or shortness of breath.
NYHA Class II	Patient has fatigue, palpitation, or shortness of breath with normal physical activity.
NYHA Class III	Patient has shortness of breath with minimal activity, including usual activities of daily living.
NHYA Class IV	Patient has shortness of breath at rest and is unable to perform any physical activity without discomfort.

CLINICAL PEARL   **STEP 2/3**

Because patients with left ventricular ejection fraction less than 35% are at increased risk of having arrhythmias leading to sudden cardiac death, they should be referred to cardiology for further intervention.

What medications are used in treatment of acute heart failure?

The following medications are used to treat acute heart failure:

- Intravenous (IV) loop diuretics are used to achieve relief of heart failure symptoms. The patient's volume status should be assessed daily by evaluating clinical signs such as daily weight as well as urine output. The goal is to achieve relief of symptoms using the lowest dose of diuretics possible. If response is not adequate, increasing the dose of diuretics is recommended, but be sure to avoid symptomatic hypotension, renal insufficiency, or marked electrolyte depletion.
- Beta blockers decrease mortality by 30% in patients with heart failure as well as decrease hospitalization. In general, beta blockers enhance the adverse effects of chronic neurohormonal activation on ventricular remodeling, reduce pulse rate, prolong diastolic filling time, and improve ventricular relaxation. In addition, new-generation beta blockers such as carvedilol also have an alpha 1 receptor, which causes vasodilation and improves the perfusion. The starting dose should be low and then the dose should be gradually increased as tolerated. Beta blockers that have been shown to have morbidity and mortality benefit in heart failure include metoprolol succinate extended release, carvedilol, and bisoprolol. During an acute decompensation, beta blockers should not be started until patients are euvolemic. For patients already taking a beta blocker, the dose may be temporarily reduced or, in severe decompensation, temporarily stopped but restarted and titrated again when patients are stable. For milder decompensations, the beta blocker dose should be continued.

CLINICAL PEARL   **STEP 2/3**

Contraindications for starting beta blockers include asthma and second- or third-degree AV block.

- Angiotensin-converting enzyme (ACE) inhibitors and angiotensin receptor blockers (ARBs) decrease mortality by 40% and reduce hospitalization as well. ACE inhibitors reduce afterload and block the adverse activation of the renin-angiotensin-aldosterone system. Other effects include arterial and venous vasodilation, decrease in left ventricle filling pressure, and prevention of ventricular remodeling. ARBs can be used in place of an ACE inhibitor for the purpose of avoiding the side effect of cough induced by ACE inhibitors. During an acute exacerbation, these agents can be continued unless the patient has acute renal insufficiency or severe hypotension.

BASIC SCIENCE/CLINICAL PEARL   **STEP 1/2/3**

Because ACE inhibitors vasoconstrict the afferent renal arteriole, a 20 to 30% increase in creatinine is expected when you start patients on an ACE inhibitor. Therefore, an initial 20 to 30% increase in creatinine is not a reason to stop the drug. Instead, closer monitoring, slower increases in dose, reduction in diuretic dose, or avoidance of other nephrotoxic agents should be considered.

- Aldosterone antagonists decrease mortality, decrease hospitalization in patients with heart failure, as well as improve NYHA functional class. Aldosterone antagonists are indicated in patients with NYHA class III through IV heart failure. Due to the risk of hyperkalemia, patients should have close monitoring of creatinine and potassium levels.
- Hydralazine and isosorbide dinitrate decrease hospitalization and mortality as well as improve the quality of life in African American patients. The combination of hydralazine and isosorbide dinitrate increases the nitric oxide availability and maximizes the vasodilation effects. This combination of medication is indicated in only two scenarios: (1) in patients who cannot tolerate ACE inhibitors or ARBs due to hyperkalemia or renal insufficiency; (2) in African American patients with NYHA class III or IV heart failure in addition to ACE inhibitors and beta blockers.
- Digoxin helps control symptoms and reduces the likelihood of hospitalization. However, digoxin has no impact on survival in patients with heart failure. Digoxin inhibits the Na-K pump, causes weak positive inotropic effects, increases parasympathetic activity, blocks the atrioventricular node, reduces vasoconstriction, and improves renal blood flow. Toxicity seems to be a problem with digoxin use, especially in patients with renal insufficiency; therefore, digoxin should be dosed at a low dose.

CLINICAL PEARL   **STEP 2/3**

Routine evaluation of electrolytes and kidney function is recommended more frequently with changes in therapy or clinical status with patients on digoxin.

The patient is started on IV Lasix 40 mg twice a day and continued on lisinopril. A beta blocker is started once the patient has little evidence of fluid retention. Due to this patient having risk factors of diabetes, dyslipidemia, and hypertension, coronary angiography is performed to rule out ischemic heart disease.

What are reasons for patients to have an acute exacerbation?
Acute heart failure can be caused by scenarios such as acute coronary syndromes, coronary ischemia, severe hypertension, atrial and ventricular arrhythmias, infections, pulmonary emboli, renal failure, and medical or dietary nonadherence.

What preventive measures should be taken for patients with heart failure upon discharge?
- Diet compliance
- Medication adherence and review of medication on discharge
- Smoking cessation counseling
- Exercise training
- Early follow-up appointment within 7 days of discharge
- Daily weight monitoring
- Symptom reporting

CLINICAL PEARL   **STEP 2/3**

Follow-up echocardiography is not indicated in patients with heart failure in the absence of changes in clinical status.

BEYOND THE PEARLS

- Because heart failure is a chronic and potentially preventable disease, early recognition and modification of risk factors can help prevent the risk of heart failure.
- In addition to diagnostic testing, physical exam findings are key to diagnosing patients in acute heart failure.
- An intracardiac device is indicated for patients with an ejection fraction less than 30% in NYHA class II and III with an overall life expectancy of greater than 1 year.
- Biventricular pacing is indicated in patients with an ejection fraction less than 35% in NYHA class I and II with a QRS >120 msec.
- All systolic heart failure patients with risk factors for coronary heart disease should undergo a stress test or coronary angiography for evaluation of ischemic heart disease.
- Inotropic drugs are used for heart failure when the patient is unresponsive to oral medications.
- Anticoagulation in heart failure patients is controversial unless the patient has atrial fibrillation, severe valvular disease, or a documented thrombus.

References

Felker GM, Lee KL, Bull DA, et al., NHLBI Heart Failure Clinical Research Network. Diuretic strategies in patients with acute decompensated heart failure. *N Engl J Med.* 2011;364(9):797-805.

Lindenfield J, Albert NM, Boehmer JP, et al. Heart Failure Society of America 2010 Comprehensive Heart Failure Practice Guideline. *J Card Fail.* 2010;16(6):e1-e194.

R. Michelle Koolaee

A 34-Year-Old Male With Chronic Bilateral Gluteal Pains

A 34-year-old male presents for outpatient evaluation of 3 to 5 years of bilateral hip pains that have become progressively worse over the past few months. The pain is located in the gluteal areas bilaterally and is worse first thing in the morning, with several hours of associated morning stiffness. It gets better as the day goes on, although it never fully resolves. The pain is worse on the right side.

Why is it important to ask about joint stiffness in the morning?
It is important to ask about joint stiffness in the morning when evaluating for an inflammatory arthritis, such as rheumatoid arthritis or ankylosing spondylitis (AS). Furthermore, you should think about a possible inflammatory arthritis in the sacroiliac (SI) joints in anyone who presents with chronic gluteal pain. The hallmark of inflammatory arthritis is the presence of joint pain that is better with activity and worse with prolonged rest. Because the joints are at rest while one is asleep, it makes sense that the joints are more painful and stiff in the morning. Morning stiffness lasting less than 30 minutes is more indicative of osteoarthritis (a noninflammatory arthritis), whereas stiffness greater than 1 hour indicates more likely an inflammatory arthritis. This patient has several hours of morning stiffness in his SI joints, concerning for an inflammatory arthritis.

CLINICAL PEARL   **STEP 2/3**

Another great clue to help figure out whether patients have an inflammatory arthritis is to ask them if the pain (particularly back pain) ever wakes them up from sleep at night.

The patient denies any other joint pains, recent infections, rashes, or blurry/painful vision. He has no nausea, vomiting, or abdominal pains. He also denies fevers, chills, weight loss, or night sweats. The remaining review of systems (ROS) is negative.

BASIC SCIENCE PEARL   **STEP 1**

When you present clinical cases to your attending, the history of present illness (HPI) should contain only the pertinent positive and negative symptoms (rather than listing every single symptom). These symptoms were chosen because they relate directly to the differential diagnosis (see below section on differential diagnosis). Your attending should have a sense of your differential diagnosis after the HPI. The ROS includes anything that does not relate directly to the HPI.

He has no previous past medical history and has had no surgeries. His family history is significant for a maternal aunt with rheumatoid arthritis (RA). He is originally from India and works as a physician. He is not married and denies any smoking or alcohol use. He has no allergies and does not take any medications.

BASIC SCIENCE/CLINICAL PEARL   **STEP 1/2/3**

In any patient for whom you are considering an autoimmune illness, it is critical to ask about family history of autoimmunity. Autoimmune diseases as a whole, particularly lupus and multiple sclerosis, frequently run in families. It is thought that a combination of genetic and environmental factors contribute to activating disease. However, people definitely can still develop autoimmune diseases without a family history of autoimmunity.

On physical exam, he is afebrile and has no rashes, nail pitting, or onychomycosis/onycholysis. His musculoskeletal exam is notable for an abnormal Schober's test (with only 2 cm of lumbo-sacral flexion) and right SI joint pain with an abnormal Patrick test on the right. His left Achilles tendon is also moderately swollen compared to the right side, with no associated warmth, tenderness, or erythema. The rest of his physical exam is normal.

What are the Schober's and Patrick tests?

The Schober's test is used to measure the degree of lumbosacral flexion. The examiner makes a mark approximately at the level of L5 (the fifth lumbar vertebrae). He or she then makes a second mark 10 cm above the first mark. The patient is asked to touch his or her toes. By doing so, the distance between the two marks should increase by ~5 cm. If the distance increases by less than 5 cm, it indicates limited lumbosacral flexion. This is typically seen in patients with AS (or any seronegative inflammatory arthritis) but can also be seen in elderly patients with severe lumbar degenerative disc disease. This test should be done in any patients (particularly young men) who present with inflammatory back or SI joint pain.

The Patrick test is performed to evaluate for pathology of the SI joint or hip. The test is performed by having the tested leg flexed, abducted, and externally rotated (a mnemonic to remember this is that the leg will look like the letter "P" when performed on the left side). It is important to make sure you ask the patient if the pain elicited with the maneuver is the same pain they presented to you with.

What is the significance of the Achilles tendon swelling?

Achilles tendon swelling could be due to a local tendonitis, although there is no history of sports/overuse, trauma, or pain in the area, which would make this less likely. This finding is most concerning for enthesitis, a common feature in the seronegative inflammatory arthritides like AS. Enthesitis is inflammation of the entheses, the sites where tendons or ligaments insert into bone. There are many different entheses that can become inflamed in autoimmune illnesses. One of the primary entheses involved in autoimmune disease is the heel, particularly Achilles enthesitis.

BASIC SCIENCE/CLINICAL PEARL   **STEP 1/2/3**

It is important to make a "problem list" once you have enough information to make a differential diagnosis (physically writing it down is very helpful). This will keep your thoughts concise when you present the case and help keep you organized (particularly with more challenging cases).

What is your differential diagnosis at this point?

Here is a sample problem list/summary for this patient: This is a young male with chronic bilateral gluteal pain with prolonged morning stiffness, abnormal Patrick and Schober's tests on the right side, and Achilles enthesitis.

The highest on the differential would be AS, which is in the family of disorders called spondyloarthropathies (SpA). These also include reactive arthritis, psoriatic arthritis, and arthritis associated with inflammatory bowel disease (Crohn's/ulcerative colitis). SpA are characterized by inflammation of the axial spine (vertebral column) and can also have associated enthesitis, uveitis, and/or dactylitis (inflammation of an entire digit, also known as "sausage digit"). They have an increased incidence of HLA-B27 positivity, as well as negative rheumatoid factor (RF) and antinuclear antibodies (ANA), hence the term *seronegative*. The presence of inflammatory SI joint/back pain (particularly bilateral disease), enthesitis, and limited spine mobility in a young male is very suggestive of AS. He has had no recent infections to suggest a reactive arthritis. He has no abdominal pain, nausea, or diarrhea to suggest inflammatory bowel disease–related arthritis. Although the majority of patients with psoriatic arthritis develop their joint symptoms after already having psoriasis, a small percentage (approximately 15%) develop psoriasis after the arthritis. So, although he does not have any rashes or nail changes (onychomycosis/onycholysis/nail pitting) to suggest psoriasis, this is a very small possibility.

Infectious causes such as tuberculosis and abscesses are less common given the chronicity of his symptoms. He also does not have any systemic features to suggest infection (he has no fevers, chills, night sweats, or weight loss). Traumatic causes such as iliopsoas bursitis, SI strain, or ischial bursitis are also unlikely given the chronicity of symptoms. Degenerative disc disease is also less likely given his young age (it also would not explain the enthesitis). RA would also be unlikely because this is usually a symmetric, small joint arthritis.

Laboratory testing reveals a negative/normal complete blood count (CBC), creatinine (Cr), liver function tests (LFTs), erythrocyte sedimentation rate (ESR), C-reactive protein (CRP), rheumatoid factor (RF), and anti-cyclic citrullinated protein (anti-CCP) antibodies.

CLINICAL PEARL   **STEP 2/3**

The ESR is a nonspecific marker of inflammation that can be elevated in many different circumstances including infection, active arthritis, postoperatively, systemic illness, and malignancy. Keep this point in mind when interpreting ESR results and always analyze the results within the right clinical context. This lab test should guide (but not dictate) your management, and clinical judgment should always take precedence. In this case, although the patient does have normal inflammatory markers, clinically his presentation is still consistent with an active inflammatory arthritis.

What would be the best first imaging test to order?

Always start with plain films (be sure to order bilateral hips and SI joints). Be mindful of medical costs when choosing lab or imaging studies. The question to ask is: "How will this test change my management?" If the x-rays are normal and you are still convinced he has sacroiliitis, you can order a magnetic resonance imaging (MRI) of the hips and pelvis. An MRI allows visualization of very detailed soft tissue structures but is much more expensive than a plain film. Patients with AS should have baseline x-rays of the entire spine in order to assess disc height and joint spaces.

X-rays of the pelvis and hips reveal bilateral sacroiliitis, worse on the right. X-rays of the entire spine show normal vertebral disc height and joint spaces.

Diagnosis: Ankylosing spondylitis

How would you proceed with treatment?

Treatment of patients with AS must be individualized. Nonsteroidal antiinflammatory drugs (NSAIDs) are the first line of treatment, unless contraindicated (i.e., history of gastrointestinal bleeds) or not tolerated. A 4-week trial of a maximally dosed standing NSAID is a reasonable start. Many patients respond dramatically well. Analgesics and opioids, when used alone, are rarely effective during active AS. The anti-tumor necrosis factor (TNF)-alpha inhibitors have dramatically improved treatment of AS. Infliximab, etanercept, adalimumab, and golimumab are approved in the United States and Europe for use in AS and have been shown to have similar efficacy. Newer retrospective studies indicate that TNF-alpha inhibitors may decrease disease progression. There are, however, no randomized controlled trials to validate this point. (AS progresses very slowly; it would be unethical to place study subjects in a control group for an extended period of time.) There is, however, unequivocal data to show that TNF-alpha inhibitors improve signs and symptoms of disease.

Systemic glucocorticoids are ineffective for these patients, as are disease modifying antirheumatic drugs (DMARDs) such as methotrexate or sulfasalazine (these can be tried in patients with peripheral arthritis).

How do you decide who needs an anti-TNF-alpha inhibitor?

This answer should be individualized for each patient. Patients with persistently high disease activity despite NSAID use can definitely benefit. There are scoring scales for AS (which are beyond the scope of this text) that can be used to guide this decision.

What tests should be ordered before considering starting someone on an anti-TNF-alpha inhibitor?

Each patient must have hepatitis B and C serologies prior to starting therapy. There are cases of fulminant hepatitis (associated with a high morbidity and mortality) in patients with hepatitis B virus infection (HBV) who concomitantly receive an anti-TNF-alpha inhibitor. They should also all have either a tuberculin purified protein derivative (PPD) skin test or a serum QuantiFERON® gold test, as both reactivation of latent infection and new infections have been reported. (Remember that these tests have no role in the diagnosis of active infection.) Anyone with either a positive PPD or QuantiFERON® gold test should be treated for latent tuberculosis (TB) for at least 4 weeks prior to starting anti-TNF-alpha therapy.

The patient has further laboratory testing, which includes negative hepatitis B and C serologies and a negative PPD skin test. He is then started on NSAIDs, which mildly improve his symptoms. After a 4-week trial, he is started on a TNF-alpha inhibitor.

BEYOND THE PEARLS

- Hallmarks of any inflammatory arthritis are prolonged morning stiffness, pain that is better with activity, and/or pain that at times awakens a patient from sleep.
- Be mindful of medical costs when ordering tests, asking, "How will this change my management?"
- NSAIDs should be part of the initial therapy of AS unless not tolerate or contraindicated.
- Anti-TNF-alpha inhibitors have revolutionized therapy in AS. They should be considered in those with very active disease.

BEYOND THE PEARLS—cont'd

- There are some emerging retrospective data showing that anti-TNF-alpha inhibitors may in fact decrease the progression of disease in AS.
- Don't forget to also order hepatitis B core antibody (anti-HBc) before initiating an anti-TNF-alpha inhibitor, in addition to hepatitis B surface antigen (HBsAg). Although rare, there have been cases reported of reactivation of the hepatitis B virus (HBV) in patients who had previous infection that has since been cleared (which would appear as anti-HBc positive but HBsAg negative).
- Osteopenia and osteoporosis may occur in patients with long-standing AS, further increasing the risk of fracture. They should be evaluated with bone mineral density testing regularly.
- Restrictive lung disease may occur in later stages of AS. This occurs as a result of costovertebral and costosternal involvement, leading to severe kyphosis and limited chest expansion. It's a good idea to order pulmonary function tests (PFTs) in patients with moderate to severe thoracic involvement in AS, particularly if they have complaints of dyspnea on exertion and/or cough.

References

Braun J, Baraliakos X, Brandt J, Sieper J. Therapy of ankylosing spondylitis. Part II: biological therapies in the spondyloarthritides. *Scand J Rheumatol*. 2005;34(3):178-190.

Braun J, van den Berg R, Baraliakos X, et al. 2010 update of the ASAS/EULAR recommendations for the management of ankylosing spondylitis. *Ann Rheum Dis*. 2011;70(6):896-904.

Mastroianni CM, Lichtner M, Citton R, et al. Current trends in management of hepatitis B virus reactivation in the biologic therapy era. *World J Gastroenterol*. 2011;17(34):3881-3887.

Son JH, Cha SW. Anti-TNF-alpha therapy for ankylosing spondylitis. *Clin Orthop Surg*. 2010;2(1):28-33.

Mark Riley ■ Patricia Lorenzo ■ John D. Carmichael

A 20-Year-Old Female With Polyuria and Polydipsia

A 20-year-old female presents to your clinic with polyuria and nocturia for the past 4 days. She states that she has been urinating every hour and wakes several times throughout the night to urinate. The urine is voluminous and clear in color. Additionally, she complains of constant thirst and has been drinking large amounts of water and an electrolyte sports drink. She has tried not to drink any fluids or caffeine products within 1 hour of bedtime, but this has not helped. During the evaluation, the patient excuses herself to urinate and get a drink of water.

Why should you ask about nocturia?
It is important to ask about the nature of nocturia when evaluating a patient with a urinary complaint. Under normal circumstances, the kidneys produce less urine during the night, allowing people to sleep through the night without having to urinate. Waking multiple times with the urge to urinate can be pathologic. When a patient presents with polyuria, nocturia, and polydipsia, you should think about the possibility of a hormonal etiology. It is also important to elucidate from the patient what and how much he or she drinks before bed. Because this patient wakes several times during the night to urinate without drinking excess fluids before bed, an endocrine disorder is likely.

The patient has no significant past medical history. She has never had surgery or been hospitalized for any reason. She does not take any medications and has no known allergies. Her parents are in good health and also have no significant past medical history. She eats a balanced diet, drinks 1 cup of coffee per day in the morning, and does not smoke, drink alcohol, or use illicit substances.

Upon review of systems, the patient admits to dry mouth and dry skin. She admits to constipation for the past several days but denies abdominal pain, nausea, and vomiting. She denies dysuria, urgency, and gross hematuria. The patient denies polyphagia, temperature intolerance, and recent weight loss. The remaining review of systems is negative.

CLINICAL PEARL   STEP 2/3

A good endocrine review of systems requires asking the patient questions that may seem unrelated to one another but are important in reaching a diagnosis. Questions to ask include changes in weight, changes in eating and drinking habits, temperature intolerance, changes in skin and hair, and changes in sweating.

On physical exam, the patient's blood pressure is 126/85 mm Hg, her pulse rate is 103/min, her respiration rate is 14/min, and her temperature is 37°C (98.6°F). She is in no acute distress. Her cardiac exam reveals mild tachycardia, regular rhythm, with clear lung sounds. Her skin is very dry with decreased turgor. Her mucus membranes and lips are dry and her abdomen is soft and nontender. Her lower extremities show no edema with intact pulses.

What tests would you order initially?

In a patient with polyuria, a urinalysis can be done to assess urine concentration and check for the presence of abnormal substances or microbes. Because the other chief complaint is polydipsia, electrolyte and serum solute status are important to know as well. These can be obtained with a basic metabolic panel. A glucose and hemoglobin A1C (HbA1C) should also be ordered to evaluate for diabetes mellitus.

Urinalysis reveals a urine osmolality of 180 mOsm/kg H_2O with no other abnormal findings. A basic metabolic panel shows a serum osmolality of 295 mOsm/kg, serum sodium of 142 mEq/L, glucose of 96 mg/dL, and calcium of 9.7 mg/dL, with all other values normal, including an absence of protein or glucose in the urine. A complete blood count is normal. The HbA1C is 5.4%.

BASIC SCIENCE PEARL	STEP 1

While the serum sodium in this patient is within the normal range (135 to 145 mEq/L), a value in the upper range of normal can still indicate existing pathology. However, sodium near the upper limit of normal usually does indicate a relative water deficit. Increased serum sodium concentration provides a stimulus for fluid intake to replenish urinary and other losses. Patients who have access to water are usually able to prevent hypernatremia. This is a natural compensatory response.

What is your differential diagnosis at this point?

A urine osmolality less than 200 mOsm/kg in conjunction with polyuria often indicates the presence of diabetes insipidus (DI). DI is a condition in which the kidneys excrete large volumes of dilute urine. Patients with untreated DI produce greater than 3 L/day but can exceed 18 L/day. This excess water loss is attributed to a problem with the normal function of vasopressin, a hormone secreted from the posterior pituitary that facilitates the reabsorption of water in the distal tubules of the kidney.

There are several forms of DI: central DI, nephrogenic DI, and primary polydipsia (also called psychogenic DI). Central DI is caused by a dysfunction in the synthesis, transport, or release of vasopressin from the hypothalamus or posterior pituitary. Nephrogenic DI is the result of resistance to the action of vasopressin by the kidneys. Primary polydipsia is the result of chronic excess fluid intake that impairs the release of vasopressin. The normal actions of vasopressin on the nephron act to conserve free water loss in the urine (Fig. 30.1). The treatment for each form of DI is different, so it is important to differentiate which form is present in this patient with further testing before proceeding with treatment. Because the patient shows no signs or symptoms of infection, a urinary tract infection would be low on the differential despite the presence of polyuria. Other conditions that can cause polyuria and polydipsia are diabetes mellitus, kidney failure, hypercalcemia, and medications such as diuretics or lithium.

It is also important to note the diagnoses that have been ruled out with the initial laboratory testing that has already been done. Uncontrolled diabetes mellitus is a common cause of polyuria. The kidneys are only able to reabsorb a certain amount of glucose and the rest is excreted in the urine. Glucose in the urine creates an osmotic gradient thereby increasing water excretion. The normal glucose on the basic metabolic panel (BMP) and HbA1C rule out diabetes mellitus. Hypercalcemia is also known to cause calcium diuresis resulting in polyuria. This was also ruled out by the BMP. Renal injury was also ruled out with normal blood urea nitrogen (BUN) and creatinine and supported by the absence of proteinuria.

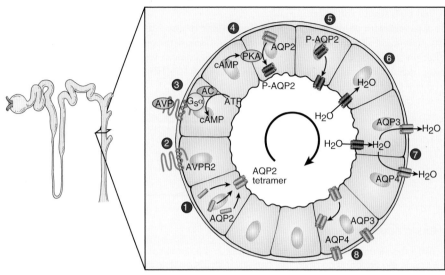

Figure 30.1 Schematic sequence of events leading to antidiuresis in response to vasopressin. Aquaporin 2 (AQP2) forms unphosphorylated tetramers (1). The vasopressin V2 receptor is a G-protein coupled 7-transmembrane receptor (2). Binding of vasopressin leads to activation of the alpha subunit of the stimulatory G protein, which in turn activates adenylyl cyclase (3). Adenylyl cyclase converts ATP to cyclic AMP (cAMP). The increase in cAMP leads to the activation of the protein kinase A pathway and, among other effects, this results in the phosphorylation of AQP2 (4). Phosphorylated AQP2 gets rapidly inserted into the apical membrane facing the luminal side (5). Water then enters the principal cell (6). At the basolateral membrane, water leaves the cell through aquaporin 3 and aquaporin 4 (7). AQP2 gets dephosphorylated and gets recycled into cytosolic compartments (8). *AC,* Adenylyl cyclase; *AQP2,* aquaporin 2; *AQP3,* aquaporin 3; *AQP4,* aquaporin 4; *AVP,* vasopressin; *AVPR2,* vasopressin V2 receptor; *cAMP,* cyclic AMP; *G$_S\alpha$,* alpha subunit of the stimulatory G protein; *P-AQP2,* phosphorylated aquaporin 2; *PKA,* protein kinase A. *(From Babey M, Kopp P, Robertson GL. Familial forms of diabetes insipidus: clinical and molecular characteristics. Nat Rev Endocrinol. 2011;7[12]:701-714, 2011. Used with permission.)*

CLINICAL PEARL   **STEP 2/3**

Determining time of onset of polyuria and polydipsia can also guide diagnosis. For example, in central diabetes insipidus, symptoms generally have an acute onset of several days, while nephrogenic DI tends to manifest over a longer period of time.

What test would you order next?

Currently, the best method for differentiating between the different types of DI is the water deprivation test. This test involves depriving the patient of all fluids to stimulate vasopressin secretion. The patient's body weight, blood pressure, urine volume, urine osmolality, serum sodium, and serum osmolality are measured hourly. The initial phase of the test ends when indices of urine concentration plateau. Once this is achieved, desmopressin (DDAVP), a synthetic vasopressin analog, is given to the patient usually as a subcutaneous injection. Urine osmolality is measured 1 and 2 hours postinjection. In patients without DI or those with primary polydipsia, the urine osmolality will be greater than the plasma osmolality in response to fluid restriction. Patients without DI usually concentrate their urine to above 500 mmol without administration of DDAVP. Furthermore, urine osmolality will show a minimal increase following DDAVP injection. With DI, urine osmolality remains less than or only mildly above plasma osmolality following fluid restriction. A rise of greater than 50% in urine osmolality after DDAVP administration is consistent with central DI. A rise of less than 50% in urine osmolality after DDAVP is consistent with nephrogenic DI.

A water deprivation test for this patient and demonstrates a 70% increase in urine osmolality.

CLINICAL PEARL   **STEP 2/3**

Patients with DI will often crave ice-cold water.

Diagnosis: Central diabetes insipidus

How would you treat this patient?

The primary goal of managing central diabetes insipidus (CDI) is the maintenance of hydration status. Patients with CDI are encouraged to drink water throughout the day. The next step is to control nocturia and polyuria during the day. First-line treatment with DDAVP at a starting dose of 10 µg at bedtime is recommended. DDAVP can be administered orally, parenterally, or as an intranasal spray. It is important to note that oral DDAVP is less bioavailable than intranasal delivery due to decreased absorption in the gut. DDAVP is generally well tolerated with few side effects. Dosage and timing should be tailored to fit each patient based on severity of symptoms and life demands.

CLINICAL PEARL   **STEP 2/3**

In patients with treated, symptomatic DI, severe increased thirst will return prior to the return of polyuria. When giving instructions to patients regarding dosing, it is helpful to guide the patient to administering the DDAVP once these symptoms recur to avoid progressive fluid retention and possible hyponatremia.

What is the long term management of CDI?

Determining the exact cause of CDI further aids in management of the condition. There are three major causes of CDI: physical damage (from a tumor, trauma, or surgery), genetic, and idiopathic. Physical damage is by far the most common cause of CDI. A magnetic resonance imaging (MRI) of the hypothalamo-neurohypophyseal region is frequently needed to determine the location and extent of damage. If a tumor is present, transsphenoidal surgery may be indicated for resection. Patients with physical damage, whether due to trauma or neurosurgical intervention, may also present with symptoms of other endocrine disorders and visual field defects. Familial CDI is exceedingly rare, and genetic mutations have only recently been discovered. Idiopathic CDI may have an autoimmune origin, but more research is needed to determine this.

BASIC SCIENCE PEARL   STEP 1

Thiazide diuretics can also be used to treat CDI, which may seem counterintuitive when considering treatment of polyuria. Thiazide diuretics decrease the reabsorption of sodium and chloride by inhibiting the Na^+/Cl^- symporter channel in the distal convoluted tubule of the nephron. The kidneys compensate by increasing the reabsorption of sodium in the proximal tubule. Therefore, by osmotic forces, water is reabsorbed. This results in a decrease in the amount of filtrate that reaches the distal tubule and thus decreased water excretion.

The patient is started on a course of 10 μg of intranasal DDAVP and responds well. She ceases nocturia almost entirely and daytime symptoms are being controlled as well.

BEYOND THE PEARLS

- The incidence of DI in the general population is 3 in 100,000 with no significant gender differences.
- If you suspect DI, it is important to ask about medications. In particular, lithium can cause nephrogenic DI. Lithium is used for the treatment of bipolar disorder and depression. At high concentrations, lithium enters the principal cells of the distal tubule via the epithelial sodium channel (ENaC). Once inside the cell, lithium impairs the action of aquaporin-2 channels, resulting in the excretion of excess water. Amiloride, a diuretic inhibiting ENaC, may be given concurrently with lithium to abate nephrogenic DI.
- Patients who undergo surgery to the pituitary gland or neighboring region are at risk of developing postoperative DI. In a large single-center study, 31% of patients who underwent transsphenoidal surgery for pituitary adenoma developed polyuria immediately postoperation. This DI is usually a transient form and ceases once water balance is corrected.
- Classically, patients who experience water-balance problems after surgery to the pituitary gland exhibit a triphasic pattern of DI. This pattern begins with an initial polyuric phase that begins within 12 to 24 hours postoperatively and can last 2 to 4 days. An antidiuretic phase then ensues usually beginning around days 5 to 10 postoperatively. Vasopressin is released inappropriately, causing water retention. A final phase of polyuria occurs around day 10. In some patients, this can lead to permanent DI, depending on the extent of degeneration of AVP-secreting neurons that occurs (Fig. 30.2).
- Nephrogenic DI (NDI), as mentioned previously, is predominantly drug-induced or genetic. Drugs such as diuretics, lithium, and antibiotics can precipitate NDI. The predominant congenital defects are V_2 receptor mutations and AQP-2 mutations. NDI does not respond to DDAVP.
- Primary polydipsia should not be treated with DDAVP. Patients with primary polydipsia must be educated that their symptoms are a normal response to their water consumption.

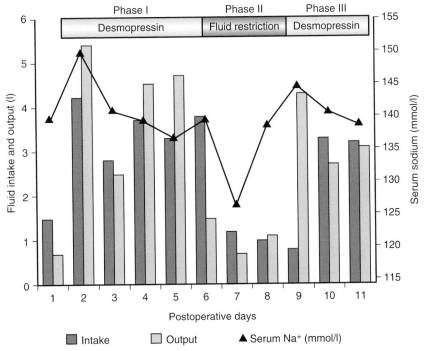

Figure 30.2 Postoperative pattern of triphasic diabetes insipidus. Fluid intake, urine output, and serum sodium demonstrate postoperative diabetes insipidus. On postoperative day 2, decreased urine output and hyponatremia signal the second phase of the syndrome of inappropriate vasopressin secretion (SIADH). On postoperative day 6, polyuria and hypernatremia return indicating diabetes insipidus on postoperative day 9. *(From Loh JA, Verbalis JG. Diabetes insipidus as a complication after pituitary surgery.* Nat Clin Pract Endocrinol Metab. *2007;3[6]:489-494. Used with permission.)*

References

Babey M, Kopp P, Robertson GL. Familial forms of diabetes insipidus: clinical and molecular characteristics. *Nat Rev Endocrinol.* 2011;7(12):701-714.

Garofeanu CG, Weir M, Rosas-Arellano MP, et al. Causes of reversible nephrogenic diabetes insipidus: a systematic review. *Am J Kidney Dis.* 2005;45(4):626-637.

Hensen J, Henig A, Fahlbusch R, et al. Prevalence, predictors, and patterns of postoperative polyuria and hyponatremia in the immediate course after transsphenoidal surgery for pituitary adenomas. *Clin Endocrinol.* 1999;50:431-439.

Lam KS, Wat MS, Choi KL, et al. Pharmacokinetics, pharmacodynamics, long-term efficacy and safety of oral 1-deamino-8-D-arginine vasopressin in adult patients with central diabetes insipidus. *Br J Clin Pharmacol.* 1996;42:379-385.

Loh JA, Verbalis JG. Diabetes insipidus as a complication after pituitary surgery. *Nat Clin Pract Endocrinol Metab.* 2007;3:489-494.

Longo DL, Fauci AS, Kasper DL, et al. *Harrison's Principles of Internal Medicine.* Vol. 1. 18th ed. McGraw-Hill, New York; 2012:340-350.

Maghnie M, Cosi G, Genovese E, et al. Central diabetes insipidus in children and young adults. *N Engl J Med.* 2000;343(14):998-1007.

Makaryus AN, McFarlane SI. Diabetes insipidus: diagnosis and treatment of a complex disease. *Cleve Clin J Med.* 2006;73(1):65-71.

Saborio P, Tipton GA, Chan J. Diabetes insipidus. *Pediatr Rev.* 2000;21(4):122-129.

Turcu AF, Erixkson BJ, Lin E, et al. Pituitary stalk lesions: the Mayo Clinic experience. *J Clin Endocrinol Metab.* 2013;98(5):1812-1818.

Steven M. Naids ▒ Ted Lyu

A 76-Year-Old Female With Eye Pain and Decreased Vision

A 76-year-old female presents to the emergency department with right eye pain that began suddenly the previous evening while she was watching television. She describes the pain as "behind the right eye" and radiating along the right side of the scalp toward the occiput. She also complains of brow ache. Acet-aminophen has not helped. She went to bed with the pain but was awoken in the middle of the night when it worsened. The vision in her right eye is blurry, which prompted her to seek attention.

What findings should point you toward an eye problem as the etiology of a headache?
Headaches are a very common presenting complaint to the emergency room. In 2008, about 2.4% of all emergency department visits in the United States were for headaches. Although headaches come in many shapes and sizes, it is important to remember that they may be the presenting complaint in patients with acute eye problems. A detailed history is important here. If there is an association with eye redness, tearing, light sensitivity, or blurry vision, an eye etiology should be high on the differential.

In addition to the persistent headache, the patient complains of worsening right eye redness and tearing. She had one episode of vomiting en route to the emergency department and is complaining of "halos" around lights.

BASIC SCIENCE/CLINICAL PEARL   **STEP 1/2/3**

An elderly female with a new-onset headache is unlikely to experience her first migraine at this age. Your clinical suspicion should be very high for another organic etiology. Remember to ask your "OPQRST" questions in regards to her headache symptoms. This acronym stands for Onset, Provocation/Palliation, Quality, Radiation, Severity, and Timing and is useful to discern reasons for a particular symptom. Pain from the front of the eye (i.e., the cornea, conjunctiva, sclera, iris, or ciliary body) can be referred to the brow, forehead, scalp, and so on.

On exam, the patient is alert but ill appearing, lying on the hospital bed with her hands over her eyes. Her pulse rate is 104/min, blood pressure is 172/89 mm Hg, and temperature is 36.8°C (98.3°F). She complains of abdominal pain in addition to her headache and begins to wretch during the encounter. You are able to get a brief look at her eye. The conjunctiva and sclera appear very injected. The right cornea is cloudier than the left, and it is more difficult to visualize the pupil. You discover that it is larger than the left pupil and not reactive to light. The patient is unable to read the "E" (20/400) on the eye chart and can only count fingers near her face. Her neurologic exam is without deficits.

Other medical history is significant for well-controlled hypertension and hyperlipidemia. She had an uneventful cataract surgery in her left eye 5 years ago. Her father had a "laser surgery" in both of his eyes many years ago.

CLINICAL PEARL

Corneal clarity is maintained by endothelial cells. When the pumping mechanism of these cells becomes overwhelmed in the setting of elevated intraocular pressure, the cornea becomes edematous, putting the corneal nerves on stretch. This is the etiology of pain in angle closure glaucoma. This also can stimulate a tremendous vagal response. Beware of the patient who presents to the emergency room with nausea and vomiting along with a headache. Always remember to check the eye!

What is your differential diagnosis at this point?
The most likely cause of this patient's symptoms is acute angle closure. This is an easy possibility to rule out in capable hands. The eye pressure should be checked before moving forward in the workup, as delaying treatment for things like computed tomography (CT) scans to evaluate the headache can result in permanent vision loss.

The differential should also include uveitis, scleritis, keratitis, endophthalmitis, orbital cellulitis, giant cell arteritis, and, of course, intracranial causes of acute headache such as subarachnoid hemorrhage, aneurysm, and so on.

The intraocular pressure is found to be 65 mm Hg in the right eye and 14 mm Hg in the left. You call the ophthalmologist to discuss your findings.

Diagnosis: Acute angle closure with pupillary block

What is the primary goal in treating this patient's angle closure?
The most frequent cause of angle closure is pupillary block. When the pupil is mid-dilated, the position of the iris against the lens may prevent the flow of aqueous humor forward from the posterior to the anterior chamber (Fig. 31.1). This produces a pressure gradient between the two chambers, resulting in the peripheral part of the iris bowing forward and sealing off the trabecular meshwork. This effectively blocks the outflow of aqueous, causing a rise in pressure.

In order to break the attack, a conduit must be created between the posterior and anterior chamber to reequilibrate the pressure and allow the angle to reopen. Laser peripheral iridotomy is the treatment of choice for angle closure caused by pupillary block.

On exam of the angle of the right eye with gonioscopy, there is enough corneal edema to obscure the view. Gonioscopy of the left eye demonstrates that it is narrow.

What types of medications can be used to lower intraocular pressure?
Lowering intraocular pressure with eye drops or oral or intravenous (IV) medications can slow the damage to the visual system. They may even break the attack. These medications work by two mechanisms: (1) by decreasing aqueous production and (2) by increasing aqueous outflow. Medications that decrease aqueous production include topical beta blockers (levobunolol, betaxolol, carteolol, metipranolol, and timolol), oral carbonic anhydrase inhibitors (acetazolamide and methazolamide), topical carbonic anhydrase inhibitors (dorzolamide and brinzolamide), and alpha-2 agonists (apraclonidine and brimonidine tartrate).

Medications that improve aqueous outflow include prostaglandin analogs (latanoprost, travoprost, bimatoprost, and unoprostone isopropyl), topical miotic agents (pilocarpine and echothiophate), and epinephrine preparations (Epifrin and Propine).

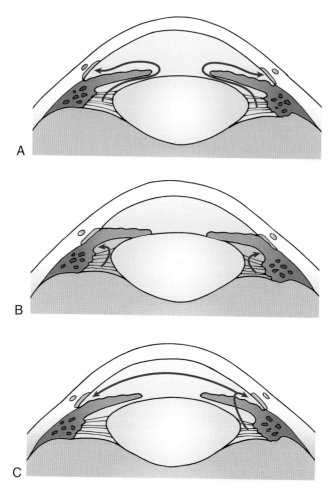

Figure 31.1   A, Normal flow of aqueous humor. The ciliary body produces the aqueous, which flows anteriorly through the pupil and out of the eye through the trabecular meshwork and Schlemm's canal. **B,** The iris has become opposed to the lens, blocking the flow of aqueous and causing it to back up in the posterior chamber. This results in peripheral iris bowing and angle closure. **C,** An iridotomy has been placed, allowing an alternate route for aqueous to flow into the anterior chamber and out of the eye through the angle.

BASIC SCIENCE/CLINICAL PEARL   **STEP 1/2/3**

There are certain important contraindications to be aware of when prescribing pressure-lowering medications, as eye drops can access the circulation via the punctual mucosa. Some points to remember: Most topical beta blockers are nonselective and can cause bronchospasm, bradycardia, central nervous system depression, and so on. The only selective topical beta blocker is betaxolol, which is not as effective as the nonselective beta blockers. Carteolol has intrinsic sympathomimetic activity, which may counteract some of the systemic beta blocking effects. Also, be aware that carbonic anhydrase inhibitors contain sulfa and are therefore contraindicated in patients with sulfa allergies. Methazolamide is primarily hepatically metabolized, making it a safer alternative than oral or IV acetazolamide in a patient with renal disease.

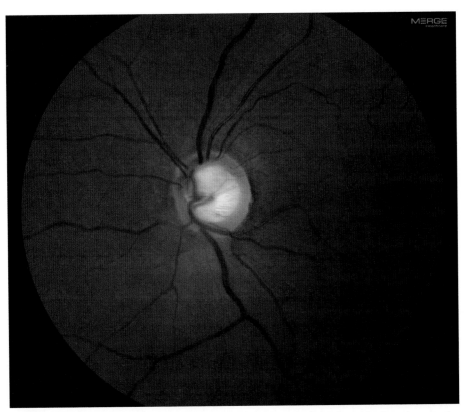

Figure 31.2   A glaucomatous-appearing optic nerve. Note the central cupping and enlarged cup-to-disc ratio.

The patient is given topical timolol, latanoprost, brimonidine, and pilocarpine, as well as oral acetazolamide. Forty-five minutes later, the intraocular pressure is 36 mm Hg, and the cornea appears to be clearer. The patient is taken to the laser room, and a peripheral iridotomy is placed at the one o'clock position. A plume of aqueous is seen through the iridotomy, and the anterior chamber begins to deepen. A short while later, she notes resolution of her headache.

What is the most important next step in this patient's management?

A laser iridotomy may spontaneously close due to tissue fibrosis, so this eye should be monitored very closely, and the patient should be warned of this possibility. Also, because of the apposition of the iris to the trabecular meshwork, the angle may become sealed due to the development of peripheral anterior synechiae. If this is the case, surgical intervention would be indicated to create an alternate pathway for the drainage of aqueous (i.e., trabeculectomy or glaucoma drainage device).

The most important next step is to look at the angle structure in the other eye with gonioscopy. If narrow, as in this patient, many ophthalmologists advocate placing a prophylactic laser iridotomy. Cataract extraction is also a good alternative to laser iridotomy in pupillary block and angle crowding, especially in the elderly.

The patient should also have a formal visual field test to establish a baseline after the attack, and the pupils should be checked for the presence of an afferent pupillary defect (Fig. 31.2).

BEYOND THE PEARLS

- The angle may seal for reasons other than pupillary block. Most commonly, a secondary angle closure can be caused by neovascular glaucoma. This is seen primarily in diabetics due to formation of neovascular vessels in the angle. Always evaluate the structure of the uninvolved eye as it can provide clues about the disease in the other eye.
- Improved intraocular pressure does not mean that the angle has reopened. High pressure can result in ciliary body ischemia, which means aqueous production decreases, but this is usually temporarily.
- Pilocarpine in concentrations greater than 2% can result in forward rotation of the ciliary body, pushing the lens-iris diaphragm anteriorly and worsening the attack.
- If an iridotomy is placed and the angle structure doesn't improve, think about plateau iris syndrome. In this case, an anteriorly rotated ciliary process pushes the peripheral iris forward, closing the angle. Other considerations would be malignant glaucoma, lens-induced glaucoma, choroidal effusion/ciliary body rotation, or even tumor.
- Without gonioscopy, the angle structures are not visible because the light reflected from the angle undergoes total internal reflection at the tear–air interface.

References

Ciofi et al. Basic and Clinical Science Course: Section 10 Glaucoma. American Academy of Ophthalmology. 2013–2014, San Francisco.

Lucado J, Paez K, Elixhauser A. Headaches in U.S. hospitals and emergency departments, 2008. Healthcare Cost and Utilization Project. May 2011. Available at <http://www.hcup-us.ahrq.gov/reports/statbriefs/sb111.pdf>. Accessed 30.12.15.

Arthur Jeng ▦ Arzhang Cyrus Javan

A 43-Year-Old Male With Left Leg Erythema and Pain

A 43-year-old male with no past medical history presents to the emergency room with a 3-day history of increasing swelling, redness, and pain of the left foot that has progressed to involve the lower leg. He has felt feverish with chills and rigors for the past day. He does not recall any trauma or animal bites to that foot. Review of systems is significant for pain and fullness in the left groin area. Vital signs reveal that his temperature is 38.3 °C (100.9 °F), pulse rate is 120/min, blood pressure is 145/84 mm Hg, and respiration rate is 16/min. Physical exam is significant for a cardiac exam showing tachycardia but regular rhythm with no murmurs, a tender 1 cm mass palpable in the left inguinal fold, and a left foot that is erythematous, edematous, warm, and tender with involvement to the shin level (Fig. 32.1). The soles of both feet show some scaling that extends between the toes. Initial laboratories are shown in Table 32.1.

What is your differential diagnosis?

In a patient who has fever and an extremity that is erythematous, swollen, warm, and tender, cellulitis should be the primary concern. Cellulitis is an infection of the dermal layers of the skin and the immediate subcutaneous tissue. The leukocytosis with left shift (immature neutrophils, such as bands) is consistent with this infectious process and the left inguinal mass represents swelling of the draining lymph node(s) (lymphadenitis), a common sequelae of cellulitis.

Other conditions for which an extremity can appear erythematous, swollen, and/or painful include:

- **Deep vein thrombosis (DVT):** Thromboses of the deep veins can cause swelling, warmth, pain, erythema, and even fevers. Clinically, DVT can be indistinguishable from cellulitis. Some of the features in this case that are less typical of DVT include the lymphadenopathy noted on the left inguinal exam and the leukocytosis with left shift. In the absence of the latter two features, a patient could have either cellulitis or DVT. Therefore, a Doppler ultrasound of the leg veins is commonly performed in the emergency department to distinguish between the two conditions.
- **Contact dermatitis:** If the patient came in contact with a substance to which the skin has an inflammatory reaction, it will appear erythematous and swollen and develop vesicles, which can ooze serous fluid that may be mistaken for pus. The latter will crust over with time. The affected areas may be pruritic but can be painful, stinging, or burning. The key features of contact dermatitis are the well-demarcated edges of the erythema (demonstrating precisely where the substance came in contact with the skin) and the lack of systemic symptoms (fever, leukocytosis, or left shift). Further questioning of the patient should reveal the offending substance the skin came in contact with.
- **Stasis dermatitis:** In patients with chronic venous insufficiency or lymphedema, the affected area can appear swollen and darker-hued and can be painful. Inflammatory papules can appear,

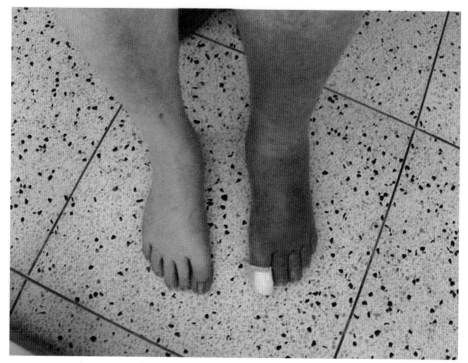

Figure 32.1 Patient's lower extremity exam.

TABLE 32.1 ▓ Initial Laboratory Tests

Leukocyte count	17,000/μL
Hemoglobin	13.8 g/dL
Platelet count	458,000/μL
Leukocyte differential	76% neutrophils, 20% bands, 4% lymphs
Serum creatinine	0.6 mg/dL
Liver function tests	Normal
Left leg x-ray	Soft tissue swelling; no bony abnormalities or gas in tissue

as can erosions and ulcerations, which can be colonized with bacteria, making superficial swabs for bacterial culture confusing to the health care provider, who will commonly attribute the findings to an infection. To distinguish from cellulitis, careful history taking should reveal a history of chronic edema of the extremity from an underlying condition (congestive heart failure, liver disease, kidney disease, proteinuria, venous insufficiency, or prior soft tissue infection of the ipsilateral extremity). Furthermore, stasis dermatitis does not cause fever, leukocytosis, nor left shift.

- **Arterial insufficiency:** With the lack of adequate blood flow to the extremities, the skin can appear shiny, atrophic, hairless, and have reactive hyperemia, where the redness blanches and abates with leg elevation. The affected area is very painful, and ulcers can develop, which are often mistaken for the nidus of infection that leads to the surrounding erythema. Detailed history may reveal claudication with use of that extremity. Demonstration that the erythema resolves with elevation of the leg can help distinguish this condition from cellulitis. As with the other conditions, fever and leukocytosis/left shift would not be seen with arterial insufficiency.

CLINICAL PEARL   **STEP 2/3**

In all of these noninfectious mimics of cellulitis, erythema, swelling, and/or pain may be present. In DVTs, even fever can be present, which makes these diagnoses clinically difficult to distinguish. The presence of leukocytosis and, especially, left shift would be a feature specific for cellulitis. Although not always seen, presence of lymphangitic spread/streaking and/or lymphadenopathy in the ipsilateral inguinal region would also clinch the diagnosis of cellulitis.

Which pathogens should you be worried about causing cellulitis?

Gram-positive bacteria cause cellulitis. Historically, beta-hemolytic streptococci (*Streptococcus pyogenes* or group A streptococcus/GAS, *Streptococcus agalactiae* or group B streptococcus/GBS, and *Streptococcus dysgalactiae* or groups C and G streptococcus/GCS/GGS) have been shown to be the primary culprits. *Staphylococcus aureus (Staph.aureus)* can also cause soft tissue infections, although in the absence of a purulent focus (such as an abscess or furuncle), it is a less common cause than streptococci. In the absence of neutropenia or specific exposure to animal bites or water, gram-negative and anaerobic bacteria are extremely uncommon causes of cellulitis.

In the presence of a purulent focus, such as an abscess or furuncle, the reverse is true, with *Staph.aureus* being the primary culprit, including methicillin-resistant *Staphylococcus aureus* (MRSA). Streptococci do not tend to form pus and therefore are less commonly involved in purulent soft tissue infections.

BASIC SCIENCE PEARL   **STEP 1**

Both streptococci and *Staph.aureus* are gram-positive cocci. The distinguishing feature on gram-stain is that when streptococci replicate, they form chains, whereas *Staph.aureus* forms clusters. Hence, a quick gram-stain from the wound (if there is any) or of colony growth from a culture plate can distinguish between these two gram-positive cocci.

Which life-threatening emergency conditions should you consider when evaluating someone with a presumptive diagnosis of cellulitis?

- **Necrotizing fasciitis:** This is a life-threatening infection of the fascial layers in the soft tissue that surrounds the muscles. In this condition, the initial symptom is severe pain, but there may be minimal visible signs of infection on the skin surface. It is thus extremely difficult to diagnose necrotizing fasciitis at this early stage. Over time, erythema will appear and may be indistinguishable from cellulitis. However, the pain is excruciating and the patient will appear very ill, often with septic physiology (tachycardia, high fevers, and, commonly, shock). Over a period of hours to days, the skin will continue to change color, becoming darker, and bullae may form, which signifies deep tissue destruction. Rapid spread, despite antibiotic administration, is a hallmark of this condition. The main cause of necrotizing fasciitis is GAS. A mixed infection comprised of non-beta-hemolytic streptococci (usually *Streptococcus viridans* group), Enterobacteriaceae family gram-negative bacilli (e.g., *Escherichia coli*, *Klebsiella* spp., *Proteus* spp.), and anaerobes can also occur; this entity is termed mixed synergistic necrotizing fasciitis. Immediate surgical debridement of all infected fascial tissue (fasciotomy with wide tissue excision) is critical for survival of the patient. Antibiotics play an adjunctive role in necrotizing fasciitis.

- **Myonecrosis:** This is a life-threatening infection of the muscle, usually caused by *Clostridium perfringens*, an anaerobic spore-forming gram-positive rod. The initial symptom is extreme pain in the muscle, which may feel wooden. However, the superficial skin exam may be unrevealing, making diagnosis at this early stage difficult. Over time, the skin will change color, and eventually bullae may develop, signifying extensive muscle destruction. Crepitus may be appreciated on exam. The key feature that differentiates clostridial myonecrosis from GAS necrotizing fasciitis is the presence of gas in tissue, which the former anaerobic bacteria produce in abundance. Management, as in necrotizing fasciitis, is immediate muscle debridement, and antibiotics play an adjunctive role.

CLINICAL PEARL   **STEP 2/3**

"Pain out of proportion with exam" is a red flag and should prompt one to consider necrotizing fasciitis and myonecrosis. Other red flags for these life-threatening conditions include rapid spread of "cellulitis," especially when the patient is on appropriate antibiotics, and/or the presence of severe sepsis/septic shock, particularly if the area of skin infection is not correspondingly severe.

BASIC SCIENCE/CLINICAL PEARL   **STEP 1/2/3**

In GAS necrotizing fasciitis, patients are usually in toxic shock syndrome (TSS) and not septic shock. TSS is caused by the many superantigens that GAS possesses (*Streptococcal pyrogenic* exotoxins or Spe), which nonspecifically recruit T-cell activation with the antigen presenting cells, causing uncontrolled inflammatory response and shock. In TSS, there is some evidence for using intravenous immunoglobulin (IVIG), the pooled antibodies of which may bind and inactivate the bacterial superantigens. Additionally, ribosomal-active antibiotics that inhibit protein production (e.g., clindamycin) can also decrease the superantigen production and are used adjunctively in GAS necrotizing fasciitis and/or TSS.

If there is no clear diagnosis after a thorough history and physical are obtained, which further testing can be performed?

- **Radiograph:** Cellulitis appears as soft tissue thickening/swelling on plain films, but this is nonspecific, as edema appears identically. However, x-rays are important in ruling out gas in tissue (Fig. 32.2). Cellulitis should not have gas in the tissue. Presence of gas may signify mixed synergistic necrotizing fasciitis or myonecrosis.
- **Computed tomography (CT) scan:** Cellulitis appears as soft tissue thickening and stranding on CT. However, this is also nonspecific and may be seen in any edematous state. CT scans can also detect gas in tissue and, most importantly, phlegmon or abscess formation. The presence of pus in tissue makes *Staph.aureus* the most likely culprit.
- **Magnetic resonance imaging (MRI):** Cellulitis appears as edema of the soft tissue, but this is nonspecific and can be seen in other edema states. Like a CT scan, an MRI can detect phlegmon or abscess, although it is not necessary to obtain an MRI for such evaluations, as CT scans are sufficient. MRIs, however, can detect joint, bone, and tendon involvement and have the best resolution of the fascial layer for visualizing necrotizing fasciitis.
- **Ultrasound:** Doppler ultrasound is primarily used to rule out DVT. However, ultrasound may also be used to detect occult abscesses, although this modality is less sensitive than a CT scan.

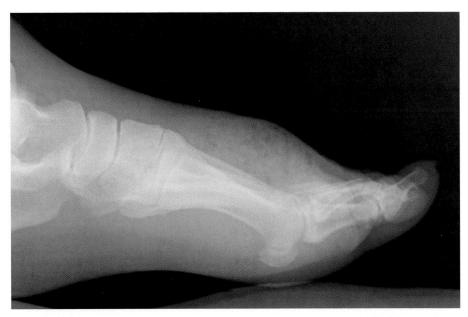

Figure 32.2   X-ray showing gas in tissue. *(Published with permission by* LearningRadiology.com.*)*

- **Blood cultures:** In nonpurulent cellulitis (i.e., it lacks a drainable focus such as an abscess), this test is the only means of isolating the bacterial pathogen. Skin aspirates and biopsies have historically been of poor yield in identifying the causative bacteria. Studies have shown that blood culture yield ranges from 0 to 24%, depending on severity of cellulitis and presence of immunocompromising conditions. Beta-hemolytic streptococci, followed less frequently by *Staph.aureus*, are the primary blood culture isolates in adults with nonpurulent cellulitis.

CLINICAL PEARL	STEP 2/3

Because the blood culture yield is higher in sicker and immunocompromised patients, two sets should be obtained in patients with cellulitis who have sepsis and who have any immunocompromising conditions.

- **Streptococcal serologies:** Antistreptolysin-O (ASO) titers are elevated in infections from GAS, GCS, and GGS and DNase-B antibodies are elevated in GAS infections. These serologies will be positive during convalescence (1 to 4 weeks after the start of infection) and therefore may not be elevated yet in the initial presentation. Generally, obtaining these serologies is not necessary but may be useful if the offending pathogen needs to be identified, such as in cases of recurrent or severe cellulitis or in cases that are not responding adequately to empiric therapy. Unfortunately, no reliable serologies exist for *Staph.aureus*.

BASIC SCIENCE PEARL	STEP 1

ASO titers have historically also been used to diagnose rheumatic fever and heart disease. These autoimmune states are felt to be from molecular mimicry between the M-protein of GAS and cardiac myosin and joint tissue. Thus, when the human immune system

Continued

BASIC SCIENCE PEARL—cont'd	STEP 1

makes antibodies against M protein, these antibodies may also attack the heart and joint tissue. DNase-B antibodies have historically been used to diagnose poststreptococcal glomerulonephritis. Similarly, antibodies to streptococci may cross react with glomerular tissue, leading to an autoimmune glomerulonephritis.

Which antibiotics would you empirically start?

This patient needs antibacterial coverage for streptococci and *Staph.aureus*. As the beta-hemolytic streptococci have never been able to acquire nor evolve resistance to the beta-lactam class of antibiotics, a gram-positive beta-lactam, such as oxacillin, nafcillin, or cefazolin, is the preferred empiric agent. These gram-positive beta-lactams do not have activity against MRSA, but MRSA has not been shown to be a significant cause of nonpurulent cellulitis. Patients with cellulitis do not need coverage for gram-negative bacteria nor anaerobes unless they have unusual exposures or conditions (e.g., animal bites, water exposure, neutropenia).

Further testing for the patient includes blood cultures that have remained negative and a lower extremity Doppler ultrasound that does not reveal DVT. The patient is begun on intravenous (IV) cefazolin 1 g every 8 hours. On the second hospital day, his fever resolves and his white blood cell (WBC) count normalizes, with a normal differential. The patient also reports significant relief in his pain. On exam, the leg appears less swollen, but some blisters have formed, and the erythema has somewhat extended beyond the pen marks outlining the borders of redness from the day of admission.

Diagnosis: Left lower extremity cellulitis

Should you be concerned about the spread of erythema beyond the borders?

All clinical signs are indicating improvement of the cellulitis, with resolution of fevers, normalization of WBC count, and relief of pain/swelling. Blisters (with clear, serous fluid) often form on the skin when edema is diminishing, so this is a sign of improvement as well. Therefore, the erythema extension is not concerning and, in fact, is known to occur with the initial treatment of cellulitis. Pathophysiologically, it is felt to be from the killing of the bacteria, with subsequent release of antigens, which may temporarily trigger an increased inflammatory response, leading to the initial, paradoxical erythema spread. Typically, the erythema will regress within the next day of treatment; extension of erythema should not progress beyond 48 hours.

If the patient's cellulitis has not definitively improved (clinically, by vitals, and/or by laboratory parameters) after 48 hours of gram-positive beta-lactam antibiotics, what is the next best step?

The concern at this point is for inadequate source control, such as an occult abscess that is not appreciable on the skin exam. Thus, a CT scan with contrast should be obtained to evaluate for a purulent focus. If a pus pocket is appreciated on imaging, it needs to be drained, as abscesses cannot be treated with antibiotics alone. The antibiotics should subsequently be changed to one that covers MRSA. A list of appropriate antibiotics with MRSA activity is shown in Table 32.2. Patients still do not need antibiotics that cover gram-negative bacteria nor anaerobes except for unusual exposure or conditions listed earlier. An algorithm on the empiric management of cellulitis is shown in Figure 32.3. Definitive oral antibiotics can be subsequently selected based on the pus culture results. A table of outpatient antibiotics active against MRSA that can be given at discharge is shown in Table 32.3.

TABLE 32.2 ▩ **Anti-MRSA Antibiotic Table for Inpatient Use**

MRSA Antibiotic	Antibiotic Class	Oral/IV	Kill Rate	Comments
Vancomycin	Glycopeptide	IV	Weakly bactericidal	Most commonly used empiric MRSA inpatient antibiotic; need to monitor levels; somewhat nephrotoxic especially with prolonged use.
Linezolid, Tedizolid	Oxazolidinone	Oral IV	Bacteriostatic	Only agents listed with oral version; activity against vancomycin-resistant enterococci (VRE). Linezolid: long-term use associated with some toxicity (thrombocytopenia, neuropathy); monoamine oxidase inhibition increases serotonin syndrome risk.
Daptomycin	Cyclic Lipopeptide	IV	Rapidly bactericidal	In vitro activity against VRE; less active with surfactant (pneumonia); monitor creatine kinase levels for rhabdomyolysis.
Telavancin, Dalbavancin, Oritavancin	Lipoglycopeptide	IV	Moderately bactericidal (Dalbavancin) to rapidly bactericidal (Oritavancin)	Telavancin: once daily, nephrotoxicity risk; Dalbavancin: once weekly dosing (×2) or one 1500 mg dose; Oritavancin: one 1200 mg dose; VRE activity.
Ceftaroline	Cephalosporin	IV	Rapidly bactericidal	Only beta-lactam to kill methicillin-resistant *Staphylococcus aureus;* also has activity against Enterobacteriaceae gram-negatives.
Tigecycline	Glycylcycline	IV	Bacteriostatic	Broad-spectrum antibiotic with gram-positive (including VRE), gram-negative (excluding *Pseudomonas aeruginosa*), and anaerobic activity; nausea/vomiting common side effect.

IV, Intravenous.

The patient is continued on cefazolin, and by hospital day 3, the erythema and swelling are now confined only to the forefoot. You decide that he is ready for discharge and write a prescription for oral cephalexin for completion of therapy. The patient asks you if he may get another bout of cellulitis and what can be done to prevent this.

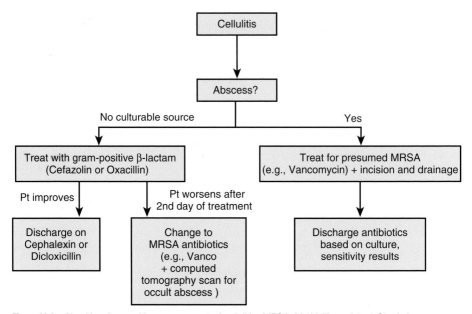

Figure 32.3 Algorithm for empiric management of cellulitis. *MRSA*, Methicillin-resistant *Staphylococcus aureus*.

TABLE 32.3 ■ **Anti-MRSA Antibiotic Table for Outpatient Use or at Discharge**

MRSA Antibiotic	Kill Rate	Comments
Trimethoprim-Sulfamethoxazole (TMP-SMX)	Weakly bactericidal	After linezolid, the highest % susceptibility for *Staph.aureus*/MRSA (>98%); poor intrinsic activity against streptococci, so need to ascertain this bacteria is not present.
Doxycycline, Minocycline	Bacteriostatic	After TMP-SMX, the next highest % susceptibility for *Staph.aureus*/MRSA (~94%); however, high rates of resistance in streptococci; skin photosensitivity side effect.
Clindamycin	Bacteriostatic	Of antibiotics listed, lowest % susceptibility for *Staph.aureus*/MRSA (80-84%), so best to use if isolate is demonstrated to be susceptible by microbiology lab; also need to test for inducible resistance. Of antibiotics listed, highest activity against streptococci (group A streptococcus resistance ≤5%) but other beta-hemolytic streptococci has appreciable resistance (*Strep.anginosus* group 11%, GBS 34-40%), with overall beta-hemolytic streptococci resistance ~14%. Ribosomal antibiotic that can inhibit protein production and often used adjunctively for this purpose.

MRSA, Methicillin-resistant *Staphylococcus aureus*.

What can be done to prevent future bouts of cellulitis?

The bacteria causing cellulitis gain access to the subcutaneous tissue via breaks in the epidermis. Thus, any condition that can cause skin disruption places one at risk for developing cellulitis. These include skin abrasions/trauma, dermatitis (atopic, stasis), psoriasis, viral skin infections (herpes simplex virus, varicella zoster virus), and tinea skin infections. This patient has scaling of the soles, with extension between the toes, classic for tinea pedis. Tinea pedis is one of the most common entry points for lower extremity cellulitis. Treatment of the feet with antifungal creams can decrease future bouts of cellulitis. Treatment of other skin conditions that may disrupt the skin integrity can help prevent cellulitis in the other conditions. Washing and keeping accidental wounds clean can help prevent entry of bacteria.

CLINICAL PEARL   **STEP 2/3**

After a bout of cellulitis, the affected extremity may remain more swollen when compared to the contralateral side due to irreversible lymphatic damage. Because of this lymphedema, that extremity is at risk for developing another bout of cellulitis, usually with beta-hemolytic streptococci.

CLINICAL PEARL   **STEP 2/3**

If the patient has numerous bouts of cellulitis afflicting the same extremity, prophylaxis with penicillin (either daily oral or monthly intramuscular shots) can help prevent future bouts. Penicillin is highly active against the most common cause of cellulitis (beta-hemolytic streptococci), and this bacteria group has never been able to acquire nor evolve resistance to any beta-lactam antibiotic. Thus, penicillin prophylaxis has been shown to be a safe, inexpensive, and effective way to prevent future bouts of cellulitis in patients with frequent attacks.

BEYOND THE PEARLS

- The bacterial etiologies of nonpurulent cellulitis are primarily beta-hemolytic streptococci, followed by *Staph.aureus.* For purulent/abscess-forming soft tissue infections, the primary pathogens are reversed: mainly *Staph.aureus* followed less commonly by streptococci.
- Although beta-hemolytic streptococci do not tend to form pus, members of the *Streptococcus anginosus* group (*Strep.anginosus, Strep.intermedius,* and *Strep. constellatus*) have a predilection for forming pus and abscesses and thus mimic *Staph.aureus.*
- Subcutaneous gas is not seen in the most common cause of necrotizing fasciitis (GAS), and therefore lack of gas on x-ray or CT scan does not rule out necrotizing fasciitis. Gas can be seen, however, in mixed synergistic necrotizing fasciitis and clostridial myonecrosis.
- For nonpurulent cellulitis, a gram-positive beta-lactam (oxacillin, nafcillin, or cefazolin) can be given empirically to cover beta-hemolytic streptococci and, secondarily, methicillin-susceptible *Staph.aureus.* Clinical trials on the treatment of nonpurulent cellulitis, comparing antibiotics with MRSA activity versus those without (linezolid vs. oxacillin-dicloxicillin, cephalexin + TMP-SMX vs. cephalexin, dalbavancin vs. cefazolin) have not shown any differences in clinical cure rates between these antibiotic types.

Continued

BEYOND THE PEARLS—cont'd

- Cat and dog bites can cause rapidly progressing cellulitis due to *Pasteurella* spp., especially *Pasteurella multocida*. Coverage for this gram-negative cocco-bacillary bacteria with a penicillin or its derivative would be optimal, such as ampicillin/sulbactam or amoxicillin/clavulanate. These penicillins also cover streptococci, and the addition of the beta-lactamase inhibitor allows coverage for *Staph.aureus* and anaerobic bacteria.
- Human bites (often from closed fist injuries to the mouth) can cause cellulitis. The infection is a mixture of oral flora, including viridans streptococci, anaerobes, and the gram-negative bacteria *Eikenella*. As with other mammalian animal bites, ampicillin/sulbactam or amoxicillin/clavulanate has comprehensive coverage of the human oral flora.
- Fresh and brackish water exposure and inoculation into the skin can allow *Aeromonas hydrophila,* a gram-negative bacilli, to cause cellulitis. This bacterium is also well known to cause necrotizing fasciitis and myonecrosis. Fluoroquinolones can be used for treatment.
- Salt water exposure, including exposure to filter-feeding mollusks (e.g., oysters, mussels, clams) can allow *Vibrio vulnificus,* a gram-negative bacilli, to cause cellulitis. In patients who are immunocompromised, ingestion of the bacteria (from the shellfish) can cause metastatic, necrotizing soft tissue infections. Doxycycline, ceftriaxone, and fluoroquinolones can be used to treat this bacterium.
- Marine mammal (e.g., whale), salt water fish slime, and swine exposure can allow *Erysipelothrix rhusiopathiae,* a gram-positive rod, to cause vesicle-forming soft tissue infections. This infection is seen in whalers, fishermen, and slaughterhouse workers. *Erysipelothrix* is one of the few gram-positive bacteria inherently resistant to vancomycin. Penicillin is effective for its treatment.
- Although patients commonly attribute their soft tissue infection to a spider bite, spiders are not known to transmit bacterial infections with their bites. Studies on the microbiology of spiders have not shown them to carry any significant pathogenic bacteria. Nearly all of these "spider bite" cases are merely furunculosis (boils), an infection of the hair shaft by *Staph.aureus.*

References

Ayoub EM, Wannamaker LW. Evaluation of the streptococcal deoxyribonuclease B and diphosphopyridine nucleotidase antibody tests in acute rheumatic fever and acute glomerulonephritis. *Pediatrics*. 1962; 29:527-538.

Baxtrom CJ, Mongkolpradit T, Kasimos JN, et al. Common house spiders are not likely vectors of community-acquired methicillin-resistant Staphylococcus aureus infections. *J Med Entomol*. 2006;43(5):962-965.

Bernard P, Bedane C, Mounier M, et al. Streptococcal cause of erysipelas and cellulitis in adults. A microbiologic study using direct immunofluorescence technique. *Arch Dermatol*. 1989;125:779-782.

Dillon HC Jr, Reeves MS. Streptococcal immune responses in nephritis after skin infection. *Am J Med*. 1974;56:333-346.

Drinker CK, Field M, Ward H, Lyons C. Increased susceptibility to local infection following blockage of lymph drainage. *Am J Physiol*. 1935;112:74-81.

Duvanel T, Auckenthaler R, Rohner P, Harms M, Saurat J. Quantitative cultures of biopsy specimens from cutaneous cellulitis. *Arch Intern Med*. 1989;149:293-296.

Goldstein B, Seltzer E, Flamm R, et al. Dalbavancin phase III skin and skin structure (SSSI) studies: pathogens and microbiological efficacy. 45th Interscience Conference on Antimicrobial Agents and Chemotherapy. Washington, DC, December 16-19, 2005 (Abstract #L-1577).

Hook EW, Hooten T, Horton C. Microbiologic evaluation of cutaneous cellulitis in adults. *Arch Intern Med*. 1986;146:295-297.

Jeng A, Beheshti M, Nathan R. The role of beta-hemolytic streptococci in causing diffuse, nonculturable cellulitis: a prospective investigation. *Medicine (Baltimore)*. 2010;89(4):217-226.

Kaul R, McGeer A, Norrby-Teglund A, et al. Intravenous immunoglobulin therapy for streptococcal toxic shock syndrome—a comparative observational study. The Canadian Streptococcal Study Group. *Clin Infect Dis.* 1999;28(4):800-807.

Liu C, Bayer A, Cosgrove S, et al. Clinical practice guidelines by the Infectious Diseases Society of America for the treatment of methicillin-resistant Staphylococcus aureus infections in adults and children. *Clin Infect Dis.* 2011;52:1-38.

Moran GJ, Krishnadasan A, Gorwitz R, et al. Methicillin-resistant S.aureus infections among patients in the emergency department. *N Engl J Med.* 2006;355:666-674.

Pallin DJ, Binder WD, Allen MB, et al. Clinical trial: comparative effectiveness of cephalexin plus trimethoprim-sulfamethoxazole versus cephalexin alone for treatment of uncomplicated cellulitis: a randomized controlled trial. *Clin Infect Dis.* 2013;56:1754-1762.

Peralta G, Padron E, Roiz MP, et al. Risk factors for bacteremia in patients with limb cellulitis. *Eur J Clin Microbiol Infect Dis.* 2006;2:619-626.

Semel JD, Goldin H. Association of athlete's foot with cellulitis of the lower extremities: diagnostic value of bacterial cultures of ipsilateral interdigital space samples. *Clin Infect Dis.* 1996;23:1162-1164.

Stevens DL, Bisno A, Chambers H, et al. Practice guidelines for the diagnosis and management of skin and soft tissue infections: 2014 update by the Infectious Diseases Society of America. *Clin Infect Dis.* 2014;59(2):e10-e52.

Stevens DL, Smith LG, Bruss JB, et al. Randomized comparison of linezolid (PNU-100766) versus oxacillin-dicloxacillin for treatment of complicated skin and soft tissue infections. *Antimicrob Agents Chemother.* 2000;44(12):3408-3413.

Stollerman GH, Lewis AJ, Schultz I, Taranta A. Relationship of immune response to group A streptococci to the course of acute, chronic and recurrent rheumatic fever. *Am J Med.* 1956;20:163-169.

Thomas KS, Crook A, Nunn A, et al. Penicillin to prevent recurrent leg cellulitis. *N Engl J Med.* 2013;368(18):1695-1703.

Emily S. Gillett ▓ Raj Dasgupta

CASE 33

A 25-Year-Old Female With Excessive Daytime Sleepiness

A 25-year-old, previously healthy female presents for outpatient evaluation of 2 to 3 years of excessive daytime sleepiness. She recently began working in a corporate firm and has been reprimanded for falling asleep during meetings with business clients. She goes to sleep at 10:00 PM and gets up at 6:30 AM. It takes only a few minutes for her to fall asleep, but she wakes up multiple times overnight and does not feel well rested in the morning. She denies symptoms of depression and anxiety as well as use of alcohol, tobacco, and illicit substances.

What are common causes of excessive daytime sleepiness in adults?

Excessive daytime sleepiness (or hypersomnolence) in adults is often due to chronic insufficient sleep from self-imposed sleep restriction (due to a "busy lifestyle"). Environmental factors (such as loud noises) or chronic medical conditions (such as joint pain or heartburn) can also cause repeated awakenings overnight and lead to nonrestorative sleep. Insomnia, defined as difficulty falling asleep or difficulty staying asleep, may be a primary problem but is often secondary to chronic medical conditions or psychiatric diagnoses, including anxiety and depression. Excessive alcohol use and abuse of illicit substances or prescription medications, such as narcotics or stimulants, may also lead to irregular sleep patterns and daytime fatigue. It is important to address these sensitive issues in confidential patient interviews and to consider drug testing when appropriate.

The patient does not think that she snores at night, but she currently lives alone.

Why might a history of snoring be medically important?

Chronic snoring may be indicative of obstructive sleep apnea (OSA), particularly in patients who are reported to have multiple short pauses (apneas) in their breathing during sleep. Obstructive apneas are often followed by a loud gasp or snort, which allows the patient to take a deep breath but also arouses him or her from sleep. Although each arousal is short, repeated arousals throughout the night lead to poor quality sleep and a decrease in the percentage of restorative slow-wave (N3) and rapid eye movement (REM) sleep. These arousals are also associated with releases of sympathetic stress hormones that cause repeated, brief increases in pulse rate and blood pressure throughout the night. Over time, untreated OSA may contribute to development of hypertension, arrhythmia, stroke, and other medical conditions. Several physical findings, including elevated body mass index (BMI), large neck circumference, large tonsils, and a small or recessed jaw (micro- or retro-gnathia), make a diagnosis of OSA more likely. One helpful screening tool is the STOP BANG questionnaire.

CLINICAL PEARL   **STEP 2/3**

The **STOP-BANG Questionnaire** is a validated screening tool for OSA. Answering "yes" to 3 to 4 questions means an individual is at intermediate risk of having OSA; answering "yes" to 5 to 8 questions is high risk for OSA.

1. **S**noring: Do you snore loudly (louder than talking or loud enough to be heard through closed doors)?
2. **T**ired: Do you often feel tired, fatigued, or sleepy during the daytime?
3. **O**bserved: Has anyone observed you stop breathing during your sleep?
4. **P**ressure: Do you have or are you being treated for high blood pressure?
5. **B**MI: Body mass index (BMI) >35 kg/m^2?
6. **A**ge: Over 50 years old?
7. **N**eck: Neck circumference >40 cm (16 inches)?
8. **G**ender: Male gender?

The patient denies history of parasomnias, including sleep walking and talking in her sleep, but she often falls asleep in the shower or at the kitchen table while eating dinner.

What are parasomnias?

Parasomnias are disruptive behaviors or distressing experiences that occur during sleep or sleep–wake transitions. Sleep deprivation may worsen the severity of any parasomnia. Parasomnias can be divided into those that are REM-related or non-REM-related. In addition to its characteristic rapid eye movements, which can be seen on electrooculogram (EOG) tracings, two important characteristics of normal REM sleep are dreams and atonic paralysis. Nightmares are the most common REM-related parasomnias, consisting of troubling or disturbing dream content that may lead to awakening. Other REM-related parasomnias involve an uncoupling of atonic paralysis from the appropriate stage of sleep. In atonic paralysis, most skeletal muscles (aside from the diaphragm) do not move, and this is important to prevent a person from acting out his or her dreams. In REM sleep behavior disorder, a person does not become atonic and physically acts out aspects of his or her dreams. In sleep paralysis, the opposite occurs and a person's mind is awake but he or she is atonic and unable to move for a few minutes after awakening. Non-REM parasomnias include night terrors, confusional arousals, teeth grinding (bruxism), sleepwalking (somnambulism), and periodic limb movement disorder (PLM-D), which is often associated with daytime symptoms of restless legs syndrome and difficulty falling asleep. A list of common parasomnias is included in Table 33.1.

The patient takes public transportation to work but will sometimes fall asleep and miss her subway stop. She stopped driving after she had a motor vehicle collision when she was 20 years old.

Why is it important to ask about driving in patients with excessive daytime sleepiness?

Drowsy driving is a significant contributing factor in many motor vehicle fatalities. It is important to counsel patients with excessive daytime sleepiness not to drive when they feel drowsy. In the interest of public safety, physicians in some jurisdictions may be required to report to local agencies those individuals with severe, refractory hypersomnia that may render them unfit to operate a motor vehicle. Drowsy driving is also an important issue for overnight shift workers and medical trainees. Surveys of medical residents have suggested that working a shift lasting over 24 hours increases the risk of having a motor vehicle collision by more than twofold. Sleep deprivation

TABLE 33.1 ▓ Common Parasomnias

REM-Related Parasomnias	Non-REM-Related Parasomnias
REM sleep behavior disorder Nightmares Sleep paralysis	Confusional arousals Night terrors Bruxism Somnambulism (sleep walking) Somniloquy (sleep talking) Periodic limb movement disorder (PLM-D)
REM, Rapid eye movement.	

can also contribute to medical errors. Most residency programs now teach trainees how to recognize signs of fatigue and encourage them to employ techniques, such as strategic napping, to mitigate fatigue and its potential impacts on education and patient care.

The patient's Epworth Sleepiness Scale score is 18 out of 24. She has normal vital signs and physical exam but is slightly overweight. She has never had a sleep study.

What is the Epworth Sleepiness Scale?

The Epworth Sleepiness Scale is a validated questionnaire that measures a patient's general level of daytime sleepiness. It has been modified for use in pediatric populations and translated into many different languages. Scores ≥9 out of 24 suggest excessive daytime sleepiness and merit evaluation by a sleep specialist.

CLINICAL PEARL   **STEP 2/3**

The **Epworth Sleepiness Scale** gives a general measure of a person's daytime sleepiness and is useful for initial screening and for following changes over time after starting therapy. A person rates from 0 to 3 how likely they are to doze off in different situations. A score of 7 to 8 is average, whereas scores ≥9 (out of 24) suggest excessive sleepiness that merits evaluation by a sleep specialist.

     0 = no chance of dozing
     1 = slight chance of dozing
     2 = moderate chance of dozing
     3 = high chance of dozing

Situation	Chance of Dozing
Sitting and reading	_____
Watching TV	_____
Sitting inactive in a public place (e.g., a theater or a meeting)	_____
As a passenger in the car for an hour without a break	_____
Lying down to rest in the afternoon when circumstances permit	_____
Sitting and talking to someone	_____
Sitting quietly after a lunch without alcohol	_____
In a car, while stopped in traffic for a few minutes	_____
	TOTAL: _____ /24

What is a sleep study?

Several different types of sleep studies exist, including home studies and daytime nap studies. One of the most common sleep studies is an overnight polysomnography (PSG) where a patient sleeps at a medical facility while his or her vital signs, breathing patterns, electroencephalography (EEG), and body movements are monitored and recorded. This type of study allows a sleep specialist to score respiratory events, such as *apneas*, in which airflow through the mouth and nose ceases, and *hypopneas*, in which airflow is significantly reduced. Information about respiratory effort is derived from expandable belts around the chest and abdomen, allowing one to distinguish *central apneas*, in which there is a pause in central respiratory drive and lack of respiratory effort from *obstructive apneas*, in which a person's chest moves but he or she is unable to overcome an upper airway obstruction.

EEG information allows for sleep staging in which one scores how an individual progresses through the different stages of sleep. Sleep stages are classified as REM and non-REM. The non-REM stages of sleep are further divided into N1, N2, and N3, and each stage has a characteristic EEG pattern (see Fig. 33.1). An individual's pattern of sleep stage progression during the night, called his or her *sleep architecture*, can be helpful in diagnosing certain sleep disorders. However, sleep architecture may also be altered by many medications, particularly antidepressants, antihistamines, and antiepileptic drugs.

> The patient is not currently taking any medications but previously used methylphenidate for attention deficit hyperactivity disorder (ADHD) during high school.

What are the treatment options for hypersomnolence?

Primary hypersomnia is a diagnosis of exclusion. The first step in treating a patient with chronic hypersomnolence is evaluation for underlying sleep disorders, including OSA, PLM-D, insomnia, circadian phase delay, and narcolepsy, as well as sleepiness due to medications or other substances. If daytime stimulants are prescribed prior to a complete diagnostic evaluation, these medications may mask daytime symptoms, prevent necessary daytime napping, and delay diagnosis of treatable sleep conditions. In addition, although stimulant medications generally produce a subjective improvement in alertness, this is not always accompanied by an objective improvement in alertness as measured by a cognitive test, such as the psychomotor vigilance test, that requires sustained attention and focus.

CLINICAL PEARL   **STEP 2/3**

It is not uncommon for patients with untreated sleep disorders, including OSA, to have a history of ADHD and/or past treatment with stimulant medication. Poor-quality sleep and sleep deprivation may lead to inattention, poor short-term memory, and poor concentration, symptoms similar to those seen in individuals with ADHD. In young children, the most common daytime symptoms related to untreated sleep disorders are irritability and hyperactivity rather than excessive sleepiness, leading to both academic and social difficulties.

> The patient is seen in a sleep center. Aside from being slightly overweight, she has normal vital signs and a normal physical exam. Based on her history and extreme level of sleepiness, the sleep specialist suspects that she may have narcolepsy. During her subsequent overnight polysomnography study, she has normal breathing during sleep and no abnormal leg movements. However, she falls asleep very quickly, entering REM within only a few minutes, and her sleep architecture is fragmented with multiple short arousals. She is asked to stay for a daytime nap study the next

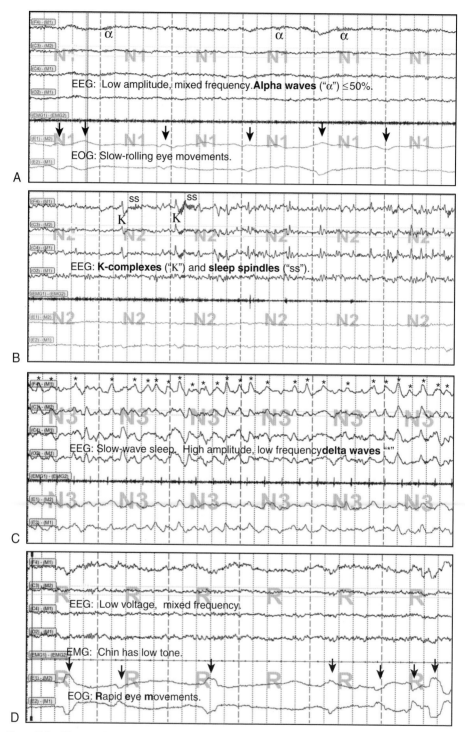

Figure 33.1 **30-second epochs from overnight polysomnography studies.** Figures depict typical electroencephalogram (EEG), electromyogram (EMG), and electrooculogram (EOG) findings during **(A)** N1, **(B)** N2, **(C)** N3 non-REM sleep, and **(D)** REM sleep.

morning, called a multiple sleep latency test (MSLT). During each of her four naps, she falls asleep 4 to 5 minutes after lying down and she enters REM sleep during two of the four naps. A urine toxicology screen collected the night of her sleep study is negative.

Diagnosis: Narcolepsy

What is narcolepsy and how is it diagnosed?

In people with narcolepsy, the switch between wakefulness and REM sleep is not properly regulated and they may enter sleep quickly and at inappropriate times. They also have difficulty maintaining their sleep continuity overnight, leading to sleep fragmentation and nonrestful sleep (see Fig. 33.2). Sleep latency, or the time from lying down with the lights out until the onset of sleep, is generally very short in people with narcolepsy both at night and during the day. During an MSLT, narcoleptics have a mean sleep latency of ≤8 minutes. In contrast, unaffected individuals with sufficient sleep have mean sleep latencies of 10 to 15 minutes. During an MSLT, REM occurring within 15 minutes of falling asleep is called a sleep-onset REM period (SOREMP). The presence of ≥2 SOREMPs during an MSLT is an essential characteristic of narcolepsy (see Fig. 33.3). Although the presence of ≥2 SOREMPs is a sensitive criterion, it is not specific to narcolepsy. Other conditions that may lead to SOREMPs include shift work disorder, recent sleep deprivation, untreated OSA, and circadian phase delay. In contrast, several medications, including stimulants and antidepressants, may suppress REM sleep leading to false-negative MSLT results.

Narcolepsy is divided into type 1 (with cataplexy) and type 2 (without cataplexy). Cataplexy is a transient weakness (generally lasting <2 minutes) in all or part of the body that is usually triggered by a strong emotion, such as laughter or excitement. In type 1 narcolepsy, a patient must have a history of daily lapses into sleep for ≥3 months. He or she must also have either a history of cataplexy AND a positive MSLT (with *both* mean sleep latency of ≤8 minutes and ≥2 SOREMPs), *OR* he or she must have a low concentration of hypocretin-1 (orexin-A) in the cerebrospinal fluid (CSF). Type 2 narcolepsy, or narcolepsy *without* cataplexy, is a diagnosis of exclusion and may not be associated with low hypocretin-1 levels. Type 2 narcolepsy requires a positive MSLT and exclusion of all alternative causes of chronic hypersomnia, including other sleep disorders and sedating medications.

The onset of narcolepsy can occur anywhere from childhood to middle age but is most often diagnosed in the teens and early 20s. In teens, symptoms of narcolepsy may be confused with delayed circadian sleep phase (a forward shift of the circadian clock to a later bedtime and wake time), which is a common finding in adolescents. Additional symptoms commonly seen in patients with narcolepsy are summarized in Table 33.2.

What is the pathophysiology of narcolepsy?

Many believe that narcolepsy is an autoimmune disorder, but the exact mechanism of this disease remains obscure. Type 1 narcolepsy is thought to result from destruction of neurons in the dorsolateral hypothalamus that produce hypocretin-1 (orexin-A), a neuropeptide hormone that promotes wakefulness through its interaction with orexin receptors in different parts of the brain. Less is known about the pathophysiology and progression of type 2 narcolepsy. Secondary narcolepsy may be seen in other disease processes that cause hypothalamic injury, including tumors of the hypothalamus or midbrain, vascular malformations, and strokes. Some paraneoplastic syndromes may also mimic narcolepsy. In general, however, patients with secondary narcolepsy usually have additional neurologic deficits.

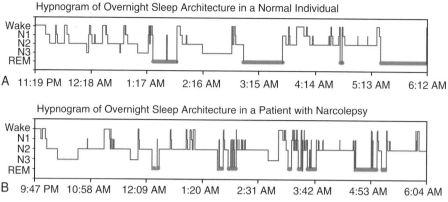

Figure 33.2 **A,** Hypnogram showing the overnight sleep architecture of a normal individual. **B,** Hypnogram showing the overnight sleep architecture of an individual with narcolepsy. Note the fragmented sleep pattern, particularly evident during rapid eye movement (REM) sleep.

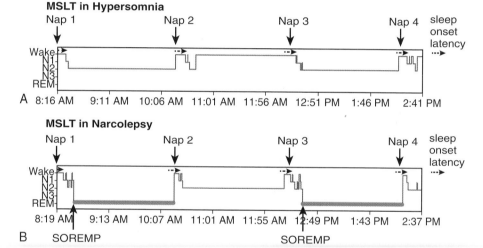

Figure 33.3 **A,** Multiple sleep latency test (MSLT) of an individual with hypersomnia. Note the short sleep-onset latency. **B,** MSLT of an individual with narcolepsy. Note the short sleep-onset latency *and* the two sleep-onset REM periods (SOREMPs).

How is narcolepsy treated?

The first line of treatment for narcolepsy is a stimulant medication, such as modafinil, methylphenidate, or dextroamphetamine. Strategic scheduled napping is important and may significantly reduce daytime sleepiness. In patients with cataplexy, sodium oxybate (Xyrem®) may be particularly helpful in treating both sleepiness and cataplexy. However, as this gamma-aminobutyric acid (GABA) derivative is related to the "date rape" drug gamma hydroxybutyrate, it is very closely regulated. Sodium oxybate rapidly produces deep sedation, and very high doses may produce respiratory depression. Patients who are prescribed sodium oxybate are followed closely, and detailed counseling is required prior to starting this medication. To avoid injury related to rapid onset of medication effects, patients are counseled not to take sodium oxybate until they are sitting in bed. They are also advised to keep the medication in a lockbox to prevent unauthorized access and potential misuse.

TABLE 33.2 ■ Common Symptoms of Narcolepsy

Inadvertent Naps	• Also called "sleep attacks," most *untreated* narcoleptics will experience ≥1 inadvertent nap each day. • The tendency to fall asleep does not correlate with a person's level of interest in an activity. • This symptom can lead to problems at work and at school, as well as socially.
Cataplexy	• Cataplexy is a sudden but transient weakness in all or part of the body triggered by a strong emotion (such as laughter, fear, or excitement). • Most attacks of cataplexy last <2 minutes. • Cataplexy is seen in type 1 narcolepsy in which patients have low levels of hypocretin-1 (orexin-A) in the cerebrospinal fluid.
Sleep Paralysis	• In sleep paralysis, a person is unable to move his or her body for several minutes after awakening. • Isolated sleep paralysis may also occur in individuals without narcolepsy.
Hypnagogic Hallucinations	• These are visual or auditory hallucinations that occur *as a person is falling asleep.* • Hallucinations occurring as a person is awakening are called *hypnopompic hallucinations.* This type of hallucination may also occur but is less specific to narcolepsy.
Weight Gain	• Mild obesity is common in narcoleptics, and significant weight gain may be seen at the onset of this disease in children.

BEYOND THE PEARLS

- Certain genetic factors may predispose an individual to developing narcolepsy. For instance, human leukocyte antigen (HLA) class II haplotype DQB1*06:02 is present in ≥90% of patients with type 1 narcolepsy with cataplexy, supporting the idea that narcolepsy is caused by an autoimmune mechanism. However, this HLA haplotype is present in between 12 and 38% of the general population, and studies in identical twins indicate that a combination of genetic and environmental factors is required to produce this disease.
- Narcolepsy is more common in patients with Prader-Willi syndrome and Niemann-Pick disease.
- Seasonal patterns in the frequency of new narcolepsy cases may be associated with cyclical patterns of communicable diseases, such as the H1N1 strain of influenza. This may be due to molecular mimicry between viral and human proteins.
- An association was noted between an increased incidence of pediatric narcolepsy cases and administration of a specific vaccine used in Northern Europe against the 2009 pandemic H1N1. This vaccine was unique in that it contained the AS03 adjuvant. An *adjuvant* is a vaccine component designed to help stimulate the host's immune response to viral proteins. It is thought that the AS03 adjuvant may have stimulated a stronger immune response than adjuvants used in other H1N1 vaccines, leading to a greater likelihood of generating an autoimmune response. In Finnish children, administration of this specific vaccine led to a >12-fold higher risk of developing narcolepsy within the next 8 months.
- The psychomotor vigilance test is designed to provide an objective measure of alertness. This cognitive test is very simple but requires sustained attention. A subject is asked to press a button in response to the repeated appearance of a dot on a computer screen.

Continued

BEYOND THE PEARLS—cont'd

Increased fatigue correlates with an increased number of "missed dots," each of which indicates a momentary lapse in attention.

- NASA studies are under way to determine the utility of a shorter version of the psychomotor vigilance test, called the reaction self-test, in monitoring fatigue among space station crew. In high-risk environments, this test may be a useful tool to assess alertness prior to beginning complex or difficult tasks.
- Living in low Earth orbit for an extended period of time produces unique challenges in terms of maintaining a normal circadian rhythm and a sleep schedule that provides adequate sleep. In addition to the physical and mental stresses of living in a confined space with microgravity and apparent weightlessness, during each 24-hour period, the astronauts on the International Space Station witness approximately 15 sunrises and sunsets. Both chronic sleep deprivation and the lingering sedative effects of sleep medications used to help regulate sleep cycles may impair cognition, judgment, and the ability to complete complex tasks critical for the safety and survival of the crew.

References

American Academy of Sleep Medicine. *International Classification of Sleep Disorders*. 3rd ed. Darien, IL: 2014.

Barger LK, Cade BE, Ayas NT, et al. Extended work shifts and the risk of motor vehicle crashes among interns. *N Engl J Med*. 2005;352:125-134.

Basner M, Mollicone D, Dinges DF. Validity and sensitivity of a brief psychomotor vigilance test (PVT-B) to total and partial sleep deprivation. *Acta Astronaut*. 2011;69:949-959.

Chung F, Yegenswaran B, Liao PM, et al. STOP questionnaire: a tool to screen patients for obstructive sleep apnea. *Anesthesiology*. 2008;108(5):812-821.

Johns MW. A new method for measuring daytime sleepiness: the Epworth Sleepiness Scale. *Sleep*. 1991;14(6):540-545.

Lockley SW, Cronin JW, Evan EE, et al. Effect of reducing interns' weekly work hours on sleep and attentional failures. *N Engl J Med*. 2004;351(18):1829-1837.

Lockley SW, Landrigan CP, Barger LK, et al. When policy meets physiology: the challenge of reducing resident work hours. *Clin Orthop Relat Res*. 2006;449:116-127.

Mignot EJ. A practical guide to the therapy of narcolepsy and hypersomnia syndromes. *Neurotherapeutics*. 2012;9:739-752.

Owens JA. Neurocognitive and behavioral impact of sleep disordered breathing in children. *Pediatr Pulmonol*. 2009;44(5):417-422.

Singh AK, Mahlios J, Mignot E. Genetic association, seasonal infections and autoimmune basis of narcolepsy. *J Autoimmun*. 2013;43:26-31.

Ward KL, Hillman DR, James A, et al. Excessive daytime sleepiness increases the risk of motor vehicle crash in obstructive sleep apnea. *J Clin Sleep Med*. 2013;9:1013-1021.

Brandon A. Miller

A 31-Year-Old Female With a Systolic Heart Murmur

A 31-year-old female comes to your office to establish care. She has not seen a physician on a regular basis since her teenage years when she was under the care of her pediatrician. She denies chronic medical problems and has no previous hospitalizations or surgeries. Both of her parents are healthy without known medical conditions. She takes no medications. She denies tobacco or illicit drug use but drinks two to three drinks per weekend night and a glass of wine one or two evenings per week. She was born in the United States and works in human resources for a tech company. She tries to stay active when she can and runs 1 to 2 miles once or twice a week.

Review of systems is positive for mild fatigue for the past year and occasional chest pain described as sharp, nonexertional, nonpositional, and not associated with eating. The pain lasts between 5 and 15 seconds and is sometimes associated with feelings of anxiousness and hyperventilation. She denies associated shortness of breath, dizziness, or sweating. These episodes occur once a month or less. She also admits to occasional palpitations described as her heart "skipping a beat" that are not associated with chest pain, lightheadedness, syncope, or near-syncope. This occurs mostly at night when lying down to go to sleep. She has not been previously evaluated for any of these symptoms.

The physical exam reveals a healthy-appearing young female of normal body habitus with normal vital signs and a body mass index (BMI) of 21 kg/m^2. The rest of the physical exam is normal with the exception a midsystolic click that occurs just prior to a nonradiating grade 2 systolic murmur best heard over the apex. Her point of maximal impulse (PMI) is nonpalpable. The patient doesn't recall ever having been told that she has a heart murmur.

What is the differential diagnosis of a systolic heart murmur? What is the most likely diagnosis in your patient?

Systolic heart murmurs are common in practice and often benign (unlike diastolic murmurs, which are usually associated with some form of pathology). In young adults, although systolic murmurs are heard in 5 to 52% of patients, the echocardiogram is normal in 86 to 100% (this number is even higher in pregnant women referred for systolic murmurs), suggesting that echocardiograms are overutilized in this population. The subject of murmurs is further complicated by the fact that general internists are quite weak at identifying the cause of murmurs. In a 1997 *JAMA* study of 314 internal medicine and family practice residents, only 20% were able to correctly identify abnormal heart sounds from recordings. In another paper in *JAMA* (from the Rational Clinical Exam series) the precision of examining a grade 2 or louder murmur in the clinical setting is poor, with a kappa statistic of only 0.30 (this includes cardiologists).

Before discussing the heart murmurs that are caused by valvular and structural heart disease, it is worth noting that blood viscosity and velocity are also factors in producing a murmur. Don't forget to think about noncardiac causes (such as anemia and thyrotoxicosis) when you hear abnormal systolic heart sounds. It's also worth noting that a thorough history is the first and most important step in assessing a murmur. A systolic murmur in a 26-year-old female with anemia and heavy menstrual periods has different implications than one in a 46-year-old male with active intravenous (IV) drug use, fevers, and weight loss.

In general, pathologic murmurs are produced from the following valvular and structural abnormalities: aortic stenosis, mitral regurgitation (including due to mitral valve prolapse [MVP]), and tricuspid regurgitation and hypertrophic cardiomyopathy (HCM). Aortic stenosis (AS) is most likely to occur in older patients with calcification of the aortic valve but can also occur in younger patients with bicuspid aortic valves. It is loudest over the aortic valve area, located over the second intercostal space just to the right of the sternum. It can radiate to the right carotid artery and is *not* associated with a click. Your patient's clinical history and murmur do not fit with AS. Tricuspid regurgitation (TR) occurs most often as a result of pulmonary pathology; however, it can rarely occur as a primary valvular problem (as when it occurs in Ebstein's anomaly). TR is loudest over the tricuspid valve area, located over the left lower sternal border and is *not* associated with a click. Again, your patient's clinical history and murmur do not fit. HCM is a heterogeneous condition of concern in a young patient as it can potentially be fatal. The vast majority of patients, though, are either asymptomatic or have nonspecific symptoms like your patient. The condition is caused most commonly by an inherited mutation in the heart muscle. The systolic murmur of HCM, especially when there is subaortic hypertrophy, is a harsh crescendo-decrescendo murmur that is best heard over the apex, located at the 5th or 6th intercostal space in the midclavicular line. It radiates to the left lower sternal border and is *not* associated with a click. Often a strong apical impulse can be palpated as well, signifying a hypertrophied left ventricle. Mitral regurgitation (MR), when it occurs as a result of MVP, is also a late systolic murmur heard loudest over the apex, occurring after a midsystolic click. The click is a distinct sound that happens as a result of the chordae tendinae suddenly tensing after the mitral valve prolapses into the left atrium.

Your patient has a distinct midsystolic click that none of the other valvular conditions have. In that same Rational Clinical Exam series article from *JAMA*, this systolic click with or without a murmur is sufficient to make a diagnosis of MVP. As we shall see soon, the rest of your patient's clinical picture is consistent with MVP as well.

BASIC SCIENCE PEARL   **STEP 1**

The kappa statistic (or kappa coefficient) is a value that measures the agreement between observers and is useful in evaluating physical exam findings or diagnostic test interpretations. A kappa of 1 indicates perfect agreement whereas a kappa of 0 indicates no agreement or that the agreement is due to chance.

CLINICAL PEARL   **STEP 2/3**

Characteristics of benign murmurs that do not require further workup include low intensity (grade 1 or 2), absence of radiation, early systolic timing, normal jugular venous pressure and carotid artery impulses, absence of cardiac symptoms, and a normal electrocardiogram (ECG) and chest radiograph.

What is MVP?

MVP is defined as a >2 mm ballooning of one or both of the mitral valve leaflets into the left atrium during systole, with or without associated mitral regurgitation. Most patients with MVP have associated MR (MVP is the most common cause of MR), though the majority of these patients have only mild or trace MR of little clinical significance. In fact, MVP is asymptomatic in most patients and is found during routine exam or on an echocardiogram performed for another reason. The most common etiology for the condition is idiopathic and due to thickening of one of the layers of the mitral valve; however, familial cases of MVP are a well-described phenomenon. Additionally, there are a number of conditions that cause secondary MVP, and these are either from connective tissue diseases affecting the valve leaflets (such as the Ehlers-Danlos and Marfan syndromes) or disruptions in the papillary muscles or chordae tendinae (which can occur in ischemic heart disease and cardiomyopathy).

The main physical exam finding of MVP is a midsystolic click followed by a late systolic murmur if mitral regurgitation is present. As noted previously, the click is generated by sudden tensing of the chordae as the mitral valve leaflets billow up into the left atrium. Most patients with the condition have a normal life expectancy, though approximately 5 to 10% have a course of progressive mitral regurgitation leading to numerous complications.

CLINICAL PEARL   **STEP 3**

Untreated severe MR results in a number of serious complications. Left ventricular dilatation and dysfunction develop as a result of the continuously increased blood volume delivered to the ventricle during diastole. This eventually leads to left-sided heart failure and pulmonary hypertension as a result of congested pulmonary vasculature. The left atrium dilates as well, making patients more prone to atrial arrhythmias such as atrial fibrillation and flutter. Both atrial fibrillation and the increased turbulence surrounding the mitral valve are major risk factors for intracardiac thrombi that can embolize to cause stroke and other complications.

What is dynamic auscultation and how can it be used to help diagnose systolic murmurs?

Dynamic auscultation refers to the change in murmur intensity (the murmur becomes either louder or softer) with certain changes in position and physical exam maneuvers. This change in intensity can help increase accuracy when trying to determine the cause of a murmur. It's important to note that no single maneuver is 100% accurate in diagnosing the cause of a systolic murmur.

In general, systolic murmurs increase in intensity when there is more blood in the heart and decrease in intensity when there is less blood. Basically, *more blood = more flow = louder systolic murmur* and vice versa. The physical exam maneuvers that cause an increased amount of blood in the heart include moving the patient from a standing to a squatting position (or simply known as squatting), laying a patient flat, or performing a passive leg raise (the examiner raises a recumbent patient's legs to a 45-degree angle). All of these maneuvers increase venous return to the heart. Allow at least 30 to 45 seconds after the change in position before assessing whether there is a change in the murmur's intensity. Inspiration, which causes a decrease in intrathoracic pressure, draws blood into the heart, thereby increasing the intensity of a systolic murmur. Maneuvers that decrease the amount of blood in the heart are having the patient stand from a seated position (at least 600 mL of blood are left pooled in the veins and therefore not returned to the heart) and instructing the patient to perform a Valsalva (which increases thoracic pressure). Expiration also causes an increase in thoracic pressure, which not only decreases venous return but forces blood out of the heart. Expiration will therefore decrease the intensity of a systolic murmur.

You decide to use dynamic auscultation to assess your patient. You perform a passive leg raise and are surprised to hear that her murmur *actually decreases in intensity*. Next you have her stand after being seated for a few minutes and you're surprised to hear that her murmur *actually increases in intensity*.

If systolic murmurs are supposed to increase with increased amount of blood in the heart and vice versa, why are you finding that the opposite is occurring in your patient?

MVP with MR does *not* follow the general rules for dynamic auscultation and systolic murmurs. The physical exam maneuvers that increase and decrease the amount of blood in the heart will actually have the *opposite* effect compared to most systolic murmurs.

Maneuvers that increase the amount of blood in the heart (squatting, laying flat, passive leg raise) *decrease* the murmur of MVP with MR. Why? Because more blood in the heart stretches the left ventricle, which causes more tension on the chordae. This condition of unusually tense chordae doesn't allow the mitral valve to prolapse as much into the left atrium during systole. Therefore, less blood flows backward across the mitral valve during systole. *More blood in the heart = less prolapse = less MR = a softer murmur and later click.*

Maneuvers that decrease the amount of blood in the heart (standing, Valsalva) will actually *increase* the murmur of MVP with MR. Why? Less blood in the heart leaves the left ventricle relatively collapsed, which results in slack chordae tendinae. Slack chordae allow the leaflets to billow up quicker and more forcefully, creating a large aperture for a regurgitant jet. *Less blood in the heart = more prolapse = more MR = a louder and longer murmur and an earlier click.*

Another maneuver that affects the murmur of MVP is handgrip. Asking your patient to make tight fists for approximately 30 seconds increases systemic vascular resistance and therefore afterload. Inflating blood pressure cuffs on a patient's arms will have the same effect. In a patient with MVP with MR, increased afterload creates an elevation in pressure in the left ventricle during systole that is transmitted backward to the mitral valve apparatus, causing an earlier and more forceful prolapse. Again, *more prolapse = more MR = a louder and longer murmur and an earlier click.*

CLINICAL PEARL   **STEP 2/3**

Hypertrophic cardiomyopathy (HCM) with subaortic stenosis is the only other murmur that does not follow the rules of dynamic auscultation and systolic murmurs. More blood in the heart will decrease the intensity of the murmur and vice versa. The only difference between MVP with MR and HCM is that handgrip will decrease the intensity of the murmur in HCM (whereas it increases the intensity of the murmur in MVP with MR).

You inform your patient that you've heard a heart murmur that sounds like the benign condition MVP. You want to take the rest of her review of systems seriously and decide to perform a basic workup for fatigue including a complete blood count (CBC) to evaluate for anemia, a thyroid-stimulating hormone (TSH) test to evaluate for thyroid disease, a human immunodeficiency virus (HIV) test, a comprehensive metabolic panel (CMP) to evaluate for liver and metabolic abnormalities, and a fasting blood sugar to evaluate for diabetes. You also order an ECG, given her murmur and report of palpitations. The labs return in a week and are completely normal. You interpret the ECG as normal sinus rhythm with a pulse rate of 62/min, no ST-T changes, normal intervals, and no evidence of chamber enlargement.

Given that you are confident that your patient's murmur is MVP, do you even have to order an echocardiogram?

Although your patient does not have any very concerning symptoms and has a normal ECG with normal intervals, the American College of Cardiology/American Heart Association (ACC/ AHA) still recommends obtaining an echocardiogram on all patients with suspected MVP even if they are asymptomatic. The purpose of the echocardiogram is to confirm the diagnosis, establish a baseline, and evaluate for the presence of factors that would suggest a course of disease that isn't typical and benign. Specifically, the echocardiogram is performed to assess the thickness of the mitral valve leaflets, the degree of MR, and the left atrial and ventricular morphology and function.

> Your patient's echocardiogram reveals 3 mm prolapse of both mitral leaflets during systole, trace MR, thickening of both leaflets (which also measure 3 mm), a left ventricular ejection fraction of 65% with normal left atrial and left ventricular morphology, and a pulmonary artery systolic pressure of 20 mm Hg.

> **Diagnosis:** Mitral valve prolapse

What follow-up is recommended for her echocardiogram findings? Does she ever need another one?

Your patient's echocardiogram findings predict a benign course of disease. She has mitral prolapse based on the ballooning of the mitral leaflets into the left atrium during systole (the echocardiogram criteria for MVP include a 2 mm or greater billowing of the mitral valves into the atrium during systole). She has only trace MR and normal left ventricular function and pulmonary artery systolic pressure. For patients with no, trace, or mild MR, no follow-up echocardiogram is required if she remains asymptomatic. The ACC/AHA recommends clinical follow up every 3 to 5 years for patients like yours. A repeat echocardiogram should be obtained only if she has a change in symptoms that suggests worsening MR or left ventricular dysfunction.

CLINICAL PEARL   **STEP 2/3**

Moderate to severe MR and mitral valve leaflets measuring more than 5 mm are predictive of future complications from MVP. Patients with these findings require closer monitoring clinically, either every 6 months or every 12 months depending on the severity of the regurgitation.

> Your patient is very concerned that she has an "abnormal heart" and is having chest pain and occasional palpitations.

What do you tell her about her diagnosis and what she can do to help her symptoms?

When a patient with MVP presents with nonspecific symptoms such as atypical chest pain, palpitations, anxiety, numbness and tingling, or fatigue this is known as *MVP syndrome*. It is a controversial diagnosis in that there is a questionable link between these symptoms and MVP. Nevertheless, patients are often concerned when they have the above symptoms, especially in the setting of having a heart murmur.

The first step in recommending a treatment plan for these sometimes vague symptoms is working them up as you would for someone without MVP. Your patient who has a normal echocardiogram without evidence of structural heart disease (other than the MVP) is predicted to have a benign course with a normal life expectancy and a low yearly rate of complications (approximately 2% per year, noncumulative). Her chest pain is very atypical for ischemic chest pain as is her personal and family history, and her ECG demonstrates no evidence of prior myocardial infarction. Her palpitations are very nonspecific and are not associated with any concerning signs. Her ECG has a normal rhythm and intervals. Patients with MVP without severe MR and no structural heart disease have a rate of arrhythmia similar to those without MVP (the most common cause of palpitations being premature atrial or ventricular beats) and should be worked up in the same way. That is, a Holter or event monitor should be obtained after an ECG if there are associated symptoms such as dizziness, lightheadedness, shortness of breath, syncope or near syncope, or the palpitations are sustained. Your patient's palpitations occur only at night when there is more opportunity to focus on them and the "skipped beat" description is typical of premature atrial or ventricular beats. There are no significant electrolyte abnormalities to suggest a cause for another arrhythmia. Her fatigue is also nonspecific and has been thoroughly evaluated with labs.

The primary treatment recommendation in this case is reassurance. Your patient is at low risk for any serious pathology. Avoidance of caffeine and alcohol, stress management, proper sleep hygiene, and aerobic exercise can help all of her symptoms as well.

CLINICAL PEARL   **STEP 2/3**

For patients with mitral valve prolapse syndrome who have persistent symptoms (chest pain, anxiety, palpitations) despite lifestyle modification, the treatment of choice is a beta blocker.

Your patient returns to your office in several months with a letter from her dentist. She is having her wisdom teeth removed and the dentist wants to know if she should receive antibiotic prophylaxis prior to the procedure.

Does your patient need antibiotic prophylaxis before going for dental procedures?

For decades, MVP was considered a strong risk factor for infective endocarditis and required prophylaxis for dental or other invasive procedures. The most recent AHA/ACC guidelines however *no longer recommend* infective endocarditis prophylaxis for patients with MVP. Instead, the guidelines recommend infective endocarditis prophylaxis only for those patients at highest risk for complications of infective endocarditis. This group includes patients with prosthetic heart valves, a history of infective endocarditis, cyanotic heart disease (repaired or unrepaired), or valvular disease in the setting of a cardiac transplant. The main rationale behind this revision is that infective endocarditis is more likely to occur with the bacteremia that occurs on a daily basis (either randomly or from activities like brushing your teeth) than from bacteremia from dental or invasive procedures. Furthermore, prophylaxis only prevents an exceptionally small number of people from getting infective endocarditis, and the risk of adverse effects from antibiotics has been shown to exceed the risk of infective endocarditis. The guidelines have also changed in that infective endocarditis prophylaxis is now recommended only for dental procedures involving manipulation of the gums or involving the periapical region of the tooth (root), and no longer for gastrointestinal or genitourinary procedures (unless there is another reason for antibiotics, such as ongoing infection).

CLINICAL PEARL   **STEP 2/3**

For those at highest risk of endocarditis from a dental procedure, the prophylactic antibiotic of choice is amoxicillin 2 g orally 30 to 60 minutes prior to the procedure. For those allergic to penicillin, alternatives include cephalexin 2 g (only if there is no history of anaphylaxis to penicillins), clindamycin 600 mg, or azithromycin 500 mg.

BEYOND THE PEARLS

- The most common ECG abnormality in patients with MVP is ST-T wave depression or T-wave inversions in the inferior leads. This can lead to false positives on exercise ECG stress testing.
- In general, for patients with MVP with severe MR, the treatment of choice is mitral valve repair, not replacement.
- Given the association of MVP with connective tissue disorders, consider MVP in patients with musculoskeletal abnormalities such as pectus excavatum and scoliosis.
- Patients with depressed ejection fraction as a result of severe MR are treated with beta blockers, angiotensin-converting enzyme (ACE) inhibitors, and loop diuretics for pulmonary congestion; this is the same as the treatment of depressed ejection fraction without MR.
- For patients with MVP who develop sudden acute worsening of MR with resulting heart failure symptoms, suspect ruptured chordae tendinae.
- Pregnant women with MVP and either no, trace, or mild MR do not require any special interventions during pregnancy. Those with severe MR should have repair prior to pregnancy. Those with severe MR and left ventricle ejection fraction <30% or with pulmonary hypertension should be counseled to avoid getting pregnant.
- The absence of a mitral area or holosystolic murmur significantly reduces the probability of having MR except in the setting of acute myocardial infarction.

References

Bonow RO, Chatterjee K, Faxon D, et al. ACC/AHA 2006 guidelines for the management of patients with valvular heart disease: executive summary. *Circulation*. 2006;114:450-527.

Bouknight DP, O'Rourke RA. Current management of mitral valve prolapse. *Am Fam Physician*. 2000;61(11):3343-3350.

Etchells E, Bell C, Robb K. Does this patient have an abnormal systolic murmur? *JAMA*. 1997;277(7): 564-571.

Freed LA, Benjamin EJ, Levy D, et al. Mitral valve prolapse in the general population: the benign nature of echocardiographic features in the Framingham Heart Study. *J Am Coll Cardiol*. 2002;40:1298.

Lembo NJ, Dell'Italia LJ, Crawford MH, O'Rourke RA. Bedside diagnosis of systolic murmurs. *N Engl J Med*. 1988;318(24):1572-1578.

Nishimura RA, Carabello B, Faxon D, et al. 2008 AHA/ACC guideline update on valvular heart disease: focused update on infective endocarditis. *Circulation*. 2008;118(8):887-896.

Shub C. Echocardiography or auscultation? How to evaluate systolic murmurs. *Can Fam Physician*. 2003;49:163-167.

Monisha Bhanote ■ Daniel Martinez

A 57-Year-Old Male With Shortness of Breath

A 57-year-old male is evaluated in the emergency department with a 1-week history of worsening shortness of breath and mildly productive cough. He has chronic obstructive pulmonary disease (COPD) and generally has some shortness of breath, but he indicates this is a dramatic change from his baseline symptoms. His medications include albuterol and ipratropium bromide inhalers as needed. He had earlier presented to an urgent care center that diagnosed him with a mild COPD exacerbation and gave him oral glucocorticoids and azithromycin. His symptoms had improved slightly, but this morning he develops hemoptysis for the first time, so he comes to the emergency room for further evaluation.

Upon more detailed questioning, he reports a 20-pound weight loss over the past 2 months and a 50-pack-year history of smoking (2 packs per day for 25 years). On physical exam, his temperature is 37.2 °C (99 °F), blood pressure is 155/92 mm Hg, pulse rate is 110/min, respiration rate is 24/min, and oxygen saturation is 92% on room air. He appears anxious and in mild respiratory discomfort. There is no jugular venous distension or lymphadenopathy. On cardiac exam, he is tachycardic with no murmurs or extra heart sounds. On pulmonary exam, there is diffuse rhonchi and diminished breath sounds in the right lower lobe. There is digital clubbing but no cyanosis or peripheral edema.

What is concerning about this presentation, and how should you proceed?
Initially the case seems to be describing a general COPD exacerbation treated with glucocorticoids and antibiotics. However, his symptoms worsened despite this treatment and he developed hemoptysis. A detailed history also discovered his weight loss and extensive smoking history. The exam was concerning for diminished breath sounds in the right lower lobe and digital clubbing. These are red flag signs and symptoms that suggest a more serious underlying pathology. Diagnoses to consider are pulmonary vasculitis, malignancy, or tuberculosis. Ultimately, a tissue biopsy of some sort is required to differentiate among the three. However, the initial workup includes basic labs and imaging directed toward evaluating abnormal physical exam findings. A complete blood count (CBC) and chest radiograph (CXR) are appropriate in this particular situation, and further imaging with a computed tomography (CT) scan may be necessary depending on the results.

The patient's CBC shows a leukocytosis of 12,000 cells/μL, hemoglobin of 11 g/dL, and mean corpuscular volume of 75 fL/cell. A CXR is done showing a solitary 2.5-cm spiculated right upper lobe mass and blunting of the right costophrenic angle. A moderate pleural effusion is confirmed by bedside ultrasound. A bedside thoracentesis is performed under ultrasound guidance, and you are able to remove 1000 mL of bloody fluid and send it to the lab. The patient now feels much better, and a postprocedure CXR is done to rule out a pneumothorax. He is admitted to the hospital for observation overnight.

TABLE 35.1 ■ **Differential Diagnosis of Solitary Pulmonary Nodules**

Malignancy	Infection	Vascular
Primary lung carcinoma	Granulomas/tuberculosis	Resolving infarctions
Metastatic carcinoma	Pneumonia	Rheumatoid nodules
		Arteriovenous malformations

TABLE 35.2 ■ **Causes of Pleural Effusions**

Transudative	Exudative
Congestive Heart Failure	Malignancy (carcinoma, lymphoma, leukemia, mesothelioma)
Nephrotic Syndrome	Infection (bacterial pneumonia, fungal disease, parasites, tuberculosis)
Cirrhosis	Connective tissue disease (Churg-Strauss, lupus, rheumatoid arthritis, Wegener granulomatosis)
Atelectasis	Post-CABG (Dressler syndrome)
Pulmonary Embolism	Pulmonary embolism

CABG, Coronary artery bypass graft.

What is the differential diagnosis for a solitary pulmonary nodule?

Pulmonary nodules are defined as solitary lesions less than 3 cm in greatest dimension completely surrounded by lung parenchyma. The differential diagnosis of a lung nodule can be divided into three main categories: malignancy, infection, and vascular (Table 35.1).

What are the basic types of pleural effusions?

Pleural effusions are an accumulation of fluid within the parietal and visceral pleura. They can be either exudative or transudative. Exudative effusions are protein rich and seen secondary to inflammation of the pleural space, whereas transudative effusions are accumulations of fluid that is normal in consistency to the fluid already present within the pleural space but seen in volume overload state (see Table 35.2). Smaller effusions can have minimal physical findings; however, effusions larger than 1500 mL may have diminished breath sounds, egophony, and dullness to percussion. Pleural fluids can be analyzed through percutaneous removal (thoracentesis). Thoracentesis can be not only diagnostic but also therapeutic, as removal of the fluid increases space in the thoracic cavity, thereby relieving difficulty in respiration. According to Light's criteria, a pleural effusion is likely exudative if at least one of the three ratios exists.

CLINICAL PEARL   **STEP 2/3**

Light's criteria:
- Pleural fluid protein/serum ratio >0.5
- Pleural fluid lactate dehydrogenase (LDH)/serum LDH >0.6
- Pleural fluid LDH >2/3 the upper limit of normal for serum

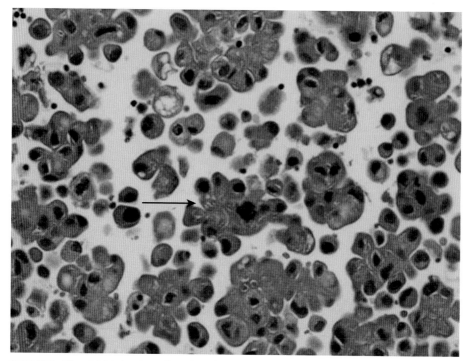

Figure 35.1 Pleural fluid showing enlarged atypical epithelioid cells forming small balls with "community borders" (see black arrow) in a cell block preparation (hematoxylin and eosin [H&E]).

BASIC SCIENCE PEARL	STEP 1

The most common causes of malignant pleural effusions are lung, gastrointestinal, ovary, breast, and lymphoid/leukemic origins.

The patient's pleural and serum protein and LDH return, indicating an exudative pleural effusion, which is consistent with the bloody nature of the fluid and the running differential diagnosis. Your attending asks you if you would like to call the lab to add any further studies now that an exudative effusion has been confirmed.

What additional testing should be performed on exudative effusions?

Thoracentesis fluid should be submitted for the following laboratory tests: cell count with differential, glucose, adenosine deaminase and acid-fast bacilli stain/culture (if tuberculosis is suspected), anaerobic and aerobic bacterial cultures (if infection is suspected), and cytology.

The tests are ordered and some preliminary results return. Glucose is low at 55 mg/dL. Cell count is slightly elevated with a lymphocyte predominance. Gram stain and acid-fast bacilli stain are negative with culture results pending. The next day cytology shows atypical epithelioid cells, highly suspicious for malignancy in the background of blood (Fig. 35.1). Now that malignancy is higher on the differential, a CT scan is ordered to better characterize the mass and look for an area to biopsy such as a lymph node.

What are the common clinical and radiologic findings that may lead to a diagnosis of malignancy over nonmalignant causes?

Malignancy is more common in patients >45 years of age who appear symptomatic. Malignant lesions tend to be >2 cm in greatest dimension with an ill-defined, spiculated, and lobulated appearance. Benign lesions are usually <2 cm in younger patients and may show well-defined smooth borders with punctate calcifications. Benign lesions may be associated with exposure to infectious organisms. Of course, there are always exceptions to the rule; therefore, malignancy should always be excluded.

What is the assessment of risk for malignancy?

Risk factors include cigarette smoking, air pollution, asbestos exposure, radiation exposure, genetic factors, and collagen vascular diseases. Of note, second-hand smoke is considered a risk factor as well.

What are the general features of a malignant effusion?

Malignant effusions are diagnosed by the presence of foreign cells and their characteristics. Normal cells found in a pleural fluid include mesothelial cells, macrophages, and inflammatory cells. Although there is no single feature diagnostic of malignancy, there are a few common characteristics of tumor types. Adenocarcinomas tend to exfoliate in cell balls or glands, whereas lymphomas and melanoma are seen as single tumor cells. The tumor cells of an adenocarcinoma tend to form "community borders," which are seen as smooth outlines to the clusters/balls (see Fig. 35.1). Malignant cells also tend to have an increased nuclear-to-cytoplasmic ratio, and the nuclei can be more hyperchromatic with prominent nucleoli. The background cells (lymphocytes or red blood cells) can be used as a reference point to size. Neoplastic cells are often five times larger than a lymphocyte.

What are some diagnostic procedures for this patient?

The patient can undergo a bronchoscopy if there is an endobronchial lesion or enlarged lymph nodes identified on imaging. If the lesion is noted to be peripheral, a CT-guided core biopsy may be indicated. If lymphadenopathy is noted, an endobronchial ultrasound (EBUS)–guided fine needle aspiration may be indicated for preop staging.

The CT scan reveals a 2.5-cm spiculated mass with no lymphadenopathy. The patient is scheduled for a transbronchial biopsy with bronchial brushing and washings as the chosen modality. No EBUS-guided biopsy is done because his CT scan of the chest shows no significant mediastinal lymphadenopathy. He undergoes the procedure without complication and is discharged with follow-up of the biopsy results.

He returns to your office the following week. You inform him that unfortunately the results came back positive for cancer. The bronchial brushing reveals an atypical population of cells, highly suspicious for non-small cell carcinoma (see Fig. 35.2), and the transbronchial biopsy confirms adenocarcinoma, a non-small cell type of lung cancer. The patient is then referred to a surgeon. The surgeon decides he is a good candidate for video-assisted thoracoscopic surgery (VATS) lobectomy as there is no disease elsewhere and his COPD is well controlled with medications. Although a wedge resection could be performed, there is a higher known risk of recurrence, and the patient opts for the lobectomy. He undergoes the procedure without complications and is sent home on day 3 postop. His lobectomy specimen is submitted to pathology for exam. You want to see what exactly is submitted, so you go to the lab and see the lobectomy specimen, which reveals a 2.5-cm mass (see Fig. 35.3).

What are the most common histologic subtypes of lung carcinoma?

Lung carcinoma is mainly divided into non-small cell carcinoma and small cell carcinoma of the lung. The three main types of non-small cell carcinoma of the lung can further be subdivided

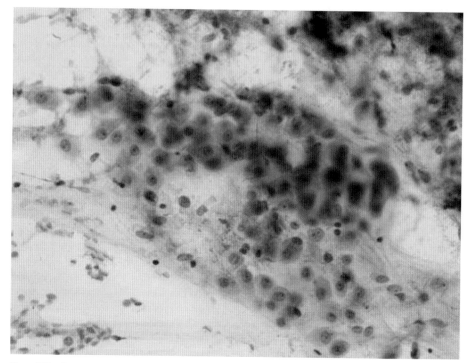

Figure 35.2 Bronchial brushing showing atypical epithelioid cells in a cohesive group with slight enlargement and prominent nucleoli, highly suspicious for non-small cell carcinoma (Pap stain).

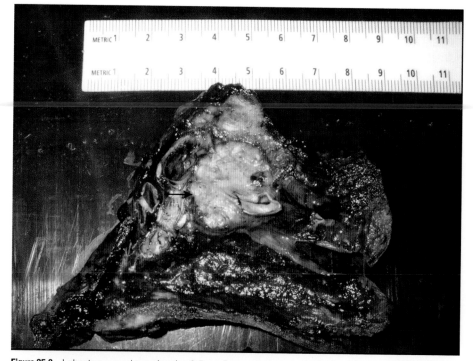

Figure 35.3 Lobectomy specimen showing 2.5-cm firm, well-circumscribed, tan mass with adjacent pink-red lung parenchyma.

into adenocarcinoma, squamous cell carcinoma, and large cell carcinoma. Although there are more subdivisions, it is important to know these main lesions. The morphology of these types of carcinomas is distinct. Adenocarcinomas have glandular differentiation and can have the presence of mucin. Squamous cell carcinomas display intercellular bridges (desmosomes) and keratinization. Small cell carcinomas tend to show molding and "salt and pepper" chromatin. The histologic features of this patient's lung carcinoma are consistent with an invasive adenocarcinoma with lipidic- and acinar-type growth pattern seen in the stroma (see Fig. 35.4). There are certain immunoperoxidase stains that can assist in differentiating types of lung carcinoma as well as distinguish primary versus metastatic disease. However, hematoxylin and eosin stain is the standard for all histology (see Fig. 35.5 and Fig. 35.6).

Diagnosis: Invasive adenocarcinoma with a lepidic and acinar growth pattern in the stroma

---

CLINICAL PEARL   **STEP 2/3**

Common immunoperoxidase stains used to differentiate different types of lung carcinoma include:
- Adenocarcinoma: Thyroid Transcription Factor 1 (TTF1) and Cytokeratin 7 (CK7) positive
- Squamous cell carcinoma: Cytokeratin 5/6 (CK5/6) and p63 positive, TTF1 and CK7 negative
- Large cell carcinoma: TTF1 negative
- Small cell carcinoma: Synaptophysin, Chromogranin, CD56, and TTF1 positive

What is the clinical significance of subtyping invasive adenocarcinoma?
Invasive adenocarcinoma subtyping is significant for prognostic impact. There are three overall prognostic groups/grades that have been identified according to 5-year disease-free survival rates. These groups are classified as low grade, intermediate grade, and high grade. The low-grade group includes adenocarcinoma in situ (AIS) and minimally invasive adenocarcinoma (MIA) and has a 100% disease-free survival. The intermediate group includes nonmucinous lepidic predominant, papillary predominant, and acinar predominant, with 90%, 83%, and 84% disease-free survival rates, respectively. The high-grade group includes solid predominant, micropapillary predominant, invasive mucinous adenocarcinoma, and colloid predominant with disease-free rates of 70%, 67%, 76%, and 71%, respectively.

What is the patient's pathologic staging of non-small cell lung cancer?
Lung cancer staging is based on the size of the primary tumor, lymph node involvement, and distant metastasis. This is known as TNM staging. This patient has a lung mass that measures 2.5 cm, which is not very large. He has no positive lymph nodes; however, his pleural fluid is involved, which makes his disease metastatic. His final pathologic stage is T4N0M1a.

What is the treatment and prognosis of his lung cancer?
Treatment and prognosis depend on the histologic type of cancer and the stage of the patient. In addition, the patient's performance stasis and overall health should be taken into account when considering treatment options. Early stage (I-II) non-small cell lung cancers are often treated with surgery and possibly adjuvant chemotherapy thereafter depending on the final pathologic stage. Late stage (IIB-IV) metastatic disease is not curable and generally treated with systemic chemotherapy. Stage IIIA non-small cell lung cancer treatment is complicated, requires a multidisciplinary approach, and is beyond the scope of a general internist. Small cell carcinoma of the lung generally responds to chemotherapy/radiotherapy.

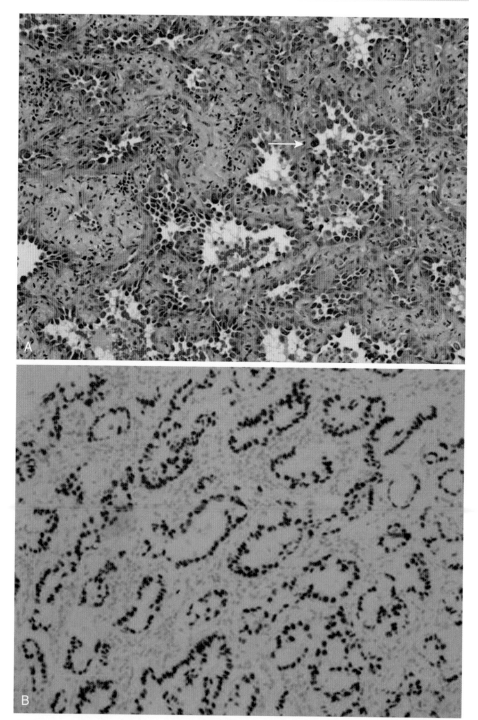

Figure 35.4 Both **A** and **B** represent histologic sections of the lung mass showing an adenocarcinoma. The arrow in **A** demonstrates lepidic spread, with an acinar growth pattern (H&E). The adenocarcinoma also shows nuclear positive staining with TTF-1, as seen in **B**.

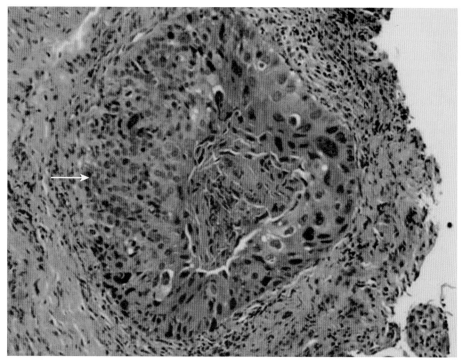

Figure 35.5 Histologic section of squamous cell carcinoma of the lung, as identified with the white arrow (H&E).

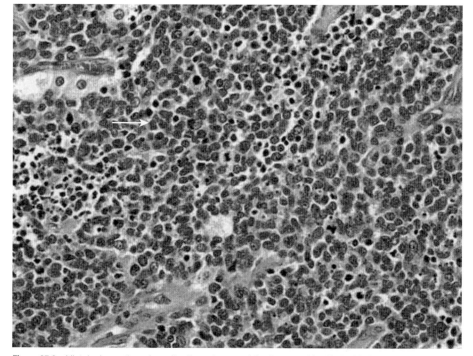

Figure 35.6 Histologic section of small cell carcinoma of the lung, as identified with the white arrow (H&E).

Prognosis can also be affected by certain gene mutations such as epidermal growth factor receptor (EGFR) and anaplastic lymphoma kinase (ALK). Molecular profiling is the first step in therapy for patients with metastatic disease. Although this patient does not have disease outside of the lung, other than the pleural fluid, EGFR and ALK mutation analysis should be performed on the resection specimen. The patient is then referred to an oncologist to follow up and get the results of his molecular testing. He follows up with the oncologist, who confirms he has an EGFR mutation, which will assist with gene therapy in the future.

What are the syndromes associated with different types of lung carcinoma?
Different types of lung tumors can be associated with different symptoms.

CLINICAL PEARL	STEP 2/3

Pancoast tumor is a type of tumor defined by its location in the apex of either lobe. It locally spreads to the adjacent soft tissues, ribs, and vertebrae, causing compression of vasculature, resulting in Horner's syndrome (miosis, anhidrosis, ptosis, and enophthalmos) when it involves the sympathetic fibers and/or Pancoast syndrome (severe pain in shoulder region, atrophy of hand and arm muscles) when it involves brachial plexus roots. Pancoast tumors tend not to display the traditional symptoms of lung tumors (cough, chest pain, etc.). They tend to present with shoulder/scapular pain.

CLINICAL PEARL	STEP 2/3

Superior vena cava syndrome (SVCS) is most commonly associated with centrally located lung tumors (most commonly small cell carcinoma) and is caused by external compression of the superior vena cava by a tumor. Patients can present with edema of the face and arms as well as traditional cancer symptoms such as shortness of breath and cough. SVCS can also be seen with lymphomas/leukemias and tuberculosis.

CLINICAL PEARL	STEP 2/3

Lambert-Eaton myasthenic syndrome (LEMS) is a paraneoplastic syndrome that occurs as a result of cancer somewhere else in the body. It results in proximal limb muscle weakness. It has been associated with small cell carcinoma of the lung.

CLINICAL PEARL	STEP 2/3

Clinical findings in common lung tumors include adenocarcinoma (hypertrophic osteoarthropathy), squamous cell carcinoma (hypercalcemia), large cell carcinoma (gynecomastia, galactorrhea), and small cell carcinoma (paraneoplastic syndromes).

What is the new classification of lung adenocarcinoma?
A new classification has been proposed to provide uniform terminology and diagnostic criteria for lung adenocarcinomas. This classification was submitted by a panel of experts including pathologists, oncologists, pulmonologists, radiologists, molecular biologists, and thoracic surgeons.

CLINICAL PEARL   **STEP 3**

New classification of adenocarcinoma of the lung:

- Atypical adenomatous hyperplasia (AAH)
  - <5 mm, usually incidental, in adjacent lung parenchyma in resected adenocarcinomas
- Adenocarcinoma in situ (AIS) (formerly nonmucinous bronchioloalveolar carcinoma [BAC])
  - Small (>5 mm and <3 cm) with growth along preexisting alveolar structures
  - ONLY lepidic growth: no stromal, vascular, or pleural invasion
- Minimally invasive adenocarcinoma (MIA)
  - <3 cm with predominantly lepidic growth pattern and ≤5 mm invasion in any one focus (may be multifocal)
  - No vascular or pleural invasion
  - No necrosis
  - If any of above are present → invasive adenocarcinoma, lepidic predominant
- Invasive adenocarcinoma
  - Lepidic predominant
  - Acinar predominant
  - Papillary predominant
  - Micropapillary predominant
  - Solid predominant with mucin production

BEYOND THE PEARLS

- Yellow nail syndrome is caused by an abnormality with the lymphatics and results in a rare triad of yellow nails, lymphedema, and pleural effusion.
- Most Pancoast tumors are non-small cell carcinomas, more specifically squamous cell carcinoma.
- A positive Pemberton sign is seen in SVCS. This is demonstrated by facial congestion, cyanosis, and respiratory distress after 1 minute of elevating both arms to touch the sides of the face.
- Implications of the classification of lung adenocarcinoma would stage AIS as "Tis" and minimally invasive adenocarcinoma would be "T1mi."
- Erlotinib, gefitinib, and afatinib inhibit tyrosine kinase at the EGFR.
- Crizotinib and ceritinib are ALK inhibitors.
- Both EGFR and ALK inhibitors are only FDA (U.S. Food and Drug Administration) approved for adenocarcinomas of the lung that are not amenable for surgical resection and metastatic disease.
- Napsin A, a new immunoperoxidase stain, is the most specific marker for pulmonary adenocarcinoma.

References

Demay RM. *Practical Principles of Cytopathology*. Chicago: American Society for Clinical Pathology; 2007.

Porcel JA, Light RW. Diagnostic approach to pleural effusion in adults. *Am Fam Physician*. 2006;73: 1211-1220.

Travis WD, Brambilla E, Noguchi M, et al. International Association for the Study of Lung Cancer/ American Thoracic Society/European Respiratory Society International Multidisciplinary Classification of Lung Adenocarcinoma. *J Thorac Oncol*. 2011;6:244-285.

Zugazagoitia J, Enquita AB, Nunez JA, Iglesias L, Ponce S. The new IASLC/ATS/ERS lung adenocarcinoma classification from a clinical perspective: current concepts and future prospects. *J Thorac Dis*. 2014;6(S5):S526-S536.

R. Michelle Koolaee

A 68-Year-Old Male With Right Knee Pain

A 68-year-old male is evaluated for a 2-year history of progressive right knee pain accompanied by morning stiffness lasting 20 minutes. He describes his pain as worse with ambulation (particularly going up and down stairs) and better with rest. He takes naproxen, which minimally relieves the pain. He works as a mail carrier and states that he has had to take several days off of work recently due to the increased severity of pain.

How does the history help to narrow your differential diagnosis?
Table 36.1 summarizes some common causes of knee pain. There are several key questions to always ask anyone who presents to you with knee pain:
- **Duration of symptoms:** This patient has chronic knee pain (>3 months), which makes a crystalline arthritis (such as gout or pseudogout) or bacterial septic arthritis (usually monoarticular) a far less likely cause of his symptoms. Both crystalline arthritis and bacterial septic arthritis present with acute knee pain.
- **Morning stiffness:** Prolonged morning stiffness (>1 hour) is a key feature of a chronic inflammatory arthritis such as rheumatoid arthritis (RA) or psoriatic arthritis (PsA). This patient has limited morning stiffness, which makes a chronic inflammatory arthritis less likely.
- **Aggravating/alleviating factors:** Chronic knee pain (in anyone over the age of 50) that is worse with weight-bearing activities (particularly stairs) and better with rest raises high suspicion for osteoarthritis (OA).
- **History of trauma:** A history of recent knee trauma or fall may raise suspicion for meniscal or ligament tears, none of which are relevant in this case.

On physical exam, vital signs are normal. Body mass index (BMI) is 29 kg/m². The right knee has a small effusion, with tenderness at the medial joint space; the knee is not erythematous or warm. There is no worsening of pain when compressing and grinding the patella upon the femur. Upon ambulation, a slight valgus deformity is noted. Range of motion of the knee elicits crepitus without any flexion contractures. Laboratory tests reveal a normal complete blood count and an erythrocyte sedimentation rate (ESR) of 6 mm/h. Synovial fluid is aspirated from the knee and reveals 750 white blood cell (WBC)/mm³.

What is your differential diagnosis?
This is a 68-year-old overweight male with no history of trauma who presents with chronic right knee pain that is worse with weight-bearing activity, medial joint space tenderness with a small effusion, and noninflammatory synovial fluid.

TABLE 36.1 ■ Common Causes of Knee Pain

Noninflammatory Arthritis (Synovial White Blood Cell Count (WBC) <2000 WBC/mm³)

Condition	Features
Osteoarthritis	Chronic pain usually in adults >50-years-old, which is worse with weight bearing and better with rest; may have crepitus or bony hypertrophy of the joint on exam
Meniscal tear	History of trauma and/or sensation that the knee may buckle or "give-out"; tenderness to palpation of the tibial femur joint and pain with twisting motions of the knee; ultrasound or magnetic resonance imaging (MRI) scan can identify tears
Anserine bursitis	Painful walking; point tenderness at the medial side of the tibia, just below the knee
Iliotibial band syndrome (common in runners)	Pain that radiates down the lateral thigh, with point tenderness around the tibial/fibular junction
Baker's cyst	Posterior knee pain that can extend to the mid/lower calf at times; ultrasound can identify cysts
Patellofemoral syndrome (common in young women)	Pain increases with stair climbing; pain over the patellofemoral joint when pressing the patella down onto the femur and "grinding" the patella up and down the femur

Inflammatory Arthritis (Synovial White Blood Cell Count >2000 WBC/mm³)

Condition	Features
Crystalline arthritis (gout or pseudogout)	Acute episodes of arthritis accompanied by warmth, erythema, and/or effusions on exam; elevated ESR or CRP common
Acute bacterial septic arthritis	Acute episode of arthritis (usually monoarticular) accompanied by warmth, erythema, and/or effusions on exam; usually due to hematogenous spread to the joint; elevated ESR or CRP common
Inflammatory arthritis (RA or PsA)	Chronic pain (>3 months); prolonged morning stiffness; synovitis and warmth on palpation; elevated ESR or CRP common

CRP, c-reactive protein; ESR, erythrocyte sedimentation rate; PsA, psoriatic arthritis; RA, rheumatoid arthritis.

Synovial fluid aspiration is a critical part of narrowing down the differential diagnosis for anyone with joint pain. Noninflammatory fluid, as in this case, is characterized by a synovial fluid WBC count of less than 2000 WBC/mm³. A WBC count of 750 WBC/mm³ essentially rules out any type of inflammatory arthritis; this includes crystalline arthritis, RA, PsA, or septic arthritis, to name a few. Even if synovial fluid analysis were not available, the chronicity of the patient's knee pain would make crystalline or acute bacterial septic arthritis unlikely. As mentioned earlier, the short duration of morning stiffness would make RA or PsA unlikely.

Table 36.1 lists common causes of knee pain with noninflammatory fluid. The clinical presentation here is most consistent with OA, although it is important to also be aware of other conditions that can often be present concurrently in someone with a history of OA. The lack of a history of trauma or sensation that the knee is going to "give out" or buckle makes the possibility of an acute meniscal or ligament tear very unlikely. The medial location of the knee pain makes iliotibial band syndrome or a baker's cyst unlikely as well. A negative patellofemoral grind test makes patellofemoral syndrome unlikely. Anserine bursitis is a cause of focal tenderness at the medial tibial plateau, just below the knee; however, this patient's pain is at the medial joint space.

CLINICAL PEARL	STEP 2/3

Musculoskeletal ultrasound can be a useful screening tool for evaluation of meniscal/ligament tears (when suspected). Although not as specific as magnetic resonance imaging (MRI), large tears can often be identified.

CLINICAL PEARL	STEP 2/3

As a cause of unexplained joint pain, always think about referred pain from pathology in either the joint one above or one below the affected joint (i.e., in someone with knee pain, think about referred pain from pathology in either the hip or the ankle joints).

Radiographs of the right knee reveal severe medial compartment joint space narrowing with subchondral sclerosis and osteophytes.

CLINICAL PEARL	STEP 2/3

When ordering knee radiographs, be sure to specify that they be weight-bearing films (otherwise the evaluation for joint space narrowing will be inaccurate). This is a common oversight, particularly in the inpatient setting.

Diagnosis: Osteoarthritis of the right knee

BASIC SCIENCE/CLINICAL PEARL	STEP 1/2/3

Plain films are not necessary to diagnose OA. In the majority of cases, history and physical exam are sufficient to establish a diagnosis.

What is the pathogenesis of OA?

Normal articular cartilage is 2 to 5 mm thick and is composed of collagen, proteins, and chondrocytes (the main "worker bee" cell of the cartilage). Chondrocytes occupy only 5% of the cartilage volume but synthesize all of the proteins needed to create the extracellular matrix (which occupies the remaining 95% of the cartilage volume). The chondrocytes also work to maintain a careful balance between the anabolic and catabolic enzymes that promote cartilage integrity. In OA, biomechanical (i.e., trauma, overuse), metabolic, and/or genetic factors lead to a weakened cartilage matrix (either by directly affecting the matrix proteins or by affecting chondrocyte function). A weak cartilage matrix, in turn, is more susceptible to damage and thus cannot sustain the same load, leading to OA. This process results in an imbalance in the proteins that regulate matrix synthesis/degradation, which leads to further cartilage damage.

BASIC SCIENCE PEARL	STEP 1

The function of articular cartilage is to provide an almost frictionless articulation and to absorb and dissipate load.

BASIC SCIENCE PEARL	STEP 1

Articular cartilage is a hypocellular, avascular, alymphatic tissue that is composed mostly (90 to 95%) of type II collagen.

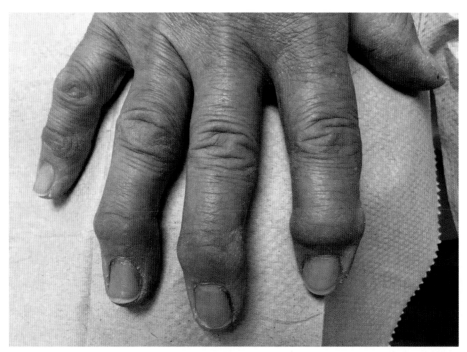

Figure 36.1 Several Heberden's nodes, most notably at the second through fourth distal interphalangeal joints. Note that on exam, these nodes feel firm and bony, in contrast to synovitis, which feels more boggy. *(From R. Michelle Koolaee, DO, CCD.)*

What are the key physical exam features of OA?
- **Bony hypertrophy:** OA is characterized by degeneration of normal articular cartilage; once cartilage is degraded, it cannot be regenerated. Beneath the articular cartilage lies subchondral bone; when cartilage is damaged, subchondral bone undergoes a remodeling process that causes new bone formation. Bony hypertrophy can be seen both on physical exam and on radiographs.
- **Joint effusions:** In contrast to the effusions seen in inflammatory arthritides, effusions in OA are not associated with warmth or erythema.
- **Heberden's and Bouchard's nodes** (in hand OA): These are bony enlargements of the distal interphalangeal (DIP) and proximal interphalangeal (PIP) joints, respectively (see Fig. 36.1).
- **Crepitus:** These are grating, crackling, or popping sounds obtained when the affected joint is passively moved with one hand while the other hand is placed on the joint.

What are the risk factors for OA?
Table 36.2 summarizes common risk factors for OA. Age and obesity are by far the strongest risk factors for the development of OA. In the United States, OA affects 13.9% of adults aged 25 years and older and 33.6% (12.4 million) of those over age 65 (2005 data). Furthermore, there were approximately 964,000 hospitalizations for OA in 2011, with a rate of 31 stays per 10,000 population. By payer, this is the second-most costly condition billed to Medicare and private insurance (2011 data). However, OA is not an inevitable outcome of aging; there are people who never develop radiographic evidence of disease as they age. Obesity is a significant epidemic in the United States and contributes significantly to both the development of OA as well as the worsening of pain symptoms.

TABLE 36.2 ■ Risk Factors for Osteoarthritis

- Advanced age
- Female gender
- Obesity
- Sports activities (repetitive high-impact exercises; however, note that regular exercise is necessary to maintain healthy joints)
- Previous joint injury
- Genetic elements

In regards to sports activities, regular joint use is beneficial and necessary for the health of joints. Repetitive exposure to high-impact exercises (i.e., professional athletics) may increase the risk for OA. Examples include:

- Gymnastics (increased risk of OA in shoulders, wrists, and elbows)
- Professional football (increased risk of OA in knees, feet, and ankles)
- Professional baseball (increased risk of OA in shoulders and elbows)

Previous joint injury is a well-established risk factor for the development of OA. This includes previous fractures, trauma, ligament tears, congenital abnormalities, and infections in joints. There are also rare genetic linkages (i.e., specific defects in the gene for type II collagen) that can be a cause of precocious generalized OA.

CLINICAL PEARL	STEP 2/3

Multiple studies have shown no increased risk for OA or premature damage of articular cartilage in long-distance runners.

How do you differentiate OA from an inflammatory arthritis?

OA is a disease characterized by a noninflammatory arthritis (synovial fluid <2000 WBC/mm^3) that occurs as a result of biomechanical (i.e., obesity, trauma), metabolic, and/or genetic derangements, which ultimately cause damage to normal articular cartilage. Common causes for inflammatory arthritis are shown in Table 36.1. Table 36.3 summarizes key distinguishing features of OA and inflammatory arthritis.

What are the radiographic features of OA?

It is important to note that the radiographic findings in OA do not correlate well with the clinical severity of OA symptoms; some patients have evidence of severe radiographic disease but do not have debilitating pain (and vice versa). Radiographic features may include osteophytes (bony overgrowth), joint space narrowing, subchondral cyst formation, subchondral sclerosis, and malalignment. Examples of radiographic changes are shown in Figure 36.2.

CLINICAL PEARL	STEP 2/3

When evaluating someone with knee pain, MRI should be ordered only when internal derangement is suspected (i.e., fractures, damage to the ligaments, menisci, or tendons) or the diagnosis is truly in question (after appropriate initial evaluation).

An intraarticular glucocorticoid injection provides moderate relief of the patient's knee pain. He is advised to wear a knee brace for additional support during work and is offered physical therapy to help strengthen his quadriceps muscles. Weight loss counseling is provided.

TABLE 36.3 ■ **Distinguishing Osteoarthritis From Inflammatory Arthritis**

Features	Osteoarthritis	Inflammatory Arthritis
Onset	Progressive	Acute or progressive
Age	Usually >50	Any age
Morning Stiffness	<30 minutes	>1 hour
Activity	Knees/hips/ankles: worse with weight bearing; worse with activity	Better with activity
Rest	Better	Worse
Crepitus?	+/−	+/−
Effusion?	+/−	+/−
Bony Hypertrophy?	+ (Heberden/Bouchard nodes)	−
Synovial Fluid Analysis	Noninflammatory	Inflammatory
Erythrocyte Sedimentation Rate	Normal	Elevated

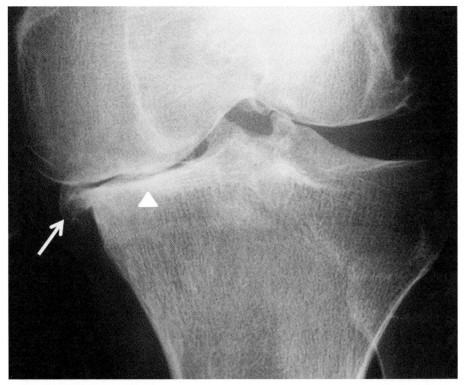

Figure 36.2 Radiographs of an osteoarthritic knee with osteophytes *(white arrow)* along with subchondral sclerosis and collapse of the medial compartment *(arrowhead)*. *(From Buckland-Wright C. Subchondral bone changes in hand and knee osteoarthritis detected by radiography.* Osteoarthritis Cartilage. *2004;12 Suppl A:S10-S19.)*

TABLE 36.4 ■ **Nonpharmacologic Therapies for Osteoarthritis**

- Weight loss
- Physical therapy: range-of-motion exercises, muscle-strengthening exercises
- Aerobic exercise programs
- Bracing devices to increase joint stability and decrease mechanical load
- Acupuncture
- Transcutaneous nerve stimulation
- Patient education

What are some pharmacologic treatments for OA?

There is unfortunately no cure at this point for OA; all available therapies help to reduce symptoms and improve quality of life (in an effort to avoid joint replacement in the future). For mild to moderate joint pain, acetaminophen is the drug of choice. There are also topical agents for pain, including methylsalicylate and menthol (found in over-the-counter pain creams) as well as capsaicin cream.

For moderate to severe pain, options include:

- Nonsteroidal antiinflammatory drugs (NSAIDs)
- Joint aspiration (if an effusion is present) with intraarticular glucocorticoid injection: The effect of these injections is variable and ranges from no relief of symptoms to indefinite relief. If effective, these injections may be performed as frequently as once every 3 months.
- Joint aspiration (if an effusion is present) with intraarticular hyaluronic acid injection: The efficacy of "viscosupplementation" through injection of hyaluronic acid is controversial, and at the present time, there are no data available to predict patients who are likely to respond to these injections. Due to high costs for these injections and questionable efficacy, many insurance companies do not reimburse for hyaluronic acid injections.
- Opioid analgesic agents
- Duloxetine

What are some nonpharmacologic treatments for OA?

Table 36.4 summarizes nonpharmacologic treatments for OA. Muscle strength and tone are significantly reduced around a joint affected by OA, so physical therapy (which incorporates isometric and aerobic exercises) is very important in these patients to help decrease symptoms of pain. If overweight (as in this case), weight loss plays a critical role in reducing symptoms, as this will help decrease mechanical load on weight-bearing joints. This can be particularly challenging for overweight/obese patients, as their pain usually limits them from exercise to begin with; water-aerobic exercises can be helpful in these instances (particularly in those with hip or knee OA).

When do you refer patients for joint replacement?

The primary considerations for the appropriateness of surgery are the severity of pain symptoms and the degree to which these OA symptoms impair normal daily function (i.e., walking short distances, bathing). The degree of radiographic OA alone is not criteria alone for joint replacement.

BEYOND THE PEARLS

- Joint pain from hip OA is usually referred to the groin, so in patients who present with hip pain, ask them to specify the exact location of the pain. On exam, pain with internal and/or external rotation that is felt in the groin represents OA. Pain felt in the lateral superior thigh likely represents trochanteric bursitis.
- The use of glucosamine and chrondroitin for OA is a controversial yet noteworthy topic because patients often ask the clinician's opinion about its use. The results of

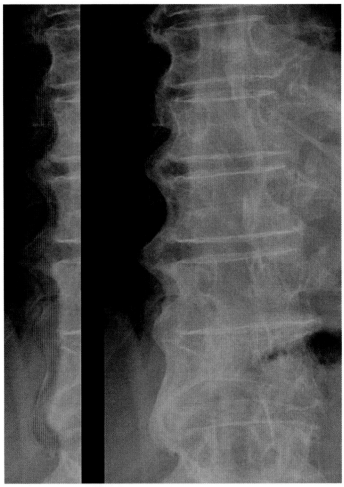

Figure 36.3   Marked ligamentous ossification of contiguous vertebrae (in a characteristic candle-wax dripping appearance) characteristic of diffuse idiopathic skeletal hyperostosis. *(From* http://commons.wikimedia.org/ wiki/File:Morbus_Forestier.jpg *and courtesy of Dr. Jochen Lengerke.)*

BEYOND THE PEARLS—cont'd

randomized trials are mixed, without definitive evidence of benefit, so many clinicians do not specifically recommend its use. However, there are few risks if any with its use so many clinicians do not object to its use.

- OA is most often a nonerosive disease; however, a very small subset of patients have erosions (which usually affect the hands). Patients with erosive OA present with flares of inflammation in the proximal and distal interphalangeal joints, associated with swelling, erythema, and severe pain. Radiographs reveal erosions of these joints.
- Diffuse idiopathic skeletal hyperostosis (DISH) is a form of noninflammatory spondyloarthropathy that is often part of the differential diagnosis in patients with OA of the spine. It is characterized by calcification of the spinal ligaments and results in very characteristic, bulky, flowing osteophytes in the spine (usually in the thoracic spine). This very classic candle-wax dripping appearance on plain films distinguishes DISH from OA or ankylosing spondylitis (see Fig. 36.3).

Continued

BEYOND THE PEARLS—cont'd

- A physical or occupational therapist can instruct patients on proper selection and use of a cane. The most common error in the use of a cane is that they are not the proper length; the cane should be held in the hand opposite the knee or hip affected by OA and the elbow should be flexed 12 to 20 degrees.
- In patients with lower extremity joint pains, pay close attention to their footwear. The use of cushioned footwear such as running or walking shoes can help to reduce pain.

References

Felson DT. The course of osteoarthritis and factors that affect it. *Rheum Dis Clin North Am.* 1993;19(3):607-615.

Hochberg MC, Altman RD, April KT, et al. American College of Rheumatology 2012 recommendations for the use of nonpharmacologic and pharmacologic therapies in osteoarthritis of the hand, hip, and knee. *Arthritis Care Res (Hoboken).* 2012;64(4):465-474.

Lane NE, Bloch DA, Jones HH, et al. Long-distance running, bone density, and osteoarthritis. *JAMA.* 1986;255(9):1147-1151.

Lawrence RC, Felson DT, Helmick CG, et al. Estimates of the prevalence of arthritis and other rheumatic conditions in the United States. Part II. *Arthritis Rheum.* 2008;58(1):26-35.

Poole AR, Kojima T, Yasuda T, et al. Composition and structure of articular cartilage: a template for tissue repair. *Clin Orthop Relat Res.* 2001;391(suppl):S26-S33.

Sohn RS, Micheli LJ. The effect of running on the pathogenesis of osteoarthritis of the hips and knees. *Clin Orthop Relat Res.* 1985;198:106-109.

Monisha Bhanote   ■   Daniel Martinez

A 20-Year-Old Female With Chronic Fatigue

A 20-year-old female presents to her primary care doctor over summer break complaining of worsening fatigue for the past 6 months. She is constantly tired and lacks the energy to do her usual summer activities with her friends. She denies associated weight loss, heat/cold intolerance, anhedonia, drug use, menorrhagia, unprotected sexual contacts, shortness of breath, skin rashes, or joint swelling. She does report mild episodes of diarrhea but it is well controlled with loperamide as needed. She states that she is a vegan since she started college to avoid the "freshman 15." Fruits, vegetables, cereals, and pastas are now the cornerstones of her diet.

What should be reasonably considered in a young female with new fatigue?
Pregnancy should be considered in any female of reproductive age with nonspecific symptoms such as fatigue. Taking a sexual history and ordering a pregnancy test is therefore important in the evaluation. Hypothyroidism is also a reasonable consideration, and a screening thyroid stimulating hormone (TSH) is generally indicated. Many rheumatologic diseases can cause fatigue, and thus a thorough review of systems and a physical exam that includes the skin, joints, and nails are also important; these will help narrow down which of the many rheumatologic tests are indicated if at all. Anemia can cause fatigue in all populations, and a complete blood count (CBC) is generally ordered.

On physical exam, the patient's temperature is 36.7 °C (98 °F), blood pressure is 110/70 mm Hg, pulse rate is 80/min, respiration rate is 14/min, and oxygen saturation is 100% on room air: body mass index (BMI) is 17 kg/m². She is a thin-appearing female in no acute distress. She has mild pallor of the conjunctiva but moist mucus membranes. The thyroid is not palpable and there is no lymphadenopathy. She has a 1/6 early systolic murmur and her lungs are clear to auscultation. Her abdomen is soft, nontender, and nondistended with no hepatosplenomegaly. There are no rashes or joint swelling.

Laboratory findings include a normal chemistry panel, normal thyroid panel, and negative urine pregnancy test. The CBC includes a white blood cell count of 8000 cells/μL, hemoglobin of 11 g/dL, mean corpuscular volume (MCV) of 114 fL/cell. You explain that her fatigue is likely due to anemia and that there are more tests that you have to order when she follows up in a week.

What are the pathologic causes of macrocytic anemia and how do you work it up?
Macrocytosis refers to the presence of abnormally large red blood cells. This can be associated without anemia as in cases of newborns or during pregnancy. It can also be associated with anemia due to many other causes (see Table 37.1).

TABLE 37.1 ■ **Pathologic Causes of Macrocytosis**

Drugs
Alcoholism
Reticulocytosis
Nonalcoholic and alcoholic liver disease
Hypothyroidism
Vitamin B12 deficiency
Folate deficiency
Multiple myeloma
Myelodysplastic syndromes
Aplastic anemia
Acute leukemia

Many of the pathologies listed have other significant clinical or laboratory abnormalities that would make the diagnosis easy to make (such as liver disease or an acute leukemia). However, in a patient with macrocytosis who has an otherwise normal clinical exam and labs, the main differential is between vitamin B12 and folate deficiency. The workup includes a peripheral smear, checking a reticulocyte count to confirm the anemia is due to decreased production, and ordering B12/folate levels. If B12 and folate levels are normal and there remains a high suspicion for deficiency, then homocysteine and methylmalonic acid levels can be ordered as they are more sensitive.

These tests are ordered and the patient returns the following week. The reticulocyte count is within normal limits. The folate level is normal but the vitamin B12 is low at 140 pg/mL. Peripheral smear shows a macrocytosis (see Fig. 37.1). The patient then asks why her B12 is so low. She wants to know if it is due to her new vegan diet.

What etiologies should be considered for a patient with vitamin B12 deficiency?
Vitamin B12 deficiency can be seen in decreased intake, poor absorption, and increased need. Therefore, vitamin B12 deficiency can happen in individuals who are vegan as well as vegetarians who do not consume enough milk, eggs, or cheese and do not supplement the vitamin in other ways. However, the average person's vitamin B12 stores can lasts several years without any signs or symptoms of deficiency. This makes it difficult for decreased vitamin intake to be the sole reason for the significant deficiency seen in this patient. A good clinician would consider other reasons for a vitamin B12 deficiency in a young person who has only been a vegan for a couple years.
   Vitamin B12 deficiency can also be seen in certain medical conditions such as atrophic gastritis, Crohn's disease, celiac disease, bacterial overgrowth, parasitic infections, immune disorders (Grave's disease or lupus), and weight loss surgery, which can cause loss of part of the gastrointestinal tract that absorbs nutrients.

You inform the patient that her fatigue is cause by an anemia due to a vitamin B12 deficiency. It is possibly due to her diet, though not definitively, and you advise her to take vitamin B12 injections weekly for 8 weeks, then once monthly thereafter. She explains that she is going on a summer trip to Europe and cannot come back to the office that frequently. Instead, you advise her to take 1 milligram (1000 μg) of vitamin B12 daily. She then returns back to school after the summer for the fall semester.

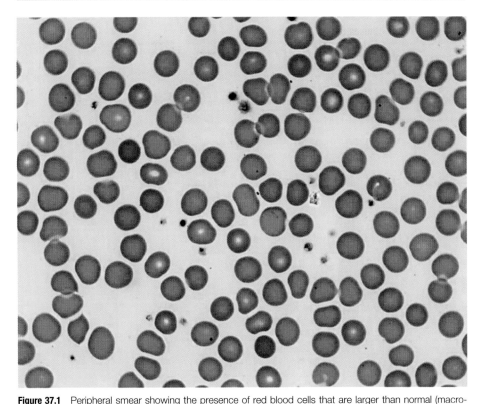

Figure 37.1 Peripheral smear showing the presence of red blood cells that are larger than normal (macrocytes). *(From* https://upload.wikimedia.org/wikipedia/commons/1/17/Macrocytosis.jpg.*)*

CLINICAL PEARL	STEP 2/3

Oral cyanocobalamin 1000 mcg provides effective maintenance therapy for vitamin B12 deficiency of all causes.

During Thanksgiving break the patient returns home and comes to your office. She reports that she is not feeling any better than this past summer. She also confirms that she is compliant with the oral vitamin B12. She now appears pale overall and has cracking around her mouth with some oral ulcers. She also complains that her diarrhea has worsened and is now associated with greasy stools and a rash on her arms. You recheck her CBC and vitamin B12 level. Her hemoglobin is now 9.5 g/dL and her vitamin B12 level is still low. Given that she did not respond to the oral vitamin supplementation, you suspect a malabsorption syndrome and refer her to a gastroenterologist.

What are common causes of malabsorption syndromes?

Malabsorption is characterized by abnormal or suboptimal absorption of nutrients (fats, vitamins, proteins, carbohydrates, electrolytes, and minerals) across the gastrointestinal tract. It can include one or multiple nutrients depending on the abnormality. Malabsorption can be subclassified into three categories: selective, partial, and total. Selective malabsorption is seen with specific nutrients such as lactose intolerance. The causes of malabsorption can be due to infective agents, structural defects, surgical changes, mucosal abnormalities, enzyme deficiencies, digestive failure, and systemic diseases (see Table 37.2).

TABLE 37.2 ■ Causes of Malabsorption

Infective agents	Parasites (giardia, fish tape worm, hookworm) Tropical sprue Whipple's disease Intestinal tuberculosis Human immunodeficiency virus–related malabsorption
Structural defects	Inflammatory bowel disease (Crohn's) Fistula/diverticula/strictures Infiltrative conditions (amyloidosis, lymphoma, eosinophilic gastroenteritis, Waldenstrom macroglobulinemia) Collagen vascular disease
Surgical structural changes	Bariatric weight loss surgery Inflammatory bowel disease surgery
Mucosal abnormality	Celiac disease Cow's milk intolerance Fructose malabsorption
Enzyme deficiency	Lactase deficiency Sucrose intolerance Intestinal disaccharidase deficiency
Digestive failure	Pancreatic insufficiency (cystic fibrosis, chronic pancreatitis) Zollinger-Ellison syndrome Bacterial overgrowth Obstructive jaundice

Systemic diseases
  affecting the
  gastrointestinal tract
	Celiac disease
	Hypothyroidism and hyperthyroidism
	Addison's disease
	Diabetes mellitus
	Hyperparathyroidism and hypoparathyroidism
	Abetalipoproteinemia

CLINICAL PEARL   STEP 2/3

Tropical sprue (also called postinfectious sprue) occurs in individuals visiting or living in tropical climates (Caribbean, India, Southeast Asia, Central and South America). The etiology is unknown, but it also causes malabsorption. Unlike celiac disease, most of the injury is distal, with abundant lymphocytes and more eosinophils. It responds to long-term, broad-spectrum antibiotic therapy. Always consider asking about travel history when considering malabsorption.

CLINICAL PEARL   STEP 2/3

Whipple's disease is a rare systemic condition involving the intestine, central nervous system, and joints. It is caused by a gram-positive actinomycete, *Tropheryma whippelii*. The small intestine mucosa demonstrates numerous macrophages containing this organism with no significant inflammation. These macrophages can also be seen in lymph nodes, joints, and the brain. In addition to malabsorption symptoms, patients can present with migratory arthritis and heart disease. It usually responds to antibiotic therapy.

The patient arrives at the gastroenterologist and explains her situation. He agrees that her worsening diarrhea, low BMI, and vitamin B12 deficiency anemia refractory to oral supplementation makes a malabsorption syndrome very likely. He schedules her for an upper endoscopy the

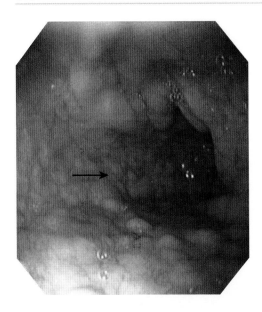

Figure 37.2 Endoscopy showing nodularity *(arrow)* in the small bowel. *(From* https://commons.wikimedia.org/wiki/File:Celiakia,_bulbus_duodena.jpg.*)*

following week. The patient tolerates the procedure well and returns for a follow-up appointment. The gastroenterologist explains that the upper endoscopy showed a normal stomach and some nodularity in the duodenum (see Fig. 37.2). At that time, the gastroenterologist had taken multiple biopsies from the stomach and duodenum and submitted them to pathology.

CLINICAL PEARL   **STEP 2/3**

Most patients with celiac disease have a normal-appearing endoscopy; however, there are five concurrent endoscopic findings that have been associated with a high specificity for celiac disease: scalloping of the small bowel folds, paucity in the folds, mosaic pattern to the mucosa "cracked mud," prominence of submucosal blood vessels, and a nodular pattern of the mucosa.

What is the histology of a normal small intestine?

The small intestine contains epithelium, which forms villi. The villi are lined by columnar absorptive cells and goblet cells. There is usually one lymphocyte per five enterocytes (columnar absorptive cells). Four normal villi in a row suggest normal villous architecture. The columnar absorptive cells have microvilli on their luminal surface (brush border) to allow absorption. Each villus contains an arteriole with capillary network, veins, and a central lymphatic with numerous nerve fibers (see Fig. 37.3).

The patient's biopsies reveal a severe mucosal lesion with abnormal villous architecture showing severe villous blunting and increased intraepithelial lymphocytes (see Fig. 37.4).

Diagnosis: Celiac disease

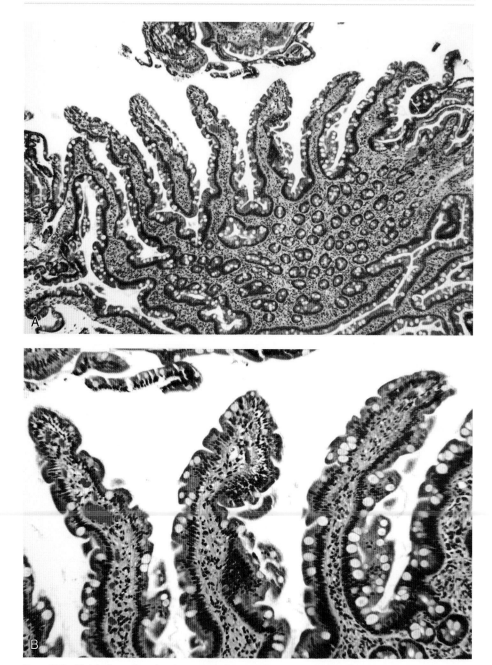

Figure 37.3   Histologic section showing normal villous architecture in the duodenum. Note the 3-5 : 1 villous to crypt ratio (**A,** low power left; **B,** high power right, hematoxylin and eosin [H&E] stain).

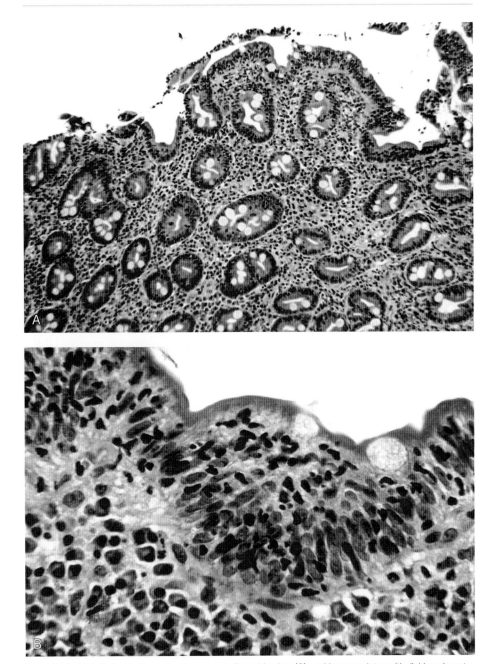

Figure 37.4 Histologic sections showing severe villous blunting **(A)** and increase intraepithelial lymphocytes **(B)**. H&E stain.

What are the histologic findings in a small intestine affected by celiac sprue?

Celiac disease, also known as gluten-sensitive enteropathy (GSE), is an immune-mediated disorder caused by gliadin, a gluten protein found in wheat and similar proteins found in barley and rye. When one is exposed to gliadin, the enzyme transglutaminase modifies the protein, and the immune system cross-reacts with the small bowel, causing an inflammatory response. This response leads to blunting (flattening) of the normal villous lining of the small intestine (villous atrophy). The atrophic villi cannot absorb nutrients effectively, thereby causing malabsorption.

CLINICAL PEARL	STEP 2/3

Celiac disease is a disorder that occurs in a genetically susceptible host. Ninety-five percent of individuals with celiac will have either genes for HLA-DQ2 or HLA-DQ8 allele. However, it should be noted that 20 to 30% of individuals carrying these genes do not have celiac disease; therefore, an additional environmental factor may be involved. One such factor that has been implicated is infection with adenovirus 12.

CLINICAL PEARL	STEP 1

The immune response to dietary gluten involves both cell-mediated injury and antibody-mediated injury.

There is a range of histologic findings in patients with celiac disease, but in general it is a disease of the proximal small intestine (duodenum and proximal jejunum). It is recommended to take biopsies distal to the duodenal bulb and to have them well oriented if possible. Because celiac can be a patchy process, the best possibility for making a diagnosis is with biopsies taken from at least two sites: the duodenal bulb and second portion of the duodenum.

CLINICAL PEARL	STEP 2/3

Findings of villous blunting and increased intraepithelial lymphocytes should always be correlated with serologic studies. *Helicobacter pylori* gastritis, peptic injury, and nonsteroidal antiinflammatory drug (NSAID) injury may show similar histologic findings.

The patient is saddened because her vegan diet depends heavily on gluten-containing foods. She asks the gastroenterologist if he is sure this is the diagnosis. He replies that her clinical history is most compatible with that diagnosis, but he will have to order some blood work to confirm the diagnosis.

What are some disorders that may show histologic overlap with celiac disease/GSE?

There are a number of entities that may show increased intraepithelial lymphocytes or villous blunting, or both (see Table 37.3). It is important to be aware of these entities and clinically exclude them before making a definitive diagnosis.

What are the clinical laboratory tests used in diagnosing celiac disease?

Enzyme-linked immunosorbent assay for immunoglobulin A (IgA) antitransglutaminase antibodies has a high degree of sensitivity (77 to 100%) and specificity (91 to 100%). This has become the serologic test of choice for celiac disease, replacing the former antigliadin and antiendomysial antibody tests.

TABLE 37.3 ■ Disorders Showing Overlap With Celiac Disease

Conditions associated with increased intraepithelial lymphocytes	*Helicobacter pylori* gastritis Viral gastroenteritis Tropical sprue Refractory sprue Bacterial overgrowth
Conditions associated with villous blunting	Crohn's disease Common variable immunodeficiency Microvillus inclusion disease Tropical sprue Refractory sprue Bacterial overgrowth Nutritional deficiencies Eosinophilic gastroenteritis Radiation or chemotherapy

The patient returns to the office, and the diagnosis of celiac disease is confirmed by positive serologic testing. The gastroenterologist explains that the only effective treatment is a lifelong gluten-free diet. The patient returns to you the following week with her test results and new diagnosis. You refer her to a dietitian to receive adequate input in eliminating her dietary intake of gluten foods as well as balancing her nutritional needs overall. Although saddened by her diagnosis, she is happy that she finally knows what is causing her symptoms and her life can get back to normal. She then asks if there is any testing that she will need in the future.

CLINICAL PEARL   **STEP 2/3**

Guidelines recommend that a total serum IgA level is checked concurrently, as patients with celiac disease and IgA deficiency can produce a false-negative serology. These patients may then benefit from immunoglobuline G-tissue transglutaminase (IgG-tTG) antibody testing.

What kind of follow-up testing is recommended for a patient diagnosed with celiac disease?
Usually there is no significant follow up as long as the patient shows clinical improvement. Repeat biopsies are unnecessary unless there is no clinical response to a gluten-free diet. In this case, other disorders such as refractory sprue, lymphoma, or infection would need to be excluded. Some patients have refractory sprue in which they have no clinical response to a gluten-free diet. This can occur when the disease has been present for so long and the small intestine cannot heal on diet alone. These patients may benefit from glucocorticoids or immunosuppressants.

BEYOND THE PEARLS

- Treatment with a gluten-free diet has been associated with improvement in the coexistent Hashimoto's hypothyroidism, with reduction of the required thyroxine doses, an effect probably related to enhanced drug absorption.
- A low level of vitamin B12 is associated with faster progression from human immunodeficiency virus (HIV) to acquired immune deficiency syndrome (AIDS). In addition, vitamin B12 (cyanocobalamin, methylcobalamin, and adenosylcobalamin) has been shown to inhibit HIV replication in vitro.

Continued

BEYOND THE PEARLS—cont'd

- Gastric antral vascular ectasia (GAVE), also called watermelon stomach, is diagnosed by endoscopy and shows dilated capillaries in the lamina propria with fibrin thrombi. These patients also demonstrate blood loss and anemia.
- Long-term use of metformin has been associated with malabsorption of vitamin B12.
- Osteopenia and osteoporosis are often present in patients with celiac disease.
- Dermatitis herpetiformis, a pruritic skin condition, has been linked to transglutaminase enzyme. It is characterized by papulovesicular lesions in a symmetrical distribution on the elbows, knees, face, scalp, neck, and trunk. It responds to a gluten-free diet.
- Patients with celiac disease are prone to certain pregnancy complications, including miscarriage, intrauterine growth retardation, low birth weight, and preterm birth.
- Celiac disease is associated with autoimmune disorders such as type 1 diabetes, hypothyroidism, primary biliary cirrhosis, and microscopic colitis.
- The Marsh classification, originally introduced in 1992 and later modified, describes the stages of development of celiac disease.
- Babies exposed to wheat, barley, or rye within the first 3 months after birth had a fivefold risk of developing celiac disease relative to babies exposed 4 to 6 months after birth.
- Nonceliac gluten sensitivity is less severe than celiac disease. These patients do not have elevations in tissue transglutaminase, endomysium, or deamidated-gliadin antibodies but experience similar physical symptoms with minimal intestinal damage. They respond to a gluten-free diet.

References

Andrès E, Noel E, Goichot B. Metformin-associated vitamin B12 deficiency. *Arch Intern Med.* 2002;162(19):2251-2252.

Aslinia F, Mazza J, Yale SH. Megaloblastic anemia and other causes of macrocytosis. *Clin Med Res.* 2006;4(3):236-241.

Ch'ng CL, Jones MK, Kingham JGC. Celiac disease and autoimmune thyroid disease. *Clin Med Res.* 2007;5(3):184-192.

Murray MT, Pizzorno J. *Encyclopedia of Natural Medicine.* Rev 2nd ed. New York: Three Rivers Press; 1997.

Odze RD. *Surgical Pathology of the GI tract, Liver, Biliary Tract, and Pancreas.* 2nd ed. Philadelphia: Saunders; 2009.

Albert Huang ■ John Khoury

A 32-Year-Old Female With Bilateral Hand Numbness

A 32-year-old female presents to an outpatient clinic with numbness in her hands. It started several days prior and was not associated with any specific incident. She describes additional tingling as pins and needle sensations. The symptoms have been constant and she is unable to identify anything that makes it better or worse.

How can occupational history contribute to the evaluation in this case?

A potential cause of hand numbness is peripheral nerve entrapments involving the radial, ulnar, or more commonly the median nerve within the carpal tunnel, also referred to as carpal tunnel syndrome (CTS). It is important to inquire about work or recreational activities that result in repetitive actions. In today's technological society, heavy use of mobile devices or poor ergonomic wrist placement while typing can result in hand numbness due to CTS. Other activities that result in median nerve damage include frequent wrist flexion while operating machinery or regularly using tools such as wrenches, screwdrivers, and even surgical instruments. Examples of occupations that can lead to repetitive wrist or hand motions include secretaries, mechanics, and surgeons.

BASIC SCIENCE/CLINICAL PEARL   **STEP 1/2/3**

The median nerve innervates both sensory and motor components of the hand. Its sensory dermatome involves the anterolateral aspect of the hand. Muscles involved cause flexion of the thumb, index, and middle fingers, as well as flexion of the wrist and pronation of the forearm. Because the sensory fibers are smaller and more sensitive to damage, sensory deficits typically occur first. The presence of weakness and motor deficits is an indication of severe median nerve damage.

What additional questions are important to ask related to the numbness and tingling in her hands?

Other common causes for upper extremity paresthesias include cervical spine pathology, such as a disc herniation or arthritic facet joint spaces leading to narrowed neuroforamen and ultimately damaged nerves exiting the cervical spine. Chronic conditions can result in damage of smaller nerves fibers distally and raise the question of hypothyroidism or diabetes mellitus. However, in this particular case, cervical spine pathology would more commonly present unilaterally and a metabolic cause is less likely considering the patient's younger age (see Table 38.1).

TABLE 38.1 ■ Differential Diagnosis of Upper Extremity Paresthesias

Central Causes
- Cerebral tumor
- Demyelinating lesions
- Cerebral ischemia
- Migraine
- Spinal cord pathology

Peripheral Causes
- Radiculopathy
- Brachial plexus lesions
- Peripheral nerve entrapment
- Polyneuropathies
  - Diabetes
  - Hypothyroidism
  - Human immunodeficiency virus
  - Guillain-Barré syndrome
  - Toxins
  - Hereditary disorders

Upon further questioning, the patient states the numbness and tingling is not associated with actual weakness and does not seem to worsen or improve with any particular movements. Inquiring about her past medical history, she mentions a visit to the emergency department for increased blurry vision in her left eye. She was diagnosed with optic neuritis at that time, and her vision returned to normal 2 weeks later. She is currently employed as a fitness instructor and unable to recall activities that require repetitive actions at her wrist. The remaining review of systems is unremarkable.

How is optic neuritis commonly tested on physical exam?

The swinging light test is commonly utilized to assess both afferent and efferent function of the optic nerves. This test is conducted by swinging a pen light from one eye to the other and assessing for symmetrical bilateral pupil dilation. Despite light being shown in only one eye, the normal response is bilateral pupil constriction. When there is unequal pupil constriction, the examiner must determine whether the cause is due to an afferent or efferent defect. If there is an afferent defect, both pupils demonstrate a symmetrical decreased constriction of the pupils when the light is shone in the affected eye. If the defect is efferent, only the affected eye demonstrates an unequal and diminished pupillary constriction when compared to the unaffected eye no matter which side the light is shone. An afferent pupillary defect is also known as a Marcus Gunn pupil and is commonly seen in cases of optic neuritis (see Fig. 38.1).

CLINICAL PEARL   **STEP 2/3**

Presence of a Marcus Gunn pupil indicates the optic nerve is still innervated despite decreased function. This dysfunction can be due to inflammation, a demyelinating process, or compression by a tumor. In this case, the affected eye will still demonstrate a bilateral pupillary constriction although decreased when compared to the unaffected side. In contrast, a complete optic nerve lesion or detachment would result in no response when light is shone into the affected eye.

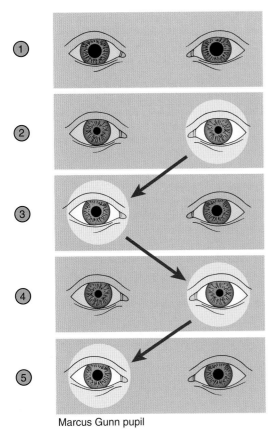

Marcus Gunn pupil

Figure 38.1   The relative afferent pupillary defect (Marcus Gunn pupil). The figure depicts a patient with an abnormal right optic nerve. Under normal room light illumination (row 1), the pupils are symmetrical. During the swinging flashlight test, the pupils constrict when the normal eye is illuminated (rows 2 and 4) but dilate when the abnormal eye is illuminated (rows 3 and 5). Although both pupils constrict or dilate simultaneously, the clinician is usually focused on just the illuminated pupil. The pupil that dilates during the swinging flashlight test has the "relative afferent pupillary defect" and is labeled the Marcus Gunn pupil. *(From McGee, S. The pupils. In: Duthie EH, Katz PR, Malone M, eds. Evidenced-Based Physical Diagnosis. 3rd ed. Philadelphia: Elsevier; 2012:161-179.)*

On exam, her temperature is 36.8 °C (98.3 °F), pulse rate is 94/min, blood pressure is 122/84 mm Hg, and respiration rate is 20/min. The cardiac and pulmonary exams are unrevealing. Sensation is present but decreased throughout her right arm and unchanged on the left. The strength in her right arm is slightly deceased to 4+/5 as compared to the left. There is also notable weakness in her legs, approximately 4–/5. Hoffman's reflex is positive on the right and negative on the left. Tinel's and Phalen's signs are negative bilaterally. Flexion of her neck results in an electric-like pain that extends down her back.

BASIC SCIENCE/CLINICAL PEARL   STEP 1/2/3

Hoffman's reflex is an upper motor sign akin to the Babinski reflex. It is elicited by holding the middle or ring finger and flicking the distal phalanx. The presence of flexion of the remaining digits is a positive sign and indicative of a possible upper motor neuron lesion. Because it can be seen in normal individuals, a positive sign is only relevant when accompanied by additional history and exam findings consistent with an upper motor neuron lesion.

What is the importance of this electrical sensation running down the back?

The presence of an electric-like sensation that runs down the back upon flexion of the cervical spine is called Lhermitte's sign. It is associated with pathology along the dorsal column of the spinal cord. The sensation itself typically starts at the cervical spine and runs down the back dorsally and can include the limbs. Lhermitte's is commonly associated with multiple sclerosis (MS) but has also been seen in other pathologies including vitamin B12 deficiency, radiation therapy, chemotherapy, Behcet's disease, and cervical cord compression related to a tumor or spondylosis.

BASIC SCIENCE/CLINICAL PEARL   **STEP 1/2/3**

The difference between a symptom and a sign is that the former is subjective and described by the patient, whereas the latter is an observable finding by the clinician and should be reproducible. Interestingly, because this electrical sensation is only describable by the patient, Lhermitte's sign is actually a symptom and not a sign as formally named.

What is your differential diagnosis at this point?

As reviewed above, numbness and tingling can represent a number of different diagnoses. Taking into account her prior hospitalization for optic neuritis, strong consideration is given for MS. Both optic neuritis and paresthesias are commonly seen in the early stages of MS. Diagnosis is based on the demonstration of lesions separated in both location and time. Review of diagnostic imaging performed at the time of her optic neuritis, specifically a magnetic resonance image (MRI) scan of her head and spinal cord, could potentially support the diagnosis if there were lesions present unrelated to her optic neuritis.

Other possibilities on the differential that should be considered include a compressive tumor centrally or peripherally, amyotrophic lateral sclerosis (ALS), injury involving the brachial plexus, sarcoidosis, and vitamin B12 deficiency.

Further diagnostic testing is performed. An MRI of her head is unrevealing on T1 and positive for hyperintense lesions on T2 (see Fig. 38.2). Gadolinium contrast enhancement with T1 shows lesions corresponding to those seen on T2 without contrast. A sample of cerebrospinal fluid (CSF) is also obtained and sent for analysis, which reveals elevated immunoglobulin levels, specifically immunoglobulin G (IgG).

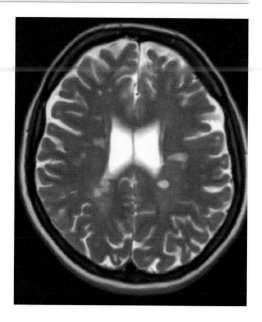

Figure 38.2 T2-weighted MRI without contrast of the brain with evidence of periventricular lesions. *(From Granziera C, Weier K, Sprenger T. MRI in clinical management of multiple sclerosis. In: Toga AW, ed. Brain Mapping. Vol 3. London: Academic Press, an imprint of Elsevier; 2012:907-912.)*

BASIC SCIENCE/CLINICAL PEARL	STEP 1/2/3

MRI is based on the creation of a strong magnetic field that causes the protons in water molecules to emit a signal, based on proton spinning and relaxation. Depending on the timing and synchronization of the magnetic field applied, different signals can be obtained. The two signals commonly provided are T1 and T2. T1-signal MRI images are useful to detect fatty (or myelinated) tissue with the brain, which appears white. T2-signal MRI images are useful to detect water in the brain (in situations where edema and/or inflammation is suspected), which also appears white. A helpful way to remember the difference between T1 and T2 signal is that T**2** highlights water, which is also known as H**2**O.

Diagnosis: Relapsing-remitting multiple sclerosis (RRMS)

What are the criteria for diagnosis of multiple sclerosis?

Diagnosis of multiple sclerosis depends on the demonstration of episodes that are separated in both time and space and referred to as the McDonald criteria (which underwent revision in 2010). Each event or attack is characterized by a neurologic disturbance that is related to demyelization and inflammation and lasts for at least 24 hours. For dissemination in time (DIT), each episode should be separated by 30 days. Dissemination in space (DIS) refers to involvement of at least two of four separate zones: periventricular, juxtacortical, infratentorial, or spinal lesions. Objective data are necessary for diagnosis and can be based on clinical signs, diagnostic imaging (MRI in particular), cerebrospinal fluid analysis, and use of visual-evoked potentials if necessary. Once a diagnosis of MS is made, it can be classified (see Table 38.2).

In addition, other possible diagnoses that could better account for the clinical picture must also be ruled out. Although rare, neuromyelitis optica (NMO or Devic's disease) should be considered when evaluating for MS. NMO typically affects vision and spinal cord function including motor and sensory impairments, all of which can be characteristic of an early MS attack. However, the spinal lesions in NMO are by definition longer than two cord segments and generally spare the brain itself.

TABLE 38.2 ▥ Multiple Sclerosis Variants

Clinically Isolated Syndrome (CIS)	Isolated neurologic event with characteristics similar to multiple sclerosis without prior evidence of the disease.
Relapsing-Remitting (RRMS)	Episodes of neurologic relapses with full recovery or minimal residual deficits between each event. There is no evidence of disease progression between each episode.
Secondary Progressive (SPMS)	Begins as relapsing-remitting MS but then converts to progressive worsening of the disease.
Primary Progressive (PPMS)	Progressive worsening of MS without periods of improvement. Individuals with this type tend to suffer greater disability when compared to the other variants.

How should she be treated acutely?

During the acute phase of a newly diagnosed or exacerbation of MS, treatment is directed toward the inflammation. Glucocorticoids are the mainstay of treatment and can be administered either orally or intravenously. A systematic review comparing the two failed to show one formulation as better than another. Admission to an acute care setting is useful to monitor for improvement of symptoms. In the event acute symptoms fail to improve with glucocorticoids, plasma exchange can also be considered.

What treatment should be initiated for chronic management?

Although there is no cure for MS, chronic treatment is based on decreasing relapse rates and slowing progression of the disease. The pharmacologic management is dependent on what form is diagnosed, relapsing-remitting (RRMS) versus progressive. Following diagnosis of RRMS and acute management, long-term treatment can be started with interferon beta-1a agents such as Avonex® or Rebif®. Common reactions to interferon therapy include site reaction, flulike symptoms, and asymptomatic hepatic dysfunction. For prevention of the latter, patients on an interferon medication are advised to avoid hepatotoxic medications or products such as alcohol. Other medications used to slow progression of RRMS are glatiramer acetate, a copolymer with amino acid components, or a human monoclonal antibody.

In the event a relapsing-remitting form progresses to secondary progressive MS (SPMS) or the patient is initially diagnosed with primary progressive MS (PPMS), a different treatment plan is considered. Whereas interferons and glatiramer are considered early mainstays of treatment for RRMS, there is little evidence to show their efficacy in progressive forms of MS. Additionally, there is little evidence for any treatment that can significantly alter the course of PPMS or SPMS. Patients are often treated with medications such as monthly intravenous (IV) dosages of glucocorticoid, rituximab, or methotrexate. However, all these treatments are considered off-label therapies, and the treatment plan is usually physician specific.

In advanced forms of MS, what symptomatic treatments are available?

In the later stages of MS, other treatments can be provided as an adjunct to disease-modifying therapy symptomatic control. Chronic impairments include paralysis, spasticity, and bowel/bladder dysfunction. The legs are most commonly affected with weakness, and patients can require assistance with braces, assist devices such as rolling walkers, or wheelchairs. Because MS is an upper motor neuron disease, uninhibited lower motor neuron activity can lead to increased spasticity, and antispasticity treatments may be considered. Baclofen is a long-acting pharmacologic option commonly used first along with a short-acting medication antispasmodic such as tizanidine. Injections with botulinum toxin (Botox®) can be considered where targeted treatment is necessary for select muscles or muscle groups. In cases where systemic side effects with oral medications are intolerable, such as increased drowsiness, an intrathecal baclofen pump can be considered. For functional retraining and adapting to new impairments, rehabilitation in an inpatient setting, acute rehabilitation center, skilled nursing home, or outpatient setting can all be utilized for continued medication adjustments and to determine optimal dosing (see Table 38.3).

CLINICAL PEARL   **STEP 2/3**

MS can result in increased heat sensitivity, referred to as Uhthoff phenomenon, where increased body temperatures can lead to exacerbations of neurologic symptoms. These exacerbations are not true MS exacerbations and are often referred to as pseudo-exacerbations, as there is no increase in lesion burden. They can be triggered via environmental increases in temperature or internal increases such as with exercise. The demyelination caused by MS leads to a decreased threshold for heat-related conduction

TABLE 38.3 ▓ Treatment Options for Various Forms of Multiple Sclerosis

Acute Event	Glucocorticoids (IV or PO) Plasma exchange
Chronic Management	
Relapsing-Remitting MS	Interferon beta-1a (Avonex®, Betaseron®, Rebif®) Glatiramer Glucocorticoids (IV; monthly dosing)
Secondary Progressive MS	Interferon beta-1a Glucocorticoids (IV; monthly dosing) Cyclophosphamide Methotrexate
Primary Progressive MS	No evidence-based proven treatment Treatment may include: • Glucocorticoids (IV; monthly dosing) • Methotrexate
Symptomatic	
Spasticity	Baclofen Tizanidine Botox® injections Orthotic bracing
Bladder Incontinence	Fluid restrictions Timed voiding Intermittent catheterization Anticholinergic medications (oxybutynin)
Bowel Dysfunction (Constipation)	Bowel regimen Senna Docusate (Colace®) Bisacodyl (Dulcolax®) suppository Manual disimpaction

IV, Intravenous; *PO,* oral.

CLINICAL PEARL—cont'd

block and increased sensitivity for those affected. Thus, it is worth advising patients with MS to avoid exposing themselves to extreme heat, such as saunas and hot baths. Fortunately, symptoms improve with cooling, and treatment can be as simple as removing the heat source and cooling the body via ice, air conditioning, or breathable clothing.

The patient is transferred and admitted to an inpatient setting where she is treated with IV glucocorticoids. Following improvement of her symptoms and completing treatment, a physical and occupational therapy consultation is requested to assess her functional skills and ability to care for herself at home. The occupational therapy evaluation notes that she is able to perform daily activities independently. The physical therapy evaluation reveals trouble with balance when walking without an assist device, but otherwise safe with transfers and walking with a cane or walker. She is recommended continued rehabilitation in a skilled nursing facility. A follow-up appointment with her neurologist is scheduled where she will likely start long-term treatment with the interferon Avonex®.

BEYOND THE PEARLS

- A patient's perception of pain and sensory deficits related to carpal tunnel syndrome may not necessarily follow a typical dermatomal distribution for the median nerve as described in textbooks. Patients may describe symptoms extending throughout the entire ring finger, posterior hand, or even proximal to the wrist. Given appropriate history and signs, it is reasonable to evaluate for carpal tunnel syndrome even if the patient's pain, numbness, and tingling complaints extend outside the median nerve dermatome.
- Although optic neuritis is commonly associated with MS, there are atypical features that would prompt consideration of a cause unrelated to acute demyelination of the optic nerve such as systemic lupus, tumor, paraneoplastic disease, sarcoidosis, Lyme disease, and Leber's hereditary optic neuropathy. These features include lack of associated pain, worsening visual loss beyond a week, and persistent visual loss beyond a month.
- Although the requirement for dispersion in time requires a separation of 30 days between events, revisions to the McDonald criteria allow for diagnosis within that time frame with MRI evidence of a separate MS-related lesion. The diagnosis can be made if a new T2 and/or gadolinium contrast-enhancing lesion is identified on a follow-up MRI after the initial baseline MRI scan. In addition, a single MRI scan that reveals both a contrast-enhancing lesion and nonenhancing lesion can confirm the diagnosis of MS as long as the nonenhancing lesion does not have another likely cause.
- In the event a diagnosis of MS is suspected but difficult to confirm with clinical history and diagnostic imaging, evoked potentials may also be utilized. This study elicits a central response to an external visual, auditory, or somatosensory stimulus. A decreased response is an indication of central nervous damage and potentially supports the diagnosis of a separate lesion in space for diagnosis of MS.
- When treating spasticity related to MS or another upper motor injury, the patient's functional status must be considered. Severe spasticity of the extremities, particularly the lower extremities, will limit movement and the ability to transfer, walk, and so on. Overtreatment of spasticity can result in weak muscles that are also unable to provide adequate function. For example, when treating spasticity in the legs, undertreating a little and allowing increased spasticity can provide additional support with standing, standing pivots, and ambulation.
- Due to the higher incidence of MS in younger females of childbearing age, these patients will likely want to discuss the effect MS will have on a potential pregnancy. In general, MS episodes tend to decrease during the pregnancy period but then increase immediately postpartum.

References

Balcer LJ. Optic neuritis. *N Engl J Med.* 2006;354(12):1273-1280.

Carmosino MJ, Brousseau KM, Arciniegas DB, Corboy JR. Initial evaluations for multiple sclerosis in a university multiple sclerosis center: outcomes and role of magnetic resonance imaging in referral. *Arch Neurol.* 2005;62:585-590.

Gutrecht JA. Lhermitte's sign: from observation to eponym. *Arch Neurol.* 1989;46(5):557-558.

Lublin FD, Reingold SC, Cohen JA, et al. Defining the clinical course of multiple sclerosis: the 2013 revisions. *Neurology.* 2014;83:278-286.

McDonald WI, Compston A, Edan G, et al. Recommended diagnostic criteria for multiple sclerosis: guidelines from the International Panel on the diagnosis of multiple sclerosis. *Ann Neurol.* 2001;50(1):121-127.

Polman CH, Reingold SC, Banwell B, et al. Diagnostic criteria for multiple sclerosis: 2010 revisions to the McDonald criteria. *Ann Neurol.* 2011;69:292-302.

Ravi Lakdawala ▓ Joseph Abdelmalek

A 22-Year-Old Male With Hematuria

A 22-year-old male presents for outpatient evaluation of 3 days of cola-colored urine that started spontaneously. He has not had any pain or burning with urination. He has also had an upper respiratory infection for the past week.

What is the significance of dark-colored urine?

When evaluating dark-colored urine, you must determine whether the etiology is blood or pigment. True hematuria signifies the presence of red blood cells and can be classified as either gross (i.e., visible to the eye) or microscopic (which requires microscopy for diagnosis). Once the presence of red blood cells is confirmed, the source of hematuria can be characterized as coming from within the kidney (intrarenal, or upper urinary tract bleeding) or from outside the kidney (extrarenal, or lower urinary tract). Intrarenal sources of bleeding include glomerulonephritis, vasculitis, pyelonephritis, and malignancy. Causes of extrarenal bleeding include nephrolithiasis, bladder or urethral infections, malignancy, or trauma.

CLINICAL PEARL   **STEP 2/3**

Pigments such as those found in hemoglobin or myoglobin, as well as in beets and carrots, can discolor urine. Patients with rhabdomyolysis or hemolysis will test positive for blood on the urinary dipstick due to the presence of myoglobin or hemoglobin, respectively, but will not have any red blood cells visible under microscopy.

The patient also denies any recent trauma or accidents, sexual intercourse, urethral discharge, urinary frequency, or urinary urgency.

CLINICAL PEARL   **STEP 2/3**

Hematuria that is associated with pain in the flanks or the groin may be associated with kidney stones or urinary tract infections. Painless hematuria in high-risk patients requires a urological evaluation including cystoscopy to evaluate for malignancy.

The patient has no prior medical history and has not had any prior surgeries. He is of Asian heritage and is currently a college student. He denies any tobacco use but endorses using alcohol occasionally. He has no allergies and does not take any medications. There is no family history of hypertension, malignancy, or renal disease.

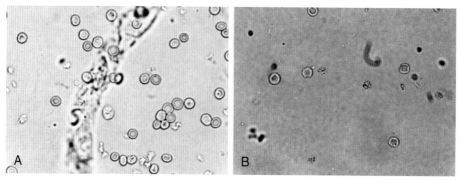

Figure 39.1 **A,** Isomorphic red blood cells. **B,** Dysmorphic red blood cells. *(From Greenberg A. Urinalysis and urine microscopy. In:* National Kidney Foundation Primer on Kidney Diseases. *Philadelphia: Elsevier; 2013:37.)*

On physical exam, he is afebrile with a pulse rate of 75/min, blood pressure of 144/87 mm Hg, and his body mass index (BMI) is 22 kg/m². He is alert and sitting comfortably. His jugular vein is not distended. His pulse rate is regular, and his lungs are clear to auscultation without any wheezes. He has no abdominal tenderness or distention. He has 1+ pitting edema in his lower extremities. His joints show no effusion or evidence of arthritis. He has no skin rashes. His neurological exam is normal.

BASIC SCIENCE PEARL   **STEP 1**

Skin findings in a patient with kidney disease may be indicative of primary or secondary small- or medium-vessel vasculitis, rheumatologic diseases such as lupus or dermatomyositis, and other immunologic diseases such as Henoch-Schonlein purpura.

What is the significance of this patient's hypertension?

About 95% of patients with hypertension have primary or essential hypertension, where blood pressure is greater than 140/90 mm Hg with no specific identifiable etiology. The likely pathogenesis for elevated blood pressure in these individuals is multifactorial, including genetics, congenital renal impairment, and renal injury leading to impaired sodium excretion with subsequent volume expansion and elevated blood pressure. Secondary hypertension can be due to renal parenchymal or glomerular diseases, renovascular disease, endocrine diseases such as Cushing syndrome and aldosteronism; preeclampsia or eclampsia, as well as obstructive sleep apnea and drug-induced causes due to sympathomimetics, glucocorticoids, nonsteroidal antiinflammatory drugs (NSAIDs), and oral contraceptives. Risk factors for a secondary cause of hypertension include the sudden onset of hypertension, very young or very old age at onset of hypertension, and resistant hypertension. Resistant hypertension is defined by the inability to control blood pressure while on at least three antihypertensive medications at the maximum tolerated dose. In this case, the presence of hypertension in a 22-year-old without a family history suggests a secondary cause.

Laboratory testing reveals a normal complete blood count, electrolytes, creatinine, and liver function. His urine dipstick is positive for 3+ blood and 2+ protein but negative for leukocyte esterase, nitrites, ketones, bilirubin, and glucose. Microscopic analysis of the urine shows >50 red blood cells per high power field, dysmorphic red blood cells (Fig. 39.1), 6 to 10 red blood cell casts per high power field (Fig. 39.2), and 0 to 3 white blood cells per high power field, with no crystals or bacteria.

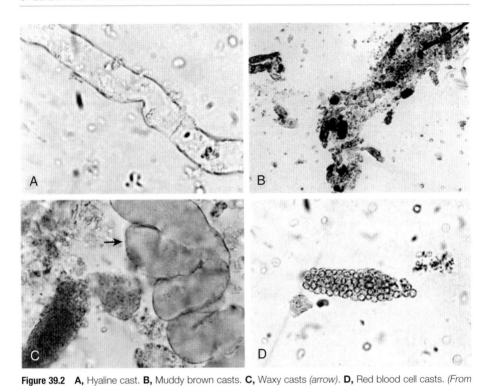

Figure 39.2 **A,** Hyaline cast. **B,** Muddy brown casts. **C,** Waxy casts *(arrow)*. **D,** Red blood cell casts. *(From Greenberg A. Urinalysis and urine microscopy. In: National Kidney Foundation Primer on Kidney Diseases. Philadelphia: Elsevier; 2013:38.)*

CLINICAL PEARL   **STEP 2/3**

As little as 1 mL of blood can cause a significant discoloration in the urine. Unless the patient has significant trauma to the urinary tract system with gross blood, it is unlikely that hematuria will cause a significant drop in a patient's hemoglobin.

BASIC SCIENCE PEARL   **STEP 1**

Normally, erythrocytes are biconcave discs about 7 micrometers in diameter, typically presenting with a central clearing. Isomorphic red blood cells are uniform in shape and size, usually originating from the lower urinary tract. Dysmorphic red blood cells, on the other hand, are erythrocytes that originated from the renal parenchyma characterized by having spicules, blebs, vesicles, and submembrane cytoplasmic precipitation.

What is your differential diagnosis at this point?
This patient is a young Asian male with dark-colored urine in the setting of a viral upper respiratory infection and hypertension. This in conjunction with the presence of numerous red blood cells under microscopy with associated dysmorphic red blood cells and red cell casts indicates glomerular injury. This presentation is most consistent with nephritic syndrome, in which there is inflammation of the glomerulus with consequent decrease in glomerular filtration rate (GFR). Characteristics of this syndrome include edema, hematuria, and hypertension. There are several glomerular diseases that may present with nephritic syndrome, including immunoglobulin A

(IgA) nephropathy, poststreptococcal glomerulonephritis (PSGN), lupus nephritis, antineutro-phil cytoplasmic antibody (ANCA) vasculitis, antiglomerular basement membrane (GBM) disease, and membranoproliferative glomerulonephritis.

What labs would you order to evaluate for specific types of glomerulonephritis?
Other lab tests that may be of value to discern causes of acute glomerulonephritis include comple-ment levels, blood and urine cultures, anti-GBM antibodies, and ANCA titers, as well as an antinuclear antibody (ANA) screen for possible lupus nephritis.

> The patient's urine protein-to-creatinine ratio is 2. Complement levels including C3 and C4 are normal. ANA, ANCA, and anti-GBM antibodies are negative. Blood and urine cultures as well as antistreptolysin O titers are negative.

BASIC SCIENCE PEARL   **STEP 1**

Urinary casts form in the renal tubules, trapping particles from the kidneys in the presence of uromodulin, or Tamm-Horsfall protein. Red blood cell casts are an indicator of glomerular bleeding. Fatty casts occur in the setting of marked proteinuria or nephrotic syndrome. White blood cell casts can be seen with pyelonephritis, interstitial nephritis, and other tubulointerstitial diseases. White blood cell casts help to distinguish pyelonephritis from a lower urinary tract infection.

When is a renal biopsy indicated?
With unrevealing labs, the only way to ascertain a diagnosis in this case is to proceed with a renal biopsy. The renal biopsy should provide further information toward a specific diagnosis, prog-nostic information, and aid in planning therapy for certain diseases. Some indications for renal biopsy include nephrotic syndrome of unknown etiology, acute kidney injury with active urine sediment, systemic disease with associated renal dysfunction, renal transplant dysfunction, as well as unexplained kidney diseases or familial disorders.

What are the contraindications to a renal biopsy?
Contraindications to a renal biopsy include uncontrolled hypertension, bleeding diathesis, hydro-nephrosis, as well as widespread cystic disease or renal malignancy.

What information can be obtained from a renal biopsy?
Once a renal biopsy is obtained, the specimen is examined under light microscopy, immunofluo-rescence, and electron microscopy. Light microscopy is used to evaluate cellularity, deposition of abnormal material, necrosis, and capillary wall thickness in the glomerulus. Light microscopy also allows for assessment of the renal tubules. Immunofluorescence allows for visualization of immunoglobulins and complement components in the glomeruli and tubules. Electron micros-copy allows for visualization of immune complexes and ultrastructural changes in the glomeruli and other parts of the kidney.

> The patient undergoes renal biopsy, which shows increased cells in the mesangial portion of the glomerulus on light microscopy (Fig. 39.3). On immunofluorescence, there is positive staining for IgA (Fig. 39.4). Electron microscopy reveals IgA immune complexes in the mesangium (Fig. 39.5). There are no crescents seen on the renal biopsy.

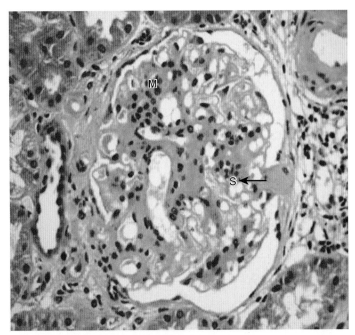

Figure 39.3   Kidney biopsy showing mesangial proliferation (M) and expansion of the mesangial extracellular matrix (S) in a patient with IgA nephropathy. A capsular adhesion can also be seen *(arrow)*. *(From Feehally J, Barratt J. Immunoglobulin A nephropathy and related disorders. In: National Kidney Foundation Primer on Kidney Diseases. Philadelphia: Elsevier; 2013:186.)*

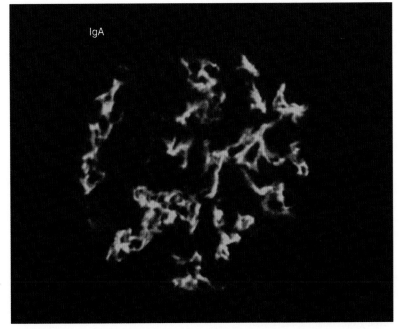

Figure 39.4   Immunofluorescence staining for mesangial IgA. *(From Feehally J, Barratt J. Immunoglobulin A nephropathy and related disorders. In: National Kidney Foundation Primer on Kidney Diseases. Philadelphia: Elsevier; 2013:186.)*

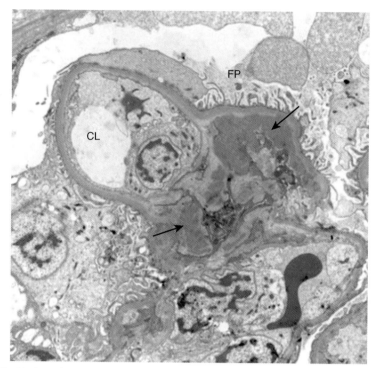

Figure 39.5 Electron micrograph showing IgA immune complex deposition within mesangium and parame-
sangium as indicated by the arrows. *CL,* Capillary loops; *FP,* normal podocyte foot processes. *(From Feehally
J, Barratt J. Immunoglobulin A nephropathy and related disorders. In:* National Kidney Foundation Primer on
Kidney Diseases. *Philadelphia: Elsevier; 2013:186.)*

Diagnosis: Immunoglobulin A (IgA) nephropathy

IgA nephropathy is the most common primary glomerulonephritis in the world, occurring in
about 25 to 50 per 10,000 people. This disease can present as asymptomatic hematuria with
normal renal function to rapidly progressive glomerulonephritis (RPGN) with renal failure in
weeks to months. This glomerular disease is more common in Asians and Caucasians, with a
peak incidence in the second and third decades of life.

BASIC SCIENCE/CLINICAL PEARL   **STEP 1/2/3**

IgA nephropathy typically presents as hematuria concurrent or within days of an upper
respiratory infection, compared to poststreptococcal glomerulonephritis, which typically
occurs 2 to 3 weeks after an upper respiratory or skin infection.

A renal biopsy typically shows the presence of immunoglobulin A in the mesangium on
immunofluorescence and electron microscopy. Patients with RPGN may have rapid loss of kidney
function with the presence of glomerular crescents on renal biopsy, which are indicative of severe
injury to the glomerular capillary wall.

What are the treatment options?

Blood pressure control is used to delay progression of renal disease with guidelines indicating a goal blood pressure of <130/80 mm Hg in those patients with proteinuria. Hypertension in glomerulonephritis occurs in the setting of sodium and water overload. Initial therapy should therefore include behavioral modification with sodium restriction, moderate exercise, weight loss, and smoking cessation. Angiotensin-converting enzyme (ACE) inhibitors and angiotensin receptor blockers (ARBs) are first-line therapies for patients with hypertension and proteinuria as they have been shown to control proteinuria independent of their effects on blood pressure. In patients with significant proteinuria or a rising creatinine, immunosuppression with high-dose glucocorticoids, and occasionally cyclophosphamide, may be added to the aforementioned supportive therapy.

The patient is counseled on a low-salt diet and is started on an ACE inhibitor, which controls his blood pressure, however he continues to have hematuria and proteinuria. He is started on glucocorticoids for 6 months with remission of his hematuria and proteinuria.

BEYOND THE PEARLS

- IgA nephropathy can present as a secondary disease indistinguishable from primary IgA nephropathy, commonly associated with chronic liver disease, celiac disease, inflammatory bowel disease, and human immunodeficiency virus (HIV). Kidney dysfunction may improve with treatment of the primary disease.
- Occurring at any age, Henoch-Schonlein purpura is a self-limiting small-vessel vasculitis that is characterized by palpable purpura and occasionally arthritis and gastrointestinal symptoms. Some patients may have transient renal involvement, which is identical to that seen in IgA nephropathy. Skin biopsy will typically show leukocytoclastic vasculitis, with immunofluorescence occasionally showing IgA deposition.
- A scoring system called the Oxford-MEST score uses parameters such as mesangial hypercellularity, endocapillary hypercellularity, segmental glomerulosclerosis, and tubular atrophy/interstitial fibrosis to predict outcomes; however, it has not been fully validated yet.
- Treatment of primary glomerular diseases typically involves both supportive therapy and occasionally immunosuppressive therapy. Supportive therapy will include intensive blood pressure control, reducing proteinuria, as well as managing the consequences of nephrotic syndrome (i.e., edema, hyperlipidemia, and occasionally hypercoagulable states).
- Omega-3 fatty acids in the form of fish oil have been studied in IgA nephropathy due to its antiinflammatory properties. The evidence for its benefit is low level; however, it is a relatively low-risk therapy.
- Nearly 25% of patients with IgA nephropathy will develop end-stage renal disease (ESRD) (i.e., require renal replacement therapy within 10 to 25 years from diagnosis, depending on severity of disease at the onset).
- Patients with ESRD who obtain a renal transplant have a high chance of developing recurrence of IgA nephropathy, with rates reaching 75% with long-term survival of the graft.
- Patients with preexisting renal dysfunction or glomerular disease should avoid exposure to nephrotoxic agents such as NSAIDs, radiocontrast agents, as well as certain antibiotics such as aminoglycosides.

328   CASE 39: A 22-YEAR-OLD MALE WITH HEMATURIA

References

Chapter 10: Immunoglobulin A nephropathy. *Kidney Int Suppl.* 2012;2(2):209-217. doi:10.1038/kisup.2012.23.

Floege J, Johnson RJ, Feehally J. *Comprehensive Clinical Nephrology*. 5th ed. Philadelphia: Elsevier Saunders; 2015.

Kincaid-Smith P, Fairley K. The investigation of hematuria. *Semin Nephrol.* 2005;25(3):127-135.

Lerma E, Nissenson A. *Nephrology Secrets*. 3rd ed. Philadelphia: Elsevier Mosby; 2012.

Nachman PH, Jennette JC, Falk RJ. Primary glomerular disease. In: Taal M, ed. *Brenner and Rector's The Kidney*. 9th ed. Philadelphia: Elsevier Saunders; 2012:1100-1191.

Salama AD, Cook HT. The renal biopsy. In: Taal M, ed. *Brenner and Rector's The Kidney*. Philadelphia: Elsevier Saunders; 2012:1006-1015.

Wyatt RJ, Julian BA. IgA nephropathy. *N Engl J Med*. 2013;368:2402-2414.

Caitlin Reed ▆ Arzhang Cyrus Javan

A 54-Year-Old Male With Chronic Cough and Weight Loss

A 54-year-old Filipino male presents to the emergency room complaining of chronic productive cough without hemoptysis, night sweats, and a 15-pound unintentional weight loss over the past 3 months. He has no known past medical history but has not seen a physician in decades. He endorses polyuria and polydipsia. Review of systems is otherwise negative.

What infection control measure should be immediately instituted?
The patient should immediately be placed in airborne isolation because pulmonary tuberculosis (TB) is in the differential diagnosis for an immigrant with chronic cough and systemic symptoms. Avoiding nosocomial transmission of TB from patients with infectious active pulmonary disease is a priority. The patient should be given a surgical mask and placed in a single room with a closed door, preferably an airborne isolation room with negative pressure. Health care personnel should wear appropriately fitted N95 masks while caring for patients under evaluation for pulmonary tuberculosis.

The patient is moved to an airborne isolation room. Additional social history is obtained. He was employed in construction but has been unable to work recently because of weakness. He immigrated from the Philippines 18 years ago. He has no known sick contacts and no known exposures to TB. He denies exposure to prisons, jails, homeless shelters, or nursing homes. He smokes one pack of cigarettes per day. He denies drinking alcohol or illicit drug use. On physical exam, he is afebrile, vital signs are normal, and he is not hypoxic; however, he is cachectic with mild bitemporal wasting. Dentition is poor. There is no oral thrush. He has scattered rhonchi in the left upper lung field and mildly decreased breath sounds bilaterally; otherwise the lungs are clear to auscultation. Cardiac exam is benign. There is no hepatosplenomegaly, ascites, or other stigmata of chronic liver disease. He has no clubbing or peripheral edema. There is onychomycosis of the toes bilaterally. There are no other notable findings.

What is the differential diagnosis of chronic cough with constitutional symptoms?
Without the night sweats and weight loss, the differential diagnosis of chronic cough is broad and includes common noninfectious etiologies such as asthma, chronic obstructive pulmonary disease, postnasal drip, and gastric esophageal reflux disease. However, this patient has significant constitutional symptoms, so we are concerned about more serious underlying diseases: pulmonary TB caused by *Mycobacterium tuberculosis*, nontuberculous mycobacteria (NTM) infection such as *Mycobacterium avium*, human immunodeficiency virus (HIV) presenting with an opportunistic infection, endemic fungal infections such as coccidioidomycosis or histoplasmosis, malignancy (especially because the patient smokes), chronic anaerobic lung abscess, interstitial lung disease, and rheumatologic diseases such as sarcoidosis and granulomatosis with polyangiitis (GPA).

What initial tests should be ordered?

A chest radiograph (CXR) is an important initial diagnostic test in evaluating chronic cough with unintentional weight loss and fevers. A sputum specimen for acid-fast bacilli (AFB) smear microscopy and culture should be obtained every 8 to 24 hours for a total of three specimens. A nucleic acid amplification test (NAAT) should be ordered on at least the first sputum specimen. NAAT tests include but are not limited to TB polymerase chain reaction (PCR), Amplicor MTB, Amplified Mycobacterium Tuberculosis Direct test, and Cepheid GeneXpert. These tests are more sensitive and specific than AFB sputum smears.

CLINICAL PEARL   **STEP 2/3**

In addition to three sputa for AFB smear and culture, order a NAAT on at least the first sputum of all patients under evaluation for pulmonary TB.

All patients under evaluation for TB should be tested for HIV. Basic laboratory testing should include a complete blood count (CBC), electrolyte panel, liver function tests (LFTs), and screening for viral hepatitis. This patient has unexplained polyuria and polydipsia, which should be evaluated with a glycosylated hemoglobin (HgbA1C) for diabetes screening. Moreover, diabetes is one of several risk factors for progression from latent TB infection to active TB disease. Additional diagnostic workup should be considered based on epidemiologic risk factors and initial findings. For example, if the CXR is abnormal and the patient has lived in the desert Southwest, serology for the endemic fungal infection coccidioidomycosis ("Valley Fever") should be ordered. Malignancy is an important consideration, especially as the patient is a smoker; however, TB must be evaluated before considering procedures such as bronchoscopy with biopsy or computed tomography (CT)-guided biopsy of a lung mass. A CT scan of the chest should be ordered if malignancy is suspected after initial workup, and sputum cytology is a noninvasive test that can be obtained as part of the evaluation.

What is the difference between latent TB infection and active TB disease?

Figure 40.1 shows the natural history of TB infection. Persons who are exposed to TB from a coughing source patient with active pulmonary TB inhale bacilli into their lungs. In most patients, the immune response contains the infection in walled-off granulomas. The person is asymptomatic and noninfectious; this state is called latent TB infection (LTBI). Bear in mind that the large majority, about 90%, of persons with LTBI never progress to active TB disease. In the United States, the majority of patients who do develop active TB disease were initially infected years and often decades prior; this is because of TB's uniquely long latent period. Active TB disease may occur because of waning of immune control of TB infection as a result of aging or other medical conditions; this presentation is referred to as reactivation TB. A small proportion of TB patients develop active disease soon after primary infection. This is more likely to occur among immunosuppressed patients, such as those with HIV/acquired immunodeficiency syndrome (AIDS).

What is the utility of a tuberculin skin test or an interferon-gamma release assay (IGRA), such as QuantiFERON-TB Gold In-Tube test, in a patient suspected of having active pulmonary TB? How do these screening tests work?

These tests are screening tests for TB infection but do not distinguish latent TB infection from active TB. These tests are of limited utility in evaluating patients suspected of having active TB. When evaluating for active TB, it is crucial to pursue diagnostic tests, including AFB smear, culture, and nucleic acid amplification tests such as TB PCR, on specimens collected at the site of disease.

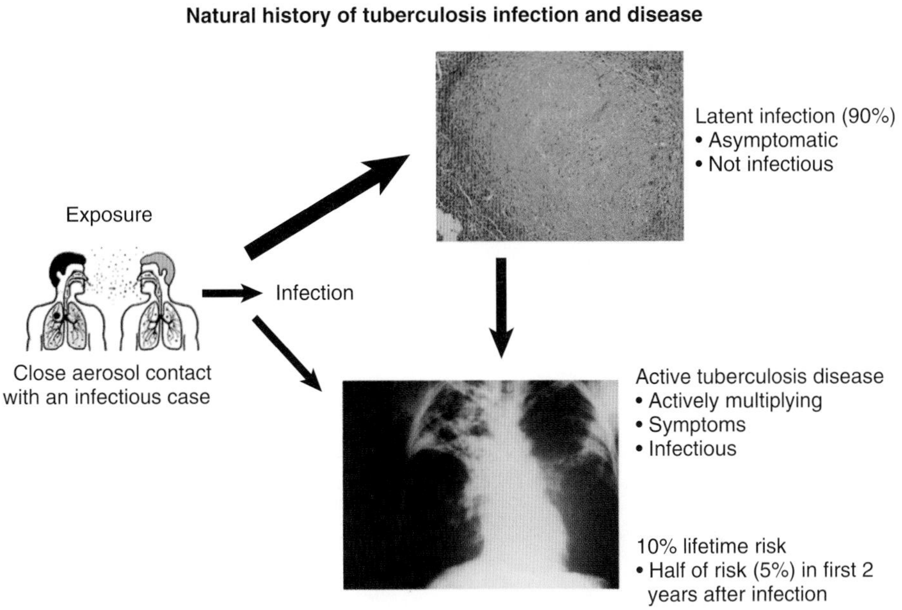

Natural history of tuberculosis infection and disease

Latent infection (90%)
• Asymptomatic
• Not infectious

Exposure

Infection

Close aerosol contact
with an infectious case

Active tuberculosis disease
• Actively multiplying
• Symptoms
• Infectious

10% lifetime risk
• Half of risk (5%) in first 2
years after infection

Figure 40.1 Schematic of the natural history of tuberculosis (TB) infection and disease. After initial infection, in most patients the immune system controls TB infection and the patient is asymptomatic. This is the latent state. A few patients, especially those with human immunodeficiency virus, may progress quickly to primary active TB disease. The large majority of patients with latent TB infection never progress to active TB disease. About 10% of latently infected patients eventually progress to active TB disease; this may occur decades after the initial infection and is referred to as reactivation. Reactivation TB occurs more frequently in immunocompromised patients. TB is an unusual organism because of its ability to persist in a latent, inactive state in the human body.

Screening tests for TB infection require an immune response to TB antigens. Patients with prior TB infection develop memory cells, so that when exposed to TB antigens again, they develop a detectable immune response. For the tuberculin skin test, the TB antigens are injected intradermally in the form of purified protein derivative (PPD). For IGRA assays, TB antigens are coated on the wall of a test tube, which is then exposed to the patient's lymphocyte-containing serum. A measurable immune response is quantified either as the size of induration at the site of the PPD injection or as the amount of interferon produced by activated lymphocytes in the IGRA tube. However, immunosuppressed patients, who are at greatest risk of progression to active TB disease, are often unlikely to mount a significant immune response to these screening tests, despite being infected with TB. Therefore, an indeterminate or negative TST or IGRA does not rule out active TB disease in patients with clinical signs and symptoms compatible with TB disease.

Initial CXR is shown in Figure 40.2. The patient has a left upper lobe cavity and signs of volume loss and apical scarring. HgbA1C is 10.4. CBC shows mild thrombocytosis. Electrolytes and LFTs are normal. Sputum is AFB smear 3+ positive. AFB sputum culture and TB PCR are pending.

What risk factors does this patient have for infection with *Mycobacterium tuberculosis*? What risk factors does he have for progression from latent infection to active TB disease?
The patient's primary risk factor for TB infection is being foreign born in a TB-endemic country, the Philippines. The top five countries of birth of foreign-born TB patients now living in the

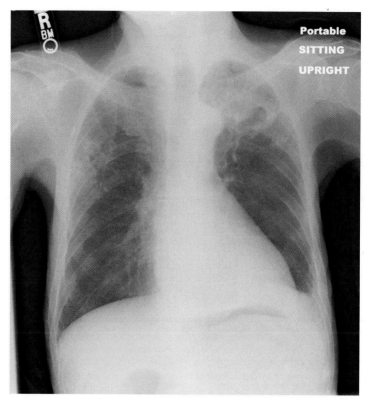

Figure 40.2   Chest radiograph of case patient, demonstrating a left upper lobe cavitary lesion.

United States in 2013 include Mexico, the Philippines, India, Vietnam, and China. All areas of Asia, Africa, South and Central America, and Eastern Europe are considered TB-endemic. Other risk factors for infection with TB include work or residence in a health care setting, homeless shelter, correctional facility, or other congregate setting, and recent close contact with an infectious TB case.

The patient's risk factors for progression from latent infection to active TB disease include poorly controlled diabetes mellitus and smoking. For progression to active TB disease, there are several important medical risk factors, as shown in Table 40.1. Of these risk factors, the two that confer the greatest risk of progression to active TB disease are HIV infection, especially among patients not taking antiretroviral therapy, and immunosuppression, especially in patients taking TNF alpha inhibitors (such as infliximab, etanercept, and others) and those on chronic glucocorticoid treatment of ≥15 mg of prednisone equivalent per day. Other notable risk factors for progression to active TB disease include recent conversion from negative to positive TST or IGRA test, substance abuse (alcohol, tobacco, and especially injection drug use), and radiographic evidence of old healed TB (fibrotic or fibronodular disease, not calcified granulomas) with no past history of TB treatment.

Does this patient have TB disease?
The patient is AFB sputum smear positive and has multiple risk factors for TB. TB disease is a likely diagnosis but should be confirmed by a nucleic acid amplification test or a sputum culture. The diagnosis is not yet confirmed because the sputum smear is not specific for *Mycobacterium*

> ### TABLE 40.1 ■ Medical Risk Factors for Progression From Latent Tuberculosis to Active Tuberculosis Disease
>
> - Human immunodeficiency virus (HIV) infection
> - Immunosuppression (TNF alpha inhibitor, ≥15 mg/day of prednisone for ≥1 month, or other immunosuppression)
> - Diabetes mellitus
> - End stage renal disease or hemodialysis
> - Smoker (current or in past year)
> - Leukemia or lymphoma
> - Silicosis
> - Cancer of head and neck
> - Intestinal bypass or gastrectomy
> - Chronic malabsorption
> - Low body weight (BMI <20)
>
> *BMI*, Body mass index; *TNF*, tumor necrosis factor.

tuberculosis; there are many other mycobacteria that are also acid fast and can cause sputum to be smear positive. For example, *Mycobacterium avium, Mycobacterium kansasii,* and *Mycobacterium abscessus* can cause cavitary disease with a similar presentation to tuberculosis disease. These other non-TB mycobacteria are collectively referred to as nontuberculous mycobacteria (NTM), atypical mycobacteria, or mycobacteria other than tuberculosis (MOTT).

CLINICAL PEARL	STEP 2/3

AFB smear-positive sputum may be caused by nontuberculous mycobacteria (NTM) such as *M. avium.*

One subcategory of NTM is known as the "rapid growers" and includes *M. chelonae, M. abscessus,* and *M. fortuitum.* These mycobacteria can cause significant pulmonary disease and usually grow on culture in 7 to 10 days, unlike *M. tuberculosis,* which usually takes 2 to 5 weeks to grow. There are also certain environmental NTM such as *M. gordonae* that are found in water systems and other environmental sources. When found, these NTM are usually considered a contaminant rather than true pathogens.

> The TB PCR (a nucleic acid amplification test) is positive on the AFB smear-positive sputum specimen.

> **Diagnosis:** Pulmonary tuberculosis

Does this confirm the diagnosis of TB? If so, what treatment should you start?
Yes, this confirms the diagnosis of pulmonary TB. You should still follow up on the culture results, which will be available in 2 to 6 weeks, and the drug susceptibility tests to confirm that the isolate is not drug resistant. Confirming that the patient's isolate is drug susceptible may take weeks because TB grows slowly in culture media. Unless you have a reason to suspect drug resistance (for example, the health department informs you that the patient is a close contact of another patient who is known to have drug-resistant TB), you should start standard treatment with the four first-line TB drugs pending results of susceptibility testing. TB is always treated with multiple medications because of the risk of selecting for drug resistance when monotherapy is used.

The four standard first-line drugs are rifampin, isoniazid, pyrazinamide, and ethambutol, often referred to as RIPE in U.S. health care settings. Pyridoxine (vitamin B6) is given along with isoniazid to help prevent peripheral neuropathy. The first 2 months are called the intensive phase of treatment. After completion of the intensive phase, pyrazinamide and ethambutol are discontinued. Rifampin and isoniazid are continued for the next 4 months, called the continuation phase of TB treatment. Although standard treatment is usually 6 months long, if the patient cannot tolerate the initial 2 months of pyrazinamide, total TB treatment duration must be extended to 9 months.

CLINICAL PEARL   **STEP 2/3**

Always start treatment for TB with multiple drugs to avoid selecting for drug resistance. The four first-line TB drugs for drug-sensitive TB are rifampin, isoniazid, pyrazinamide, and ethambutol. Never add a single drug to a failing TB regimen.

The drug dosing for RIPE is weight-based, and TB patients are often underweight, so check the patient's weight and calculate dosages. Be aware that rifampin is metabolized by the liver and upregulates the cytochrome p450 enzyme system, increasing the rate of clearance of other drugs. There are potential serious drug interactions with warfarin, antiretroviral medications, hormonal contraceptives, and other medications. Always check the medication list carefully for drug interactions. Rifabutin has less effect on the p450 system and sometimes may be substituted for rifampin when drug interactions are a concern.

CLINICAL PEARL   **STEP 2/3**

Rifampin is metabolized by the liver and has many drug interactions, including with warfarin, antiretroviral therapy, antifungal azoles, and oral contraceptives. Always check for interactions. Where interactions cannot be avoided, consider substituting rifabutin for rifampin.

Why should you be cautious about using fluoroquinolones for community-acquired pneumonia when TB is also in the differential diagnosis?

A common pitfall is treatment of a patient with pulmonary infiltrates and chronic cough for presumptive community-acquired pneumonia with a fluoroquinolone, such as levofloxacin or moxifloxacin, only to find later that the diagnosis was actually TB. Fluoroquinolones have good activity against *M. tuberculosis*. Treatment with quinolone monotherapy often leads to initial clinical improvement until the patient relapses with TB disease that has become resistant to quinolones. A better choice when treating empirically for bacterial pneumonia in a patient who is also a TB suspect is a macrolide such as azithromycin or, for inpatients, a beta-lactam antibiotic such as ceftriaxone and a macrolide.

What is TB treatment failure? What are some reasons for treatment failure?

Patients who fail to convert from TB culture positive to negative after 4 months of treatment are classified as failing treatment. Some reasons for treatment failure include patient nonadherence to the TB regimen, malabsorption of TB drugs, and baseline or acquired TB drug resistance. If it appears that your patient is failing treatment or is not improving clinically (for example, failing to gain weight, cough not improving or resolving), you should consult with an experienced TB clinician for guidance. An important principle is "never add a single drug to a failing regimen." This adage reminds us to avoid taking actions that could select for additional drug resistance.

TABLE 40.2 ■ Diagnostic Interpretation of Acid-Fast Bacilli (AFB) Sputum Smear and Nucleic Acid Amplification Test (NAAT) Results

	AFB Smear Positive	AFB Smear Negative
NAAT Positive	Tuberculosis	Tuberculosis, likely with a low burden of disease; repeat to confirm and follow-up culture
NAAT Negative	If confirmed on repeat specimen: nontuberculous mycobacteria	Unlikely tuberculosis, but collect additional specimens; could still be tuberculosis if high clinical suspicion or inadequate specimen collection

Another patient on your medicine service is under evaluation for TB because of an abnormal CXR and chronic cough with weight loss. He has three negative sputum smears. Is the diagnosis of TB excluded? What other tests should be ordered?

It is still possible that this patient has TB, despite the negative smears. Although three negative sputum smears are referred to as a "TB rule out" in many hospitals, this is a misnomer because it does not rule out TB. However, it does exclude *highly infectious* TB disease. This is because AFB smear-positive patients have a higher bacillary burden of TB organism in their sputum, and therefore are considerably more infectious to others than smear-negative patients.

CLINICAL PEARL   **STEP 2/3**

Although often called a "TB rule out," three negative AFB sputum smears do not exclude the diagnosis of TB. Smears are negative in about 40% of patients with culture-confirmed TB disease. However, the finding of three negative smears does rule out highly infectious TB.

The best test to order is a NAAT (including but not limited to TB PCR, Amplicor MTB, Amplified *Mycobacterium tuberculosis* Direct test, or Cepheid GeneXpert) on at least the first sputum specimen collected from a patient under evaluation for TB. For guidance on how to interpret the combination of AFB sputum smear and NAAT result, refer to Table 40.2. It is important to note that a negative NAAT test on an AFB sputum smear-negative specimen does not exclude TB. This is because among culture-confirmed TB cases, AFB sputum smear-negative patients have low numbers of organisms ("low bacillary burden") and therefore NAAT tests are less sensitive at detecting TB in these patients. Culture remains the gold standard for diagnosis. Clinical judgment is important in interpreting the results of all TB tests.

BEYOND THE PEARLS

- For most patients, lifetime risk of progression from latent TB infection to active TB disease is about 10%; however, in patients with advanced HIV/AIDS, risk of progression is about 5 to 10% *annually.*
- TB may be found in any organ, and extrapulmonary disease can be difficult to diagnose. For example, peritoneal TB resembles malignancy with ascites and peritoneal implants.
- A standard regimen for TB is 2 months of RIPE followed by 4 months of rifampin and isoniazid. However, treatment may be extended for severe disease or extrapulmonary disease such as TB meningitis or osteomyelitis.

Continued

BEYOND THE PEARLS—cont'd

- Avoid use of fluoroquinolones such as levofloxacin and moxifloxacin for empiric treatment of bacterial pneumonia in patients who might have TB in order to avoid giving monotherapy that could select for drug resistance.
- There are new rapid molecular tests for TB drug resistance that can predict resistance in <24 hours. These tests compare the TB isolate's genetic sequence to a library of known mutations that correlate with drug resistance.
- Glucocorticoids are not contraindicated for TB patients receiving effective TB therapy and are recommended for treatment of TB meningitis and TB pericarditis.
- Multidrug resistant (MDR) TB is resistant to both rifampin and isoniazid. Extensively drug resistant (XDR) TB is resistant to rifampin, isoniazid, at least one fluoroquinolone (ciprofloxacin, moxifloxacin, or levofloxacin), and at least one injectable agent (amikacin, capreomycin, or kanamycin).
- For patients with drug-resistant TB or intolerance to first-line TB drugs, traditional second- and third-line TB drugs include fluoroquinolones such as moxifloxacin, injectables such as amikacin and capreomycin, linezolid, cycloserine, ethionamide, and paraaminosalicyclic acid (PAS).
- Bedaquiline, the first new drug for treatment of drug-resistant TB in many years, was FDA (U.S. Food and Drug Administration)-approved in 2012, and another new drug, Delamanid, was recently approved in Europe.

References

American Thoracic Society; Centers for Disease Control and Prevention; Infectious Diseases Society of America. American Thoracic Society/Centers for Disease Control and Prevention/Infectious Diseases Society of America: Controlling tuberculosis in the United States. *Am J Respir Crit Care Med.* 2005;172(9):1169-1227.

Centers for Disease Control and Prevention. Latent Tuberculosis Infection: A Guide for Primary Health Care Providers. Available at <http://www.cdc.gov/tb/publications/LTBI/default.htm>. Accessed 28.05.15.

Davies P, Gordon S, Davies G. *Clinical Tuberculosis.* 5th ed. Boca Raton: CRC Press; 2014.

Getahun H, Matteelli A, Chaisson R, Raviglione M. Latent *Mycobacterium tuberculosis* infection. *N Engl J Med.* 2015;372(22):2127-2135.

Brandon A. Miller

A 57-Year-Old Male With Exertional Chest Pain

A 57-year-old male who you see every 1 to 2 years for a physical exam presents to your office for a checkup. He has a past medical history of hypertension, prediabetes, and hypercholesterolemia. He is a former smoker with a 20-pack-year history. He has a family history of heart disease in his father, who had a myocardial infarction (MI) at age 65, and type 2 diabetes in his mother. His medications include lisinopril and atorvastatin. He admits to using sildenafil (which he borrows from his brother) for erectile dysfunction on average once per week. He works as a mechanical engineer.

He feels well in general but reports that he gets a discomfort in his chest that he describes as a "squeezing" sensation that has been occurring over the past year. The squeezing sensation is located in the middle of his chest and does not radiate to his arms, neck, back, or jaw. There is no associated diaphoresis or vomiting, but he admits that occasionally he feels slightly "winded" and mildly nauseated. The discomfort is brought on by heavy exertion such as hiking with his sons, riding a stationary bike, and moving heavy objects (he reports that the pain occurred once while helping his son move and once when loading equipment onto his boat). The discomfort lasts for approximately 5 minutes, and after reaching a peak in intensity, it gradually eases after he stops whatever activity he is doing. He has not visited the emergency department on any of these occasions because the pain went away on its own. The pain does not ever occur at rest.

The physical exam reveals a slightly overweight middle-aged male with truncal obesity. Cardiopulmonary exam is unremarkable, and there are good distal pulses.

In the outpatient setting, what are the most likely causes of chest pain?
Approximately 1 to 2% of primary care visits are for chest pain, and it is always important to consider a cardiac etiology given that heart disease is the number one cause of death in the United States. It is also important to keep in mind that the majority of outpatient visits for chest pain involve noncardiac etiologies, with approximately 36% of cases involving a musculoskeletal condition, 19% involving a gastrointestinal condition, 8% involving a psychosocial or psychiatric condition, 5% involving a pulmonary condition, and 16% involving nonspecific chest pain (or chest pain of unclear etiology). This leaves about 16% of cases with a serious cardiac etiology, either stable coronary artery disease (angina in about 10% of cases) or unstable coronary artery disease (unstable angina, pulmonary embolism, heart failure comprising the other 6%). Compare this to the approximately 50% of patients in the emergency department setting that present with chest pain from serious cardiovascular etiology (either acute coronary syndrome, stable angina, pulmonary embolism, heart failure, or aortic dissection).

CLINICAL PEARL	**STEP 2/3**

Acute coronary syndrome (ACS) is a term that applies to the following conditions: unstable angina, non-ST elevation myocardial infarction (NSTEMI), and ST-elevation myocardial infarction (STEMI).

What features of the patient's presentation are consistent with chest pain of cardiac origin?
The patient has several risk factors for coronary disease, including hypertension, prediabetes, hypercholesterolemia, a significant smoking history, and a family history of coronary artery disease. Given the patient's underlying risk, you should hold a high level of suspicion for heart disease. The patient has many symptoms of typical (or classic) angina, including a midsternal location, a squeezing quality, a relatively predictable onset with exertion, a duration lasting between 2 and 15 minutes (usually 2 to 5) with a crescendo–decrescendo pattern and abatement with rest. If he had been prescribed sublingual nitroglycerin in the past for his symptoms and this resulted in relief, this is also a typical feature.

Although the patient has many typical features, there are other features of stable angina that he doesn't have but that are worth noting. These include a description of the discomfort as a heaviness, burning, pressure, weight, or ache (typical cardiac discomfort is rarely described as an outright pain). Although the onset of pain is usually with exertion, it can occur with emotion (frustration, anger, sadness) or eating a large meal (due to a "steal-like" phenomenon as blood is diverted to the gastrointestinal [GI] tract to aid in digestion). The discomfort can also radiate, usually to the shoulders, neck, jaw, inner arm (can be down to the ulnar forearm), lower chest, or back. Discomfort associated with coronary artery disease is rarely located below the umbilicus or above the jaw.

It is also important to understand that there also exists a category of atypical symptoms that can be associated with stable coronary artery disease. These should be considered in elderly patients, women, and diabetics and are known as "anginal equivalents." Patients may describe fatigue, nausea, dyspnea, lightheadedness, and diaphoresis that occur with exertion or strong emotions.

Patients who describe their pain as pleuritic, sharp, pricking, stabbing, or choking are less likely to have coronary artery disease as the etiology for their pain. Similarly, those who describe their pain as either originating in the inframammary region, lasting for only seconds, or made worse with palpation are not likely to have an underlying cardiac etiology.

BASIC SCIENCE PEARL   **STEP 1**

Nitroglycerin works mainly as a systemic venodilator but dilates the coronary arteries as well. Its metabolism to nitric oxide in smooth muscle cells leads to an increase in cyclic guanosine monophosphate (cGMP), which causes relaxation of the blood vessel walls. This works in a similar fashion to the phosphodiesterase inhibitors prescribed for erectile dysfunction, and the combination of these two drugs can cause life-threatening episodes of hypotension.

CLINICAL PEARL   **STEP 2/3**

Due to its vasodilator properties, nitroglycerin can cause a headache from dilation of cerebral vessels. For this reason, nitroglycerin is contraindicated in hospitalized patients with elevated intracranial pressure.

Diagnosis: Stable angina

What medications should you prescribe and what tests should you order at this visit?
Given the patient's typical anginal symptoms, the stability of the symptoms over time, his lack of chest pain at this visit, and his underlying risk factors for coronary artery disease, you give a diagnosis of stable angina from coronary artery disease until proven otherwise.

Stable angina refers to the symptoms patients have when they have atherosclerotic plaques in the coronary arteries that obstruct blood flow, resulting in regional myocardial ischemia occurring during times of increased myocardial oxygen demand (usually exertion or emotional stressors that cause tachycardia). The severity of the symptoms does not correlate with the severity of coronary artery disease seen on cardiac catheterization, and one or more vessels can be involved with any degree of symptoms. Usually, an epicardial coronary artery needs to be at least 70% stenosed to cause symptoms.

At this visit, you advocate lifestyle modifications such as increased exercise as tolerated, smoking cessation, and weight loss through improved dietary practices. Given the diagnosis of stable angina, you start the patient on low-dose aspirin and give him a prescription for sublingual nitroglycerin (either tablets or a spray) that he can take to help relieve his symptoms faster when they occur. You instruct him that if he develops symptoms with exertion, he can take one tablet or spray every 5 minutes as needed to resolve the pain. He can also take the nitroglycerin 5 minutes prior to any planned strenuous activity. You instruct him not to use any phosphodiesterase inhibitors (sildenafil, vardenafil, etc.) for his erectile dysfunction within 24 hours of using nitroglycerin. You order an electrocardiogram (ECG) as a baseline and to look for evidence of prior MIs. You can also use the ECG to determine the best stress test for the patient, as we will soon see. You order a stress test to confirm the diagnosis and to determine whether a cardiac catheterization is warranted.

Lastly, you warn the patient of the signs and symptoms of MI and unstable angina and tell him to call 911 immediately if he experiences any of these.

CLINICAL PEARL   **STEP 2/3**

Distinguishing between stable and unstable angina is of utmost importance and has drastic implications on treatment and mortality. Unstable angina should be suspected in any patient with previously typical angina symptoms that are now occurring more severely or more frequently, lasting longer, or occurring at rest. These patients need to be sent to the emergency department, given antiplatelet agents and anticoagulation, and admitted.

The patient is sent to another room for his ECG and returns. Your interpretation of the ECG is as follows: normal sinus rhythm with a rate of 76/min, no significant Q-waves are present, normal PR and QTc intervals, and no ST elevations. You do note, however, deep S-waves in leads V2 and V3 and tall R-waves in leads V5 and V6 with associated downsloping ST segments and T-wave inversions consistent with left ventricular hypertrophy (LVH) with a "strain pattern" that you surmise is due to long-standing hypertension (see Fig. 41.1).

Is an exercise ECG stress test recommended for this patient?

There are several types of stress tests available that internal medicine doctors and cardiologists use to evaluate patients for coronary artery disease. Though the array of stress tests that exist can seem daunting at first, you really only need to decide on two things before selecting the proper one for your patient. First, you need to decide *how you will stress your patient's heart*. Your choices here are either using exercise or drugs (otherwise known as a pharmacologic stress test). For pharmacologic stress tests, the drugs most commonly used are dobutamine (which increases pulse rate) or vasodilators (such as adenosine and dipyramidole, which do not increase pulse rate; rather, they dilate the coronary arteries to mimic the effects of exercise). Next, you need to decide *how you will look for the ischemia*. Here your choices are either utilizing ECG tracings or some form of imaging (either with echocardiography or the use of nuclear tracers and positron emission

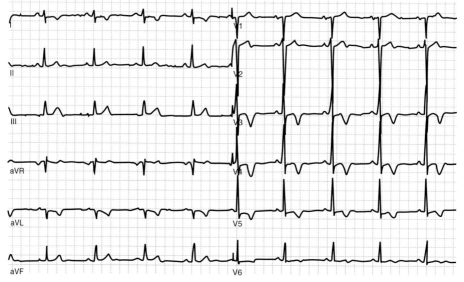

Figure 41.1 An electrocardiogram demonstrating left ventricular hypertrophy with a strain pattern; note the ST-T changes in the lateral leads V5 and V6.

tomography). It's that simple. The best choice for a patient depends on his or her baseline characteristics.

The most commonly ordered stress test is the exercise ECG stress test. Patients walk on a treadmill that gradually increases in speed and incline in a protocolized fashion. ECG tracings and blood pressure measurements are obtained before, during, and after the test. If patients are not able to reach 85% of their maximum pulse rate with exercise for whatever reason (i.e., orthopedic issues, vertigo, severe lung disease, symptomatic aortic stenosis, pulmonary hypertension, pulmonary embolism, congestive heart failure, etc.), this test is not the best option.

An exercise ECG stress test is considered positive when the patient develops new horizontal or downsloping ST depressions (at least 1 to 2 mm) during exercise. Once the patient develops symptoms or ST depressions, the test is stopped. Additional reasons for halting the test include a decrease in systolic blood pressure >10 mm Hg with increasing exertion and the development of an arrhythmia (though this does not necessarily qualify as a positive test). Patients who develop severe anginal symptoms or ST depressions at low levels of exertion or ST depressions that persist for greater than 5 minutes after the test ends are more likely to have severe coronary disease.

As with any diagnostic test, it is important to know the sensitivity (65 to 70%) and specificity (70 to 75%) and the circumstances in which false positives and false negatives may arise with an ECG stress test. False negatives can be seen in patients with disease of the left circumflex artery, and a negative test in a patient at otherwise high risk with continued symptoms should prompt consideration of further testing. False positives are most likely to occur when patients have a low pretest probability for coronary disease such as those under 40, those without symptoms, and those without risk factors. False positives are also more likely to occur in patients with baseline ECG abnormalities such as left bundle branch block (LBBB), preexcitation, ST or T wave changes (due to repolarization abnormalities and electrolyte disturbances), or LVH (which can cause abnormal repolarization abnormalities). Either alternative testing or the combination of an ECG stress test with some form of imaging should be performed.

The patient's ECG demonstrates LVH and resting ST-T changes, which would make an exercise ECG stress test difficult to interpret. Therefore, he should **not** be referred for this test. He requires an exercise stress test with imaging, either exercise stress echocardiography or exercise myocardial perfusion testing with nuclear tracers.

BASIC SCIENCE PEARL   **STEP 1**

The normal physiologic response to exercise is increased pulse rate, increased systolic blood pressure, and decreased diastolic blood pressure.

BASIC SCIENCE PEARL   **STEP 1**

Beta 1 receptors are inotropic and chronotropic adrenergic receptors in the heart. Beta blockers decrease pulse rate by inhibiting these receptors and should be discontinued before a stress test to allow the heart to reach maximum pulse rate and stress.

CLINICAL PEARL   **STEP 2/3**

Exercise puts more stress on the heart than the drugs used in a pharmacologic stress test and gives the clinician a chance to observe the relation of chest pain to a more "real life" situation. If your patient can perform physical activity, order an exercise stress test (remember, there are exercise stress tests other than exercise ECG stress tests).

Which stress tests are acceptable and which should be avoided if the patient has a left bundle branch block?

A baseline LBBB, as we just reviewed, makes interpreting an exercise ECG stress test difficult and can cause false positives. This is also true in the case of stress echocardiograms. Both of these stress tests involve an echo before and immediately after exercise or the administration of dobutamine to look for wall motion abnormalities. Because the conduction abnormality from the LBBB can cause baseline wall motion abnormalities, stress echos are also not recommended in patients with LBBB.

Myocardial perfusion single photon emission computed tomography (SPECT) stress tests (Fig. 41.2) involve the injection of a nuclear tracer, a stressor (either exercise or a vasodilator), and imaging before and after the stress. Nuclear medicine stress tests (both exercise and pharmacologic) have the best sensitivity (80 to 90%) and specificity (80 to 90%) of all the stress tests. As with other imaging stress tests, they provide direct visualization to allow for a more accurate determination of the size of an ischemic area (which can have important implications for treatment). Nuclear medicine stress tests are the best to perform in patients with an LBBB.

What if the patient has a pacemaker?

Pacemakers have the same implications for stress testing as LBBBs; therefore, nuclear medicine stress tests are the test of choice. If the patient can exercise, order an exercise nuclear medicine stress test. If not, order a pharmacologic nuclear medicine stress test.

What if the patient has chronic obstructive pulmonary disease (COPD)?

Though patients with COPD or severe asthma may have difficulty with exercise stress tests, these should be attempted if the patient doesn't have active wheezing. If there is difficulty exercising in these patients, consider a dobutamine stress echo. Avoid a pharmacologic nuclear medicine stress test as these tests use vasodilators (either dipyridamole or adenosine) to mimic the coronary

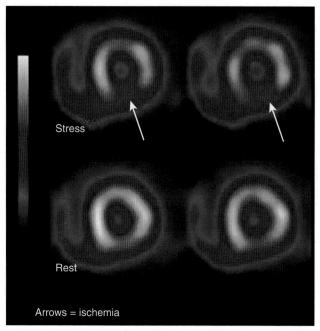

Figure 41.2   A nuclear medicine stress test; note that ischemic areas of myocardium (as seen in the arrows) are represented by a different color than healthy areas.

artery vasodilation that occurs with exercise. Vasodilators can cause severe bronchoconstriction in patients with reactive airway disease and should be avoided.

CLINICAL PEARL	STEP 2/3

The principle behind nuclear medicine stress tests is that diseased segments of coronary arteries will not dilate as well as healthy ones and therefore the nuclear tracer doesn't flow as well to the myocardium, which results in perfusion defects on imaging.

False negatives can occur in nuclear medicine stress tests when there is diffuse coronary disease. These imaging tests rely on detecting relative perfusion defects (that is, areas of myocardium that are ischemic relative to healthy areas). If all areas are ischemic due to diffuse coronary disease, there is no relative difference, and the test comes out looking negative.

Your patient is able to exercise but has baseline ECG ST-T abnormalities. You realize you need an imaging component to the test and decide to order an exercise stress echocardiogram. The patient has the test done approximately a month from his last visit with you. He has had no emergency department visits or hospitalizations since that time. You receive the results of the patient's test, which is significant for a small area of segmental wall motion abnormality in the anterior wall of the left ventricle after meeting his maximum pulse rate on the treadmill. The preexercise and postexercise left ventricular ejection fractions are 60 to 70%. You have him return to your office to discuss the results and to check in on his symptoms. He continues to have symptoms with exertion only and is interested in increasing the amount of exercise he can do because he would like to lose weight and be healthier overall. He continues to take lisinopril, aspirin, atorvastatin, and sublingual nitroglycerin as needed for chest pain.

In addition to reviewing lifestyle modifications with him again, what medications are indicated to better control his angina?
In general, there are three classes of antianginal medications: beta blockers, calcium channel blockers, and nitrates. These can be used in combination to control symptoms from stable angina; however, certain combinations should be avoided in order to prevent significant hypotension or bradycardia. No single class has been shown to be superior to another in head-to-head trials and thus it is reasonable to start with any class.

Beta blockers work by decreasing myocardial oxygen demand by slowing pulse rate and lowering blood pressure and myocardial contractility. Although they have been shown to decrease mortality in patients who have had an acute ST segment elevation MI or non-ST segment elevation MI, there are no large trials demonstrating that they decrease significant coronary events or morality in patients with stable angina. Potential side effects include depression, bradycardia, hypotension, fatigue, loss of libido, erectile dysfunction, and bronchospasm (in patients with reactive airway disease).

Calcium channel blockers are systemic vasodilators, and it is through this vasodilatory effect on the coronary arteries that they increase coronary blood flow. There are two distinct categories of calcium channel blockers: dihydropyridines and nondihydropyridines. In general, dihydropyridines have more of a vasodilatory effect than nondihydropyridines and less effect on pulse rate and contractility. Common examples of dihydropyridines include amlodipine, nifedipine, and nicardipine. Nondihydropyridines also have a vasodilatory effect, but less so, and work by decreasing myocardial oxygen demand through negative inotropy and chronotropy. As such, they are contraindicated in patients with congestive heart failure with reduced ejection fraction. Common examples of these medications include diltiazem and verapamil.

Nitrates, as discussed earlier, are also systemic vasodilators that work mainly on the venous side but also on the coronary arteries. The venodilation decreases blood return to the heart and therefore cardiac work, and the coronary artery vasodilation increases coronary blood flow. Short-acting nitrates (sublingual tablets and sprays) are used before exercise and as needed for chest pain, and longer-acting nitrates (tablets and transdermal patches) are used on a daily basis.

CLINICAL PEARL   **STEP 2/3**

The combinations most likely to cause significant bradycardia or hypotension are beta blockers and nondihydropyridine calcium channel blockers, and dihydropyridine calcium channel blockers and long-acting nitrates.

BASIC SCIENCE PEARL   **STEP 1**

Arterial vasodilators such as dihydropyridine calcium channel blockers cause a decrease in arterial blood pressure that is sensed by baroreceptors in the carotid sinus and aortic arch. This activates the sympathetic nervous system to increase the pulse rate in order to maintain cardiac output and is otherwise known as "reflex tachycardia."

You explain the three classes of antianginal medications to the patient and decide together to start him on a calcium channel blocker (because of his concern of his erectile dysfunction possibly worsening with beta blockers). He finds that he is able to exercise longer without having to use nitrates as often. He does not report any significant adverse effects from the medicine.

Given the result of his stress test, does your patient need a cardiac catheterization (coronary angiography)?

Though it is the gold standard for diagnosing coronary artery disease and allows for percutaneous intervention (stenting or ballooning a severely obstructed vessel), cardiac catheterization is invasive, can have life-threatening complications, and may miss extraluminal coronary artery plaques. Moreover, not all patients with stable angina and positive stress tests require cardiac catheterization.

There are many indications for undergoing a cardiac catheterization, but some of the most common (excluding acute coronary syndrome [ACS]) are severe symptoms uncontrolled with an appropriate medication regimen, positive imaging stress tests with large or multiple areas of ischemia, positive exercise ECG stress tests with symptoms at low levels of exertion or ST segment depressions of greater than 1 to 2 mm at low levels of exertion, and in patients with angina and depressed left ventricular ejection fraction. Also, consider cardiac catheterization in patients with angina symptoms, multiple risk factors for coronary disease but negative stress tests, and, interestingly, in patients with an occupation in which they are responsible for the lives of others, such as firefighters and airline pilots. As your patient has only a small area of ischemia in a single coronary artery territory, has symptoms that are predictable and well controlled with a calcium channel blocker, and does not have a high-risk occupation, he does not need a catheterization at this time.

When patients do undergo catheterization and coronary artery disease is visualized, a decision must be made about revascularization. This entails either percutaneous intervention (PCI; stenting or ballooning) or coronary artery bypass grafting (CABG; "open-heart surgery"). In general, PCI is preferred in patients with one- or two-vessel disease with easily visualized "culprit" lesions. CABG is preferred when there is left main disease, two-vessel disease (if one of the lesions is a proximal left anterior descending [LAD] lesion) or three-vessel disease, depressed left ventricular ejection fraction, or diabetes. CABG has been associated with better relief of anginal symptoms but is associated with a higher rate of stroke and early mortality due to the invasiveness of the procedure. However, the rates of death and MI in CABG compared with PCI (bare metal stents) after 5 years are similar. PCI is changing due to the use of better drug-eluting stents, which are associated with lower rates of restenosis and improved symptom control. Comparison of drug-eluting stent placement to CABG is still being studied. As with any major procedure, shared decision making with the patient is an important component when deciding on CABG versus PCI. The quality and experience of the interventional cardiologist and surgeons who will be performing the procedures are important factors to consider as well.

CLINICAL PEARL   **STEP 3**

When reviewing the report of a cardiac catheterization, do not focus only on areas with severe disease that were stented or ballooned. Make sure to review the entire report as there may have been several plaques that were not severe but still present and that can cause symptoms or rupture, leading to a STEMI in the future.

BEYOND THE PEARLS

- Levine's sign is an eponymous term for when a patient holds a clenched fist over their midchest to indicate the presence of a squeezing midsternal chest discomfort.
- Chest pain that radiates to the trapezius is more associated with pericarditis than with angina.
- Patients who use sublingual nitroglycerin very frequently develop a tolerance to its effects. To avoid this, it is recommended to have 12 hours each day free of nitrates.

BEYOND THE PEARLS—cont'd

- Atherosclerotic plaques tend to remain external to the lumen when they are growing. This is known as remodeling or the "Glagov effect." It is not until they reach a larger size that they begin to extend into the lumen and can cause symptoms of angina.
- Patients on chronic beta blocker therapy can develop rebound hypertension and tachycardia when the drugs are withdrawn suddenly. It is recommended to taper them down rather than abruptly discontinue them, especially in patients with heart disease.
- Angina decubitus describes anginal symptoms that occur when the patient is laying flat. This is due to increased return of blood to the heart, which causes increased end diastolic volume leading to wall tension and increased myocardial oxygen demand.
- CABGs are sometimes not able to be performed in patients with diffuse coronary disease who do not have adequate "targets." Targets refer to the segments of the native coronary arteries that are not diseased and allow for connection of bypass grafts.
- Arteries (i.e., the internal mammary artery) are better blood vessels to use for anastomosis in CABG. They are the preferred vessel for bypassing a diseased left main or proximal left anterior descending artery.
- Ranolazine is an FDA (U.S. Food and Drug Administration)-approved medication for second-line medication treatment of stable angina. It works as an inhibitor of sodium channels, which eventually decrease intracellular calcium, and has a similar mechanism of action to calcium channel blockers. It is contraindicated in patients with prolonged QTc and those with liver disease.
- For patients with continued angina despite having "clean coronaries" on catheterization, in addition to suspecting noncardiac causes, consider microvascular angina, myocardial bridging (in this condition, portions of an epicardial coronary artery run through the myocardium and are compressed, especially when there is a strong myocardial contraction), coronary artery vasospasm, or altered cardiac pain receptors.

References

Abrams J. Chronic stable angina. *N Engl J Med*. 2005;352:2524-2528.
Antman EM, Selwyn AP, Loscalzo J. Heart failure and cor pulmonale. In: Longo D, Fauci A, Kasper D, et al. *Harrison's Principles of Internal Medicine*. 18th ed. New York: McGraw Hill; 2012:1998-2014.
Cayley W. Diagnosing the cause of chest pain. *Am Fam Phys*. 2005;72(10):2012-2021.
Gibbons RJ, Abrams J, Chatterjee K, et al. ACC/AHA 2002 guideline update for the management of patients with chronic stable angina—summary article. *J Am Coll Cardiol*. 2003;41:159-168.

Rachel Ramirez

A 45-Year-Old Female With Fatigue and Headache

A 45-year-old female presents to the office as a new patient to establish primary care after switching insurance plans. Her biggest concern is fatigue, which she has been experiencing for the past several months.

How should you begin to evaluate fatigue?

A good way to evaluate fatigue is to first establish its timing or chronicity. Is the fatigue of recent onset (i.e., in the past few days)? Or has it been present for weeks to months? As you take the patient's history, it is important to use open-ended questions and clarifying statements such as "What is it that you mean when you say 'I'm feeling tired'?" or "Describe for me the fatigue you feel."

Additional history gathering should include the following:
- Onset (insidious or abrupt)
- Duration (days to weeks or months)
- Course (intermittent, improving, or worsening)
- Exacerbating or alleviating factors (e.g., activities and rest)
- Impact on daily life (whether the fatigue is interfering with work, home, or social activities)
- Accommodations the patient or family have made to adjust to the symptoms

The differential diagnosis for fatigue is very broad, and the etiology is often multifactorial (see Table 42.1).

On further questioning, the patient reveals that her fatigue has been progressively worsening. It is present each day to varying degrees, depending on the day's activities. She is able to commute to work and back but she no longer goes to the park with her children and dog. The patient also notes shortness of breath and a feeling of her heart pounding in her chest when she climbs stairs. She complains of an intermittent headache that is dull, diffuse, and pounding with no preceding aura. It resolves with over-the-counter acetaminophen or ibuprofen.

When asked about her past medical history, the patient recalls being told she has fibroids in her uterus. Her surgical history includes a caesarian section for the birth of her only child.

The patient is married and works in real estate part time. She lives at home with her husband, her biological son, two stepsons, and a dog. She has never used tobacco; she drinks a glass of wine once a week and has never used illicit drugs. She eats an average American diet that includes meat and vegetables. She does not specifically avoid any items.

In addition, the patient reveals that she has been told by her dentist that she has "terrible enamel" and admits to having a craving for ice all the time and chewing it throughout the day.

TABLE 42.1 ■ **Differential Diagnosis of Fatigue***

Type

Sleep Disorders:
Sleep apnea, insufficient sleep syndrome, insomnia

Infections (Both Acute and Chronic Infections):
Bacterial infections, mononucleosis, hepatitis, and HIV

Malignancy

Psychologic Illness:
Depression, anxiety

Chronic Autoimmune Illnesses:
Rheumatoid arthritis, lupus, scleroderma, systemic vasculitis

Endocrine/Metabolic Disorders:
Hypothyroidism, diabetes mellitus type 1 and 2, adrenal dysfunction, electrolyte abnormalities

Drugs and Medications:
Antidepressants, muscle relaxants, opiate drugs, antipsychotic drugs

Anemia
Iron deficiency anemia, thalassemia, anemia of chronic disease, B12 deficiency

*This list is by no means everything—there are so many different causes—this is just a glimpse of some
    common causes.
CHF, Congestive heart failure; *COPD,* chronic obstructive pulmonary disease; *HIV,* human immunodeficiency
    virus; *ILD,* interstitial lung disease.
(Modified from Seller RH, Symons AB. *Differential Diagnosis of Common Complaints.* 6th ed. Philadelphia:
    Elsevier; 2011.)

You note no neck swelling or symptoms of adenopathy and no rashes. Her weight is stable, and she denies dark or bloody stools, abdominal pain, nausea or vomiting. She has no swallowing complaints. Her nails are thin and break easily. Her menstrual periods are heavy and long lasting, with her cycles falling between 28 and 30 days. She has painful cramps that sometimes limit her ability to work on the first day of her menses. She soaks up to eight pads a day and has to "double up" at night.

She has no musculoskeletal complaints, nor other neurologic complaints. She has no urinary tract complaints.

What are the key elements to this patient's fatigue history that help narrow down the differential diagnosis? What questions do you want to ask further?
The patient's history reveals a number of important elements:
• "Progressive and daily": This suggests the fatigue is not resolving on its own.
• "Depending on activities": This prompts the clinician to inquire, "What activities make it worse?"

- "No longer does [physical activity]": This may mean the fatigue is exertional fatigue.
- "Shortness of breath": This suggests pulmonary symptoms, prompting the clinician to ask "Is there cough? Do you have chest tightness? Do you have trouble breathing when at rest? Do you have trouble breathing when laying down flat? Do you have to take many deep breaths or are your breaths small and rapid?"
  - Cough would aim toward an alveolar or infiltrative process.
  - Tightness may indicate bronchoconstriction as in asthma.
  - Breathlessness at rest can be a sign of severe congestive heart failure.
  - Breathlessness when recumbent can be a sign of congestive heart failure, pericardial effusion, pleural effusion, or compression by a neoplasm.
  - The timing and depth of breathing can indicate infiltrative process such as interstitial lung disease (rapid shallow breathing) or physical deconditioning (deep breathing).
- "Heart pounding": This suggests cardiovascular effects, prompting the clinician to ask "Is it a regular or irregular pounding?"
  - Regular rhythm that is rapid (tachycardia) can indicate supraventricular tachycardia or atrial tachycardia.
  - Irregular heart rhythm may be atrial fibrillation, atrial flutter, or premature ventricular contractions.
- "Headache": The differential for headache is broad and diverse. However, in the context of fatigue, shortness of breath, absence of focality or classic migraine pattern, a primary neurologic finding is unlikely.

The patient provides a tremendous amount of information that can help narrow down the differential. Of the above history, a few key phrases can direct us toward the diagnosis:

- "Fibroid uterus": Fibroids are also known as uterine leiomyomas; they are the most common pelvic tumor in women. They can lead to anemia from excessive menstrual blood loss.
- "Terrible enamel": This is a dental finding that is not often shared with the clinician. The loss of enamel in adulthood is usually due to salivary inadequacy, excess organic acids, local, repeated trauma, or inadequate fluoride. Inadequate enamel can lead to dental caries and decay.
- "Long heavy menstrual periods": This can lead to anemia, primarily iron deficiency. The average female loses about 15 mg of elemental iron per month. If her loss is greater and intake is less than the loss, the net result is gradual iron deficiency.

On physical exam, the blood pressure is 90/58 mm Hg, her pulse rate is 88/min, respiration rate is 16/min, and the body mass index (BMI) is 23.38 kg/m². In general, she is a well-developed, well-nourished African American female showing no distress.

She has pale conjunctivae and pale sublingual mucosa. Her thyroid is normal in size and texture and she has no lymphadenopathy. Her cardiopulmonary exam is normal. Her abdomen has normal active bowel sounds and is soft and nontender. A firm, nontender mass is appreciated in the left lower quadrant. Her pelvic exam reveals normal external genitalia with no vaginal or cervical discharge. A bimanual exam reveals an enlarged, nontender uterus. Her ovaries are not palpated and no cervical motion tenderness is noted. Her rectal exam reveals a normal sphincter tone and brown stool negative for occult blood. Her neurologic exam reveals that her cranial nerves are intact, her reflexes are symmetric, and strength and gross sensory testing are normal. The patient possesses normal insight, orientation, judgment, and thought processes. The results of laboratory testing are shown in Table 42.2 and Table 42.3. The peripheral blood smear is reviewed and pictured in Figure 42.1.

What are the next steps in evaluating this patient's anemia?

Anemia is defined as a reduction in red cell mass. Blood volume is usually at a relatively constant level. The degree of anemia is measured by either the hemoglobin concentration in the plasma (Hb) or the volume of red cells indicated as a percentage (Hct).

TABLE 42.2 ■ Patient's Serum Chemistry Results

Name	Value	Reference Range
Glucose	87	70-100 mg/dL
Blood urea nitrogen	15	0-23 mg/dL
Creatinine	0.74	0.00-1.11 mg/dL
Sodium	137	135-145 mEq/L
Potassium	4.1	3.5-5.1 mEq/L
Chloride	110	98-110 mEq/L
Carbon dioxide	16	20-31 mEq/L
Aspartate aminotransferase	13	5-34 U/L
Alanine aminotransferase	<6	0-55 U/L
Alkaline phosphatase	91	40-150 U/L
Total bilirubin	0.4	0.2-1.2 mg/dL
Calcium	8.9	8.5-10.7 mg/dL
Albumin	4.4	3.3-4.7 g/dL
Total protein	7.9	6.4-8.3 g/dL
Thyroid stimulating hormone	1.382	3.50-5.50 mIU/L

TABLE 42.3 ■ Patient's Complete Blood Count

Name	Value	Reference Range
White blood cells	4.1	4.0-12.0 k/μL
Red blood corpuscles	3.66	4.2-5.4 M/μL
Hemoglobin	5.3	12.0-16.0 g/dL
Hematocrit	18.9	37-47%
Mean corpuscular volume	51.5	81-99 fL
Mean corpuscular hemoglobin concentration	28.1	32-36%
Red cell distribution width	28.9	11.5-15%
Platelet	192	140-400 k/μL
Mean platelet volume	10.1	7.4-10.4 fL
Neutrophils	61	%
Lymphocytes	33	%
Monocytes	4	%
Eosinophils	2	%
Basophils	0	%
Absolute neutrophils	2.2	1.8-9.0 k/μL
Absolute lymphocytes	1.5	1.5-3.2 k/μL
Absolute monocytes	0.1	0.0-0.9 k/μL
Absolute eosinophils	0.1	0.0-0.5 k/μL
Absolute basophils	0.0	0.0-0.2 k/μL

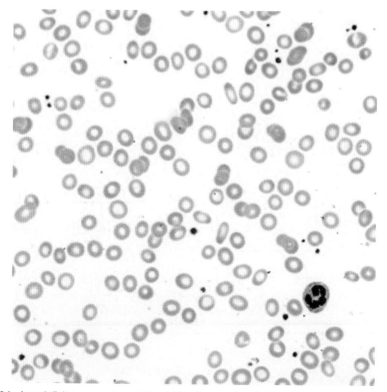

Figure 42.1 Iron deficiency anemia peripheral blood smear. Iron deficiency typically results in hypochromic, microcytic red blood corpuscles (findings are demonstrated throughout the entire field). This type of anemia often results in an increased platelet count, as shown. Other morphological features of iron deficiency not shown on this smear include target red blood corpuscles. Magnification, 20×; stain, Wright–Giemsa. *(From Torres R, Tormey CA, Smith, BR. Hematology in clinical pathology. In: McManus LM, Mitchell RN, eds.* Pathobiology of Human Disease. *San Diego: Academic Press; 2014:3269-3286.)*

CLINICAL PEARL	STEP 2/3

Hemoglobin/hematocrit values change depending on gender and geographic altitude of the patient. People who live at high altitudes (low oxygen tension) tend to have a higher hemoglobin.

The degree of anemia and the rate at which it develops influence the symptoms the patient may feel. For example, one may feel lightheaded and weak immediately after donating a pint of blood for a local blood drive, whereas a patient who develops anemia over a longer period of time (i.e., females with anemia due to menorrhagia) may develop symptoms of fatigue and/or lightheadedness more gradually.

Once you determine that the patient is anemic, the next step is to evaluate the red cell morphology. Defining the anemia based on red cell morphology is the most important aspect of the anemia workup. The mean corpuscular volume (MCV) included in the complete blood count (CBC) is a good first place to start. The MCV is useful in evaluating hypoproliferative anemia. Hypoproliferative anemia, defined as anemia due to a lack or impairment of red blood cell (RBC) production, is further organized in Table 42.4.

TABLE 42.4 ■ **Causes of Hypoproliferative Anemia**

Microcytic	Normocytic	Macrocytic
Iron deficiency	Bone marrow failure (aplastic anemia)	Vitamin B12 deficiency
Thalassemia	Myelophthisis	Folate deficiency
Sideroblastic	Anemia of chronic disease	Myelodysplasia
Anemia of chronic disease	Early iron deficiency	Liver disease
		Chronic alcoholism

The peripheral blood smear remains a crucial piece to the anemia puzzle. Although the automated cell counters in the lab provide timely and measurable information, the smear provides immediate and direct visualization of the patient's blood. Asking your laboratory to prepare a peripheral smear is a simple call that will help you save time, energy, and resources. The main cell you will see on the patient's smear is the RBC, which you observe for its shape and size.

Another important laboratory test to obtain in the workup of the patient is the reticulocyte count. Reticulocytes are the most immediate RBC precursors. On average, the reticulocytes occupy about 1% of the circulating RBCs in the patient's periphery. However, in the setting of bone marrow stimulation from erythropoietin, the reticulocyte percentage increases. Erythropoietin acts on the erythroid colony forming units (CFU-E) group of erythroid precursor cells.

BASIC SCIENCE PEARL   **STEP 1**

Reticulocytes take about 1 day to mature in the peripheral circulation when the hematocrit is >45%. When the hematocrit is lower (<30%), it can take up to 3 days to mature.

BASIC SCIENCE PEARL   **STEP 1**

Erythropoietin is a hormone that is produced in the peritubular cells of the kidneys and in the fetal liver. There is a group of specialized interstitial cells of the inner cortex and outer medulla of the kidney that respond to oxygen levels of the blood. This stimulates erythropoietin production and secretion.

Finally, evaluation of the bone marrow can complete the workup for anemia if the initial evaluation does not provide conclusive evidence. This is particularly important if the patient's reticulocyte count is inappropriately low for the hemoglobin. A variety of causes for hypoproliferative anemia can be found on the bone marrow. For example, megaloblastic changes will be evident. Infections with organisms such as mycobacteria, cytomegalovirus, and histoplasma can be cultured or found via stains. Iron staining will confirm iron deficiency or identify ring sideroblasts. Take note that bone marrow evaluation is usually not helpful in the setting of an adequate reticulocyte response to anemia, because a healthy marrow with normal red cell precursor production manifests reticulocytes appropriately.

BASIC SCIENCE/CLINICAL PEARL   **STEP 1/2/3**

Sideroblasts are normal in iron-sufficient bone marrow. Ring sideroblasts are abnormal cells that have iron-containing granules surrounding the nucleus of the cell. This is due to an inability, whether congenital or acquired, to process iron in the erythroblast.

As we consolidate the patient's information and integrate her laboratory studies, we find that she has a profound microcytic anemia. Her history of leiomyomatous uterus can certainly predispose her to heavy menstrual periods and excessive iron loss. As noted earlier, the patient has an insatiable craving for ice, which, when it is abnormally frequent and excessive, is known as pagophagia. This is part of a cluster of symptoms known as pica.

CLINICAL PEARL   **STEP 2/3**

Pica is repeated eating for more than 1 month of nonfood substances that are inappropriate to the patient's developmental level or culturally inappropriate. Common substances that are ingested are clay, ice, chalk, cloth, coal, gum, dirt, hair, metal, paint, paper, pebbles, soap, string, and wool.

What is the evaluation of microcytic anemia?

Microcytic anemias are part of the hypoproliferative group of anemias. Table 42-4 lists the differential diagnosis. The most common hypoproliferative microcytic anemia is iron deficiency. Evaluating iron deficiency should begin with the following question: "Is enough iron being consumed, or is too much iron being lost?"

Causes for inadequate intake, including malabsorption, are varied. Inadequate intake of dietary iron commonly occurs throughout the world. Dietary iron occurs in two forms: heme and nonheme iron. Heme iron is found in meat, poultry, and fish. It is more readily absorbed and utilized than nonheme iron. Nonheme iron is found in vegetables, fruit, legumes, and iron-fortified products. It is not as bioavailable because it is found in the presence of phytate (in cereals and grains), which chelates iron and prevents its absorption. A low iron status will facilitate increased nonheme iron absorption.

Malabsorption of iron occurs in patients who have other conditions such as gastric bypass procedures (achlorohydria), celiac disease (gluten sensitivity), *Helicobacter pylori* gastritis, atrophic gastritis, or other generalized malabsorption syndromes.

Blood loss is the most common cause of iron-deficiency anemia. The most common source of blood loss in men and postmenopausal women is from the gastrointestinal (GI) tract. There are two types of blood loss from the GI tract: acute (obvious) and occult (not so obvious). Acute blood loss includes hematemesis (vomiting bright red blood), hematochezia (stool with acute, undigested blood), and melena (dark, tarry, partially digested blood). These are clinical emergencies.

Occult blood loss is more difficult to determine the source, as it is not nearly as voluminous as the acute forms. Blood is usually detected by finding anemia and then checking stool for blood via biochemical reaction (stool Guaiac) or fecal immunoglobulin testing (FIT).

Any blood loss from the GI tract can be broken down into different categories:
1. Ulcerative or erosive
   a. Esophagitis
   b. Peptic ulcer disease
   c. Gastric ulcer
   d. Gastritis

2. Portal hypertension driven
    a. Esophageal, gastric varices
    b. Portal hypertensive gastropathy
3. Vascular malformations
    a. Arteriovenous malformation
    b. Hereditary hemorrhagic telangiectasia
4. Postsurgical or traumatic
    a. Mallory-Weiss tear
    b. Foreign body ingestion
    c. Aortoenteric fistula
5. Tumors (benign or malignant)
6. Anatomic
    a. Diverticulosis
    b. Hemorrhoids
    c. Ischemia
7. Infectious or inflammatory
    a. Infectious colitis
    b. Inflammatory bowel disease

Premenopausal women lose blood from menstruation, pregnancy, childbirth, and lactation. A careful history of the patient's menses often reveals that she has significant menorrhagia. Menstruation results in about 15 mg of elemental iron loss per month. About 900 mg of elemental iron is utilized during pregnancy and childbirth because iron is transferred to the fetus and placenta and lost during postpartum bleeding.

Occasionally, other rarer causes of blood loss occur via hematuria or pulmonary hemorrhage. Pulmonary hemosiderosis is also an uncommon situation found in Goodpasture's syndrome and antiglomerular basement membrane antibody disease where the pulmonary macrophages sequester iron, making it unusable to the body.

Not uncommonly, there is on occasion increased demand for iron that can cause a relative deficiency in the setting of rapid increases in growth in infants, children, and adolescents.

In addition, it is important to ask in the history if the patient donates blood frequently as this may not be obvious in the usual history taking.

Finally, there is a state of relative iron deficiency when iron is delivered to the erythroid precursors but is not effectively utilized due to "iron sequestration." This commonly occurs in the setting of infection, inflammation, autoimmune disorders, chronic kidney disease, and cancer.

Other causes of hypoproliferative microcytic anemia include thalassemia, a group of syndromes that manifest inherited defects of one or more of the globin chain subunits of hemoglobin. The α-chain coding is found on chromosome 16, whereas the β-chain coding is found on chromosome 11. The phenotypes of thalassemia vary in severity depending on which subunit is affected. The worst is homozygous α-thalassemia, where none of the four α chains are produced, and thus patients die in utero or shortly after birth (hydrops fetalis). Silent carriers make three of the four α subunits and have no clinical syndromes. When two α subunits are produced, the patient manifests mild microcytic anemia. This is often erroneously treated with iron.

β-thalassemia is a spectrum of mutations for the β-globulin chain. More than 100 mutations have been described. These thalassemias are further defined by the defect (minor, intermedia, and major). Minor β-thalassemia has a trait, one mutation on one chromosome, and shows a mild microcytic anemia. Intermedia β-thalassemia is a combination of two inherited mutations. The syndrome manifests as microcytic anemia that is not transfusion dependent. Major β-thalassemia is also called "Cooleys" anemia and manifests as severe hemolysis, ineffective erythropoiesis, skeletal abnormalities, hepatosplenomegaly, and iron overload.

The pathogenesis of β-thalassemia is twofold: 1. There is ineffective erythropoiesis. 2. The reticuloendothelial system breaks down the abnormal RBCs that have abnormal hemoglobin, which precipitates within the cells.

Diagnosing thalassemia occurs by hemoglobin electrophoresis when there is a clinical suspicion.

CLINICAL PEARL   **STEP 2/3**

Thalassemia is most common in areas of the world historically afflicted by malaria, including the Mediterranean region, the Arabic peninsula, Turkey, Iran, India, and Southeast Asia. This is thought to be because the RBCs of heterozygotes are relatively resistant to infection with the malaria parasite.

Sideroblastic anemia can be congenital or acquired. Congenital syndromes are numerous and are genetically detected. Acquired sideroblastic anemia usually occurs from an underlying comorbidity like alcoholism, lead poisoning, or copper deficiency or is drug induced. Another cause of acquired sideroblastic anemia is a defect in clonal differentiation as in myelodysplastic syndromes. Diagnosing sideroblastic anemia begins with a CBC, peripheral smear, and iron studies. There will be evidence of iron overload. Bone marrow evaluation will show erythroid hyperplasia with cytoplasm that is poorly hemoglobinized. Ring sideroblasts are the hallmark of the disorder. Macrophages within the marrow have iron in them as well.

What are the first labs to send out in a patient with microcytic anemia? What is important to know about iron-deficiency anemia?

The next step in evaluating a patient who has microcytic anemia is to evaluate his or her serum ferritin, iron, and transferrin saturation (or iron-binding capacity). These labs measure the patient's iron stores indirectly. Iron is transported and bound to a plasma-binding protein called transferrin. The complex binds to membrane receptors and is taken into RBCs. Ferritin is an intracellular protein that stores iron in a nontoxic form to be mobilized at the time of need. Ferritin is the most sensitive and specific indicator of iron deficiency. The main sites of iron storage are the liver (hepatocytes and macrophages), bone marrow, spleen, and muscle. The ratio of iron/iron-binding capacity should be about 20%. Iron deficiency reduces the ratio by decreasing iron and increasing the binding capacity.

BASIC SCIENCE/CLINICAL PEARL   **STEP 1/2/3**

Ferritin is the most sensitive and specific indicator of iron deficiency.

In this context, it is important to understand iron metabolism by the body. The body recycles iron very efficiently as RBCs are broken down. Additionally, the body does not have an effective mechanism to excrete iron. Because iron levels can be toxic, the body absorbs only about 1 to 2 mg per day. Most of the daily iron needed (25 mg) is acquired through recycling of aged RBCs via macrophage phagocytosis. Absorption and phagocytosis of RBCs are regulated by the hormone hepcidin. As mentioned above, in the human diet, iron exists in either heme or nonheme form. Heme iron is more readily absorbed than nonheme iron. Absorption of iron is primarily regulated by mucosal cells of the proximal small intestine via the effect of hepcidin.

Together, ferritin, iron, and iron-binding capacity are indirect measures of iron deficiency. To make a definitive diagnosis of iron deficiency, an iron stain of a bone marrow aspirate can be performed. If iron is not present, this is iron deficiency. However, this is often not necessary.

TABLE 42.5 ■ Patient's Iron Studies

Ferritin	2	5-204 ng/mL
Iron	12	25-156 µg/dL
Iron-binding capacity	481	240-450 µg/dL
Iron saturation	2	23-59%

Iron studies are added to the patient's labs drawn the day before (see Table 42.5).

Using Figure 42.2 as a guide, it is clear the patient is likely iron deficient.

Diagnosis: Iron deficiency anemia due to menorrhagia

How is iron deficiency anemia managed?

Patients with iron deficiency are managed with iron supplementation. The severity of the patient's symptoms dictates the mode of correction. Before correction is performed, however, one must always answer the question "Why is the patient iron deficient?" Answering that will help prevent further episodes of deficiency once the hard work of correction is accomplished.

The patient's total body iron deficit can be calculated with the following equation:

$$1850 \text{ mg} = (13 - 5.3) \times 50 \text{ kg} \times 2.21 + 1000$$

$$\text{Iron (mg)} = (\text{normal Hb} - \text{patient Hb}) \times \text{weight (kg)} \times 2.21 + 1000$$

She requires nearly 2 grams of replacement iron.

There are three main ways to correct iron deficiency in its simplest form:
1. Oral iron supplementation.
2. Parenteral iron (intravenous)
3. Red cell transfusion

If patients exhibit signs of cardiovascular insufficiency such as heart failure or angina, a red cell transfusion is indicated. Each unit of packed red blood cells contains approximately 200 mg of iron.

Oral iron therapy is safe, inexpensive, and relatively well tolerated. Iron sulfate is the most common iron salt administered. Patients should receive between 100 to 200 mg of elemental iron per day in divided doses (2 to 4 times per day). Coadministration of oral iron with oral vitamin C 250 mg facilitates absorption. It may take up to 6 months to replete the patient's iron stores. A reticulocyte count can be checked several days after beginning therapy. A rise in the reticulocytes will be evident and the amount will peak at about 10 days after initiation of therapy. Patients may experience some side effects from oral iron, with nausea, stomach upset, and constipation being the most common symptoms. Administering the iron with food and adding stool softeners such as docusate can mitigate these symptoms. Iron causes dark stools but does not cause false-positive occult blood tests. On the occasion that oral iron fails (and the patient was adherent to the therapy) consider evaluating for *H. pylori* infection or gluten intolerance.

Parenteral iron replacement should be reserved for patients who cannot tolerate oral therapy; those who have a malabsorption syndrome, ongoing blood loss, chronic kidney disease, or personal objections to blood transfusions; or those who need a more rapid correction of iron deficiency. Numerous versions of the iron salt are safe for intravenous (IV) use. The most common

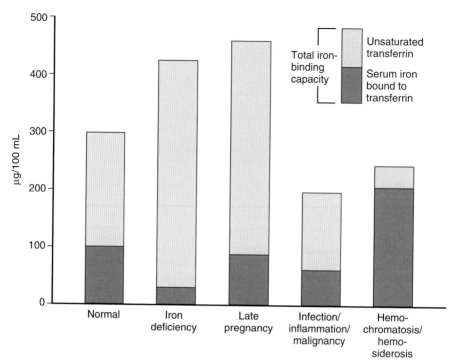

Figure 42.2 Description of iron levels.

is ferric gluconate. Dosing is typically 100 mg per day or 200 mg every other day with a usual goal of 1000 mg total. Side effects of IV iron include nausea, vomiting, pruritus, flushing, headache, myalgia, and arthralgia. Hypersensitivity reactions are increasingly rare because IV formulations have changed in recent years.

Red cell transfusion therapy is the last option with the highest costs and risks associated with it. Caution must be used in patients who have blood volume–sensitive conditions such as chronic heart failure, as packed red cells carry an oncotic load and may increase blood volume past what the patient can handle in the short term.

> The patient's symptoms of fatigue, headache, pica, and shortness of breath are all due to iron deficiency from chronic menorrhagia due to uterine fibroids. Although she had strikingly low hemoglobin and very low iron stores, she remained clinically stable. She is successfully managed with IV iron loading and subsequent oral iron therapy. Her symptoms improve drastically after 2 weeks of therapy. She is referred to gynecology for evaluation of the menorrhagia.

BEYOND THE PEARLS

- Hepcidin is the peptide hormone that regulates the absorption and utilization of iron. It is produced in the liver, is an acute phase reactant, and fluctuates with plasma iron levels.
- Total body iron deficit can be calculated with the following equation: Iron (mg) = (normal Hb – patient Hb) × weight (kg) × 2.21 + 1000.
- Each unit of packed red blood cells has about 200 mg of iron.
- Some patients with iron-deficiency anemia may develop restless leg syndrome. This is a disorder that causes a strong urge to move the legs, mainly at rest during the night.

References

Bottomley SS. Clinical aspects, diagnosis, and treatment of the sideroblastic anemias. Available at <http://www.uptodate.com/home/index.html>; 2015. Accessed 08.01.16.

Bottomley SS. Pathophysiology of the sideroblastic anemias. Available at <http://www.uptodate.com/home/index.html>; 2015. Accessed 08.01.16.

Camaschella C. Iron-deficiency anemia. *N Engl J Med*. 2015;372:1832-1843.

Doubeni C. Tests for screening for colorectal cancer: stool tests, radiologic imaging and endoscopy. Available at <http://www.uptodate.com/home/index.html>; 2015. Accessed 08.01.16.

Fosnocht KM, Ende J. Approach to the adult patient with fatigue. Available at <http://www.uptodate.com/home/index.html>; 2015. Accessed 08.01.16.

Saltzman JR. Approach to acute upper gastrointestinal bleeding in adults. Available at <http://www.uptodate.com/home/index.html>; 2015. Accessed 08.01.16.

Schrier SL. Approach to the adult patient with anemia. Available at <http://www.uptodate.com/home/index.html>; 2015. Accessed 08.01.16.

Schrier SL. Causes and diagnosis of iron deficiency anemia in the adult. Available at <http://www.uptodate.com/home/index.html>; 2015. Accessed 08.01.16.

Travis AC, Saltzman JR. Evaluation of occult gastrointestinal bleeding. Available at <http://www.uptodate.com/home/index.html>; 2015. Accessed 08.01.16.

Monisha Bhanote ∎ Wen Chen ∎ Daniel Martinez

A 55-Year-Old Male With Fever and Abdominal Pain

A 55-year-old homeless male with no known past medical history presents to the emergency room for 3 days of fever, chills, and abdominal pain. The pain is sharp, 7/10 in intensity, diffuse, nonradiating, and associated with nausea but no vomiting. He reports heavy alcohol drinking for the past 5 years since he lost his job and got divorced. He has been living on the streets and drinking up to "a fifth" (around 750 mL) of vodka a day. However, he says he has not had a drink in the past few months because it started to make him "feel sick." He also noted that his skin was "more yellow" than normal and that his "belly was getting big." He denies any episodes of vomiting, diarrhea, hematemesis, hematochezia, or melena.

On physical exam, his temperature is 38.8 °C (101.9 °F), pulse rate is 109/min, blood pressure is 90/50 mm Hg, and oxygen saturation is 94% on room air. The patient is in mild discomfort and noticeably jaundiced throughout. He has a strong and sweet smell to his breath, and there is mild parotid gland enlargement bilaterally. He has no jugular venous distension or lymphadenopathy. There are multiple spider angiomata on his upper chest, and gynecomastia is present. He is tachycardic with 1/6 systolic ejection murmur, and his lungs are clear to auscultation. His abdomen is soft and diffusely tender to palpation with mild guarding. It is also very distended with a positive fluid wave and shifting dullness to percussion. A palpable spleen is noted in Traube's (semilunar) space (see Fig. 43.1). He has palmar erythema, proximal nail bed pallor, but no asterixis. His sclera appear icteric (see Fig. 43.2).

What is concerning about his physical exam?

There are many classic physical exam findings associated with cirrhosis, and this vignette is designed to illustrate most of them. These are important to put to memory because recognizing them helps to make a bedside diagnosis, and they are also common questions that an attending may ask. Patients with cirrhosis can also have many acute and life-threatening complications. Knowing early on that a patient likely has cirrhosis can help you place these pathologies on your initial differential diagnosis and affect your initial workup and management (see Table 43.1).

Knowing that he has a decent chance at having cirrhosis based on exam, how would you approach this patient?

Being able to assess and differentiate between acute, chronic, and acute on chronic pathologies is a necessary skill to be a good clinician. This is especially the case in a patient with many chronic comorbid conditions that can flare up. The patient likely has a chronic diagnosis of cirrhosis, but this alone does not explain his acute presentation (3 days of abdominal pain, fevers, and nausea). It is important not to let a chronic diagnosis detract you or mislead you from the acute presentation.

Patients with cirrhosis can get acute appendicitis, cholecystitis, and cholangitis like anyone else, so these should be on the differential. With his drinking history, he can also have acute

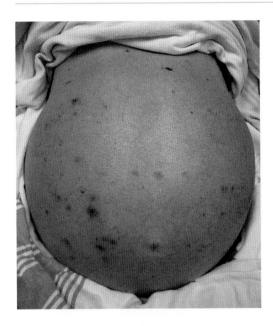

Figure 43.1 Patient's abdomen showing distension by ascites fluid. *(From James Heilman, MD.* https://commons.wikimedia.org/wiki/File :Hepaticfailure.jpg#/media/File:Hepatic failure.jpg.*)*

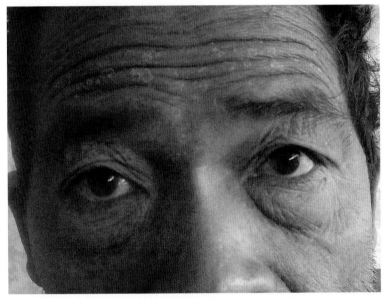

Figure 43.2 Patient's sclera showing yellowing/jaundice. *(From Bobjgalindo* https://commons.wikimedia.org/ wiki/File:Jaundice_of_the_sclerotic.JPG#/media/File:Jaundice_of_the_sclerotic.JPG.*)*

pancreatitis like anyone else. However, keeping cirrhosis in mind, the differential expands to other acute pathologies such as spontaneous bacterial peritonitis, portal venous thrombosis, or even gastrointestinal (GI) bleeding.

In the emergency room setting, the workup should include labs and imaging directed at evaluating these life-threatening pathologies. An abdominal ultrasound with Doppler would be

TABLE 43.1 ▪ **Physical and Laboratory Exam Findings in Chronic Liver Disease**

Physical Findings	Laboratory Findings
Ascites	Elevated partial thromboplastin time, prothrombin time, international normalized ratio
Spider angiomas	Macrocytic anemia
Asterixis	Thrombocytopenia
Splenomegaly	Acanthocytosis on peripheral smear
Palmar erythema	Elevated blood urea nitrogen and creatinine
Dupuytren's contracture	Hyperbilirubinemia
Testicular atrophy	Hypoalbuminemia
Gynecomastia	Aspartate aminotransferase/alanine aminotransferase variable

very helpful as it could evaluate for cholecystitis, appendicitis, cholangitis, cirrhosis, portal vein thrombosis, and the presence of ascites. A complete blood count (CBC), blood cultures, hepatic function panel, basic metabolic panel (BMP), lipase, and prothrombin time would also be helpful for the differential diagnosis.

Two large-bore intravenous (IV) lines are placed, and the patient is given a 2-liter normal saline bolus; his blood pressure and pulse rate improve. Labs are drawn during this time, and the patient is sent for a STAT abdominal ultrasound. You then call the radiologist for a preliminary read. It shows no evidence of cholecystitis, appendicitis, or biliary ductal dilatation. However, it does reveal a nodular liver surface, splenomegaly, and large ascites.

What is cirrhosis and how is it diagnosed?

Cirrhosis is the last stage of progressive liver fibrosis due to chronic liver damage and is characterized by a coarsening of the liver architecture and the formation of regenerative nodules.

BASIC SCIENCE PEARL   **STEP 1**

Histologically, cirrhosis is characterized by hepatic architecture distortion and the formation of regenerative nodules with fibrosis.

The gold standard for the diagnosis of cirrhosis is a liver biopsy, but a presumptive diagnosis of cirrhosis can be made if the patient has a constellation of physical exam findings, laboratory abnormalities, or imaging studies suggestive of cirrhosis.

Obvious physical exam findings in cirrhosis include scleral icterus, jaundice, spider angiomata, caput medusa, ascites, palmar erythema, and splenomegaly. More subtle findings include parotid gland enlargement, fetor hepaticus, gynecomastia, and two classes of nail pallor (Muehrcke's nails and Terry's nails). Common laboratory abnormalities in cirrhosis include anemia, thrombocytopenia, elevated prothrombin time, low fibrinogen, hypoalbuminemia, mildly elevated transaminases, and increased direct and indirect bilirubin (see Table 43.1, Fig. 43.3, and Fig. 43.4).

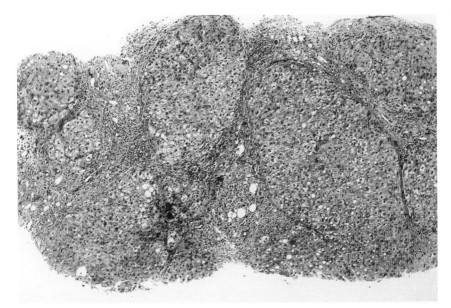

Figure 43.3 Liver core biopsy shows hepatocytes surrounded by fibrosis highlighted with a trichrome stain *(blue)*. *(From* https://commons.wikimedia.org/wiki/File:Cirrhosis_of_the_liver_[trichrome_stain]_[5690946257].jpg.*)*

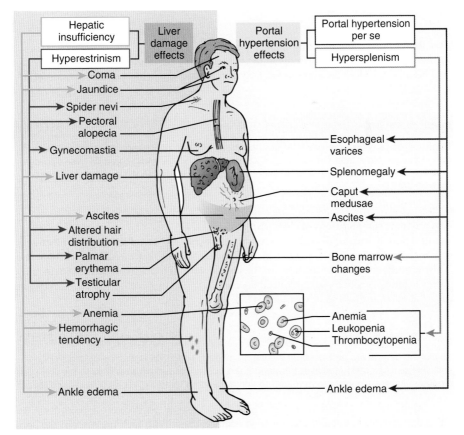

Figure 43.4 Clinical manifestations of cirrhosis. *(From Floch MH, Floch NR, Kowdley KV, and Pitchumon CS.* Netter's Gastroenterology. *Page: 576.)*

TABLE 43.2 ■ Major Causes of Cirrhosis

Chronic hepatitis	Hepatitis B and C Autoimmune hepatitis
Fatty liver disease	Alcoholic liver disease Nonalcoholic steatohepatitis
Chronic biliary diseases	Primary biliary cirrhosis Primary sclerosing cholangitis
Inherited diseases	Hemochromatosis Wilson's disease Alpha-1 antitrypsin storage disorder
Hepatic venous outflow obstruction	Budd-Chiari syndrome
Drug-induced	Amiodarone Methotrexate Acetaminophen Isoniazid

Common imaging tests used to diagnose cirrhosis include a right upper quadrant ultrasound, which can show a nodularity of the surface of the liver and evidence of portal hypertension such as ascites and splenomegaly. A computed tomography (CT) scan of liver may also show similar findings (see Fig. 43.5).

What are the most common causes of cirrhosis?
The most common causes of cirrhosis in the United States are chronic viral hepatitis (hepatitis B and hepatitis C), alcoholic liver disease, fatty liver disease, and hemochromatosis (see Fig. 43.6 and Table 43.2).

CLINICAL PEARL   **STEP 2/3**

Nonalcoholic fatty liver disease (NAFLD) occurs when fat is deposited (steatosis) in the liver due to causes other than excessive alcohol use. NAFLD is the most common liver disorder in Western industrialized nations. Nonalcoholic steatohepatitis (NASH) is the most extreme form of NAFLD.

What are some complications of cirrhosis?
Most of the complications of cirrhosis develop from either the loss of the intrinsic functions of the liver or the development of portal hypertension due to poor flow through the cirrhotic liver.

The intrinsic functions of the liver can be broken down into the synthesis of certain crucial proteins (clotting factors and albumin) and the conjugation or metabolism of certain compounds such as bilirubin, toxins, and drugs (Table 43.3).

BASIC SCIENCE PEARL   **STEP 1**

All clotting factors are produced by the liver; however, factor VIII is also produced by endothelial cells outside the liver throughout the body. This protein circulates in the bloodstream in an inactive form bound to von Willebrand factor.

Portal hypertension can also cause myriad complications. With high pressures in the portal circulation, circulating blood is shunted through collateral veins, which have a relatively lower

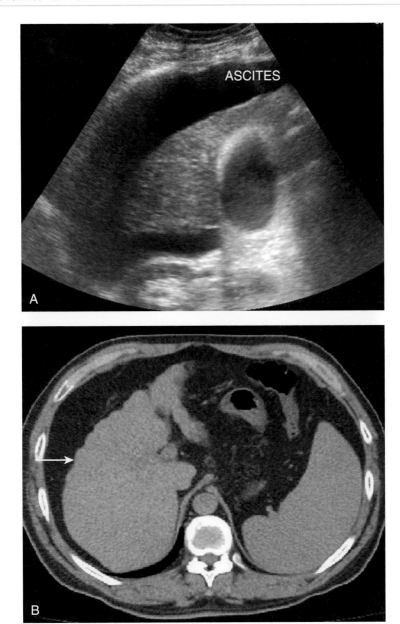

Figure 43.5 **A,** Ultrasound image showing a coarsened cirrhotic liver surround by ascites. **B,** Computed tomography (CT) image showing a nodular cirrhotic liver and splenomegaly. *(A from* https://commons .wikimedia.org/wiki/File:Ascites_ultrasound_2.JPG; *B from* https://commons.wikimedia.org/wiki/File:Liver _cirrhosis.JPG.*)*

pressure. This can cause varices to form in the esophagus and stomach, which can lead to life-threatening bleeding. Collateral flow through the splenic veins specifically can also cause splenic enlargement and lead to the sequestration of platelets, causing thrombocytopenia.

Other complications of cirrhosis include portal venous thrombosis and hepatocellular carcinoma.

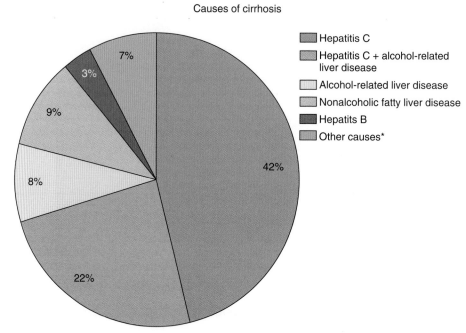

Causes of cirrhosis

- Hepatitis C
- Hepatitis C + alcohol-related liver disease
- Alcohol-related liver disease
- Nonalcoholic fatty liver disease
- Hepatits B
- Other causes*

7%
3%
9%
8%
22%
42%

Figure 43.6 Proportion of cirrhosis by the most common causes. Other causes include hemochromatosis, primary biliary cirrhosis, autoimmune hepatitis, cryptogenic chronic liver disease, primary sclerosing cholangitis, granulomatous disease, and drug-induced liver disease. *(Data from Bell BP, Manos MM, Zaman A, et al. The epidemiology of newly diagnosed chronic liver disease in gastroenterology practices in the United States: results from population-based surveillance. Am J Gastroenterol. 2008;103[11]:2727-2736.)*

TABLE 43.3 ■ Complications of Loss of Intrinsic Function of Liver

Coagulopathy	Due to a failure to synthesize an adequate amount of clotting factors
Jaundice	Due to the inability to conjugate and excrete bilirubin
Spontaneous bacterial peritonitis	Likely caused by the translocation of intestinal flora into the protein-deficient ascites fluid
Portal venous thrombosis	Likely due to portal vein stasis and unbalanced hemostasis
Variceal hemorrhage	Due to portal hypertension and unbalanced hemostasis
Hepatic encephalopathy	Due to the inability to metabolize urea causing a buildup of ammonia
Hepatorenal syndrome	Due to the inability to adequately metabolize certain vasodilatory agents leading to peripheral and splanchnic vasodilation and leading to poor perfusion of the kidneys
Hepatopulmonary syndrome	Due to the inability to metabolize vasodilatory agents, mainly nitric oxide, in the blood causing small shunts to develop in the lung causing deoxygenated blood to be able to bypass the lung
Portopulmonary hypertension	Caused by vasoactive agents in the blood not being metabolized and leading to pulmonary arterial vasoconstriction and pulmonary hypertension

While the patient is at ultrasound, the labs results come back. The white blood cell count is 15,000 cells/µL, hemoglobin is 10 g/dL, platelets are 100,000/µL (100 × 10^9/L), and mean corpuscular volume is 105 fL/cell. Sodium is 130 mEq/L, chloride is 92 mmol/L, CO_2 is 18 mmol/L, blood urea nitrogen (BUN) is 45 mg/dL, and creatinine is 1.5 mg/dL. Albumin is 2.8 g/dL, aspartate transaminase (AST) is 65 U/L, alanine transaminase (ALT) is 60 U/L, and total bilirubin is 6 mg/dL. Prothrombin time is 20 seconds. Your attending asks what you think about the lab results and how you want to proceed.

How do you interpret these results, and how should you proceed?

The leukocytosis in the setting of a fever, tachycardia, and hypotension in an ill-appearing patient is concerning for sepsis. This is further supported by the anion gap metabolic acidosis seen on the BMP (which is likely from a lactic acidosis). Sepsis should be treated with aggressive IV fluid resuscitation, drawing blood cultures, lactate, and prompt initiation of an empiric but reasonable IV antibiotic regimen based on the likely source of infection.

The macrocytic anemia, thrombocytopenia, hypoalbuminemia, and elevated prothrombin time in the context of the patient's history, physical exam, and ultrasound findings enables you to make the diagnosis of cirrhosis.

This new diagnosis will help guide how you should proceed with regard to management of his sepsis. His new ascites and peritonitis on exam in the setting of an otherwise normal ultrasound make the diagnosis of spontaneous bacterial peritonitis (SBP) highly likely. An immediate diagnostic paracentesis should be performed.

You tell your attending that you are concerned about SBP and would like to proceed with a diagnostic paracentesis. Your attending agrees and asks what you would like to order on the ascites fluid to make the diagnosis.

How is SBP diagnosed?

SBP is diagnosed through the analysis of peritoneal fluid obtained via a paracentesis.

A paracentesis is a procedure that consists of removing a sample of ascites fluid from the abdomen using a large bore needle. By analyzing the ascites fluid, the cause may be narrowed and the presence of infection identified. Common laboratory studies to request on ascites fluid include a cell count and differential, total protein, albumin, Gram stain with culture, and cytology. The albumin from the fluid is typically compared with the serum albumin in order to calculate the serum-ascites albumin gradient (SAAG).

In ascites caused by cirrhosis, one typically sees a high SAAG (greater than 1.1 g/dL) because the ascites in cirrhosis is a direct cause of portal hypertension. Other causes of a high SAAG include heart failure, Budd-Chiari syndrome, and portal vein thrombosis. Causes of a low SAAG include malignancy, tuberculosis, and pancreatitis.

Because SBP is an infection of the peritoneal fluid, it is associated with a high cell count, with a high proportion of polymorphonuclear leukocytes (PMNs) as well as a positive Gram stain or culture. The diagnostic criteria for SBP and indication for treatment is a positive Gram stain or culture of the ascites fluid or a PMN count ≥250 cells/mm^3.

CLINICAL PEARL	**STEP 2/3**

Low protein levels in ascites fluid is a strong predictor of developing the first episode of SBP due to low levels of immunoglobulins and complement levels in the peritoneum.

CLINICAL PEARL   **STEP 2/3**

For patients with cirrhosis who have SBP, 70% are Child-Pugh class C.

You perform the diagnostic paracentesis, obtain 1500 mL of clear yellow fluid, and send the fluid to the lab. While you wait for the results, your attending asks what empiric antibiotics you would start, given that the patient is septic and unstable.

How is SBP treated?

Gram-negative organisms such as *Escherichia coli* and *Klebsiella* make up the majority of organisms found in patients with SBP. However, infections with gram-positive organisms such as *Staphylococcus* and *Streptococcus* are also commonly seen. SBP is typically treated empirically with a broad-spectrum third-generation cephalosporin such as cefotaxime or ceftriaxone as soon as the patient is diagnosed using the results of a paracentesis. However, if the patient is unstable and septic, empiric treatment can be warranted like in this case. The antibiotic coverage is tailored based on the patient's clinical response and data from the bacterial cultures.

CLINICAL PEARL   **STEP 2/3**

Three fourths of SBP infections are caused by aerobic gram-negative infections (half of those are due to *E. coli*), and the remainder by aerobic gram-positive organisms, particularly streptococcal species. Anaerobic organisms are rare because of high oxygen tension of ascites fluid.

IV albumin is also commonly used in patients with SBP as its use has been associated with improvement in renal function and even mortality. It is still unclear exactly which of the many types of patients with SBP would benefit from albumin administration. It is also unclear exactly how much albumin should be given. However, it is reasonable to give albumin to patients who already present with renal dysfunction like in this case.

Once a patient has been diagnosed with SBP, the patient is at a much higher risk of developing SBP in the future and needs to be on lifelong SBP prophylaxis. Common antibiotics used for SBP prophylaxis are sulfamethoxazole and trimethoprime combination or the fluoroquinolones; they have excellent gram-negative and gram-positive coverage. Another indication for SBP prophylaxis is a total protein concentration in the ascites fluid of less than 1.5 g/dL.

CLINICAL PEARL   **STEP 2/3**

An alternative for prophylactic use in SBP includes the nonabsorbable antibiotic rifaximin, which appears to reduce the incidence of bacterial peritonitis in patients with advanced liver cirrhosis without promoting antibiotic resistance.

The patient is started on IV cefotaxime and IV albumin. An hour later some test results from the ascites fluid come back. The SAAG is 1.5 g/dL, the PMN count is 300 cells/µL, and you are able to confirm the diagnosis of SBP. You admit the patient to the hospital for further management of his sepsis.

TABLE 43.4 ■ West Haven Grades of Hepatic Encephalopathy

Grade 0: Minimal	Minimal impairments in memory, concentration, and intellectual functioning
Grade 1: Mild	Decreased attention, irritability, depression, and alterations in the sleep–wake cycle
Grade 2: Moderate	Poor memory, slurred speech, inappropriate behavior, tremors
Grade 3: Severe	Loss of orientation, somnolence
Grade 4: Coma	Unconscious

Over the next 48 hours, the patient decompensates. On the morning of his second day of admission, the nurse notes that the patient is acting "confused." On physical exam, his temperature is 36.7°C (98.0°F), pulse rate is 80/min, blood pressure is 110/85 mm Hg, and oxygen saturation is 92% on room air. The patient is lethargic, oriented only to self, thinks the year is 1975, and demonstrates asterixis.

Diagnosis: Spontaneous bacterial peritonitis/alcoholic cirrhosis/hepatic encephalopathy

What are some signs and symptoms of hepatic encephalopathy?

Signs of hepatic encephalopathy include inattention, poor concentration, confusion, disorientation, and asterixis. The first signs of hepatic encephalopathy are usually poor sleep and an alteration of the patient's normal sleep–wake cycle. The severity of hepatic encephalopathy is graded on a scale of 1 to 4, with grade 4 encephalopathy being the most severe (see Table 43.4).

Hepatic encephalopathy is treated with urea-reducing agents such as lactulose and rifaximin. Lactulose prevents ammonia (NH_3) by transforming it into ammonium (NH_4), which cannot be reabsorbed in the bloodstream. Rifaximin, on the other hand, kills the colonic bacteria that produce ammonia.

CLINICAL PEARL   **STEP 2/3**

Rifaximin is now generally preferred over neomycin based on the ototoxicity and renal toxicity of the aminoglycoside class of antibiotics.

The dosage and frequency of lactulose is titrated to achieve two to three soft stools daily, as well as an improvement in mental status. Approximately 70 to 80% of patients with hepatic encephalopathy improve after correction of the precipitating cause, such as gastrointestinal bleed, hypovolemia, and infection.

You suspect that the patient has hepatic encephalopathy triggered by his SBP. You start lactulose and he begins to have regular bowel movements. His mental status also dramatically improves over the next 48 hours. His renal dysfunction, leukocytosis, and hemodynamics all normalize as well. The ascites fluid culture comes back as *Escherichia coli* that is sensitive to most antibiotics. The original blood cultures also come back with no growth to date. You discharge him in stable condition with follow-up with a primary care doctor and hepatologist. When he arrives at the hepatologist, he asks if he is a candidate for a liver transplant.

What is the role of transplant in cirrhosis?

Once cirrhosis has developed, it is irreversible. All patients with cirrhosis should be evaluated for possible transplant candidacy early in the course of their disease. However, due to the limited supply of livers available for transplant, the sickest patients are usually given priority. The Model for End-Stage Liver Disease (MELD) score is now used by the United Network for Organ Sharing (UNOS) to prioritize allocation of liver transplants instead of the Child-Pugh score, which is used to assess the prognosis of cirrhosis and was originally used in predicting mortality during surgery.

CLINICAL PEARL   **STEP 2/3**

Without transplant, patients who have decompensated alcoholic cirrhosis who continue drinking have a 5-year survival rate of 30% compared to 60% for those who quit drinking.

While waiting for transplant, patients are typically treated or screened for the complications of cirrhosis, which may cause discomfort or reduce their life expectancy. Patients are considered to have decompensated cirrhosis when complications such as ascites, hepatic encephalopathy, or portal hypertension develop. Patients with portal hypertension refractory to medical therapy may require placement of a transjugular intrahepatic shunt to establish communication between the portal vein and hepatic vein to decompress the portal circulation.

CLINICAL PEARL   **STEP 2/3**

A low complication of TIPS is development or worsening of hepatic encephalopathy based on the elimination of first-pass clearance of nitrogen from the gut.

BEYOND THE PEARLS

- A rare physical exam finding in cirrhosis is the Cruveilhier-Baumgarten murmur, a venous hum that can be auscultated in the epigastrium caused by blood flowing through collateral connections between the portal system and a remnant of the umbilical vein.
- Childs-Pugh score is based on clinical and lab criteria, which numerically categorize patients into classes A, B, and C, giving points based on encephalopathy, ascites, bilirubin, albumin, and prothrombin time (PT)/international normalized ratio (INR).
- Model for End-Stage Liver Disease (MELD) score is used to allocate donor livers to patients waiting for transplant. The score is calculated using three parameters: total bilirubin, INR, and serum creatinine.
- Mental status changes in a patient with cirrhosis have a broad differential, which includes infection, uremia, electrolyte disturbances, alcohol intoxication/withdrawal, and hypoglycemia.
- Dysfunction of the urea cycle (ornithine cycle) is the main etiology of hyperammonemia in cirrhosis, resulting in encephalopathy.
- Most cirrhotic patients regardless of etiology tend to be acidemic secondary to dysfunction of the Cori (lactic acid) cycle, resulting in accumulation of lactic acid.
- The presence of spider angiomas noted on physical exam in a patient with cirrhosis is secondary to decreased metabolism of nitric oxide resulting in vasodilation.

References

Grant A, Neuberger J. Guidelines on the use of liver biopsy in clinical practice. *Gut.* 1999;45(suppl 4):1-11.

Huang YW, Yang SS, Kao JH. Pathogenesis and management of alcoholic liver cirrhosis: a review. *Hepat Med.* 2011;3:1-11.

Moore KP, Aithal GP. Guidelines on the management of ascites in cirrhosis. *Gut.* 2006;55(suppl 6):vi1-vi12.

Rimola A, García-Tsao G, Navasa M, et al. Diagnosis, treatment and prophylaxis of spontaneous bacterial peritonitis: a consensus document. *J Hepatol.* 2000;32(1):142-153.

Runyon BA. Low-protein-concentration ascitic fluid is predisposed to spontaneous bacterial peritonitis. *Gastroenterology.* 1986;91(6):1343-1346.

Salerno F, Navickis RJ, Wilkes MM. Albumin infusion improves outcomes of patients with spontaneous bacterial peritonitis: a meta-analysis of randomized trials. *Clin Gastroenterol Hepatol.* 2013;11(2):123.

Sort P, Navasa M, Arroyo V, et al. Effect of intravenous albumin on renal impairment and mortality in patients with cirrhosis and spontaneous bacterial peritonitis. *N Engl J Med.* 1999;341(6):403.

Sundaram V, Shaikh OS. Hepatic encephalopathy: pathophysiology and emerging therapies. *Med Clin North Am.* 2009;93(4):819-836.

CASE 44

Seth Politano ■ Eric Hsieh

A 28-Year-Old Female With Difficult-to-Control Hypertension

A 28-year-old female presents to you to establish care. She has a previous history of high blood pressure on amlodipine 10 mg daily, atenolol 100 mg daily, and lisinopril 40 mg daily. She has no other medical problems, but her family history is significant for type 2 diabetes mellitus in her mother, who uses insulin. Review of systems is positive for fatigue, intermittent headaches, diaphoresis, and palpitations. Vital signs reveal a blood pressure of 180/110 mm Hg in the right arm, 182/110 mm Hg in the left arm, and a pulse rate of 104/min. Her physical exam is otherwise normal.

When should you be concerned about secondary hypertension?

Essential hypertension is responsible for the majority of patients with hypertension (>90%). There are a number of features, however, that would clue you in to suspect a cause of secondary hypertension:

- Disease onset in a young patient (<30 years of age)
- A sudden increase in blood pressure in a patient who has hypertension usually controlled on antihypertensive medication
- Hypertensive emergency in a patient without a prior history of hypertension, or repeated hypertensive urgencies/emergencies in a patient with hypertension
- Difficult to control hypertension (on three or more medications, making sure that the patient is adherent to medications)
- Clinical features suggestive of an underlying cause

CLINICAL PEARL	STEP 2/3

Make sure to verify correct blood pressure measurement. This includes ensuring appropriate cuff size and making sure the measured arm is at heart level. Check blood pressure in both arms, repeat measurements, and consider the possibility of white-coat hypertension.

In this younger patient with uncontrolled hypertension on three agents at maximum dosage, and clinical features suggestive of a secondary cause, secondary hypertension should be considered.

What are the causes of secondary hypertension? What clues should you look for on history or physical exam?

Table 44.1 summarizes the causes of secondary hypertension and key clinical findings.

CLINICAL PEARL	STEP 2/3

In patients with suspected secondary hypertension, testing should be performed as guided by clinical suspicion for causes, instead of a battery of all possible tests.

TABLE 44.1 ■ **Causes of Secondary Hypertension and Key Physical Exam/Historical Findings**

Condition	Hints to Obtain from History/Exam/Workup
Hyperaldosteronism	Hypokalemia and metabolic alkalosis.
Pheochromocytoma	Palpitations, headache, diaphoresis, anxiety.
Cushing's syndrome	Dorsocervical fat pad ("buffalo hump"), central obesity, moon facies, striae of the abdomen and thighs. Fatigue, easy bruising, myopathy, amenorrhea. Use of corticosteroids, smoker, and/or chronic lung disease suggesting an ectopic source.
Chronic kidney disease	Elevated potassium, serum creatinine, low serum bicarbonate, uremic symptoms.
Renal artery stenosis	Patient with atherosclerotic risk factors and with other atherosclerotic diseases (coronary artery disease, cerebral vascular accident, peripheral vascular disease). Renal bruit. Hypokalemia. Can present with sudden pulmonary edema and acute renal failure especially after starting angiotensin-converting enzyme in bilateral renal artery stenosis.
Fibromuscular dysplasia	Young female with headache, pulsatile tinnitus. Epigastric, renal, carotid bruits.
Coarctation of the aorta	Systolic blood pressure is >20 mm Hg higher in arms compared to legs. Absent or delayed femoral pulses. Chest radiograph with rib notching and/or "3" sign.
Thyroid diseases (both hyperthyroidism and hypothyroidism)	Fatigue, weight gain/loss, tremor, tachycardia/bradycardia, heat/cold intolerance, menstrual irregularities, bowel irregularities, warm/dry skin.
Obstructive sleep apnea	Excessive daytime somnolence, large neck circumference, snoring and apneic events reported by partner.
Acromegaly	Visual changes, fatigue, headaches. Observed change in appearance including jaw enlargement and coarse facial features. Change in hat/shoe/glove/ring size. Can have visual disturbances, secondary diabetes, sleep apnea.
Hyperparathyroidism	Fatigue, osteoporosis, nephrolithiasis, abdominal pain, constipation, nausea, anorexia, altered mental status, lethargy.

CLINICAL PEARL   **STEP 2/3**

Medications and substances that can contribute to hypertension include oral contraceptives, decongestants, nonsteroidal antiinflammatory drugs, thyroid supplementation, corticosteroids, cyclosporine, erythropoietin, triptans, ergotamine, alcohol, cocaine, methamphetamine, and phencyclidine (PCP) use.

On further questioning, the patient reveals that she gets "anxious" frequently throughout the day, worries about this occurring, and this prevents her from performing her job to previous standards.

Does this finding increase your suspicion for any causes of the patient's hypertension?

Drugs of abuse (including cocaine or methamphetamine) as well as withdrawal from certain medications (i.e., alcohol and benzodiazepines) should be considered as they can cause both hypertension and anxiety. In addition, medical causes such as pheochromocytoma should be considered in this setting as they induce anxiety as well as hypertension.

The patient denies the use of any illicit drugs or alcohol. Given her clinical findings, including headache, diaphoresis, palpitations, resistant hypertension, and anxiety disorder, you are concerned for pheochromocytoma.

What is the epidemiology of pheochromocytomas?

Pheochromocytomas are rare tumors of the adrenal medulla that derive from neural crest cells. Incidence ranges from 1 to 10 patients per million. They are present in from 0.1 to 1% of hypertensive patients. They usually present in patients between 30 and 40 years of age.

What is the pathophysiology of the disease?

Chromaffin cells can produce norepinephrine (most common), epinephrine, dopamine (more common with malignant tumors), and other substances such as vasoactive intestinal peptide and somatostatins. These are responsible for the clinical findings in patients and the variability of clinical presentation.

BASIC SCIENCE/CLINICAL PEARL   **STEP 1/2/3**

There are other tumors that arrive from the same neural crest, such as neuroblastomas and gangliomas, and therefore may present with symptoms similar to those of pheochromocytoma.

What are the risk factors for pheochromocytoma? What other conditions are associated with pheochromocytoma?

Risk factors for pheochromocytoma include a family history of a genetic syndrome known to be associated with the disease. Table 44.2 lists disease associations with pheochromocytoma.

TABLE 44.2 ■ **Disease Associations With Pheochromocytoma**

Condition	Clinical Hints/Findings
MEN IIA	Pheochromocytoma, hyperparathyroidism, and medullary carcinoma of the thyroid.
MEN IIB	Pheochromocytoma, medullary carcinoma of the thyroid, marfanoid appearance, mucosal neuromas.
Von Hippel Lindau syndrome	Headaches, vertigo, balance disturbances. Retinal and cerebral hemangioblastomas, renal cell carcinoma, cystic disease of kidneys and pancreas, endolymphatic sac tumors in the middle ear.
Neurofibromatosis type 1	Café-au-lait macules, axillary/inguinal freckling, dermal neurofibromas, Lisch nodules, optic gliomas, seizures, skeletal deformities.

MEN, Multiple endocrine neoplasia.

Where are pheochromocytomas located?

You can remember the general "rule of 10s" to get a sense of certain features of the disease: Only 10% are extraadrenal and 10% are bilateral. The rule also applies to their malignant potential (10%) and inheritance pattern (only 10% are inherited). With this being said, the "rule of 10s" does not accurately reflect true findings, as some observational studies have shown that some of these features may be present anywhere from 5 to 25%.

BASIC SCIENCE PEARL   **STEP 1**

Although rare, the location of these extraadrenal paragangliomas include the bladder, heart, carotid arteries, and the organ of Zuckerkandl (around the area of aortic bifurcation).

How do pheochromocytomas commonly present?

The presentation can be variable depending on which catecholamine is in excess and the quantity of catecholamine being produced. Intermittent symptoms last approximately 30 minutes and may be precipitated by stress, surgery, exertion, or movement of abdominal organs. The classic clinical triad of periodic headache, palpitations, and diaphoresis is very sensitive (up to around 90%) but has variable diagnostic specificity (ranging from 60 to 95%). Out of these, headache is most common and is seen in most patients. You can use the absence of the clinical triad in a hypertensive patient without any other suspicion for the disease to exclude the possibility of pheochromocytoma.

As mentioned in the above case, anxiety can be present. Some patients may have panic attacks. Patients may also complain of nausea, tremor, pallor, fever, constipation, abdominal pain, and symptoms of hypercalcemia and/or hyperglycemia. Most patients (>90%) have both systolic and diastolic hypertension as well as tachycardia. These findings are paroxysmal in up to half of patients and sustained in the other half. The vasoconstriction that causes this can be so severe that patients may complain of cold extremities and may have decreased pulses/cool extremities on physical exam. Keep in mind that patients can develop intermittent orthostatic hypotension when the tumor also secretes epinephrine, often alternating with hypertension. A sudden surge in catecholamines can cause arrhythmias or coronary ischemia, sometimes leading to sudden death. Rarely, pheochromocytomas can secrete other substances that cause systemic symptoms including vasoactive intestinal peptide (which causes diarrhea) and adrenocorticotropic hormone (ACTH; which causes Cushing's syndrome).

What should your approach be to workup?

Workup first consists of laboratory testing for catecholamine excess and then imaging to localize the tumor.

What is the best test to initiate a workup?

There are many potential approaches to the workup of suspected pheochromocytoma. Each biochemical test has variable diagnostic sensitivity and specificity (see Table 44.3), and this changes from laboratory to laboratory.

Any level above two times the upper limit of normal is seen in general catecholamine excess, with levels usually at least three times the upper limit seen in pheochromocytoma. It is not necessary to send every test in order to workup a patient suspected of having the disease; the initial choice for biochemical workup depends on a variety of factors. Twenty-four-hour urine testing is often the first option for those patients with a lower pretest probability. The best initial urine diagnostic is fractionated metanephrines. Plasma fractionated metanephrines is the initial test in patients with a higher pretest probability (i.e., those with familial syndromes). In these patients,

TABLE 44.3 ■ **Approximate Sensitivity and Specificity of Laboratory Investigation for Pheochromocytoma**

Test	Sensitivity	Specificity
Plasma-free metanephrines	99%	89%
Plasma catecholamines	84%	81%
24-hour urine total metanephrines	77%	93%
24-hour urine fractioned metanephrines	97%	69%
24-hour urine catecholamines	86%	88%

TABLE 44.4 ■ **Medications and Conditions That Can Alter Laboratory Testing for Pheochromocytoma**

Falsely Raising Levels in Testing (Possibly Causing a False Positive)
Tricyclic antidepressants, monoamine oxidase inhibitors, buspirone, alpha-1 antagonists, beta blockers, methyldopa, levodopa, radiographic contrast agents, sleep apnea, hypoglycemia, exercise, caffeine, nicotine, amphetamines, alcohol, and clonidine withdrawal

Falsely Lowering Levels in Testing (Possibly Causing a False Negative)
Alpha-2 agonists, calcium channel blockers

normal values portend a good negative predictive value. Keep in mind, however, that unless the values are many times the upper limit of normal, elevated plasma fractionated methanephrines need to be followed up by the more specific urine testing. There are many other factors that influence the initial test of choice.

CLINICAL PEARL	STEP 2/3

Urine testing is usually easier to analyze than plasma testing due to concentration levels, but it is difficult to analyze in children, cannot be used in those with renal failure, is harder to collect from patients, and is more difficult to control for influences on situations that can falsely raise levels.

Are there any special precautions to take when sending this workup?
Refer to Table 44.4 for a list of some conditions that can interfere with biochemical testing for pheochromocytoma.

24-hour urine metanephrines are sent, and they are greater than four times the upper limit of normal.

Given the elevated levels, what should your approach be to imaging studies? What are the radiographic features of the disease?
Initial imaging is usually a computed tomography (CT) scan of the abdomen and pelvis, noting attention to adrenal masses. Magnetic resonance imaging (MRI) can also be sent and has similar sensitivity (>95%) and specificity (70%) but can also be used for detection of local metastasis. An metaiodobenzylguanidine (MIBG) scan (this is more specific but less sensitive than CT or MRI) is a nuclear medicine scan that can be performed when suspecting extraadrenal disease, for example when biochemical testing is positive but CT or MRI is negative.

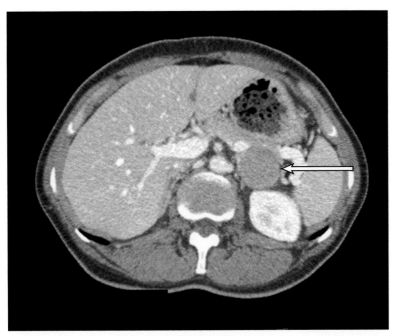

Figure 44.1   Computed tomography (CT) scan of the abdomen/pelvis of a patient with a left adrenal mass *(see arrow).*

CT scan of the abdomen reveals a heterogeneous 3.3 cm by 3.2 cm mass in the left adrenal gland (see Fig. 44.1).

Diagnosis: Pheochromocytoma

How should you treat the patient?

The approach to treatment is oral medications to control blood pressure, then surgical resection. Alpha blockers (such as phenoxybenzamine or prazosin) are given approximately 2 weeks preoperatively to lower the blood pressure to <140/90 mm Hg. Another sign of adequate alpha blockade is reflex tachycardia. Once this is obtained, beta blockers are administered—usually a few days prior to surgery. These usually help with the tachycardia and potential tachyarrhythmias that occur from alpha blockade. These steps are taken to prevent postoperative hypotension and intraoperative catecholamine crisis. It is important that alpha blockers are started before beta blockers because beta blockade alone leads to unopposed alpha receptor mediated vasoconstriction and hypertensive crisis. Calcium channel blockers can also be used in addition to, or in place of, alpha and beta blockers in the preoperative management stage. It is important to maintain an adequate intravascular status, and normal saline infusions are given before and after surgery.

CLINICAL PEARL   **STEP 2/3**

Upon initiating beta blockage preoperatively, some patients may develop pulmonary edema, reflecting underlying catecholamine-induced cardiomyopathy.

There are various surgical procedures for resection, but the laparoscopic adrenalectomy is usually the preferred approach. In those with familial syndromes, however, bilateral adrenalectomy is often performed or varied depending on the clinical syndrome. After surgery, it can take up to 2 weeks for a patient to become normotensive.

CLINICAL PEARL   **STEP 2/3**

Despite adequate preoperative treatment with alpha and beta blockade, it is not uncommon for arrhythmias and hypertension to occur during surgery, especially with anesthetic introduction and manipulation of the mass. Elevations in pressure during surgery may require agents such as nicardipine, nitroprusside, and phentolamine. Postoperative hypoglycemia and hypotension can occur as well, sometimes requiring vasopressor support.

The patient is started on phenoxybenzamine followed by propranolol with subsequent stabilization of blood pressure and resolution of symptoms. After an uncomplicated surgical resection of the adrenal mass, the patient returns to see you in 2 weeks. She is off all antihypertensives and has a blood pressure of 126/84 mm Hg. She denies headaches or palpitations. She reports marked improvement in her anxiety symptoms.

BEYOND THE PEARLS

- Pheochromocytoma may present clinically with an elevation in blood pressure and pulse after starting monoamine oxidase inhibitors, tricyclic antidepressants, and during surgical procedures or anesthesia induction.
- Another rare familial syndrome that includes pheochromocytomas is the Carney complex of pheochromocytoma, gastrointestinal stromal tumors, and pulmonary chondromas (females) or Leydig tumors (males).
- Consider genetic testing for multiple endocrine neoplasia (MEN) syndromes, neurofibromatosis, and Hippel-Lindau syndrome in patients with a family history of pheochromocytomas, bilateral disease, extraadrenal/metastatic disease, diagnosis at a young age, or if there are clinical findings suggestive of a syndrome.
- Malignant pheochromocytomas are usually indolent. Sites of metastasis include the liver, lung, bone, and regional lymph nodes. Unfortunately, the treatment is usually palliative in nature. Because the tumors are not chemosensitive, surgical therapy followed by medication (such as ^{131}I-MIBG) is the treatment of choice. Radiation therapy does not improve the course of the tumor and is usually used for palliation of bony metastases.
- Vanillylmandelic acid (VMA) testing should not be performed in the biochemical workup for pheochromocytoma due to low positive predictive value and poor sensitivity compared to metanephrines testing.
- To minimize the possibility of obtaining false-positive results during plasma testing, the patient should have an intravenous (IV) line placed then lay in the supine position for at least 30 minutes before drawing the sample.
- In cases of suspected pheochromocytoma where the clinical suspicion is high but laboratory testing is not conclusive (i.e., elevated levels but not in the range you would expect for pheochromocytoma), send a serum chromogranin A level (elevated) or perform a glucagon stimulation test or clonidine suppression test. When IV glucagon is administered, patients with pheochromocytoma have a rise in blood pressure or plasma catecholamine levels. In the clonidine suppression test, baseline serum norepinephrine and epinephrine is measured. Clonidine is administered, and serum norepinephrine and epinephrine are measured at hourly intervals for 3 hours. In patients with essential

BEYOND THE PEARLS—cont'd

hypertension, the administration of clonidine suppresses the levels of circulating catecholamines after administration but the levels usually increase in those with pheochromocytoma.

- One must do a full medication screen when MIBG scanning is performed in order to reduce the possibility of false-positive testing.
- After surgery, patients should undergo repeat biochemical testing in a week to ensure normalization of levels. This is then repeated annually to monitor for reoccurrence, and the duration of monitoring is influenced by the presence or absence of familial syndromes.
- It may be difficult to diagnose pheochromocytoma in pregnant patients because it could be confused with preeclampsia. In addition, pregnant patients can present with supine hypertension (as the uterus will push against the tumor).

References

Amar L, Bertherat J, Baudin E, et al. Genetic testing in pheochromocytoma or functional paraganglioma. *J Clin Oncol.* 2005;23(34):8812-8818.

Amar L, Servais A, Gimenez-Roqueplo AP, et al. Year of diagnosis, features at presentation, and risk of recurrence in patients with pheochromocytoma or secreting paraganglioma. *J Clin Endocrinol Metab.* 2005;90(4):2110-2116.

Lenders JW, Eisenhofer G, Mannelli M, et al. Pheochromocytoma. *Lancet.* 2005;366(9486):665-675.

Lenders JW, Pacak K, Walther MM, et al. Biochemical diagnosis of pheochromocytoma: which test is best? *JAMA.* 2002;287(11):1427-1434.

Motta-Ramirez GA, Remer EM, Herts BR, et al. Comparison of CT findings in symptomatic and incidentally discovered pheochromocytomas. *Am J Roentgenol.* 2005;185(3):684-688.

Pacak K, Eisenhofer G, Ahlman H, et al. Pheochromocytoma: recommendations for clinical practice from the First International Symposium. October 2005. *Nat Clin Pract Endocrinol Metab.* 2007;3(2):92-102.

Sawka AM, Jaeschke R, Singh RJ, et al. A comparison of biochemical tests for pheochromocytoma: measurement of fractionated plasma metanephrines compared with the combination of 24-hour urinary metanephrines and catecholamines. *J Clin Endocrinol Metab.* 2003;88(2):553-558.

Sinclair AM, Isles CG, Brown I, et al. Secondary hypertension in a blood pressure clinic. *Arch Intern Med.* 1987;147(7):1289-1293.

Joseph Meouchy ■ Joseph Abdelmalek

A 35-Year-Old Female With Subacute Progressive Bilateral Lower Extremity Edema

A 35-year-old African American female, previously healthy, presents to clinic for worsening swelling of her feet, legs, and thighs. She first noticed she was not able to put her shoes on 2 weeks prior to her presentation and reports a 20-pound weight gain despite regular exercise and decreased appetite.

She denies any dysuria, hematuria, frequency, and urgency but reports that her urine has appeared foamy lately.

What is the significance of foamy urine?

Foaming occurs because albumin has a soaplike effect that reduces the surface tension of urine. It is generally thought that foamy urine may be an early sign of renal disease and, thus, that patients with this condition should be further evaluated. To note, foamy urine is subjective and is not always pathologic.

She also denies any chest pain, palpitations, shortness of breath, skin rashes, arthralgias, or joint swelling. She denies any use of over-the-counter medications including nonsteroidal antiinflammatory drugs (NSAIDs).

Family history is unremarkable for any renal disease.

Her body mass index (BMI) is 30 kg/m², and her vitals are significant for a blood pressure of 155/72 mm Hg. The exam is notable for mild periorbital edema with bilateral +1 pitting edema of her hands, feet, legs, and thighs. The rest of the physical exam is normal.

What is the differential diagnosis of systemic edema (anasarca)?

Differential diagnosis includes congestive heart failure, cirrhosis (systemic venous hypertension and decreased plasma oncotic pressure from reduced protein synthesis), renal disease (nephrotic syndrome, renal failure), malabsorption/protein-calorie malnutrition, pregnancy and premenstrual edema (increased plasma volume), and allergic reaction/angioedema (increased capillary permeability).

Laboratory exam reveals a serum creatinine level of 1.1 mg/dL, serum albumin of 2.9 g/dL, total cholesterol of 282 mg/dL, and hemoglobin A1C of 6.1%.

What is an easy and quick test to perform to evaluate for proteinuria?
Dipstick urinalysis is a convenient and quick method to detect proteinuria, but false-positive and false-negative results are not unusual. The main cause for a false-positive test is alkaline, concentrated urine. A false-negative test can be seen with acidic, dilute urine. Because the dipstick detects only albumin, nonalbumin protein (such as that seen with monoclonal gammopathies) does not cause a positive dipstick test.

BASIC SCIENCE/CLINICAL PEARL   **STEP 1/2/3**

The reagent on most dipstick tests is sensitive to albumin but may not detect low concentrations of γ-globulins and Bence Jones proteins. In patients with monoclonal gammopathy, the dipstick may be negative even when excreting high amount of nonalbumin protein.

Urinary dipstick is performed and shows 3+ protein with negative glucose, negative leukocyte esterase/nitrates, and negative blood.

What is the significance of 3+ protein on urinary dipstick? What is the best way to quantify the amount of protein excreted?
Dipstick tests for "trace" amounts of protein are positive at concentrations of around 5 to 10 mg/dL—lower than the threshold for clinically significant proteinuria. A result of 1+ corresponds to approximately 30 mg/dL of protein and is considered positive; 2+ corresponds to 100 mg/dL, and 3+ to 300 mg/dL. Nephrotic range proteinuria typically corresponds to dipstick proteinuria of 3+ to 4+.

Measurement of the protein content in a 24-hour urine sample is the definitive method of establishing the presence of abnormal proteinuria. However, the process of urine collection is cumbersome. Studies have shown a strong correlation between spot urine protein/creatinine ratio and 24-hour urine total protein excretion in proteinuria levels from 300 mg/day to 3499 mg/day.

Urine microscopy shows 0 to 1 white blood cell (WBC), 2 to 3 red blood cells (RBC), 1 to 5 epithelial cells, 0 casts, and 24-hour urine collection estimated 6.2 g of protein.

What is the definition of nephrotic syndrome?
Nephrotic syndrome is defined as protein excretion of more than 3.5 g over 24 hours, hypoalbuminemia (<3 g/dL), hyperlipidemia, and edema.

Normally, the kidneys do not excrete high amounts of protein (<150 mg/day) because serum proteins are excluded from the urine by the glomerular filter both because of their large size and their net negative charge. The appearance of significant proteinuria heralds glomerular disease, with disruption of its normal barrier function. Nephrotic syndrome is defined by excretion in the urine of over 20 times the upper limit of normal protein excretion.

Proteinuria causes a fall in serum albumin, and if the liver fails fully to compensate for urinary protein losses by increased albumin synthesis, plasma albumin concentrations decline, leading to edema formation. Interstitial edema is then a result of either a fall in plasma oncotic pressure from urinary loss of albumin or from primary sodium retention in the renal tubules.

What is the differential diagnosis?
Nephrotic syndrome is divided in two main categories: primary (idiopathic) and secondary glomerular disease.

The following are characteristics of primary (idiopathic) glomerular disease:
- Membranous nephropathy (the most common cause in white patients)
- Focal segmental glomerulosclerosis (FSGS; the most common cause in African American patients [50 to 57% of cases])
- Minimal-change nephropathy (the most common cause of proteinuria in children)
- Hereditary nephropathies
  The following are characteristics of secondary glomerular disease:
- Diabetic nephropathy (the most common cause secondary to the increasing prevalence of diabetes)
- Amyloidosis and immunoglobulin (Ig) light chain nephropathy (account for 10%)
- Medications including NSAIDs, antibiotics, lithium, tamoxifen, and captopril
- Infections (mainly human immunodeficiency virus [HIV], hepatitis B and C [HBV/HCV], and syphilis)
- Congenital causes (rare)

CLINICAL PEARL   **STEP 2/3**

When nephrotic syndrome is suspected, it is crucial to note features suggestive of systemic disease, drug history, acute or chronic infections, and cancer. For example, the onset of membranous nephropathy in a patient over 50 years of age often is associated with underlying malignancy. FSGS can be associated with HIV infection and certain medications.

C-reactive protein (CRP), erythrocyte sedimentation rate (ESR), serum and urine protein electorphoresis, antinuclear antibody (ANA) screen, serum complement levels (C3 and C4), hepatitis B/C panel, HIV, and rapid plasma reagin (RPR) are sent. The patient is instructed to follow up in 2 weeks.

She returns to the office 1 week later because of right calf pain that started 1 day prior to her presentation. Her pain is aggravated by exertion and mildly relieved by rest.

What is Homans' sign?
Described by John Homans in 1944, it is defined by pain in the calf and popliteal region in response to a forced dorsiflexion of the ankle when the knee is flexed. However, a diagnosis based solely on the evaluation of this clinical sign has proven unreliable.

What are the possible complications of nephrotic syndrome?
The following are possible complications:
- Thromboembolic (deep vein thrombosis [DVT] or renal vein thrombosis): This is due to urinary loss of anticoagulant proteins, such as antithrombin III and plasminogen, along with simultaneous increase in clotting factors (mainly I, VII, VIII, and X).
- Infection: The most common are bacterial cellulitis, pneumonia, and peritonitis. Increased risk of infection may be secondary to immunoglobulin losses and loss of complement factor.
- Hyperlipidemia: This is the typical feature rather than a complication. It is related to hypoproteinemia and low serum oncotic pressure, which leads to reactive hepatic protein synthesis, including lipoproteins, in addition to a reduction of lipoprotein lipase and decreased metabolism. Some of the lipoproteins are filtered at the glomerulus, leading to lipiduria and oval fat bodies and fatty casts in the urine sediment.
- Vitamin D deficiency: This results from urinary loss of vitamin D-binding proteins, which may lead to reduced intestinal calcium absorption. Hypocalcemia is usually caused by low serum albumin rather than true hypocalcemia.

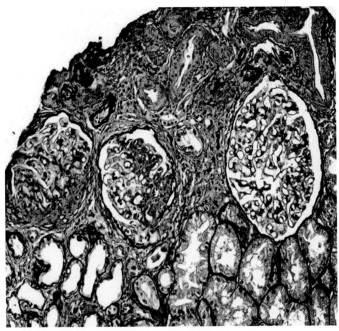

Figure 45.1   Focal segmental glomerulosclerosis (FSGS). There are more advanced segmental sclerotic lesions affecting two of the three glomeruli in this field, with surrounding proportionate tubulointerstitial fibrosis. The sclerosis is characterized by increased matrix and obliteration of capillary lumens (Jones silver stain, ×200). *(From Fogo AB, Kashgarian M.* Diagnostic Atlas of Renal Pathology: A Companion to Brenner & Rector's The Kidney. *2nd ed. Philadelphia: Elsevier/Saunders; 2012.)*

- Acute renal failure: This may indicate underlying glomerulonephritis but is more often precipitated by hypovolemia. Edema of the kidneys that causes pressure-mediated reduction of glomerular filtration rate (GFR) has been hypothesized.

> Lower extremity ultrasound reveals a right lower extremity DVT. The patient is started on anticoagulation.
>   She subsequently undergoes a renal biopsy that shows 22 normal-sized glomeruli, 2 globally sclerosed glomeruli, and 3 glomeruli showing scarring limited to the hilar region of the glomerulus (hilar variant of FSGS). Electron micrograph shows 70% foot process effacement and no electron-dense deposits (see Figs. 45.1 and 45.2).

What is FSGS?

The term *focal segmental glomerulosclerosis* is truly a pathologic description. *Focal* means that <50% of the glomeruli are affected, and *segmental* means that only part of an individual glomeruli is damaged. Thus, FSGS is a pattern of histologic injury rather than a disease. It is the most common primary glomerular histologic lesion associated with high-grade proteinuria and end stage renal disease (ESRD). Separation into primary and secondary FSGS is not easy but is critical not only for diagnostic but also therapeutic purposes.

Primary FSGS is a progressive disorder with <5% spontaneous remission and a 50% ESRD rate over a period of 5 to 8 years from the time of biopsy in patients who are either unresponsive to treatment or not treated.

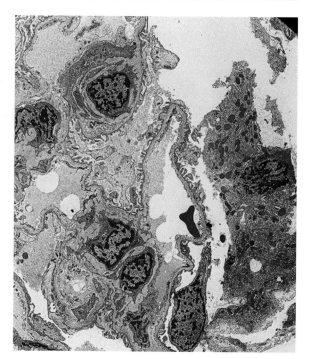

Figure 45.2 Focal segmental glomerulosclerosis (FSGS). By electron microscopy, there is extensive foot process effacement in FSGS. However, it may not be complete, as illustrated here. If there is less than approximately 50% foot process effacement, the diagnosis of primary FSGS is in doubt. There is also mesangial matrix expansion, without immune deposits (transmission electron microscopy, ×3000). *(From Fogo AB, Kashgarian M. Diagnostic Atlas of Renal Pathology: A Companion to Brenner & Rector's The Kidney. 2nd ed. Philadelphia: Elsevier/Saunders; 2012.)*

Causes of secondary FSGS include drugs (analgesics, intravenous heroin, pamidronate, lithium), infections (mainly HIV and HBV), hemodynamic factors with or without reduced renal mass (solitary kidney, renal dysplasia, vesicoureteral reflux, massive obesity), malignancies, and sickle cell disease.

The most current histologic classification, also known as the Columbia classification, includes classic FSGS (the most common variant), collapsing, tip (the most favorable prognosis), perihilar (more commonly associated with secondary FSGS, mediated by an adaptive response to increased glomerular capillary pressures and flow rates), and cellular types.

CLINICAL PEARL   **STEP 2/3**

One of the most challenging areas in FSGS is to determine whether the patient has secondary forms of FSGS, where immunosuppressive therapy would not be helpful. This patient has some clues that might indicate a secondary form of FSGS (obesity, hilar histologic variant).

What is the FSGS variant associated with HIV?

HIV is associated with the collapsing variant of FSGS. It carries the worst prognosis. The collapsing variant may also be associated with pamidronate, captopril, and parvovirus infection.

Diagnosis: Primary FSGS

How should you proceed with treatment?

The goal of therapy is to induce a complete remission of proteinuria, which will lead to better long-term preservation of renal function. Achieving partial remission is not optimal but slows the progression of kidney disease and substantially improves renal survival.

Regardless of the cause, all patients should be managed with renin-angiotensin system inhibitors, a low-salt diet, and diuretics unless contraindicated.

Initial treatment of primary FSGS consists of prednisone 1 mg/kg daily given for 4 to 16 weeks, as tolerated, or until complete remission.

CLINICAL PEARL   **STEP 2/3**

The distinction between minimal-change disease and FSGS is difficult given the histologic similarities and the possibility of missing diseased glomeruli with the biopsy sample. Response to glucocorticoid treatment remains the clinical gold standard.

BEYOND THE PEARLS

- Hematuria occurs in over half of FSGS patients, and approximately one third of patients have some degree of renal insufficiency at presentation. Gross hematuria is more commonly seen in FSGS than in minimal change glomerulopathy.
- Susceptibility of African Americans to FSGS has been linked to a polymorphism in the *APOL1* gene on chromosome 22. Its variants are associated with 17-fold higher odds for FSGS and 29-fold higher odds for HIV-associated nephropathy. Of interest, it is believed that *APOL1* variants protect patients against *Trypanosoma brucei,* the parasite that causes sleeping sickness.
- In patients with FSGS, angiotensin-converting enzyme (ACE) inhibitors decrease proteinuria while maintaining GFR and renal plasma flow.
- The degree of proteinuria and the achievement of remission in response to treatment are predictors of long-term clinical outcome.
- After transplantation, approximately 20 to 30% of patients develop recurrent FSGS. The risk factors for recurrence of FSGS include childhood onset and age <15 years, rapid progression of the initial FSGS to ESRD, recurrence of FSGS in a previous allograft, diffuse mesangial hypercellularity in the native kidney, collapsing FSGS, and podocin gene mutation.
- De novo FSGS also develops in approximately 10 to 20% of allografts, chronic transplant glomerulopathy, and calcineurin inhibitor toxicity.

References

Bose B, Cattran D, Toronto Glomerulonephritis Registry. Glomerular diseases: FSGS. *Clin J Am Soc Nephrol.* 2014;9(3):626-632.

Fogo AB, Kashgarian M. *Diagnostic Atlas of Renal Pathology: A Companion to Brenner & Rector's The Kidney.* 2nd ed. Philadelphia: Elsevier/Saunders; 2012.

Freedman BI, Kopp JB, Langefeld CD, et al. The apolipoprotein L1 (APOL1) gene and nondiabetic nephropathy in African Americans. *J Am Soc Nephrol.* 2010;21(9):1422-1426.

Hull RP, Goldsmith DJ. Nephrotic syndrome in adults. *BMJ.* 2008;336(7654):1185-1189.

International Society of Nephrology. Kidney disease improving global outcomes (KDIGO): clinical practice guideline for glomerulonephritis. *Kidney Int Suppl.* 2012;2(2):142.

Kang KK, Choi JR, Song JY, et al. Clinical significance of subjective foamy urine. *Chonnam Med J.* 2012;48(3):164-168.

Shimizu A, Higo S, Fujita E, et al. Focal segmental glomerulosclerosis after renal transplantation. *Clin Transplant.* 2011;Suppl 23:6-14.

Simerville JA, Maxted WC, Pahira JJ. Urinalysis: a comprehensive review. *Am Fam Physician.* 2005;71(6): 1153-1162.

Taal MW, Chertow G, Marsden PA, et al. *Brenner & Rector's The Kidney.* 9th ed. Philadelphia: Elsevier Health; 2012.

Nicholas Landsman ■ Kelly Walsma ■ Raj Dasgupta ■ Richard Snyder

A 40-Year-Old Female With Facial Rash and Persistent Cough

A 40-year-old female presents with a chief complaint of a persistent, dry cough for several weeks with associated dyspnea. She also complains of increasing fatigue during this time and finds that daily activities have become more difficult. A facial rash has been progressively worsening over the course of several months, and erythematous, painful patches of skin on her lower extremities are causing distress.

What are the most common etiologies of a chronic cough?

Chronic cough is an extremely common complaint seen in the outpatient setting. Knowing the most common causes of a chronic cough can eliminate unnecessary tests that increase health care costs. The four most common causes of cough include gastroesophageal reflux disease (GERD), asthma, angiotensin-converting enzyme (ACE) inhibitors, and upper airway cough syndrome. A detailed and focused history can lead to a diagnosis quickly (see Table 46.1).

A diagnostic algorithm for chronic cough has been proposed by the American College of Chest Physicians, and practice guidelines have been developed and published.

CLINICAL PEARL   **STEP 2/3**

Aside from a detailed history and physical exam, a chest radiograph (CXR) is recommended in all patients with chronic cough, unless a cause is readily identified and effectively treated.

The patient denies family history of rheumatologic disease, lung disease, or cancer; she notes a two-pack-year smoking history in her early 20s, yet otherwise no illicit drug or alcohol use. She is employed as a loan officer at a local bank. She denies acid reflux or wheezing associated with her cough.

Physical exam reveals a fatigued-appearing female in no acute distress. She is afebrile, normotensive, with oxygen saturation at 99% on room air. Her pulse rate is 85/min and regular. Her lungs are clear to auscultation, there is no lower extremity edema or elevated jugular venous pressure (JVP). No clubbing or cyanosis is appreciated.

Skin exam findings include a patchy, nodular, plaquelike erythematous facial rash over the forehead, nasal, and nasolabial areas bilaterally, yet sparing the nasolabial folds. On exam of her lower extremities, you note tender, erythematous subcutaneous nodules up to 1 cm in size (see Fig. 46.1).

How does the patient's skin exam affect the differential diagnosis?

The facial rash and presence of erythema nodosum is most likely a sign of systemic disease. Although infectious etiologies such as tuberculosis (TB) are still within the differential, the

TABLE 46.1 ■ **Etiologies of Chronic Cough**

Diagnosis	Presentation
Upper airway cough syndrome (UACS)	Previously postnasal drip syndrome; history of nasal congestion, rhinorrhea, recurrent throat clearing Associated with sinusitis, allergies, vasomotor rhinitis
Asthma	Shortness of breath, decreased exercise tolerance, wheezing, dyspnea Cough-variant asthma with cough as dominant feature; may occur in absence of wheeze
Nonasthmatic eosinophilic bronchitis (NAEB)	Chronic cough associated with atopic findings; may be indistinguishable from cough-variant asthma initially
Gastroesophageal reflux disease (GERD)	Heartburn, acid/sour taste in mouth, acid-reflux symptoms are worse at night A variant of GERD: laryngopharyngeal reflux, with hoarseness, dysphagia
Chronic obstructive pulmonary disease (COPD)	Generally due to chronic bronchitis, productive cough for most days for at least 3-month period over 2 consecutive years, without alternative etiology
Postinfectious	Recent viral/bacterial upper respiratory tract infection or pneumonia; cough generally only lasts 8 weeks yet may persist longer
Opportunistic infections (i.e., mycobacterial infections, *Pneumocystis jiroveci*)	Immunocompromised patient due to human immunodeficiency virus (HIV)/acquired immunodeficiency syndrome (AIDS), immune deficiency syndromes; organ transplant or autoimmune disease patients on chronic immunosuppressive therapy
Medication induced	Most notable is angiotensin-converting enzyme (ACE) inhibitor use, usually within 1 week yet may be delayed up to 6 months
Lung cancer/metastatic disease	Current or former smoker, yet increasingly among nonsmokers Generally large central airway bronchogenic carcinoma; new or change in chronic "smoker's cough" persistent after smoking cessation; hemoptysis in absence of infection Metastatic disease or bulky lymphadenopathy from lymphoma are rare etiologies

patient's lack of productive cough and known risk factors (institutionalization, immunosuppression, exposure history) argue against this diagnosis. The rash is not typical of rheumatologic disease such as systemic lupus erythematosus (SLE), which is generally a malar or discoid facial rash. Although the patient is young with a limited smoking history, a primary lung malignancy or metastatic disease cannot be excluded. The cutaneous and pulmonary manifestations are consistent with sarcoidosis, and this should be at the forefront of the differential diagnosis. Nevertheless, sarcoidosis is a diagnosis of exclusion, and other granulomatous diseases and malignancies such as lymphoma, lung cancer, metastatic disease, infection, carcinoid tumors, vasculitides, and collagen vascular diseases must be ruled out.

Complete blood count (CBC) reveals normal hemoglobin concentration, renal function, and electrolytes, except for elevated serum calcium levels with a normal albumin level. CXR reveals bilateral hilar prominence (see Fig. 46.2).

What is the most likely diagnosis? How can this be confirmed?
The diagnosis of sarcoidosis is confirmed by three essential clinical characteristics, including evidence on CXR, clinical features as noted above with suspicion for sarcoidosis, and nonnecrotizing

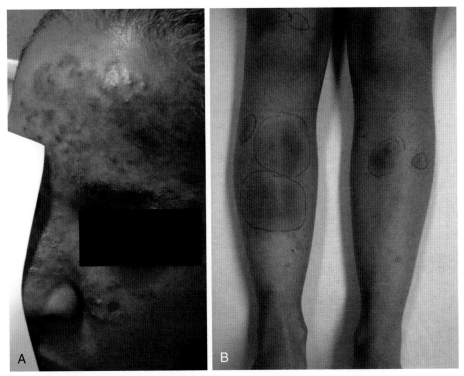

Figure 46.1 Erythematous, maculopapular facial rash and erythema nodosum. A, Erythematous, plaquelike, nodular facial rash. **B,** Erythema nodosum. Note the erythematous subcutaneous nodules that are tender to palpation. *(B from Wikipedia Commons: James Heilman, MD; Licensed under Creative Commons Attribution-Share Alike 3.0 Unported license.)*

granulomata on biopsy of an affected organ in the absence of an alternative etiology. Table 46.2 provides an overview of the clinical manifestations of sarcoidosis. Peripheral blood samples have been shown to have elevated tumor necrosis factor (TNF) alpha levels in sarcoidosis patients, yet assays have not yet been standardized or tested for routine clinical efficacy to date.

CLINICAL PEARL   **STEP 2/3**

Bilateral hilar lymphadenopathy, erythema nodosum, and arthralgia are pathognomonic for Lofgren's syndrome without the need for a biopsy to demonstrate granulomatous disease.

There is currently no widely accepted or consensus guideline available for workup of suspected sarcoidosis. If sarcoidosis is suspected based on presentation and imaging, then a biopsy of the suspected organ involved should be pursued. A minor salivary gland biopsy, transbronchial needle aspiration, endobronchial ultrasound lymph node biopsy, or transbronchial lung biopsy is warranted in the absence of a peripheral lymph node or skin biopsy site.

CLINICAL PEARL   **STEP 2/3**

There is no role for biopsy of erythema nodosum because it is not a granulomatous finding; histology is nonspecific and will demonstrate an inflammation of the septa in the subcutaneous fat tissue (septal panniculitis).

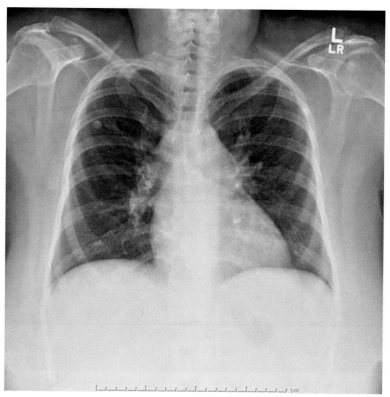

Figure 46.2   Chest radiograph (CXR) showing hilar prominence that may represent hilar/mediastinal lymphadenopathy versus pulmonary arterial dilation as seen in pulmonary hypertension.

Endobronchial ultrasound is performed in order to obtain a biopsy from the hilar lymph nodes, which demonstrates nonnecrotizing granulomas (see Fig. 46.3). Acid-fast bacilli (AFB) smear is negative, and AFB cultures are negative for TB after 6 weeks.

Diagnosis: Sarcoidosis

Why is it important to check the AFB smear and culture in this case?

The granulomas of TB tend to contain necrosis, but nonnecrotizing granulomas may also be present. A definitive diagnosis of TB requires identification of the organism by microbiologic cultures. It is important to consider TB as part of the differential diagnosis because immunosuppressive therapy (the treatment for sarcoidosis, to be discussed later) can be detrimental if initiated in a patient who actually has TB. The clinical suspicion for TB is low, but ruling this out definitively is valuable nonetheless.

What illnesses can mimic the clinical presentation of sarcoidosis?

Chronic beryllium disease is another granulomatous disease, primarily of the lung, most associated with occupational exposure. A type IV delayed hypersensitivity reaction due to beryllium

TABLE 46.2 ■ Clinical Manifestations of Sarcoidosis

The clinical presentation of various manifestations in sarcoidosis patients. Recommended workup considerations are noted for each manifestation/presentation.

Organ Involvement (Prevalence %)	Typical Presentations
Skin (15)	Lupus pernio, erythema nodosum, macules, plaques, subcutaneous nodules, scar infiltration
Ocular (10-30)	Anterior, intermediate, posterior uveitis, nodular conjunctiva, retinal vascular disease, enlarged lacrimal gland with chronic dry eyes
Pulmonary (>90)	Cough, dyspnea on exertion, and pulmonary arterial hypertension; chest imaging may reveal bilateral hilar adenopathy
Cardiac (2-5)	Conduction abnormalities, ventricular tachycardia/fibrillation, congestive heart failure, cardiac arrest due to lethal arrhythmia, palpitations, orthopnea
Liver/spleen (10-30)	Usually asymptomatic; hepatosplenomegaly, cytopenias, abnormal liver tests, cholestasis
Lofgren's syndrome	Bilateral hilar lymphadenopathy, erythema nodosum, and arthralgia
Heerfordt's syndrome	Clinical syndrome of parotitis, uveitis, fever, facial palsy
Nervous system (5)	Cranial nerve palsies, optic neuritis, peripheral neuropathy, seizures, cognitive deficits
Renal (2)	Hypercalcemia, hypercalciuria, nephrolithiasis, nephritis, renal insufficiency
Nasopharyngeal (5)	Anosmia, epistaxis
Gastrointestinal/genitourinary (GU) (1)	May involve any part of alimentary tract; generally asymptomatic; any GU organ can be involved
Peripheral lymphadenopathy (10-30)	Cervical, supraclavicular, inguinal, axillary lymphadenopathy
Skeletal muscle (1)	Muscle weakness, poor negative inspiratory force

(Adapted from Valeyre D, Prasse A, Nunes H, et al. Sarcoidosis. *Lancet.* 2014;383:1155-1167; Valeyre D, Bernaudin JF, Uzunhan Y, et al. Clinical presentation of sarcoidosis and diagnostic work-up. *Semin Respir Crit Care Med.* 2014;35[3]:336-351.)

exposure also characterizes chronic beryllium disease. The noncaseating, epithelioid granulomata found in the lung are indistinguishable histopathologically from sarcoidosis. A detailed history is essential to its diagnosis, and if uncertainty or ambiguous history is noted, then a peripheral blood beryllium lymphocyte proliferation test (BeLPT) is necessary to distinguish chronic beryllium disease from pulmonary sarcoidosis.

Common variable immunodeficiency, characterized by hypogammaglobulinemia with absent or decreased levels of specific antibody production leading to recurrent infections, also mimics sarcoidosis. Granulomatous and lymphocytic interstitial lung disease has been reported in up to 20% of patients with common variable immunodeficiency, and like sarcoidosis can involve multiple organs. Key differences include recurrent infections, autoimmunity, and extrapulmonary manifestations favoring liver and spleen in common variable immunodeficiency compared to sarcoidosis. High-resolution computed tomography (CT) scans of the lungs favor predominantly lower lobe disease with significant nodularity in common variable immunodeficiency.

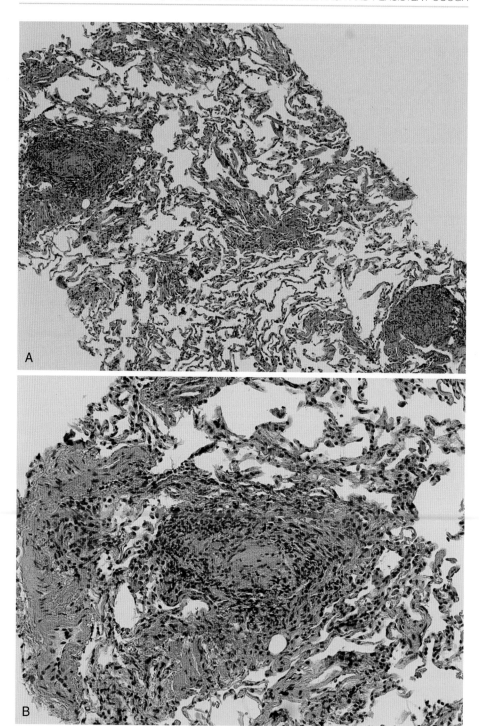

Figure 46.3 Endoscopic transbronchial lung biopsy demonstrating nonnecrotizing granulomas. **A,** Transbronchial biopsy showing nonnecrotizing granuloma *(upper left)* among the background of normal appearing lung alveolar parenchyma (10× magnification). **B,** Granuloma of multinucleated giant cells and lymphocytes (hematoxylin and eosin, 40× magnification).

TABLE 46.3 ■ **Chest Radiograph Scoring System for Sarcoidosis: Scadding Classification**

Although there is little prognostic value to stages 0 to 3, stage 4 disease is associated with poor prognosis, as fibrosis and likely severe symptomatic restrictive lung disease may be irreversible.

Scadding Classification	Findings on Chest Radiograph
Stage 0	Normal chest radiograph
Stage 1	BHL only
Stage 2	BHL and pulmonary infiltrates
Stage 3	Pulmonary infiltrates without BHL
Stage 4	Pulmonary fibrosis

BHL, Bilateral hilar lymphadenopathy.

What is the CXR scoring system for sarcoidosis?
Table 46.3 reviews the Scadding Classification, which is the scoring system for CXRs in sarcoidosis.

What are the clinical manifestations of sarcoidosis?
Sarcoidosis is a systemic, multiorgan disease characterized by the formation of noncaseating (otherwise known as nonnecrotizing) granulomas in a yet incompletely understood inflammatory process. Perhaps the most common symptom at presentation is fatigue, which may be seen in up to 80 to 90% of patients at presentation. Pulmonary involvement is also very common. However, the diagnosis is often delayed, as initial symptoms of fatigue and vague pulmonary symptoms are nonspecific and therefore patients may progress to subacute dyspnea or severe fatigue over the course of multiple office visits prior to diagnosis. Extrathoracic disease is also common and may present in a variety of ways (see Table 46.2).

Clinical manifestations of sarcoidosis include pulmonary, ocular, dermatologic, hepatic, splenic, cardiac, central and peripheral nervous system, peripheral lymphatic, renal, glandular, muscular, skeletal, nasal, and laryngeal involvement. Gastrointestinal involvement is exceedingly rare yet generally asymptomatic (see Table 46.2).

As noted, fatigue is very common, and other constitutional symptoms such as fever and weight loss have been noted in Lofgren's and Heerfordt's syndromes, in multiorgan disease, and elderly-onset disease. Aside from fatigue, pulmonary manifestations are the most common, noted in approximately 90% of cases, and include chronic cough, dyspnea on exertion, and rarely wheezing or pleuritic chest pain. Chronic dyspnea generally occurs only in late, stage 4 disease due to pulmonary fibrosis. Up to 65% of patients may have airflow limitation on pulmonary function tests (PFTs), with reduced forced vital capacity (FVC) and forced expiratory volume in 1 second (FEV1) on spirometry. However, 50% of patients may have obstructive airway disease with air-trapping, with a reduced FEV1:FVC ratio. Hyperreactive airways are also common. Diffusing capacity of the lung for carbon monoxide (DLCO) may be impaired, especially during exercise. Maximal inspiratory and expiratory respiratory pressures have also been shown to correlate with disease severity and may represent a reliable evaluation tool. Six-minute walk testing may show decreased distance that correlates with impairments on spirometry. However, PFTs with ple-thysmography are necessary to evaluate for restrictive lung disease, due to fibrosis or bronchiectasis, to determine any decrease in functional residual capacity (FRC) and total lung capacity (TLC).

Cutaneous involvement may cause significant morbidity for patients, especially in the case of scarring disease such as lupus pernio, yet the varying manifestations may be quite treatable and reversible. Generally, variants of cutaneous sarcoidosis include papular rash, plaques, lupus pernio, psoriasiform, annular, subcutaneous nodules (asymptomatic, nontender nodules felt only on palpation), and scar hypertrophy or infiltration. Erythema nodosum is a nonspecific presentation that generally portends a benign disease course with favorable prognosis, as in the case of Lofgren's syndrome. Cutaneous involvement occurs in 25 to 35% of patients.

Ocular involvement has been reported in 30 to 60% of patients with sarcoidosis. Anterior, intermediate, or posterior uveitis is common, and they may coincide as in diffuse uveitis in 10 to 15% of patients with ocular involvement. Symptoms include redness, pain, photophobia, blurred vision, and decreased vision. Although symptoms may be acute, chronic uveitis is common and can lead to eventual blindness. Vitreous opacities may develop, and surgical intervention may be warranted if topical or systemic therapies fail. Dry eyes are also common due to lacrimal gland granulomatous inflammation.

> Urine studies are obtained and show elevated 24-hour calcium excretion.

What is the significance of hypercalcemia and hypercalciuria in this patient?
Hypercalcemia and hypercalciuria are common among patients with sarcoidosis. Sarcoidosis can present as renal calculus disease. Hypercalciuria is more common, presenting in up to 50% of sarcoidosis patients, with hypercalcemia in up to 20% of patients.

BASIC SCIENCE PEARL   **STEP 1**

Activated pulmonary macrophages may produce calcitriol in sarcoidosis, as they contain 25-hydroxyvitamin D-1-alpha-hydroxylase, which converts 25-hydroxyvitamin D to 1,25-dihydroxyvitamin D (calcitriol).

Such extrarenal production of calcitriol is independent of parathyroid hormone, which should be suppressed by elevated calcium levels in peripheral blood and decrease the amount of calcitriol made in the proximal tubule of nephrons. Hypercalciuria may lead to renal calculi and subsequent renal insufficiency; therefore, all sarcoidosis patients should have a 24-hour calcium excretion measured.

What type of neurologic involvement is seen in sarcoidosis?
Neurologic involvement may include the central or peripheral nervous system. Generally less than 10% of patients present with neurologic symptoms, yet autopsy studies have shown up to 25% of patients with sarcoidosis have central nervous system involvement. In order of incidence, cranial nerve palsies (such as Bell's palsy involving cranial nerve VII), headache, ataxia, cognitive deficits, weakness, and seizures have been documented. Neurosarcoidosis is rare yet may present with profound dementia in the elderly. Some patients may present with monocular vision loss and oligoclonal bands in cerebrospinal fluid, making differentiation from multiple sclerosis difficult. Contrast-enhanced magnetic resonance imaging (MRI) is of clinical utility to evaluate neurosarcoidosis inflammatory processes and response to treatment. Bony lesions have been noted on positron emission tomography scans, yet are usually asymptomatic and may be mistaken for metastatic disease. High-resolution computed tomography (HRCT) is an essential tool in evaluating disease activity and progression in sarcoidosis. Identifying accessible hilar lymph node targets for endobronchial ultrasound biopsy and demonstrating pulmonary parenchymal inflammation or

developing fibrosis and the degree of restrictive lung disease are valuable assessments in managing sarcoidosis patients. HRCT may soon replace the Scadding Classification system for staging of sarcoidosis and has been shown to correlate well with severity of disease on both PFTs and pathology specimens, in contrast to significantly limited correlation with CXR.

CLINICAL PEARL   **STEP 2/3**

Contrast chest imaging is not necessary unless pulmonary hypertension, malignancy, or embolic disease is suspected.

CLINICAL PEARL   **STEP 2/3**

At a minimum, all patients with sarcoidosis should have a detailed history and exam with special attention to family and occupational/exposure history, CXR, PFTs with plethysmography and DLCO measurements, CBC, routine chemistry panel, liver tests, urine studies, serum protein electrophoresis (SPEP), electrocardiogram, routine ophthalmologic exam, purified protein derivative placement or interferon-gamma release assays, with regular follow-up (depending on the severity of disease).

What are the mainstays of treatment for sarcoidosis?

Treatment of sarcoidosis generally depends on disease severity and specific organ involvement. Systemic glucocorticoid therapy is the mainstay of treatment. Glucocorticoid-sparing immuno-suppressive, cytotoxic agents are becoming more commonly utilized, yet there are no established guidelines on their use at present. Table 46.4 shows various treatment regimens and considerations based on the organ systems involved, severity of disease, or intolerance to glucocorticoids.

The patient is diagnosed with sarcoidosis and is treated with high-dose glucocorticoids with good initial response. She is tapered to a dose of prednisone 5 mg daily after 6 months and followed every 2 to 3 months. However, a few months later she develops increased dyspnea on exertion and lower extremity edema.

What etiologies or organ-specific involvement of sarcoidosis may best explain her new symptoms?

The new onset progressive dyspnea and lower extremity edema suggest possible cardiac sarcoidosis or pulmonary hypertension. Pulmonary inflammation progressing to fibrosis should be considered, and HRCT of the chest is necessary. Routine transthoracic echocardiography is essential, and additional diagnostic modalities may be warranted for adequate detection of cardiac disease activity. Pulmonary hypertension is well documented in sarcoidosis due largely to fibrosis of lung parenchyma yet has also been noted in patients with normal CXR and HRCT. The latter is thought to be due to granulomatous involvement of pulmonary vasculature and hypoxic vasoconstriction effects. Cardiac catheterization is warranted if estimated right ventricular systolic pressures or pulmonary artery pressures are elevated out of proportion to left ventricular systolic dysfunction.

CLINICAL PEARL   **STEP 2/3**

Cardiac MRI or serial cardiac MRI and PET imaging have recently been evaluated with some promising results for early detection of cardiac involvement in sarcoidosis, yet they are not currently routinely employed.

TABLE 46.4 ■ Treatment Regimens for Sarcoidosis Based on Organ Involvement

Glucocorticoid sparing, cytotoxic agents include methotrexate, azathioprine, leflunomide, thalidomide, mycophenolate; may be used as indicated below or when systemic glucocorticoids are not tolerated.

Organ System	Local Therapy	Systemic Therapy
	Pulmonary	
Cough	Inhaled glucocorticoids	
Dyspnea (with pulmonary function test abnormalities)		Oral glucocorticoids Methotrexate, azathioprine, leflunomide, or mycophenolate if unable to tolerate glucocorticoids; consider TNF-alpha inhibitors or repository corticotropin injection (Acthar® Gel) if refractory disease
Pulmonary hypertension (World Health Organization class V)		Endothelin receptor antagonists, phosphodiesterase-5 inhibitors
	Skin	
Limited papules/ plaques	Topical glucocorticoids	
Papules/plaques and nodules	Intralesional triamcinolone	
Disfiguring, diffuse lesions, lupus pernio, ulcerations		Oral glucocorticoids Anti-TNF alpha or methotrexate for lupus pernio; hydroxychloroquine if patient cannot tolerate oral glucocorticoids
	Ocular	
Anterior uveitis	Ophthalmic glucocorticoids	
Posterior uveitis		Oral glucocorticoids Methotrexate, azathioprine, leflunomide, or mycophenolate if unable to tolerate glucocorticoids; consider TNF-alpha inhibitors or repository corticotropin injection (Acthar® Gel) if refractory disease
	Neurologic	
Cranial nerve palsy		Oral glucocorticoids
Neurologic deficits, seizures		Oral glucocorticoids
	Cardiac	
Congestive heart failure		Oral glucocorticoids, concurrent heart failure medications (angiotensin-converting enzyme inhibitor, beta blocker, +/− aldactone, statin, aspirin)
Complete heart block		Pacemaker
Ventricular arrhythmias		Automatic implantable cardioverter-defibrillator
	Renal	
Hypercalcemia, hypercalciuria		Oral glucocorticoids or hydroxychloroquine

TNF, Tumor necrosis factor.

(Adapted from Baughman RP, Lower EE. Medical therapy of sarcoidosis. *Semin Respir Crit Care Med.* 2014;35[3]:391-406 and Valeyre D, Prasse A, Nunes H, et al. Sarcoidosis. *Lancet.* 2014;383:1155-1167)

What is the prognosis for patients with sarcoidosis?

Prognosis of patients with sarcoidosis is variable, and there are few clinical predictors of disease persistence and severity. As previously noted, patients with Lofgren's syndrome generally have a favorable prognosis with over 80% of patients symptom free at 24 months, whereas patients with severe cutaneous manifestations, such as lupus pernio, tend to have a more chronic and progressive course. Transplantation of failed organs is possible and well studied in sarcoidosis, where lung transplant due to severe pulmonary fibrosis is most common. Furthermore, comorbid conditions and complications, such as pulmonary hypertension, dramatically worsen prognosis.

BEYOND THE PEARLS

- When presented with a CXR or chest CT with predominately upper lobe disease, the reviewer should think of sarcoidosis, TB, cystic fibrosis, ankylosing spondylitis, silicosis, and Langerhans cell histiocytosis in the differential. Lower lobe predominant disease favors bronchiectasis, chronic aspiration, drug-induced pneumonitis, asbestosis, scleroderma, collagen vascular disease, and idiopathic pulmonary fibrosis with usual interstitial pneumonia (UIP).
- Immune reconstitution during antiretroviral therapy for HIV/AIDs has been shown to result in underlying sarcoidosis that was essentially "dormant" due to helper T-cell depletion.
- Although likely to be less significant with the advent of protease inhibitor therapy for hepatitis C, prior treatment regimens containing interferon therapy for hepatitis C were reported to be associated with the onset of granulomatous disease such as sarcoidosis.
- Paradoxically, the use of TNF-alpha antagonists for treatment of Crohn's and rheumatologic disease has been shown to "unmask" sarcoidosis or sarcoidlike granulomatous disease. In such cases, higher dosing or an alternate TNF-alpha inhibitor may be effective for resolution, or the class of drug may need to be stopped altogether. Etanercept and adalimumab are most associated with sarcoidosis in this class.
- Although historically with conflicting data, there are reported statistically significant increased relative risks of malignancy in sarcoidosis; skin and hematologic malignancies have the highest relative risk (up to twofold).
- ACE levels have not been shown to be of use clinically. ACE levels have a low sensitivity and specificity, are altered by the use of ACE inhibitors, and are not prognostic of disease activity.

References

Alsalek M, Baydur A, Louie SG, Sharma OP. Respiratory muscle strength, lung function, and dyspnea in patients with sarcoidosis. *Chest.* 2001;120(1):102-108.

Baughman RP, Lower EE. Medical therapy of sarcoidosis. *Semin Respir Crit Care Med.* 2014;35(3):391-406.

Baydur A, Alavy B, Nawathe A, et al. Fatigue and plasma cytokine concentrations at rest and during exercise in patients with sarcoidosis. *Clin Respir J.* 2011;5:156-164.

Bonifazi M, Bravi F, Gasparini S, et al. Sarcoidosis and cancer risk. *Chest.* 2015;147(3):778-791.

Craido E, Sanchez M, Ramirez J, et al. Pulmonary sarcoidosis: typical and atypical manifestations at high resolution CT with pathologic correlation. *Radiographics.* 2010;30(6):1567-1586.

Gobel U, Kettritz R, Schneider W, Luft FC. The protean face of renal sarcoidosis. *J Am Soc Nephrol.* 2001;12:616-623.

Goldberg HJ, Fiedler DF, Webb A, et al. Sarcoidosis after treatment with interferon-alpha: a case series and review of the literature. *Respir Med.* 2006;100:2063-2068.

Haimovic A, Sanchez M, Judson MA, Prystowsky S. Sarcoidosis: a comprehensive review and update for the dermatologist: part I. Cutaneous disease. *J Am Acad Dermatol.* 2012;66(5):699, e1-e18.

Iannuzzi MC, Rybicki BA, Teirstein AS. Sarcoidosis. *N Engl J Med.* 2007;357(21):2153-2165.

Kojima K, Maruyama K, Inaba T, et al. The CD4/CD8 ratio in vitreous fluid is of high diagnostic value in sarcoidosis. *Ophthalmology*. 2012;119(11):2386-2392.

Lynch JP III, Hwang J, Bradfield J, et al. Cardiac involvement in sarcoidosis: evolving concepts in diagnosis and treatment. *Semin Respir Crit Care Med*. 2014;35(3):372-390.

Marcellis RGJ, Lenssen AF, Kleynen S, De Vries J, Drent M. Exercise capacity, muscle strength and fatigue in sarcoidosis: a follow up study. *Lung*. 2013;191:247-256.

Mayer AS, Hamzeh N, Maier LA. Sarcoidosis and chronic beryllium disease: similarities and differences. *Semin Respir Crit Care Med*. 2014;35(3):316-329.

Morris DG, Jasmer RM, Huang L, et al. Sarcoidosis following HIV infection. *Chest*. 2003;124:929-935.

Ors F, Gumus S, Aydogon M, et al. HRCT finding of pulmonary sarcoidosis; relation to pulmonary function tests. *Multidiscip Respir Med*. 2013;8:8.

Shino MY, Lynch JP III, Fishbein MC, et al. Sarcoidosis-associated pulmonary hypertension and lung transplantation for sarcoidosis. *Semin Respir Crit Care Med*. 2014;35(3):362-371.

Valeyre D, Bernaudin JF, Uzunhan Y, et al. Clinical presentation of sarcoidosis and diagnostic work-up. *Semin Respir Crit Care Med*. 2014;35(3):336-351.

Valeyre D, Prasse A, Nunes H, et al. Sarcoidosis. *Lancet*. 2014;383:1155-1167.

Verbsky JW, Routes JM. Sarcoidosis and common variable immunodeficiency: similarities and differences. *Semin Respir Crit Care Med*. 2014;35(3):330-335.

Wendling D, Prati C. Paradoxical effects of anti-TNF-alpha agents in inflammatory diseases. *Expert Rev Clin Immunol*. 2014;10(1):159-169.

Wijnen PA, Cremers JP, Nelemans PJ, et al. Association of the TNF-alpha G-308A polymorphism with TNF-inhibitor response in sarcoidosis. *Eur Respir J*. 2014;43:1730-1739.

Zissel G. Cellular activation in the immune response of sarcoidosis. *Semin Respir Crit Care Med*. 2014;35(3):307-315.

Dawn Piarulli ■ R. Michelle Koolaee

A 63-Year-Old Male With Acute Polyarticular Arthritis

A 63-year-old male with a past medical history significant for obesity, type 2 diabetes, hypertension, hyperlipidemia, chronic kidney disease (CKD), and heart failure is admitted with an episode of acute decompensated systolic heart failure. His home medications include lisinopril, carvedilol, aspirin, atorvastatin, hydrochlorothiazide, and sitagliptin. He is treated with aggressive intravenous (IV) diuresis with furosemide. Three days into his admission he begins to complain of severe bilateral wrist, elbow, and right knee pain. On exam, he is febrile to 38.22 °C (100.8 °F). His cardiopulmonary exam is significant for an S3 heart sound, bibasilar crackles, and pitting pedal edema of the lower extremities bilaterally. Musculoskeletal exam reveals tenderness and swelling of the wrists and elbows; there is a moderate effusion in the right knee with associated warmth and tenderness. There are nodules on the extensor surface of the right 3rd and 5th metacarpophalangeal (MCP) joints, as well as both olecranon bursae.

What is the differential diagnosis for this patient's joint pain?
This is a patient presenting with an acute polyarticular inflammatory arthritis. The causes of polyarticular arthritis include but are not limited to:
- Viral infection (especially parvovirus B19 but also hepatitis B/C and human immunodeficiency virus [HIV] among others)
- Reactive arthritis (i.e., *Chlamydia trachomatis, Yersinia, Salmonella, Shigella, Campylobacter, Escherichia coli, Clostridium difficile,* and *Chlamydia pneumonia*)
- Bacterial arthritis (i.e., *Neisseria gonorrhoeae* [gonorrhea], poststreptococcal arthritis, *Staphylococcus aureus*)
- Other infections (i.e., tubercular and fungal organisms, *Borrelia burgdorferi* [Lyme disease])
- Crystal-induced arthritis (i.e., gout, pseudogout, calcium oxalate, hydroxyapatite)
- Systemic rheumatic disease (i.e., rheumatoid arthritis [RA], systemic lupus erythematosus [SLE], Sjögren's syndrome, inflammatory myositis)
- Systemic vasculitis
- Spondyloarthropathies (i.e., psoriatic arthritis, ankylosing spondylitis, inflammatory bowel disease–related arthritis, reactive arthritis)
- Endocrinopathies (i.e., hyperparathyroidism, hyperthyroidism, hypothyroidism)
- Malignancy (metastatic cancer, multiple myeloma)

The acuity of his symptoms makes causes such as crystal-induced arthritis very likely (especially gout, given his comorbidities, along with use of diuretics; calcium oxalate crystals is less common but is seen exclusively in patients with CKD). An infectious arthritis is also possible, given the acuity of the symptom. A systemic rheumatic illness is unlikely; these tend to present with chronic inflammatory arthritis.

How does the physical exam in this case help to narrow the differential diagnosis?

This patient has multiple nodules of the extensor surfaces of his joints. The differential diagnosis of nodules includes xanthoma (history of hyperlipidemia), rheumatoid nodules (multiple joints involved), sarcoidosis (usually located on the lower rather than upper extremities), tumors (less likely to be present in multiple locations superficially), and tophi (which are due to deposition of monosodium urate crystals in and about the joints of a gout patient). Given the location of the nodules, along with the acuity of his arthritic symptoms, his nodules likely represent tophi (nodules in RA and sarcoidosis would be associated with a chronic inflammatory arthritis). Figure 47.1 represents examples of gouty tophi.

CLINICAL PEARL   **STEP 2/3**

It is far more common to see tophi in the olecranon bursae than on the ears.

CLINICAL PEARL   **STEP 2/3**

Fevers are not specific for an infectious arthritis; in fact, it is not common for patients with crystal-induced arthritis to also present with fevers.

Furthermore, based on his comorbidities (obesity, type 2 diabetes, CKD, and hypertension; all of which are associated with gout), likely tophi in the elbows, and the onset of symptoms during hospitalization for diuretic therapy, the most likely diagnosis is acute polyarticular gout. Table 47.1 highlights the common risk factors for gout flares.

What is the single best test to help determine the diagnosis?

The best way to determine the etiology of any arthritis with effusion is arthrocentesis. Synovial fluid analysis is a valuable tool to help in the diagnostic workup.

CLINICAL PEARL   **STEP 2/3**

A diagnosis of gout can never be made based on the uric acid level alone. Furthermore, the uric acid level does not correlate with the severity of the gout flare (some patients have severe polyarticular flares with only modest elevation in the serum uric acid).

Laboratory tests reveal a serum creatinine of 1.5 mg/dL (at baseline) and uric acid level of 9.6 mg/dL. 15 mL of straw-colored synovial fluid is aspirated from the patient's right knee. Synovial fluid leukocyte count is 42,000/μL ([42 × 10^9/L], 82% polymorphonuclear cells). Polarized light microscopy reveals several needle-shaped, negatively birefringent crystals. Gram stain and cultures are negative.

Diagnosis: Acute polyarticular gout flare

CLINICAL PEARL   **STEP 2/3**

You should be able to read newspaper print if it is placed behind a sample of normal synovial fluid. The more inflammatory the fluid becomes, the cloudier it will be, and the more difficult it will be to read the print.

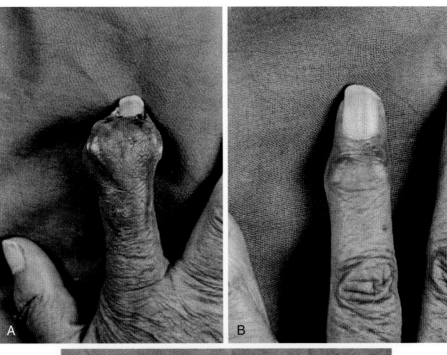

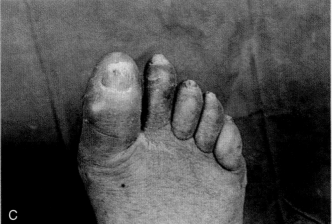

Figure 47.1 **A,** Ulcerating tophus of the right index finger. **B,** Tophi along the fourth distal interphalangeal joint of the left hand. **C,** Tophus along the interphalangeal joint of the right hallux. *(From van der Klooster JM, Peters R, Burgmans JPJ, Grootendorst AF. Chronic tophaceous gout in the elderly. Netherlands J Med. 1998;53[2]:69-75.)*

CLINICAL PEARL   **STEP 2/3**

Only one drop of fluid is need for crystal analysis using polarized light microscopy (more fluid is necessary for cell count and fluid culture).

TABLE 47.1 ■ Risk Factors for Gout Flare

- Trauma
- Surgery
- Starvation
- Purine-rich animal-based foods (red meat and seafood especially)
- Alcohol (beer and spirits)
- Dehydration
- Diuretics (thiazide due to decreased uric acid excretion) and loop diuretics (due to fluid shifts/dehydration)
- Hyperuricemia
- Aspirin
- Many drugs, especially posttransplant medications (i.e., cyclosporine)

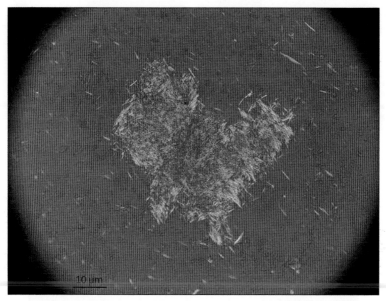

Figure 47.2   Compensated polarized microscopy of numerous negatively birefringent, needle-shaped monosodium urate crystals. *(From Richette P, Bardin T. Gout.* Lancet. *2010;375[9711]:318-328.)*

How do you interpret the synovial fluid analysis results?

The leukocyte count above 2,000/mm^3 confirms the presence of inflammatory fluid.

Figure 47.2 demonstrates monosodium urate (MSU) crystals, which have the characteristic needle-shaped appearance and are negatively birefringent on polarized light microscopy; this is the definitive way to diagnose gout. Septic arthritis can rarely occur simultaneously as an acute gout flare, but the leukocyte count is usually over 50,000/mm^3. Table 47.2 compares synovial fluid findings in patients with inflammatory versus noninflammatory arthritis.

See Table 47.3 for a summary of risk factors for septic arthritis. Although this patient has type 2 diabetes and gout, both risk factors for septic arthritis, this diagnosis would be highly unlikely given that he presented with a polyarticular arthritis (bacterial septic arthritis usually presents as a monoarticular arthritis).

TABLE 47.2 ▓ **Synovial Fluid Analysis**

Specimen	Normal	Noninflammatory*	Inflammatory	Septic
Clarity	Transparent	Transparent	Translucent/cloudy	Cloudy
Color	Slightly yellow	Yellow	Yellow to opalescent	Yellow to green
White blood cell, per mm^3	<200	200-2000	2000-100,000	15,000† >100,000
Polymorphonuclear leukocytes %	<25	<25	≥50	≥75
Culture	(−)	(−)	(−)	Often (+)

*Noninflammatory fluid is commonly seen in effusions due to osteoarthritis.
†Lower numbers can occur among immunosuppressed patients, those with partially treated infections, or during infection with low virulence organisms.

TABLE 47.3 ▓ **Risks Factors for Septic Arthritis**

- Age >80
- Diabetes
- Rheumatoid arthritis
- Prosthetic joint
- Recent joint surgery
- Joint glucocorticoid injection or instrumentation in general
- Bacteremia (skin infections, ulcers, endocarditis, recent dental work, etc.)
- Intravenous drug use
- History of gout or pseudogout
- Prior trauma to joint

CLINICAL PEARL   **STEP 2/3**

Synovial fluid should be analyzed for cell count very soon after aspiration, as the leukocyte count will be artificially reduced the longer one waits. Also, when interpreting the synovial fluid cell count, note whether the patient received glucocorticoids prior to aspiration; this may also decrease the leukocyte count and lead to inaccurate results.

What are the treatment options for this patient with acute gout?

In general, the treatment options for attacks of acute gouty arthritis include nonsteroidal antiinflammatory drugs (NSAIDs), intraarticular glucocorticoid injections, systemic glucocorticoids, and colchicine. Agents that inhibit interleukin-1 (IL-1) have shown some benefit in treating acute flares, with a role in patients with contraindications to traditional therapeutic measures.

BASIC SCIENCE PEARL   **STEP 1**

Colchicine inhibits cell mitosis by inhibiting microtubule polymerization. It binds to tubulin (one of the main constituents of microtubules), thereby rendering the microtubule inactive. Colchicine also inhibits neutrophil motility and activity, which leads to an overall antiinflammatory effect.

BASIC SCIENCE PEARL	STEP 1

The inflammasome is a multiprotein oligomer that promotes inflammation through release of IL-1. The NOD-like receptor family, pyrin domain containing 3 (NLRP3) inflammasome, represents a subset of proteins that promote the release of IL-1. MSU crystals activate the NLRP3 inflammasome in macrophages, leading to the production of IL-1β. This is why IL-1 inhibitors are used to decrease inflammation in very select cases of acute gout.

This patient has CKD, which makes the use of NSAIDs less desirable. Because the patient has type 2 diabetes, systemic glucocorticoids may not be the best option for his polyarticular flare (they are not an absolute contraindication though and can still be given in someone whose blood glucose levels are not dramatically elevated with glucocorticoids). Colchicine, which may be used carefully in patients with renal impairment, is reasonable to consider. Colchicine is also an excellent abortive agent, which when taken at the first sign of a gout attack can often modulate the inflammatory response and help resolve the symptoms of attack faster than if no treatment is given. Although an intraarticular glucocorticoid injection is the preferred treatment for a monoarticular gout attack, it is less favorable in oligoarticular or polyarticular gout due to the need for multiple injections.

The patient's flare improves with the use of low-dose colchicine for several days, his heart failure is treated, and he is discharged home. Upon further questioning, the hospitalist notes that he has had several prior distinct episodes of pain and joint swelling for which he had not sought medical attention prior to the current admission. He has had three prior episodes this year alone. He is counseled on reducing his alcohol intake and decreasing his red meat and shellfish consumption. His hydrochlorothiazide is switched to a calcium channel blocker upon discharge to avoid aggravating his gout. He presents to his primary care physician 1 month after discharge feeling well with complete resolution of the flare. His laboratory tests reveal a serum creatinine of 1.3 mg/dL and uric acid of 9.1 mg/dL.

What drug would you start for this patient?

The patient has hyperuricemia with multiple distinct episodes of painful joint swelling consistent with attacks of gout (he has what rheumatologists refer to as "crystal proven gout"). It is a clinical judgment when to initiate chronic uric acid–lowering therapy, but it is reasonable to consider in someone who has had two or more attacks in a year. Allopurinol is the initial choice in most cases; it is best to start at a low dose and titrate gradually to higher doses, while checking uric acid levels prior to each dose adjustment. Allopurinol inhibits xanthine oxidase, the enzyme responsible for the conversion of hypoxanthine to xanthine to uric acid; it acts on purine catabolism, reducing the production of uric acid without disrupting the biosynthesis of vital purines.

CLINICAL PEARL	STEP 2/3

Probenecid is not frequently prescribed in recent years due to its multiple-daily dosing regimen, contraindication in patients with nephrolithiasis (it increases urinary calcium excretion in patients with gout), and frequent gastrointestinal upset.

How should allopurinol therapy be monitored and what is the goal of therapy?

The usual goal is to reduce the serum uric acid level to below 6 mg/dL (and often lower than 6 mg/dL in patients with tophi, as in this case). This can be achieved by gradually increasing the allopurinol dose while checking uric acid levels prior to each office visit.

CLINICAL PEARL	STEP 2/3

When up-titrating the allopurinol dose, the repeat uric acid level can be rechecked as early as 1 week after the allopurinol dose has been increased.

The 6 mg/dL number was derived from studies of uric acid solubility. Uric acid crystalizes at a serum concentration of approximately 6.5 mg/dL. As such, it was decided that a uric acid goal of <6 mg/dL would be reasonable to prevent precipitation of uric acid into the crystal form and maintain it in the liquid state. Of note, as a patient is started on allopurinol and uric acid stores are in flux, acute episodes of gout can and often do occur. This is why most patients are on a low dose of colchicine (with reduced doses for moderate to severe renal impairment) until the uric acid level is at goal. Once at goal, colchicine is stopped, and maintenance includes the uric acid–lowering therapy (i.e., allopurinol) alone.

BASIC SCIENCE PEARL	STEP 1

Lesch-Nyhan syndrome is an X-linked disorder caused by an inborn error in purine metabolism, which results from deficiency of hypoxanthine-guanine phosphoribosyltransferase (HGPRT). The patients have hyperuricemia, poor muscular control, intellectual disability, and a very striking manifestation of self-mutilating behavior.

CLINICAL PEARL	STEP 2/3

Any abrupt increase or decrease in the serum uric acid level can precipitate or worsen a gout flare. That is why when a patient presents with a gout flare and is already on allopurinol, the allopurinol should not be stopped (and by the same token, allopurinol should not be first started during an acute flare).

What are the safety concerns with allopurinol?

Allopurinol is associated with a number of hypersensitivity reactions (some of which can be severe), particularly in patients with CKD or end-stage renal disease (ESRD). For this reason, many clinicians mistakenly believe allopurinol is nephrotoxic, when in fact nephrotoxicity (in the form of an interstitial nephritis) is exceedingly rare. In patients with decreased ability to excrete the compound (which is renally cleared), allopurinol can increase the chances of these hypersensitivity reactions. These are reactions that vary from a rash to more severe reactions like drug reaction with eosinophilia and systemic symptoms (DRESS; this is potentially life threatening) and Stevens-Johnson syndrome. As such, it is the authors' preference to stop allopurinol in anyone who develops even an isolated rash from the drug.

The patient is started on allopurinol 100 mg daily and colchicine 0.6 mg daily; allopurinol is titrated to a dose of 300 mg daily after 2 months. His uric acid level lowers to 7.2 mg/dL (which is not at the goal of <6 mg/dL) and he continues to have periodic flares. His allopurinol is increased to 400 mg daily, and 2 weeks later the patient presents with a rash and malaise. Allopurinol is discontinued.

What is another treatment option in this patient?

Febuxostat is also a xanthine oxidase inhibitor and (with caution) is useful in patients who have hypersensitivity to allopurinol, who do not achieve the uric acid goal with allopurinol, and/or who have moderate renal insufficiency (there is no dose adjustment for those with a creatinine

TABLE 47.4 ■ Comparison of Allopurinol to Febuxostat

	Allopurinol	Febuxostat
Mechanism	Xanthine oxidase inhibitor	Xanthine oxidase inhibitor
Dosing (Oral)	Start at 50-100 mg and titrate up to 800 mg daily	Fixed at 40 mg and 80 mg daily
Renal Impairment	Titrate cautiously in patients with CKD (increased risk of hypersensitivity reactions); not a contraindication in CKD	No dose adjustment CrCl ≥30: not studied with CrCl <30
Cost	Inexpensive	Very expensive
Adverse Reactions	Hypersensitivity reactions (some severe), nausea, rash	Hypersensitivity reactions (some severe), liver function test abnormalities, thromboembolic events

CKD, Chronic kidney disease; CrCl, creatinine clearance.

clearance [CrCl] of ≥30 mL/min). Febuxostat is much more expensive than allopurinol, which is why it is not a first-line option for therapy. Table 47.4 highlights some main differences between the two xanthine oxidase inhibitors.

CLINICAL PEARL   **STEP 2/3**

Patients need to stay on uric acid–lowering therapy (i.e., allopurinol) indefinitely; do not let patients stop their allopurinol even if they have had no flares for years. Their gout flares will inevitably return if you do.

The patient is started on febuxostat 40 mg daily along with colchicine 0.6 mg daily. After several months his gout attacks stop, his tophi shrink, and his uric acid lowers to 5.2 mg/dL. His febuxostat is continued indefinitely and his colchicine is stopped.

What are other crystals that can cause arthritis?

Calcium pyrophosphate (CPPD) crystals can lead to flares of pseudogout. This is usually a monoarthritis (the knee is very common) but can also be oligoarticular or polyarticular; older age is strongly associated with pseudogout. These crystals are weakly positively birefringent, rhomboid-shaped, and are often more difficult to visualize on polarized microscopy than MSU crystals. Radiographs may reveal chondrocalcinosis, which is due to deposition of CPPD crystals. Conditions associated with CPPD disease include hyperparathyroidism, hemochromatosis, hypophosphatemia, hypomagnesemia, Gitelman syndrome, hypothyroidism, gout, x-linked hypophosphatemic rickets, familial hypocalciuric hypercalcemia, and hemosiderosis. Figure 47.3 shows the appearance of CPPD crystals under polarized microscopy.

Uncommonly seen are calcium oxalate crystals, which cause arthritis in patients with ESRD on dialysis. Also less frequently seen are basic calcium phosphate (hydroxyapatite) crystals, which are characterized by large effusions with hemorrhagic, noninflammatory synovial fluid. These can cause joint destruction and are the crystals associated with the Milwaukee shoulder syndrome. Both of these crystals are difficult to visualize and require a special stain (an Alizarin red stain) to be seen.

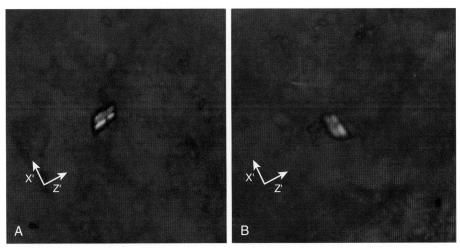

**Figure 47.3   Calcium pyrophosphate (CPPD) crystal appears rhomboid-shaped with positive birefrin-
gence. A,** When the long axis of the crystal is parallel to the Z′ axis (parallel to the axis of the compensator),
the color of the crystal is blue. **B,** When the long axis of the crystal is parallel to the X′ axis (perpendicular
to the axis of the compensator), the color of the crystal is yellow. *(Ryu K, Iriuchishima T, Oshida M, et al.
The prevalence of and factors related to calcium pyrophosphate dihydrate crystal deposition in the knee
joint.* Osteoarthritis Cartilage. *2014;22[7]:975-979.)*

BEYOND THE PEARLS

- Colchicine is a rare cause of myopathy, usually in patients with renal insufficiency.
- Hyperuricemia is an independent risk factor for coronary artery disease.
- Allopurinol should be avoided in patients on azathioprine. The combination of the two
  can cause life-threatening bone marrow suppression. Concomitant use requires
  extremely close monitoring and dose reduction of azathioprine by at least 25% of the
  recommended dose.
- Allopurinol can be safely up-titrated to a dose of 800 mg per day in patients with normal
  renal function despite the myth that the maximum dose should be 300 mg per day.
- The goal serum urate for tophaceous gout is 4 to 5 mg/dL as opposed to the goal of
  6 mg/dL for typical gout.
- Milwaukee shoulder syndrome is a rare destructive crystal arthritis manifestation that
  usually occurs in elderly females after a recent trauma to the affected joint. The crystal is
  basic calcium phosphate.
- Pegloticase (Krystexxa®) is recombinant uricase and is approved to treat severe,
  tophaceous gout. The mechanism of action is reduction of urate to allantoin (which is
  much more soluble), thereby decreasing the chances of crystal formation. Pegloticase is
  similar in mechanism of action to rasburicase (approved for tumor lysis syndrome); it is
  PEGylated however, and so its half-life is increased from 8 hours to 10 to 12 days.
- When conventional therapy fails or is contraindicated, IL-1 inhibitors can be used in
  severe gout (although they are not FDA (U.S. Food and Drug Administration) approved
  for this indication). These agents include anakinra (daily subcutaneous [SQ] injection),
  rilonacept (weekly SQ injection), and canakinumab (SQ injection every 8 weeks).
- On December 22, 2015, the FDA approved lesinurad, a new oral agent to treat
  hyperuricemia associated with gout. Lesinurad is a urate anion exchanger 1 (URAT1)
  inhibitor. URAT1 is a protein localized to the membrane of the renal proximal tubular
  cells and mediates the reabsorption of uric acid (thereby regulating blood uric acid
  concentrations).

References

Baker D, Schumacher HR. Acute monoarthritis. *N Engl J Med*. 1993;329(14):1013-1020.

Kashina AS, Rogers GC, Scholey JM. The bimC family of kinesins: essential bipolar mitotic motors driving centrosome separation. *Biochim Biophys Acta*. 1997;1357(3):257-271.

Li-Yu J, Clayburne G, Sieck M, et al. Treatment of chronic gout. Can we determine when urate stores are depleted enough to prevent attacks of gout? *J Rheumatol*. 2001;28:577-580.

Puig JG, Torres RJ, Mateos FA, et al. The spectrum of hypoxanthine-guanine phosphoribosyltransferase (HPRT) deficiency. Clinical experience based on 22 patients from 18 Spanish families. *Medicine (Baltimore)*. 2001;80(2):102.

Richette P, Bardin Y. Gout. *Lancet*. 2010;375(9711):23-29, 318-328.

Ryu K, Iriuchishima T, Oshida M, et al. The prevalence of and factors related to calcium pyrophosphate dihydrate crystal deposition in the knee joint. *Osteoarthritis Cartilage*. 2014;22(7):975-979.

Sholter D, Russell A. Synovial fluid analysis. Up-To-Date. 2013. Available at <www.uptodate.com>. Accessed 25.05.15.

van der Klooster JM, Peters R, Burgmans JPJ, Grootendorst AF. Chronic tophaceous gout in the elderly. *Neth J Med*. 1998;53(2):69-75.

CASE 48

Patrick E. Sarte ■ Seth Politano ■ Eric Hsieh

A 67-Year-Old Male With Syncope

A 67-year-old male presents with a complaint of syncope after carrying a bag of groceries up a flight of stairs. He has a 20-year history of hypertension and has an 80-pack-year smoking history. He had a heart attack 7 years ago and has been medically managed with enalapril and simvastatin daily.

What are the considerations for the differential diagnosis of this patient's presenting symptom?

In a patient presenting with syncope, one can divide up the etiology into broad categories, of which the majority are cardiac and neurologic in origin. However, as can be seen in Table 48.1, other causes include pulmonary, vascular, and even psychiatric.

On physical exam, the patient's blood pressure is 160/96 mm Hg, pulse rate is 84/min, respiration rate is 14/min, and oxygen saturation is 100% on room air. There are no orthostatic changes in blood pressure or pulse. The patient is alert and without pallor. Lungs are clear to auscultation bilaterally. The cardiac exam reveals a nondisplaced apical impulse. There is a crescendo–decrescendo systolic murmur heard best in the aortic area with radiation to the carotids. The intensity of the murmur decreases with the Valsalva maneuver. There is no lower extremity edema or cyanosis, and capillary refill is less than 2 seconds. The neurologic exam is grossly normal, with no motor or sensory deficits.

Given this physical exam, what do you think is the most likely cause of this patient's syncope?

The presence of a murmur on cardiac exam suggests a cardiac etiology, particularly a valvular disorder. In addition to the patient's age, the description and location of the murmur are most consistent with aortic stenosis. A definitive diagnosis is established with echocardiogram.

CLINICAL PEARL   **STEP 2/3**

Aortic sclerosis is thickening of the valve causing turbulent flow but no stenosis. The murmur may be similar to that of aortic stenosis but without radiation to the carotids or supraclavicular area. Similarly, a flow murmur (in a hyperdynamic state such as thyrotoxicosis, infection, or anemia) can be a systolic murmur similar to aortic stenosis but without the characteristic crescendo–decrescendo pattern or radiation.

407

TABLE 48.1 ▮ **Causes of Syncope**

Cardiac	Arrhythmias
	Ischemia
	Valvular disease
	Pericardial disease
	Heart failure
	Hypertrophic obstructive cardiomyopathy
Vascular	Subclavian steal syndrome
	Vasculitis
	Pulmonary embolism
	Aortic dissection
Neurologic	Cerebrovascular accident
	Autonomic neuropathy
	Carotid sinus sensitivity
	Multisystem atrophy
	Situational syncope
	Vasovagal syncope
Other	Dehydration/orthostasis
	Anemia
	Hypoglycemia
	Hypothyroidism
	Hypoxia
	Psychological disorders
	Drug-induced/intoxication

What are the physical exam findings of aortic stenosis?

Aortic stenosis classically has a systolic ejection murmur with a crescendo–decrescendo quality heard best in the aortic area (i.e., the right second intercostal space) with radiation to the carotids. When severe, there is a characteristic delay and decrease in the intensity of the pulse, which is also referred to as *pulsus tardus et parvus*. Patients may also have an audible S4 and laterally displaced point of maximal cardiac impulse because they develop concentric left ventricular hypertrophy as a compensatory response by the left ventricle to pump blood across a stenotic aortic valve to maintain systemic perfusion pressures. The patient may likewise have the same physical findings of congestive heart failure such as elevated jugular venous distension, bibasilar rales on pulmonary auscultation, and/or lower extremity pitting edema in advanced cases of aortic stenosis.

BASIC SCIENCE PEARL	STEP 1

Other auscultatory findings for aortic stenosis include a soft or absent S2.

BASIC SCIENCE/CLINICAL PEARL	STEP 1/2/3

The grade of the murmur does not reflect the severity of the stenosis. However, severe aortic stenosis may present with a delayed S2 or reversed split S2 (P2 precedes A2).

What maneuvers are performed to accentuate or diminish the murmur associated with aortic stenosis, and why do they have that effect?

The typical maneuvers that are performed and that affect the murmurs of valvular disorders are the Valsalva maneuver, passive leg raise, and hand grip (Table 48.2). The Valsalva maneuver is

TABLE 48.2 ■ **Effect of Maneuvers on the Murmur of Aortic Stenosis and Hypertrophic Obstructive Cardiomyopathy**

	Valsalva Maneuver	Passive Leg Raise	Hand Grip
Aortic Valve Stenosis	Decreases intensity	Increases intensity	Decreases intensity
Hypertrophic Obstructive Cardiomyopathy	Increases intensity	Decreases intensity	Decreases intensity

performed by asking the patient to bear down, which causes an increase in intrathoracic pressure and thus a decrease in venous return. The passive leg raise is performed by the examiner on the patient in the supine position, and this results in an increase in venous return. The hand grip is performed by the patient, and this causes an increase in afterload. During a Valsalva maneuver, as the venous return decreases, the gradient across the stenotic aortic valve also decreases, and thus the magnitude of the murmur decreases as well. The opposite effect on the aortic stenosis murmur is achieved when a passive leg raise is performed, which increases the venous return to the heart and increases the pressure gradient across the stenotic aortic valve. Finally, as mentioned above, the hand grip leads to an increase in afterload, which causes a decrease in the pressure gradient across the stenosed aortic valve, and this results in a diminishment of murmur intensity.

CLINICAL PEARL   **STEP 2/3**

Hypertrophic obstructive cardiomyopathy (also known as idiopathic hypertrophic subaortic stenosis) can present with the same type of murmur as aortic stenosis. However, the Valsalva maneuver and passive leg raising have the opposite effect on the murmur, whereas performing the hand grip has the same effect on the murmur for both aortic stenosis and hypertrophic obstructive cardiomyopathy. These maneuvers can clinically distinguish a murmur due to subaortic stenosis from that due to stenosis of the aortic valve. Because the stenosis in hypertrophic obstructive cardiomyopathy is subaortic, a decrease in venous return due to the Valsalva maneuver narrows the left ventricular outflow tract by the hypertrophied interventricular muscle wall and accentuates the murmur. An increase in venous return from a passive leg raise opens up the left ventricular outflow tract and diminishes this murmur. The effect of an increase in afterload as the result of the hand grip maneuver has the same effect on the pressure gradient and murmur in both types of stenoses because this effect is downstream from both stenoses.

This patient presents with syncope. What are other presenting symptoms of aortic stenosis, and what are their implications on prognosis?
As with any valvular disorder, patients can present with shortness of breath or dyspnea on exertion, and many patients may be asymptomatic until stenosis of the aortic valve progresses to a severity that poses a significant obstruction to left ventricular outflow (Fig. 48.1). If aortic stenosis is discovered incidentally before symptoms develop, patients have a survival similar to that of the general population. However, if the patient presents with angina, syncope, or heart failure, these patients have a mean survival of less than 5 years, 3 years, or 1 to 2 years, respectively, if no valvular replacement is undertaken. (**ASH** is a helpful mnemonic to remember this.)

Why do these symptoms develop in aortic stenosis?
Angina occurs when oxygen demand is greater than the supply. Aortic stenosis causes angina because there is an increase in oxygen demand by a hypertrophied left ventricle that must work

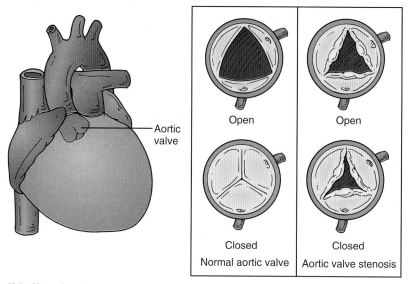

Figure 48.1 Normal aortic valve and aortic valve stenosis. With aortic valve stenosis, because the valve does not open as wide, the heart must work harder to pump blood through the valve. *(From Cribier A. Development of transcatheter aortic valve implantation [TAVI]: a heart-warming adventure.* Europ Geriat Med. *2013;4[6]:401-406.)*

harder to generate forward blood flow through a stenotic aortic valve (Fig. 48.2). Furthermore, this demand is not met by diminished blood flow through the coronary arteries due to lower pressures generated beyond a stenosed aortic valve. Because blood pressures beyond a stenotic valve are lower, cerebral perfusion may be compromised and cause syncope. This occurs especially during physical exertion because exercise causes a drop in total peripheral resistance, and the stenotic aortic valve limits the ability of the heart to compensate with an increase in cardiac output. Both systolic and diastolic heart failure can ensue after long-standing aortic stenosis. As aortic stenosis progresses, the left ventricle is not able to generate an adequate ejection fraction due to the worsening outlet obstruction, and the hypertrophied left ventricle is also less capable of generating a contractile force sufficient to move blood forward. In addition to decreasing the chamber size of the left ventricle, the hypertrophied walls of the left ventricle become stiff and less compliant. These physical features lead to poor left ventricular filling and hence diastolic dysfunction.

BASIC SCIENCE PEARL   **STEP 1**

Another mechanism for syncope in patients with aortic stenosis is increased baroreceptor stimulation due to pressure overload. This response causes reflex vasodilation and bradycardia.

What causes aortic stenosis, and what are the risk factors?

Aortic stenosis usually develops in the seventh decade of life as a result of calcification and inflammation of the endothelial surface of an otherwise normal aortic valve in a similar manner to how plaques form in the walls of coronary arteries of patients who have coronary artery disease. Therefore, the risk factors of advanced age, hypertension, hyperlipidemia, and tobacco use are

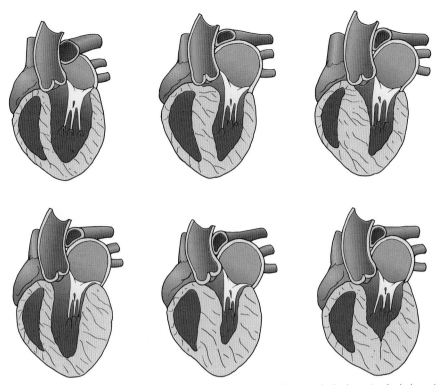

Figure 48.2 Schematic representation of the variable distribution of left ventricular hypertrophy in hypertrophic cardiomyopathy. The upper left is the normal heart for comparison. *(From Ommen SR. Hypertrophic cardiomyopathy. Curr Probl Cardiol. 2011;36[11]:409-453.)*

the same for both diseases. Furthermore, patients who develop aortic stenosis usually have a concomitant coronary artery disease.

Bicuspid aortic valves are the most common congenital cardiac abnormality and occur in approximately 1% of the population (Fig. 48.3). They are often associated with coarctation of the aorta (about 50% of cases of coarctation of the aorta have a bicuspid aortic valve) and Turner syndrome. Bicuspid aortic valves by themselves do not compromise hemodynamic flow, but they are predisposed to earlier degeneration and calcification. Aortic stenosis usually develops in patients with bicuspid aortic valves about 20 years earlier than would occur in patients with otherwise normal tricuspid aortic valves.

Rheumatic heart disease as a late complication of *Streptococcal* pharyngitis, due to group A beta-hemolytic *Streptococcal* infection such as from *S. pyogenes*, is a rare cause of aortic stenosis.

How is aortic stenosis confirmed?

The confirmatory diagnostic test of choice is echocardiography. The echocardiogram can visualize the valves and measure the aortic valve area directly as well as determine the gradient across the valve by measurement of Doppler flow. This is used in grading the severity of the disease. Other tests that have low sensitivity and specificity for determining whether a patient has aortic stenosis are electrocardiography and chest radiograph (CXR). The electrocardiogram (ECG) might show voltage criteria for left ventricular hypertrophy and possibly demonstrate left atrial enlargement.

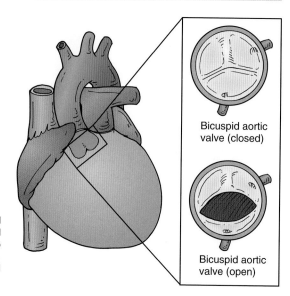

Bicuspid aortic valve (closed)

Bicuspid aortic valve (open)

Figure 48.3   Schematic of the bicuspid aortic valve. Depicted is the abnormal bicuspid valve. Figure illustration by Rob Flewell. *(From Siu SC, Silversides CK. Bicuspid aortic valve disease.* J Amer Coll Cardiol. *2010;55[25]:2789-2800.)*

The CXR might show calcifications at the aortic valve, atherosclerotic changes of the aortic arch and aortic valve annulus, or an enlarged cardiac silhouette. Despite these nonspecific findings on ECG or CXR, none of these findings actually demonstrate aortic stenosis, whereas the echocardiogram has the combination of both high sensitivity and specificity for detecting this disorder. Nevertheless, after an echocardiogram detects aortic stenosis, patients would also undergo cardiac catheterization before any intervention is undertaken because coronary artery disease commonly coexists. It is important to note that exercise stress testing is contraindicated in patients with symptomatic aortic stenosis.

The patient's ECG shows Q-waves consistent with his old myocardial infarction, but it also shows left ventricular hypertrophy and normal sinus rhythm. The echocardiogram reveals moderate concentric hypertrophy of the left ventricle, ejection fraction of 55%, and severe aortic stenosis. CXR reveals atherosclerotic changes of the aorta.

Diagnosis: Aortic stenosis

What is the treatment for aortic stenosis?

Aortic valve replacement is the only definitive treatment for aortic stenosis and is especially indicated for symptomatic individuals. In patients with poor operative risk, recent advances in nonsurgical techniques have made percutaneous transcatheter aortic valve replacement (TAVR) a feasible alternative option with similar success rates as surgical intervention without the need for open-heart surgery. Historically, before TAVR was available, patients who were poor surgical candidates for open-heart surgery had a balloon aortic valvotomy performed, which would resolve the aortic stenosis but cause aortic insufficiency, and the patient would still be at high risk for restenosis. Moreover, the procedure would only palliate symptoms and not improve survival.

CLINICAL PEARL   STEP 2/3

Whereas medical therapy does not delay the need for surgery, patients should be treated for risk factors for aortic stenosis. Hypertension should be treated but with monitoring because hypotension can develop due to preload dependence. For this reason, venodilators should be used with caution.

The patient is referred to cardiology and cardiothoracic for consideration of aortic valve replacement as indicated by his symptoms and the severity of his aortic stenosis. He undergoes aortic valve replacement and is discharged home 5 days postoperatively without any complications.

BEYOND THE PEARLS

- On physical exam, the presence of an opening snap with a murmur of aortic stenosis may represent a bicuspid valve.
- The Gallavardin phenomenon is a separation of the auscultatory sounds heard during aortic stenosis. The musical component can be heard at the apex, and the harsh component at the right upper sternal border. This can be misinterpreted as the murmur of mitral insufficiency. This could be differentiated by the lack of radiation to the axilla with aortic stenosis.
- Rarely, presenting features of aortic stenosis can be syncope when extension of the calcification causes atrioventricular block or stroke from embolization of a calcified valve.
- An intraaortic balloon pump can support hemodynamics in patients with severe aortic stenosis and severe left ventricular dysfunction manifesting as cardiogenic shock.
- Class I indications for aortic valve replacement include severe aortic stenosis with symptoms by history, decreased ejection fraction of <50%, or when undergoing other cardiac surgery such as coronary artery bypass grafting.
- According to revised guidelines from the American Heart Association in 2007, no endocarditis prophylaxis is indicated for patients with aortic stenosis, including those patients with a bicuspid aortic valve or rheumatic valve disease. These recent guidelines do not recommend antibiotic prophylaxis for patients with native valvular lesions. However, if the patient undergoes aortic valve replacement, then the presence of a prosthetic cardiac valve is an indication for endocarditis prophylaxis, but such prophylaxis is only indicated for all dental procedures involving manipulation of gingival tissue or the periapical region of teeth, or perforation of the oral mucosa. Prophylaxis is not necessary for genitourinary or gastrointestinal procedures with or without biopsies.
- For those adult patients requiring oral endocarditis prophylaxis, acceptable regimens include amoxicillin, or clindamycin, azithromycin, or cephalexin in penicillin-allergic patients.
- 3-hydroxy-3-methyl-glutaryl-CoA (HMG-CoA) reductase inhibitors are not used in the prevention of progression of calcific aortic stenosis.

References

Cuculich P, Kates A, eds. *The Washington Manual of Cardiology Subspecialty Consult*. 3rd ed. New York: Lippincott Williams & Wilkins; 2014.

Goldman R, Schafer A, eds. *Goldman's Cecil Medicine*. 24th ed. Philadelphia: Saunders-Elsevier; 2011.

Kasper D, ed. *Harrison's Principles of Internal Medicine*. 19th ed. New York: McGraw-Hill Education; 2015.

Nishimura RA, Otto CM, Bonow RO, et al. 2014 AHA/ACC guideline for the management of patients with valvular heart disease: executive summary. *Circulation*. 2014;129(23):2440-2492.

Rosendorff C, ed. *Essential Cardiology: Principles and Practice*. 3rd ed. New York: Springer; 2013.

Walter Chou ▪ Raj Dasgupta ▪ Ahmet Baydur

A 63-Year-Old Male With a Unilateral Pleural Effusion

A 63-year-old male presents to the emergency department with 3 months of progressive dyspnea on exertion, nonproductive cough, night sweats, and 15 pounds of unintentional weight loss. He denies lower extremity edema, chest pain, hemoptysis, fevers, chills, or animal contact. He has no known past medical history. He has a 30-pack-year history of smoking. He has recently emigrated from Vietnam. On physical exam, his blood pressure is 128/72 mm Hg, pulse rate is 90/min, respiration rate is 20/min, and oxygen saturation is 97% on room air. He has dullness to percussion and decreased breath sounds of the right lower chest. The rest of his physical exam is normal. A chest radiograph (CXR) reveals a moderate right-sided opacity of the right lower lung consistent with a pleural effusion (see Fig. 49.1).

What can cause pleural effusions?

A pleural effusion is an excess of fluid in the pleural space between the parietal and visceral pleura of the thorax. A variety of clinical conditions, particularly infection and malignancy, can cause a pleural effusion. Classifying a pleural effusion as exudative or transudative often aids in the diagnosis of the cause of a pleural effusion. Causes of both exudative and transudative effusions are summarized in Table 49.1. Light's criteria, which use pleural fluid lactate dehydrogenase (LDH), pleural fluid protein, serum LDH, and serum protein levels, are used to evaluate for exudative effusions.

BASIC SCIENCE PEARL   **STEP 1**

Light's criteria are used to differentiate between exudative and transudative pleural effusions. If any of the following are present, the pleural effusion is likely to be an exudate:
- Protein ratio: pleural fluid protein/serum protein >0.5
- LDH ratio: pleural fluid LDH/serum LDH >0.6
- Pleural LDH level: pleural fluid LDH level >2/3 upper limit of normal serum LDH

Given the various causes of pleural effusions, a thorough history and physical exam often play a key role in diagnosing the etiology of pleural effusions. Congestive heart failure (CHF) usually causes bilateral pleural effusions and can be accompanied by other signs of volume overload such as lower extremity edema, orthopnea, and elevated jugular venous distension. Hepatic cirrhosis, often with concomitant abdominal ascites, can cause a unilateral, typically right-sided, pleural effusion. Various malignancies can cause pleural effusions, either as a primary presentation or in conjunction with other symptoms. Pneumonia can lead to a parapneumonic effusion, which can be simple or complicated. If left untreated, these can lead to frank pus in the pleural space, also called an empyema.

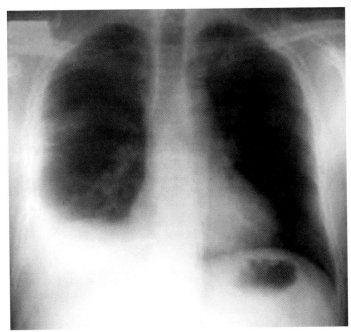

Figure 49.1   Chest radiograph demonstrating a right-sided pleural effusion. *(From* http://commons.wikimedia. org/wiki/File:Tbc.jpg, *ErikH at Dutch Wikipedia.)*

TABLE 49.1 ■ **Causes of Pleural Effusions**

Transudates	
Congestive heart failure Renal failure Cirrhosis Atelectasis Urinothorax Pulmonary embolism (usually an exudate)	
Exudates	
Infection	Parapneumonic, tuberculous, fungal, viral, parasitic
Malignancy	Lung, lymphoma, metastatic, mesothelioma
Abdominal	Pancreatitis, hepatitis, postsurgical
Collagen Vascular Disease	Rheumatoid arthritis, systemic lupus erythematosus, granulomatosis with polyangiitis (formerly Wegener's granulomatosis), Sjögren's syndrome, eosinophilic granulomatosis with polyangiitis (formerly Churg-Strauss syndrome), familial Mediterranean fever

BASIC SCIENCE/CLINICAL PEARL   **STEP 1/2/3**

Simple parapneumonic effusions are exudative effusions predominantly made up of neutrophils. They resolve with treatment of the underlying pneumonia.

A *complicated parapneumonic effusion* is the result of bacterial entrance into the pleural space. The fluid is exudative, often with high LDH values (>1000 IU/L), neutrophil

Continued

BASIC SCIENCE/CLINICAL PEARL—cont'd

predominance, and often with low glucose and pH. Despite the presence of bacteria, cultures are usually negative.

An *empyema* is diagnosed when frank pus is aspirated from the pleural space or when a Gram stain of the fluid is positive for bacteria. A positive fluid culture is not needed for the diagnosis.

When should a thoracentesis be performed?

A thoracentesis can be both therapeutic and diagnostic but is not always indicated. Relative contraindications include small volume (<10 mm on ultrasound or decubitus radiograph), positive pressure ventilation, systemic anticoagulation or coagulopathies, altered mental status, or an overlying cutaneous infection at the proposed entry site. A therapeutic thoracentesis is indicated to relieve symptoms of dyspnea but should not be performed in patients where previous thoracentesis has not improved their symptoms.

A diagnostic thoracentesis should be performed whenever the cause of an effusion is unclear. For example, if a patient is known to have an acute CHF exacerbation and has bilateral pleural effusions, observation with appropriate therapy is acceptable. However, if that same patient's effusion does not resolve despite 3 days of appropriate therapy, is unilateral, or the patient has atypical features like fever or chest pain, a diagnostic thoracentesis is indicated.

What tests should be performed on pleural fluid?

There are many options for laboratory testing of pleural fluid (Table 49.2). Like most of medicine, a "shotgun" approach is usually cumbersome, wasteful, and time consuming. For most effusions, at minimum, the laboratory components of Light's criteria should be evaluated to differentiate between exudate and transudate. Laboratory tests should be aimed at ruling out differential diagnoses, which are generated based on each patient. For example, if you suspect a patient has a parapneumonic effusion, common tests include cell count with differential, glucose, pH, LDH, protein, and appropriate cultures and stains.

How can cell differential aid in the diagnosis of pleural effusions?

A cell count and differential is a simple test that can be very useful in interpreting pleural fluid etiology. A neutrophil-predominant fluid (>50%) indicates an acute pathologic process affecting the pleura. Examples of these include effusions due to pneumonia or pulmonary embolism. Monocytes tend to dominate in fluid where the pleural injury is more remote.

Nucleated cell counts >50,000/mm^3 are found in complicated parapneumonic effusions or empyemas. Nucleated cell counts >10,000/mm^3 are found in bacterial parapneumonic effusions, acute pancreatitis, and lupus pleuritis. Chronic exudates like tuberculous pleurisy or malignancy typically have nucleated cell counts <5000/mm^3.

Lymphocytosis can suggest tuberculous pleurisy, lymphoma, sarcoidosis, chronic rheumatoid pleurisy, chylothorax, or yellow nail syndrome as a cause.

Eosinophilia (>10% of nucleated cells) is usually due to air or blood in the pleural space.

Mesothelial cells are usually high in transudates and can be low, normal, or high in exudative effusions. Having more than 5% mesothelial cells in an exudate makes tuberculosis unlikely.

When should a tube thoracotomy (chest tube) be performed for a pleural effusion?

There are several indications for tube thoracotomy, or chest tube, drainage of pleural effusions. Most of these indications are aimed at avoiding complications of certain pleural effusions, such as loculation or persistent infection. A chest tube is also placed for hemothoraces, both traumatic and postsurgical, to monitor and control hemorrhage.

TABLE 49.2 ■ Diagnostic Testing of Pleural Fluid

Test	If Transudate	If Exudate	Comments
Nucleated cell count	Normal differential	Often elevated	The white cell differential can be useful in evaluating exudative effusions
LDH	Low	>0.6 of the serum LDH or >2/3 the upper limit of normal serum LDH	Elevated due to cell breakdown
Protein	Low	>0.5 of the serum protein	Can be elevated after diuresis of a transudative effusion; use the albumin gradient instead; levels of 8-9 g/L are seen in multiple myeloma and Waldenström's macroglobulinemia (lymphoplasmacytic lymphoma)
pH	Normal (~7.4)	Low (<7.3)	Congestive heart failure often causes an elevated pleural fluid pH (>7.4)
Glucose	>60 mg/dL or >1/2 serum glucose	Normal or low	If glucose is very low (<30), likely cause is rheumatoid pleurisy or empyema
Albumin	Low	Normal	A serum to pleural fluid albumin difference of >1.2 g/dL helps differentiate transudative effusions after diuresis better than protein
Triglycerides	Low	Elevated	In chylothorax, triglycerides are often >110 mg/dL
Cholesterol	Low	Normal or elevated	Pleural cholesterol >45 mg/dL suggests exudate; pleural cholesterol >250 mg/dL diagnostic of pseudochylothorax or cholesterol effusion
Amylase	Low	Elevated (pleural to serum ratio >1.0)	If elevated, acute pancreatitis, chronic pancreatic pleural effusion, esophageal rupture, and malignancy are the most likely causes
ADA	Low	Elevated	In a lymphocytic, exudate effusion, an elevated adenosine deaminase level suggests tuberculous pleurisy
NT-proBNP	Low or normal	Elevated	Measuring serum or pleural NT-proBNP is equally effective; an elevated level can help diagnose a pleural effusion due to heart failure after diuresis

ADA, Adenosine deaminase; *LDH,* lactate dehydrogenase; *NT-proBNP,* N-terminal pro-brain natriuretic peptide.

A chest tube should be placed to drain all empyemas or complicated parapneumonic effusions. Pleurodesis, the joining of the parietal and visceral pleura, eliminates the pleural space and usually requires the placement of a chest tube for adequate drainage of the pleural space. It is usually considered for effusions that are expected to be recurrent, such as malignancy-associated effusions. It is achieved after adequate drainage of the pleural fluid by infusing irritants, such as talc, into

TABLE 49.3 ■ Pleural Fluid and Serum Laboratory Results for Case

Appearance	Serosanguineous
Serum LDH	145 IU/L
Pleural fluid LDH	440 IU/L
Serum protein	5.7 g/L
Pleural fluid protein	4.2 g/L
Cell count and differential	4250 cells/mm³, 70% lymphocytes
Pleural fluid pH	7.35
Bacterial stain/culture	Negative stain and culture
Acid-fast bacteria stain/ culture	Negative stain and culture

LDH, Lactate dehydrogenase.

the pleural space. Like thoracentesis, a chest tube placed for malignant pleural effusion should be placed only if there is demonstrated relief of symptoms and the malignancy is not expected to improve with treatment.

CLINICAL PEARL   **STEP 2/3**

Malignant effusions that are chemotherapy responsive include small-cell lung cancer, breast cancer, lymphoma, and prostate, ovarian, thyroid, and germ-cell tumors.

A thoracentesis is performed on the patient. Fluid and serum characteristics are displayed in Table 49.3.

How would you characterize the pleural fluid in this case? What is your differential diagnosis?
At this point, you have a patient who presents with dyspnea, weight loss, night sweats, and chronic nonproductive cough, who is found to have a right-sided, exudative, serosanguineous, lymphocytic pleural effusion. Given his recent immigration from an area where tuberculosis is endemic, tuberculous pleurisy should be high on his differential. Given his age, weight loss, and history of smoking, malignancy is also a possibility; fluid cytology should be evaluated, and if testing for tuberculosis is negative for tuberculosis, a chest computed tomography (CT) study would likely aid in his diagnosis.

BASIC SCIENCE/CLINICAL PEARL   **STEP 1/2/3**

When tuberculosis is highly suspected in a patient, certain pleural fluid tests can help distinguish a tuberculous exudate from other causes of exudative effusions. Typical results include a lymphocytic exudate, often with high protein levels. Acid-fast bacilli cultures tend to be negative in >70% of cases. Adenosine deaminase (ADA) is almost never low in a tuberculosis effusion. Pleural fluid interferon-gamma >240 pg/mL is highly specific and sensitive for pleural tuberculosis. Pleural fluid lysozyme >15 mg/dL is seen in the large majority (80%) of tuberculous effusions but is also elevated in bacterial empyemas. Demonstration of the presence of mycobacterium tuberculosis in the fluid, either by culture, polymerase chain reaction (PCR), or pleural biopsy, is also diagnostic. A biopsy is usually considered only if pleural fluid studies are inconclusive.

The patient has a polymerase chain reaction (PCR) that is positive for *Mycobacterium tuberculosis* and is diagnosed with tuberculous pleurisy. He is started on antituberculosis medications, such as rifampin, isoniazid, pyrazinamide, and ethambutol (RIPE therapy), with eventual resolution of his pleural effusion.

Diagnosis: Tuberculous pleurisy with pleural effusion

BEYOND THE PEARLS

- Pleural effusions are commonly seen on CXR and are typically separated into transudative or exudative effusions based on Light's criteria.
- The workup of an exudative effusion depends on the clinical scenario. Fluid cytology for malignancy, special testing for tuberculosis, and serologic tests for collagen vascular diseases are indicated based on the clinical indicators.
- Not every effusion needs to be aspirated, but fluid analysis is essential for a definitive diagnosis. Certain effusions, such as empyemas, need drainage as part of their treatment.
- For non-small cell lung cancers, positive pleural fluid cytology is a negative prognostic indicator.
- Malignant pleural effusions should be drained only for symptomatic relief or if the malignancy is not expected to respond to treatment; in this case, attempts should be made at pleurodesis.
- Using ultrasound marking reduces complication rates in thoracentesis.
- Pleural biopsies can be valuable for diagnosing malignant, tuberculous, or rheumatoid effusions. They can also evaluate for foreign particles such as asbestos. They can be obtained via blind, percutaneous closed biopsy or through video-assisted thoracoscopic surgery (VATS).
- Reexpansion pulmonary edema refers to a rare complication of thoracentesis, where clinical findings of crackles and radiographic consolidations can be seen after a thoracentesis. Risk factors include young age, a collapsed lung for a long duration, and rapid reexpansion. The treatment is largely supportive.
- Loculated pleural effusions, in which pleural fluid is trapped in fixed pockets rather than free-flowing, are treated with catheter drainage and instillation of intracavitary fibrinolytics.

References

Anthony VB, Loddenkemper R, Astoul P, et al. Management of malignant pleural effusions. *Am J Respir Crit Care Med.* 2000;162:1987-2001.

Bartter T, Santarelli R, Akers SM, Pratter MR. The evaluation of pleural effusion. *Chest.* 1994;106(4):1209-1214.

Bielsa S, Porcel JM, Castellote J, et al. Solving the Light's criteria misclassification rate of cardiac and hepatic transudates. *Respirology.* 2012;17:721-726.

Burgess LJ, Martiz FJ, Le Roux I, Taljaard JJF. Use of adenosine deaminase as a diagnostic tool for tuberculous pleurisy. *Thorax.* 1995;50:672-674.

Houston MC. Pleural fluid pH: diagnostic, therapeutic, and prognostic value. *Am J Surg.* 1987;154:333-337.

Laws D, Neville E, Duffy J. BTS guidelines for insertion of a chest drain. *Thorax.* 2003;58(suppl II):ii53-ii59.

Light RW. Pleural effusion. *N Engl J Med.* 2002;346(25):1972-1977.

McGrath EE, Anderson PB. Diagnosis of pleural effusion: a systematic approach. *Am J Crit Care.* 2009;20(2):119-127.

Moulton JS, Moore PT, Mencini RA. Treatment of loculated pleural effusions with transcatheter intracavitary urokinase. *AJR Am J Roentgenol.* 1989;153:941-945.

Perricone G, Mazzarelli C. Reexpansion pulmonary edema after thoracentesis. *N Engl J Med.* 2014;370(12):e19.

Carla LoPinto-Khoury ■ John Khoury

A 55-Year-Old Male With Hand Tremors

A 55-year-old male presents to your office with complaints of his hands shaking. The tremor has been noticeable in the past 6 months and is getting worse.

What is the initial differential diagnosis of tremor, and what parts of the history are important?

Tremor has a wide differential diagnosis. Medications can cause tremor, especially psychotropic medications. Metabolic tremors can be from hepatic or renal disease, including Wilson's disease, and tremor can be a complication of rheumatic fever. A common cause of tremor is benign essential tremor, which may be familial, but Parkinson's disease and related disorders are of course on the list. Therefore, it is important to obtain the past medical, psychiatric, and family history for these patients.

When narrowing down the diagnosis in the history, it is helpful to define the extent of the tremor: is it in the hands only, or does it extend to the head, voice, or even legs? Is it symmetric, or does it favor one side? Does it seem to occur at rest or when the patient is moving or trying to accomplish tasks? Does alcohol seem to relieve the tremor (as is the case with benign essential tremor)? Associated symptoms to ask about include any problems with balance or gait, sense of smell, small handwriting, hypophonia (as in Parkinson's disease), or behavioral problems (as in Huntington's disease).

CLINICAL PEARL   **STEP 2/3**

In benign essential tremor, alcohol consumption reduces tremor significantly.

The patient reports that the tremor is worse in his right hand. The tremor does not bother him, but he finds that other people notice it. In addition, he has also had a fall and reports problems with balance in the last few months.

What are the cardinal features of Parkinson's disease?

Parkinson's disease is a hypokinetic movement disorder characterized by bradykinesia, rigidity, resting tremor, postural instability, and a masked face.

What is the expected tremor for Parkinson's disease?

Tremor is generally asymmetric and in early disease unilateral, although patients may not seek treatment until symptoms are more severe and bilateral. The tremor is low frequency, 4 to 6 Hz, and is "pill rolling" (supination-pronation movement). It usually involves the distal extremities and affects the upper limbs more than the lower limbs. Tremor is worse with distraction and can commonly be seen when patients are walking or when given a distracting task (such as counting down from 100 by 7 [serial 7's task]).

CLINICAL PEARL   **STEP 2/3**

Jaw tremor is highly specific for Parkinson's disease, and this feature should not be confused with head tremor associated with benign essential tremor.

On physical exam, the patient has a low frequency pill-rolling tremor of the right greater than left hand at rest. On gait testing he has a slow, shuffling gait with decreased arm swing on the right side. His tone is increased in the right arm with "cogwheeling." On a pullback test he is unable to right himself with one step after being pulled backward. Magnetic resonance imaging (MRI) of the brain is normal.

Diagnosis: Parkinson's disease

What is an appropriate treatment for Parkinson's disease? What categories of medications can be used to treat him?

He appears to have early to moderate stage Parkinson's disease, and therefore treatment with levodopa/carbidopa is appropriate as it will help his symptoms and improve his mobility and quality of life. Levodopa replaces dopamine in the substantia nigra, and carbidopa is a catechol-O-methyl transferase (COMT) inhibitor that inhibits the systemic effect of dopamine outside of the brain and thus reduces side effects such a nausea, vomiting, and hypotension.

Other classes of medications for Parkinson's disease include dopamine agonists. Side effects of these medications are similar to dopamine. Older versions in the ergot class include pergolide and bromocriptine, which have severe potential cardiac side effects and are no longer used. Commonly used nonergot dopamine agonists include pramipexole, ropinirole, and rotigotine.

Monoamine oxidase B (MAO-B) inhibitors include selegiline and rasagiline. These "dopamine-sparing" agents are preferred in early Parkinson's disease as they offer benefit with minimal side effects. Additionally, in one study published in the *New England Journal of Medicine,* 1 mg of rasagiline daily may in fact offer neuroprotection and slow down the course of disease.

Trihexyphenidyl (Artane) and benztropine (Cogentin) can also reduce tremor. For severe Parkinson's disease with freezing, apomorphine can be used.

BASIC SCIENCE PEARL   **STEP 1**

Parkinson's disease is caused by the degeneration of dopaminergic cells in the substantia nigra pars compacta.

Your patient is treated with rasagiline and ropinirole, but the patient's wife reports to you that he has been spending a significant amount of time online gambling and has blown tens of thousands of dollars at casinos.

How do you treat this problem?

All dopamine agonists can cause behavioral problems such as hypersexuality, excessive gambling, and compulsive shopping. Stopping the agent is recommended; however, the side effect is dose dependent, and lower doses may be effective without causing behavioral disturbances.

> On a follow-up visit, the patient's wife tells you that the patient has been acting out his dreams at night. These enactments occur in the later part of the night. The patient can describe the dreams in detail and states that the dreams tend to be violent and he is trying to fight off random attackers from him or his wife.

What stage of sleep do these attacks occur in?

These dream enactments are classic descriptions of rapid eye movement (REM) behavior disorder (RBD). RBD is a parasomnia that is highly associated with Parkinson's disease and Lewy body dementia. The disorder can in fact be seen in patients a decade or longer before symptoms start.

CLINICAL PEARL	STEP 2/3

Stage 3 sleep disorders include sleep walking, sleep talking, sleep eating, and night terrors. These disorders usually do not have dream recall and occur in the earlier part of the evening. Contrast these disorders with RBD that occurs in the latter part of the night with vivid dream recall. Although night terrors or sleep talking do not need to be treated, the other disorders can be effectively treated with clonazepam to prevent the parasomnias.

What are other nonmotor symptoms that need to be addressed by both neurologists and primary care physicians in patients with Parkinson's disease?

Patients with Parkinson's disease are at increased risk of depression, constipation, and sexual dysfunction.

> After you treat the patient for over 10 years with varying medicines including escalating doses of levodopa/carbidopa, his wife complains that he is staring off into space trying to speak to his deceased sister. In addition to mild memory problems, the patient reports seeing little children running around the house who are not there.

What single intervention should be done to help in the diagnosis?

Levodopa/carbidopa may cause hallucinations, and the medicine should be decreased. If holding the levodopa/carbidopa improves symptoms, then these hallucinations are simply drug side effects. If they still persist, antipsychotics such as quetiapine may help.

Other than medication, what can cause behavioral changes and memory problems in a patient with Parkinson's disease?

Lewy body dementia (LBD) eventually effects up to 80% of patients with Parkinson's disease. The diagnosis can only be 100% confirmed on autopsy. However, clinically the patient can be diagnosed with *probable LBD* or *possible LBD*. The presence of dementia must be seen with two of the core features in Table 50.1 for a diagnosis of *probable LBD* or with one core and one suggestive feature. For a diagnosis of *possible LBD*, dementia should be present with either a core or suggestive feature.

TABLE 50.1 ■ Lewy Body Dementia

Core Features
1. Fluctuating cognition with pronounced variation in attention and alertness
2. Recurrent visual hallucinations (typically well formed and detailed)
3. Spontaneous features of parkinsonism

Suggestive Features
1. Rapid eye movement (REM) sleep behavior disorder
2. Severe neuroleptic sensitivity
3. Low dopamine transporter uptake in basal ganglia demonstrated by SPECT or PET imaging

PET, Positron emission tomography; *SPECT,* single-photon emission computed tomography.

BASIC SCIENCE PEARL   **STEP 1**

The pathologic finding of dementia with Lewy bodies is the presence of eosinophilic intracytoplasmic accumulations of alpha-synuclein (Lewy bodies).

BEYOND THE PEARLS

- Deep brain stimulation is a reasonable treatment option for both refractory essential tremor and Parkinson's disease. In Parkinson's disease, it is best used on patients who respond well to dopamine but have too many side effects such as dyskinesia.
- Parkinson plus syndromes include diagnoses such as the following:
  - Multisystem atrophy is characterized by parkinsonism with autonomic dysfunction or cerebellar symptoms. Parkinsonism plus more pronounced autonomic dysfunction has previously been referred to as Shy-Drager syndrome.
  - Cortical basal degeneration should be considered in patients who do not respond to levodopa and is characterized by asymmetric rigidity, bradykinesia, and apraxia.
  - Progressive supranuclear palsy is also not responsive to levodopa and is characterized by falls, postural instability, paralysis of vertical gaze, and dementia.
- The medications used to treat benign essential tremor are propranolol, primidone, and topiramate.

References

Bain P, Brin M, Deuschl G, et al. Criteria for the diagnosis of essential tremor. *Neurology.* 2000;54(suppl 11):S7.

Boeve BF, Lang AE, Litven I. Cortical basal degeneration and its relationship to progressive supranuclear palsy and frontotemporal dementia. *Ann Neurol.* 2003;54(suppl 5):S15-S19.

Gagnon JF, Bedard MA, Fantini ML, et al. REM sleep behavior disorder and REM sleep without atonia in Parkinson's disease. *Neurology.* 2002;59(4):585-589.

Olanow CW, Rascol O, Hauser R, et al. for the ADAGIO Study Investigators. A double-blind, delayed-start trial of rasagiline in Parkinson's disease. *N Engl J Med.* 2009;361:1268-1278.

Poston KL. Overview of rare movement disorders. *Continuum (Minneap Minn).* 2010;16(1):49-76.

CASE 51

Arzhang Cyrus Javan ▪ Andrea Censullo

A 35-Year-Old Male With Fatigue and Rash

A 35-year-old male from Massachusetts with no significant past medical history presents to your urgent care clinic in July with complaints of mild fatigue and a slowly expanding rash near his axilla that appeared 6 days ago. Review of systems is otherwise negative. He embarked on a hike in the woods near his home 3 weeks prior to his visit but denies any animal or insect bites. He is single and has had no recent sexual activity. He denies drug use.

Vital signs are normal. There are no pertinent positives on physical exam besides his rash (see Fig. 51.1).

What is your differential diagnosis?
Erythema migrans (EM), the rash caused by Lyme disease, is high on the differential. EM begins at the site of a tick bite and is frequently homogenously red during the first few days. Sometimes the centers of early lesions become intensely erythematous and indurated, vesicular, or necrotic. The red outer borders slowly expand over the course of several days to create a large annular lesion, while the center of the rash may partially clear, hence the terms "target" or "bull's-eye" that are often used to describe this rash. Occasionally, the expanding lesion remains an evenly intense red, several red rings can be found within the larger outside ring, or the central area turns blue before the lesion clears. The lesion is warm and is often described by patients as burning. It can sometimes be pruritic or even painful. EM can be accompanied by mild constitutional symptoms such as fatigue and malaise.

Other etiologies to consider in the differential diagnosis for EM are cellulitis, hypersensitivity (allergic reaction) to tick bite saliva, a skin manifestation of a spider bite, tinea (ringworm) infections, and erythema multiforme. Cellulitis typically expands more rapidly, lacks central clearing, and is usually painful. Hypersensitivity (allergic reaction) to tick bite saliva also typically expands very rapidly and lacks central clearing. Spider bites can cause a lesion with a necrotic center and are often quite painful. Tinea (ringworm) lesions are, like EM, annular with central clearing, but they characteristically have peripheral scales. Multiple EM lesions (this can be observed in later stages of Lyme disease and will be described shortly) can resemble erythema multiforme. The distinguishing feature of erythema multiforme is that it can blister and cause lesions on the palms, soles, and mucous membranes.

What further testing needs to be performed to help establish a diagnosis?
No further tests are warranted as the patient's history and physical exam highly suggest a diagnosis of early Lyme disease (i.e., stage 1 or localized infection).

This is the only stage of Lyme disease in which the diagnosis should be made on the basis of the clinical picture alone. Testing serologies (i.e., antibodies) isn't warranted in this stage because significant circulating antibody levels may not have had time to develop. All other stages of Lyme disease require laboratory confirmation.

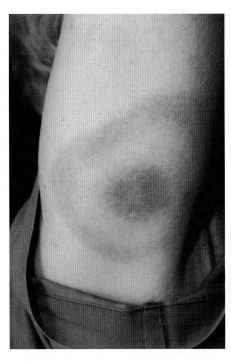

Figure 51.1 Classic rash of erythema migrans (EM). *(From* https://commons.wikimedia.org/wiki/Category :Erythema_migrans#/media/File:Erythema _migrans_-_erythematous_rash_in_Lyme _disease_-_PHIL_9875.jpg*)*

CLINICAL PEARL	STEP 2/3

In a patient with the classic EM rash who lives in or has recently traveled to an area endemic for Lyme disease, do not perform any further laboratory testing; empirically treat based on clinical diagnosis alone.

What is the etiology of Lyme disease?

Lyme disease is the most common tick-borne illness in North America and Europe. Lyme disease is caused by the spirochete bacteria *Borrelia burgdorferi* and can be transmitted to humans by various tick species with unique geographic distributions. The *Ixodes scapularis* tick (deer tick) is the primary vector in the United States and is found throughout New England, the Mid-Atlantic states, and also in Wisconsin, Michigan, and Minnesota. The majority of Lyme disease cases in the United States occur in these regions. *Ixodes pacificus* is another tick species that can infrequently transmit Lyme disease in the coastal regions of Oregon and northern California.

Is it unusual that the patient does not recall a tick bite?

No. Even though a tick must be attached for at least 24 hours to transmit Lyme disease, the tick in its nymphal stage, which is the period in its life cycle in which it infects humans, is quite small and often goes unnoticed. Therefore, the absence of a reported tick bite should not deter the clinician when considering Lyme disease as a diagnosis.

CLINICAL PEARL	STEP 2/3

In a patient with exposure to a Lyme endemic area with a clinical picture suggestive of Lyme disease, inquiring about the *possibility* of tick exposures is imperative and can aid in diagnosis, even in the absence of a known tick bite.

TABLE 51.1 ▓ **Clinical Manifestations of Lyme Disease With Recommended Therapy**

Stage	Clinical Manifestations	Preferred Route of Therapy
Stage 1 (Localized)	*General:* mild flulike symptoms *Skin:* EM	Oral (14-21 days)
Stage 2 (Disseminated)	*General:* malaise, fatigue, fever, headache *Skin:* multiple EM *Rheumatologic:* migratory arthralgias/myalgias *Neurologic:* cranial nerve palsy (especially facial nerve palsy) *Cardiac:* first- and second-degree heart block, myocarditis	Oral (14-21 days)
	Neurologic: mononeuritis multiplex, myelitis, aseptic meningitis	IV (14-28 days)
	Rheumatologic: oligoarthritis	Oral (28 days)
	Cardiac: third-degree or complete heart block	IV until advanced block resolved, then switch to oral (14-21 days total)
Stage 3 (Persistent)	*General:* fatigue *Skin:* acrodermatitis chronica atrophicans	Oral (14-28 days)
	Rheumatologic: recurrent oligoarthritis of large joints	Oral (28 days) or IV (14-28 days)
	Neurologic: subtle cognitive disturbances, polyradiculopathy, ataxic gait	IV (14-28 days)

EM, Erythema migrans; *IV,* intravenous.

What are the clinical stages of Lyme disease?

Lyme is classified into three clinical stages, but there can be some overlap between them. Refer to Table 51.1 for a detailed description of these stages:

- Early Infection: Stage 1 (Localized Infection): Occurs after an incubation period of 3 to 32 days.
  - An EM rash characterizes this stage in about 80% of patients and can be accompanied by regional lymphadenopathy and mild constitutional symptoms such as fatigue and malaise.
- Early Infection: Stage 2 (Disseminated Infection): Begins within days to weeks after the onset of EM. Some of the neurologic manifestations within this stage begin within weeks to months after the onset of EM.
  - A plethora of signs and symptoms may develop in stage 2, but the focus here will be on some of the more noteworthy findings. Initially, patients often develop multiple annular secondary skin lesions as a result of hematogenous dissemination. They appear similar to the initial EM lesion but are smaller and do not have indurated centers. EM and these stage 2 lesions usually disappear within 3 to 4 weeks. Severe constitutional symptoms such as fevers and chills, fatigue and malaise, myalgias, and headache are often present early in this stage and are the initial symptoms of infection in 18% of patients. Migratory arthralgias and myalgias may also develop. After several weeks to months, about 15% of untreated patients develop neurologic abnormalities such as meningitis, encephalitis, cranial neuritis, motor and sensory radiculoneuritis, mononeuritis multiplex, cerebellar ataxia, or myelitis. A few weeks after Lyme disease symptoms begin, about 5% of untreated patients develop cardiac disease. The most typical cardiac findings are first-degree atrioventricular (AV) block, Wenckebach, or complete heart block.

- Late Infection: Stage 3 (Persistent Infection): Occurs months after initial symptoms.
  - This stage is often characterized by arthritis, with large joints more commonly involved than small joints. Other late manifestations of Lyme disease include Lyme encephalopathy, where subtle cognitive disturbances can be seen, and peripheral neuropathies. Acrodermatitis chronica atrophicans is a late skin manifestation that primarily occurs in Lyme disease acquired in Europe and Asia.

How is Lyme disease diagnosed?
In contrast to stage 1 Lyme disease, the diagnosis of Lyme disease in the later stages is made by a combination of clinical features and laboratory testing.

BASIC SCIENCE/CLINICAL PEARL   **STEP 1/2/3**

The Centers for Disease Control and Prevention (CDC) currently recommends a two-step serologic testing approach to detect antibodies (immunoglobulin G [IgG] and immunoglobulin M [IgM]) against *Borrelia burgdorferi*. An enzyme-linked immunosorbent assay (ELISA) is performed first, with positive or indeterminate results confirmed by Western blot.

As noted earlier in the case, serologic testing is often negative in early Lyme disease because antibodies can take up to 1 month to develop. To minimize false-positive and false-negative results, only patients who have a high pretest probability should have the two-step serologic testing performed; this requires the presence of symptoms of early disseminated or late Lyme disease, recent exposure to an endemic area for Lyme disease, and risk factors for tick exposure.

Furthermore, do not use serologic testing to screen asymptomatic patients who live in an endemic area nor those with chronic, nonspecific subjective symptoms such as fatigue or myalgias.

CLINICAL PEARL   **STEP 2/3**

To confirm the diagnosis of Lyme arthritis, synovial fluid can be sent for *Borrelia burgdorferi* polymerase chain reaction (PCR) testing.

CLINICAL PEARL   **STEP 2/3**

In Lyme meningitis, cerebrospinal fluid (CSF) studies show a lymphocytic pleocytosis of about 100 cells/mm^3, and CSF Lyme antibodies are positive. The protein is often elevated and the glucose is normal.

How should this patient be treated? If he had presented with other manifestations of Lyme disease, how would treatment differ?
The treatment of Lyme disease is based on clinical manifestations and the stage of disease. With a few exceptions described below, oral doxycycline 100 mg twice daily for 14 to 21 days is generally the preferred treatment for patients 8 years or older with early localized or early disseminated disease because it also has activity against some other tick-borne pathogens. Other oral options are amoxicillin and cefuroxime; amoxicillin should be used in pregnant patients and in children younger than 8 years of age.

For patients with objective neurologic disease such as meningitis, a 2- to 4-week course of intravenous (IV) ceftriaxone is commonly used for treatment. However, cranial nerve palsy alone is typically treated with oral doxycycline as opposed to IV ceftriaxone. Advanced heart block such as that found in third-degree or complete heart block should be treated with IV ceftriaxone for

TABLE 51.2 ■ Recommended Antibiotics for the Treatment of Lyme Disease

	Preferred	Alternative
Oral Agents	Doxycycline* 100 mg oral twice daily Amoxicillin 500 mg oral three times daily Cefuroxime 500 mg oral twice daily**	Erythromycin
Intravenous (IV) Agents	Ceftriaxone 2 grams IV daily	Cefotaxime 2 grams IV every 8 hours Penicillin G 4 million units IV every 4 hours

*Doxycycline is contraindicated in pregnant women and children <8 years old; use other options.
**Although all three oral agents are considered first line, doxycycline is preferred for early localized or disseminated Lyme disease due to its activity against other tick-borne pathogens (i.e., human granulocytic anaplasmosis).

14 to 21 days. Arthritis in stage 3 Lyme disease is typically treated with oral doxycycline for a longer course, typically 30 to 60 days, or with IV ceftriaxone for a 14- to 28-day course (see Table 51.2).

CLINICAL PEARL   **STEP 2/3**

Advanced (third-degree or complete) heart block caused by Lyme disease should be initially treated with IV therapy. Once the advanced heart block resolves, therapy can be completed with an oral agent. Insertion of a pacemaker is not necessary.

The patient is sent home with doxycycline but returns to your urgent care clinic a week later with new fevers, chills, and worsened malaise.

On physical exam, temperature is 38.2 °C (100.8 °F), blood pressure is 110/64 mm Hg, pulse rate is 96/min, respiration rate is 16/min, and oxygen saturation is 98% on room air.

There is slight improvement in the original EM rash. No other new findings are noted on physical exam.

Results of laboratory testing are shown in Table 51.3. A Giemsa-stained thin blood smear reveals parasites in a tetrad-form ("Maltese cross") formation.

Diagnosis: Stage 1 localized Lyme disease, with concomitant babesiosis

What is the most likely etiology of these findings? What further testing should be performed?

In a patient with Lyme disease who fails to improve or worsens despite appropriate treatment, the possibility of coinfection with another tick-borne pathogen of *Ixodes* should be high on your radar. This patient most likely has concomitant babesiosis, a disease caused by the tick-borne parasite *Babesia microti*. Human granulocytic anaplasmosis (HGA), caused by *Anaplasma phagocytophilum,* is another possibility but is less likely because doxycycline is also used to treat this disease.

The clinical manifestations of babesiosis vary greatly depending on the degree of parasitemia, ranging from asymptomatic infections to severe infections with a significant potential for death. In mild infections, fever is the most common finding. Sweats and chills are also frequently encountered. Other less frequent findings include headache, myalgia, anorexia, nausea, and arthralgias. Severe disease, associated with many systemic complications, is associated with parasitemia levels of >4% and warrants hospitalization. Risk factors for severe disease include male

TABLE 51.3 ■ **Results of Laboratory Testing**

	(reference range in parentheses)
White Blood Cell Count (WBC)	$5.8 \times 10^3/\mu L$ ($3.8-10.8 \times 10^3/\mu L$)
Hemoglobin	9.6 g/dL (13.3-17.7 g/dL)
Platelet Count	110,000/μL (150,000-450,000/μL)
Alanine Aminotransferase (ALT)	65 units/L (7-40 units/L)
Total Bilirubin	3.5 mg/dL (0.1-1.2 mg/dL)
Direct Bilirubin	2.5 mg/dL (0.1-0.3 mg/dL)
Lactate Dehydrogenase (LDH)	350 units/L (122-222 units/L)
Haptoglobin	12 mg/dL (43-212 mg/dL)
Reticulocyte Count	6.5% (0.5-2.0%)

gender, age greater than 50, asplenia, human immunodeficiency virus (HIV), malignancy, and immunosuppression.

Babesiosis often causes hemolytic anemia, which typically presents with a low hemoglobin and hematocrit, along with an elevated reticulocyte count and lactate dehydrogenase (LDH). Low platelets and elevated liver enzymes are also commonly encountered in patients with babesiosis.

BASIC SCIENCE PEARL   **STEP 1**

Diagnosis of babesiosis is made on Giemsa-stained thin blood smears. Trophozoites typically appear as rings. Tetrads of merozoites, commonly referred to as the "Maltese cross," are essentially diagnostic of babesiosis.

Further testing should include microscopic exam of a thin blood smear. Serum PCR should be performed along with serologies to confirm the diagnosis of babesiosis if there remains a high clinical suspicion despite a negative thin smear.

Treatment is warranted in symptomatic patients. First-line treatment for patients with mild disease is a 7- to 10-day course of oral atovaquone plus azithromycin. Second-line treatment is clindamycin plus quinine. Patients with severe infection should be treated with IV clindamycin plus oral quinine for at least a 7- to 10-day course. Some patient populations require an extended duration of treatment.

How could these tick-borne diseases have been prevented?

The best way to prevent tick-borne diseases is to avoid tick-infested areas. If this is not possible, patients with possible tick exposure should be advised to use insect repellants containing diethyltoluamide (DEET), wear protective clothing such as long pants, and perform periodic tick checks with prompt removal of ticks if found.

Prophylactic antibiotics for Lyme disease after a tick bite are recommended if all of the following criteria are met:
- The tick is identified as *I. scapularis.*
- The tick has been attached for >36 hours.
- Local rates of infection of ticks with *B. burgdorferi* is >20% (which occurs in endemic regions).
- Prophylaxis is given within 72 hours of tick removal.
- Doxycycline is not contraindicated.

If all the above criteria are met, a single dose of doxycycline 200 mg has been shown to help prevent Lyme disease. There is currently no vaccine available to prevent Lyme disease.

There is no babesiosis vaccine available and there is no role for antibiotic prophylaxis for babesiosis.

The patient asks you if he should be worried about developing "chronic Lyme disease."

After successful treatment for Lyme disease, some patients continue to have subjective symptoms including fatigue, myalgias, and arthralgias. These symptoms usually improve on their own, but if they persist for >6 months, this is referred to as "post-Lyme disease syndrome" or "chronic Lyme disease"; the latter is actually a misnomer because it implies chronic infection with *B. burgdorferi* despite the use of antibiotics. Although the etiology is not known, at this time there is no evidence to suggest that these chronic nonspecific symptoms represent continued infection with *B. burgdorferi*; therefore, further antibiotic treatment is not recommended. Randomized controlled trials have also failed to demonstrate a benefit of repeat or prolonged antibiotic treatment for chronic Lyme disease.

CLINICAL PEARL   **STEP 2/3**

In patients with chronic, nonspecific symptoms lasting >6 months after treatment for Lyme disease, it is important to look for other possible causes of the symptoms such as fibromyalgia, depression, or obstructive sleep apnea.

BEYOND THE PEARLS

- Lyme disease was first discovered in 1976 after a cluster of children in Lyme, Connecticut, were thought to have juvenile rheumatoid arthritis (JRA).
- In addition to transmitting *Borrelia burgdorferi*, *I. scapularis* can carry *Babesia microti* and *Anaplasma phagocytophilum,* the agents of babesiosis and human granulocytic anaplasmosis (HGA), respectively. Doxycycline is the treatment of choice for Lyme disease and HGA, but does not treat babesiosis.
- Southern tick-associated rash illness (STARI) causes a lesion identical to erythema migrans, and is transmitted by the Lone Star tick *(Amblyomma americanum)* in the southeastern United States. The causative agent of this disease has not yet been identified.
- Early in Lyme disease, IgG and IgM will be positive, but after 2 months only IgG should be positive, so in a patient presenting over 2 months after infection, a positive IgM is likely to be a false-positive result.
- The CDC criteria for Lyme disease considers an IgM Western blot positive if 2 out of 3 bands are present. An IgG is considered positive if 5 out of 10 bands are present.
- Within the first 24 hours of therapy for Lyme disease, about 15% of patients develop transient worsening of symptoms from a Jarisch-Herxheimer-like reaction. This is the body's immune response to the antigens released when spirochetes are killed. This reaction also can occur in secondary syphilis.
- Serologic testing for Lyme disease should not be used to screen asymptomatic patients in endemic regions for Lyme disease or patients with chronic nonspecific subjective symptoms such as myalgias and fatigue. Serologic testing should also not be performed in patients with EM, as these patients should be treated based on clinical diagnosis alone.

BEYOND THE PEARLS—cont'd

- *B. burgdorferi* can be cultured from Barbor-Stoenner Kelley (BSK) medium for definitive diagnosis. It should be noted that this has only been reliably performed using tissue from EM biopsies.
- Doxycycline is relatively contraindicated in pregnant women and children under 8 years old. The preferred treatment of Lyme disease in these cases is amoxicillin. Doxycycline may cause permanent tooth discoloration in children, and if used during pregnancy may cause problems with tooth and skeletal development in the fetus.

References

Shapiro E. Lyme disease. *N Engl J Med.* 2014;370(18):1724-1731.

Steere A. Lyme borreliosis. In: Kasper DL, Fauci AS, eds. *Harrison's Infectious Diseases.* 2nd ed. New York: McGraw-Hill Medical; 2013:720-727.

Steere A. Lyme borreliosis. In: Longo DL, Fauci AS, Kasper DL, et al., eds. *Harrison's Principles of Internal Medicine.* 17th ed. New York: McGraw-Hill Medical; 2008:1055-1059.

Steere A. Lyme disease (Lyme borreliosis) due to *Borrelia burgdorferi*. In: Bennett JE, Dolin R, Blaser MJ, eds. *Mandell, Douglas, and Bennett's Principles and Practice of Infectious Diseases.* 8th ed. Philadelphia: Saunders; 2015:2725-2735.

Tugwell P, Dennis D, Weinstein A, et al. Guidelines for laboratory evaluation in the diagnosis of Lyme disease. *Ann Intern Med.* 1997;127(12):1106-1107.

Vannier E, Gelfand F. Babesiosis. In: Kasper DL, Fauci AS, eds. *Harrison's Infectious Diseases.* 2nd ed. New York: McGraw-Hill Medical; 2013:1174-1176.

Wormser G, Dattwyler R, Shapiro E, et al. The clinical assessment, treatment, and prevention of lyme disease, human granulocytic anaplasmosis, and babesiosis: clinical practice guidelines by the Infectious Diseases Society of America. *Clin Infect Dis.* 2006;43(9):1089-1134.

Daniel Martinez

A 45-Year-Old Female With Nausea, Vomiting, and Abdominal Pain

A 45-year-old female with a past medical history of type 1 diabetes mellitus (DM1) presents to the emergency room with 2 days of progressive nausea, vomiting, and abdominal pain. The patient is from Brazil and moved to the United States 3 years ago. Unfortunately, she lost her job and health insurance earlier this year, and she is recently homeless. During the past year, she was not able to eat well and ran out of insulin 1 week ago. She describes her abdominal pain as 5/10, pressurelike, generalized, nonradiating, and mildly worse with eating. In the emergency room, her blood pressure is 90/55 mm Hg, pulse rate is 125/min, respiration rate is 28/min, and temperature is 37.2 °C (99 °F). Her height is 5′4″ and weight is 120 pounds. She appears unwell, has dry mucus membranes, and has normal heart and lung sounds. Her abdomen is soft, mildly tender to palpation, but without rebound or guarding.

What is concerning about this presentation?

The patient's history is very concerning for diabetic ketoacidosis (DKA). Her history of DM1 with decreased oral intake and a lack of insulin places her at high risk for DKA. Other causes of DKA include infection/sepsis, intoxication (alcohol/drugs), myocardial infarction, stroke, and pancreatitis.

BASIC SCIENCE PEARL	STEP 1

Patients with type 1 diabetes mellitus (DM1) are more at risk for developing DKA than patients with type 2 diabetes mellitus (DM2). This is because the pathophysiology of DKA involves severe insulin deficiency, which is rarer with DM2. This is because DM2 involves insulin resistance and relative insulin deficiency more so than an actual lack of insulin in the body. However, patients with DM2 can and do develop DKA during extreme conditions.

How should you begin workup of this patient?

There are three basic requirements to diagnose someone with DKA. There needs to be a plasma glucose >250 mg/dL, an anion gap acidosis with pH <7.3, and ketosis. The basic evaluation of DKA thus involves measuring a glucose finger-stick, a basic metabolic panel, arterial blood gas, and urinalysis.

You start a 2-liter normal saline bolus because she appears severely dehydrated on exam. Your nurse reports that the finger-stick blood glucose level is 550 mg/dL, which raises your suspicion for DKA. You then give 10 units of insulin intravenous (IV) push. Lab results become available: sodium 135 mEq/L, potassium 3.5 mEq/L, chloride 98 mEq/L, bicarbonate 15 mmol/L, blood urea nitrogen 25 mg/dL, creatinine 1.2 mg/dL, and glucose 600 mg/dL. The pH on the blood gas is 7.25, and ketones are found in the urinalysis. You then start an insulin drip, continue high-rate isotonic IV fluid resuscitation, and admit the patient to the medical intensive care unit.

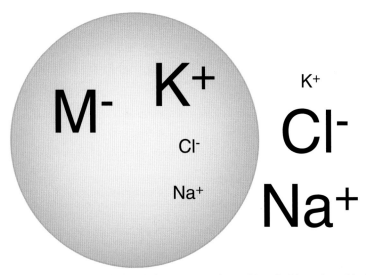

Figure 52.1   A graphic depiction of the relative concentrations of ions inside and outside the typical human cell. Note that potassium is mainly an intracellular ion, so it is difficult to gauge how much potassium is in the body simply by measuring how much is in the extracellular fluid. *(From* http://aups.org.au/ Proceedings/42/19-28/Figure_1.jpg.)

Diagnosis: Diabetic ketoacidosis

What other abnormalities are found in DKA?

The pathophysiology of DKA involves far more than hyperglycemia and anion gap ketoacidosis. Another major pathology is the osmotic diuresis that occurs when blood glucose levels are consistently that high. As glucose is filtered into the renal tubules, it pulls in water and other important electrolytes with it. This causes severe polyuria/polydipsia, dehydration, hypokalemia, and hypomagnesemia. The treatment of DKA therefore commonly involves aggressive replacement of fluids and electrolytes.

BASIC SCIENCE/CLINICAL PEARL   **STEP 1/2/3**

Hypomagnesemia is a cofactor for reactions that utilize adenosine triphosphate (ATP). Most importantly, hypomagnesemia therefore causes sodium-potassium-ATPase pump dysfunction, which can lead to dangerous cardiac arrhythmias. You will notice that it is a commonly ordered electrolyte on the wards.

Why isn't the patient's potassium very low?

It is important to remember that potassium is mainly an intracellular electrolyte, and therefore a serum potassium level is not always an accurate representation of total body potassium (see Fig. 52.1). A thorough understanding of the causes of hypokalemia and a detailed history that screens for these causes is the best way to estimate a patient's total body potassium. That is the only way to manage a patient's potassium levels effectively.

What are the causes of hypokalemia?

Causes of hypokalemia can be classified into four major categories. The first category is a decreased intake of potassium; second is potassium loss via the gastrointestinal tract; third is

TABLE 52.1 ▥ Evaluation of Hypokalemia

Etiology of Hypokalemia	Transtubular Potassium Gradient	History
Decreased intake	Low	Nausea/vomiting/restriction of oral food and fluids (NPO)
Gastrointestinal losses	Low	Diarrhea
Renal losses	High	Variable
Transcellular shifting	Variable	Alkalemia/insulin excess/ beta-2 agonists

potassium loss via the renal system; and fourth is a transcellular shift of potassium into cells (see Table 52.1).

It is rare for a healthy individual to develop hypokalemia simply by not eating enough as there is a sufficient amount of potassium in the normal Western diet. However, this is a very common reason for hospitalized patients to develop hypokalemia. Many patients have severe nausea/vomiting and cannot tolerate a regular diet. Other patients are instructed not to eat or drink for a procedure or as a therapeutic modality for an underlying illness (ileus, pancreatitis, etc.). It is also common for postoperative patients not to be able to eat for many days following a surgery. This is why potassium is added to maintenance IV fluids when patients are not able to eat in the hospital. Depending on their condition, patients may need between 40 and 80 mEq of potassium chloride (KCl) a day (which is why you will commonly see patients get about 2 to 3 liters of maintenance fluids per day, with 20 to 40 mEq of KCl added per liter).

Diarrhea is a common cause for relatively minor levels of hypokalemia. It is not a cause of hypokalemia that requires a significant workup to rule in as it is evident from the patient's history. It is more important to understand that when patients are having diarrhea, it is helpful to keep a close eye on their serum potassium and appropriately replace it. Furthermore, the presence of diarrhea does not itself rule out other causes of hypokalemia, and they should be investigated when clinically indicated.

The definitive workup of potassium losses from the kidneys is complicated and will be discussed later in this chapter. However, the initial step to evaluate whether the kidneys are involved as an etiology for hypokalemia is very simple: A spot urine potassium concentration can be used. If urine potassium is >15 mEq/L, the kidneys are likely playing a role in the patient's hypokalemia. In a state of hypokalemia, normal functioning kidneys are very good at minimizing renal potassium losses, and this dramatically lowers the urine potassium concentration. Therefore, if the potassium is found at a normal to high concentration in the urine, there is likely something going wrong with the kidneys themselves, and further workup is indicated.

Different physiologic states and medications can cause a transcellular shift of potassium into cells without actually altering the total body potassium. Most commonly, this includes an alkalemic state and beta-2-agonist or insulin administration. Alternatively, an acidemic state or a lack of insulin can cause a transcellular shift of potassium out of the cells. A "normal" serum potassium concretion in this instance can mislead physicians to presume a patient's total body potassium is relatively normal when in fact a patient can be severely total body potassium depleted.

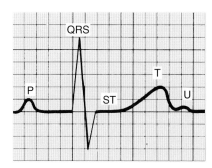

Figure 52.2   An electrocardiogram (ECG) sample of the U wave, which is defined as the deflection following the T wave. *(From Goldberger AL, Goldberger ZD, Shvilkin A. Clinical Electrocardiography: A Simplified Approach. 8th ed. Philadelphia: Elsevier; 2012.)*

CLINICAL PEARL	STEP 2/3

Transcellular shifting is responsible for seemingly normal serum potassium levels in patients with DKA who are in fact severely total body potassium depleted. The acidemic state and lack of insulin cause a transcellular shift of potassium outside of the cells. However, as the acidemic state is corrected and insulin is replaced, this can cause a rapid and dangerous drop in serum potassium levels. This is why most DKA treatment protocols include potassium in the IV fluid resuscitation, with frequent serum electrolyte checks. Attendings commonly ask questions to make sure you understand this very important concept.

CLINICAL PEARL	STEP 2/3

The symptoms of hypokalemia can be very nonspecific. They include nausea, vomiting, and vague abdominal pain. However, as the hypokalemia worsens, patients can develop muscle weakness/cramps (including weakness of the diaphragm) and rhabdomyolysis. Hypokalemia can also cause electrocardiogram (ECG) changes. Patients can develop a classic U wave on ECG (see Fig. 52.2), which can be seen in other conditions as well. Patients can also develop a prolonged QT interval and a variety of arrhythmias, including ventricular tachycardia/fibrillation.

In the medical intensive care unit, the insulin drip and aggressive IV fluid resuscitation are continued with frequent monitoring of electrolytes, anion gap, and pH. By breakfast time the next day, the patient's glucose is 180 mg/dL, the anion gap has closed, and the patient is feeling hungry. She is given her regular weight-based subcutaneous insulin, and she eats her breakfast readily. A couple hours later the insulin drip is stopped and the anion gap remains closed. The patient is then transferred to the floor that afternoon. A third-year medical student on the team is given the patient to follow on the floor over the next few days for social discharge planning. However, the student notices that the patient's serum potassium is still low at around 3.2 mEq/L despite aggressive repletion, and she is mildly hypertensive to 165/85 mm Hg. The patient is eating well, has no diarrhea, and is currently without any metabolic abnormalities. The judicious student suspects a renal cause for the patient's hypokalemia and decides to do a workup.

How do you confirm renal potassium losses?

The first step in the workup is to confirm the kidneys are inappropriately secreting potassium into the urine. As discussed previously, a spot urine potassium concentration should be less than 15 mEq/L in a normal functioning kidney during a hypokalemic state. If the urine potassium concentration is >15 mEq/L, the kidneys are likely inappropriately secreting potassium into the urine and contributing to the patient's hypokalemia. This is a simple screen, but it has some

TABLE 52.2 ▪ Evaluation of Renal Causes of Hyperkalemia

Renal Causes of Hyperkalemia	Blood Pressure	Acid-Base
Mineralocorticoid excess	High	Metabolic alkalosis
Diuresis (increase sodium/ fluid delivery to distal tubules)	Low-Normal	Contraction alkalosis
Type 1 or 2 renal tubular acidosis	Low-Normal	Nongap metabolic acidosis

limitations. Specifically, it does not take into account free water reabsorption, which can deceptively increase the concentration of potassium in the urine. This can lead a clinician to believe incorrectly that a kidney is excessively secreting potassium, when in fact it is just excessively reabsorbing free water.

This problem is one of the reasons why the transtubular potassium gradient calculation was developed. The calculation takes into account both potassium and free water reabsorption in the kidneys and compares the two. The equation is $(U_K/P_K)/(U_{osm}/P_{osm})$. However, because it is essentially a ratio of ratios, it is difficult to understand at first glance. Breaking it down, the numerator (U_K/P_K) is comparing the concentration of potassium in the urine (U_K) to the concentration of potassium in the serum (P_K). The ratio is high when the concentration of potassium in the urine is higher than in the serum. This means the kidneys are either dumping potassium into the urine or reabsorbing water back into the body. This ambiguity is why the numerator must be compared and standardized against the water reabsorption activity of the kidneys, which is represented by the denominator (U_{osm}/P_{osm}). This second ratio compares the overall osmolality of the urine (U_{osm}) to the osmolality of the serum (P_{osm}). If this denominator ratio equals 1, it means the kidneys are not actively reabsorbing free water, and the value of the numerator (U_K/P_K) is not affected and can be trusted. If this denominator ratio is greater than 1, it means that the kidneys are reabsorbing free water, which also deceptively elevates U_K. To correct this deceptive elevation, the high denominator value is placed into the equation $(U_K/P_K)/(U_{osm}/P_{osm})$, which will appropriately lower the overall value of the transtubular potassium gradient.

There are no standard interpretations for the values of the transtubular potassium gradient. However, it is generally accepted that if this ratio is >7 during a hypokalemic state, the kidneys are abnormal and likely playing a role in the patient's hypokalemia. A normally functioning kidney should have a ratio <3 during a hypokalemic state.

What are the different types of renal potassium losses?
There are three main reasons why the kidneys may be inappropriately wasting potassium (see Table 52.2), and they generally work by manipulating the principal cell in the distal tubule of the nephron (see Fig. 52.3). The principal cell is the key modulator of potassium in the kidneys, and it works by absorbing sodium while secreting potassium (see Fig. 52.4).

The first reason involves excessive mineralocorticoid activity. Principal cells are under direct, positive control of mineralocorticoids like aldosterone. Thus, if a patient is found to be hypertensive (due to excessive sodium reabsorption) and to have renal potassium wasting, hyperaldosteronism should be considered as an etiology. The workup includes testing renin and aldosterone levels in the serum (aldosterone can also be measured in a 24-hour urine sample) to evaluate for primary or secondary causes of hyperaldosteronism. Conn syndrome is the classic primary hyperaldosteronism, which would have a high aldosterone but low serum renin level. However, reno-

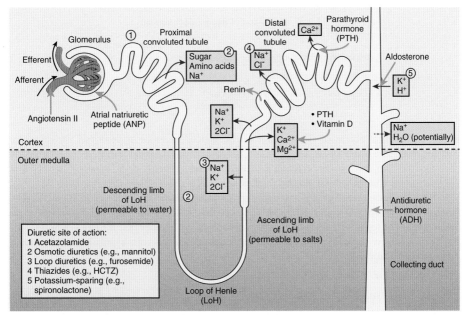

Figure 52.3 A graphic depiction of the typical nephron illustrating which electrolytes are reabsorbed and secreted at various parts of the nephron and which hormones are responsible for regulating this movement. It also illustrates the mechanism of action of each of the diuretic medications by pointing out where and how they act upon the nephron. *HCTZ,* Hydrochlorothiazide. *(From* http://www.pathophys.org/wp-content/uploads/2013/02/MPR-nephron.png.*)*

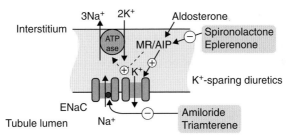

Figure 52.4 A graphic depiction of a principal cell in the distal nephron illustrating how it functions to reabsorb sodium and secrete potassium into the urine. It also illustrates that this action is under direction positive control of aldosterone and that spironolactone functions by blocking aldosterone and thus sodium reabsorption. *ENaC,* Epithelial sodium channel. *(From Waller DG, Sampson AP. Medical Pharmacology and Therapeutics. 4th ed. Philadelphia: Elsevier; 2014:213-223, Fig. 14.2.)*

vascular disease or a renin-secreting tumor can cause a secondary hyperaldosteronism, which would have both high aldosterone and renin levels (see Table 52.3).

Second, changes in the nephron proximal to the principal cell can cause excessive potassium secretion. Specifically, increasing the flow of fluid or increasing the delivery of sodium to the principal cell can cause it to secrete more potassium. These two changes are commonly seen with diuretic use (loop and thiazide) and the analogous genetic disorders Bartter syndrome and Gitelman syndrome. Also, both loop diuretics and Bartter syndrome directly block the absorption of potassium in the thick ascending loop of Henle (Fig. 52.3), causing hypokalemia through that mechanism as well. Because these patients are undergoing active diuresis, they tend to be

TABLE 52.3 ■ Evaluation of Hyperaldosteronism

Hyperaldosteronism	Renin Level	Aldosterone Level
Primary hyperaldosteronism	Low	High
Secondary hyperaldosteronism	High	High

hypotensive to normotensive. This is unlike the hyperaldosteronism described earlier where patients tend to be hypertensive. Furthermore, because these patients are relatively intravascularly depleted, they can develop a contraction alkalosis as well. Hypotension and alkalosis are therefore very important clues when diagnosing these conditions.

Third, hypokalemia is common in both type 1 and type 2 renal tubular acidosis (RTA). The exact pathophysiology of hypokalemia in RTA is beyond the scope of a general internist as there are many postulated mechanisms. It is more important to remember that if there is a normotensive or hypotensive patient who has a nongap metabolic acidosis with hypokalemia, you should entertain the diagnosis of RTA.

CLINICAL PEARL   **STEP 2/3**

Medical exams love to test systemic pathologies that cross multiple organ systems. Making questions that test the causes of RTA and their effects is one way to do this. For example, autoimmune diseases such as Sjögren syndrome and rheumatoid arthritis can cause a type 1 RTA, while amyloidosis and multiple myeloma can cause a type 2 RTA.

BASIC SCIENCE PEARL   **STEP 1**

Three medications are notorious for causing a type 1 RTA: ifosfamide, amphotericin B, and lithium. Again, a question involving these medications and RTA can cross three different medical specialties at once and would be a good test question.

The third-year medical student orders the tests necessary to calculate a transtubular potassium gradient. The ratio comes back at >7, and this confirms that excess renal losses are a component of the patient's persistent hypokalemia. The student then notices that the patient has a normal pH and is mildly hypertensive. The student finds it unusual that a patient with type 1 diabetes who does not have the metabolic syndrome would be so hypertensive. The student therefore suspects a hyperaldosteronism and orders a morning serum renin and aldosterone level. To the surprise of the supervising resident, the renin level is very low and the aldosterone level is very high (aldosterone/renin ratio >20). Primary hyperaldosteronism is confirmed with a sodium load suppression test (3-day oral salt load with a 24-hour urine aldosterone level, which is not suppressed). A computed tomography (CT) scan of the abdomen is then ordered and a 7-cm solitary left adrenal mass is found (see Fig. 52.5). Further tests are ordered and exclude a glucocorticoid-secreting tumor, an estrogen/testosterone-secreting tumor, and a pheochromocytoma. Adrenal vein sampling confirms a unilateral cause of hyperaldosteronism. The patient then proceeds to surgical resection of the mass, and pathology reveals an adrenal adenocarcinoma with clean margins. With the aid of hospital financial services, the patient is able to follow-up with an outside primary care physician. Since discharge, her diabetes has been well controlled on her new insulin regimen and her hypertension and hypokalemia have resolved since resection of the mass.

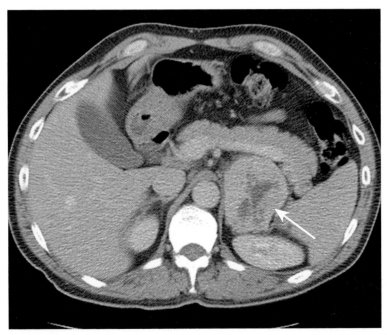

Figure 52.5   A cross-sectional computed tomography (CT) scan of an abdomen illustrating a large left-side adrenal mass (as indicated by the arrow) found in the patient in this case. *(From* http://radiology.casereports .net/index.php/rcr/article/viewFile/770/1070/11016.*)*

Diagnosis: Diabetic ketoacidosis, primary hyperaldosteronism, and adrenal adenocarcinoma

---

BEYOND THE PEARLS

- Although adrenal adenocarcinomas are exceedingly rare, people from southern Brazil have 15 times the risk of the general population.
- Adrenal adenocarcinomas have been seen to have a bimodal age distribution: the first before age 5 and the second in ages 40 to 50.
- The U wave (an ECG deflection that comes after the T wave) was first described by Willem Einthoven in 1903. It was not part of the original five deflections he originally described in 1896 (P, Q, R, S, T waves) (see Fig. 52.2).
- Although U waves can be seen in hypokalemia, hypertension is the most common cause (about 40% of U waves).
- Because magnesium is used as a cofactor in many enzymatic reactions, it is very difficult to replete potassium without also replacing this electrolyte.

References

Agus MS, Agus ZS. Cardiovascular actions of magnesium. *Crit Care Clin.* 2001;17(1):175-186.
Batlle D, Moorthi KMLST, Schlueter W, Kurtzman N. Distal renal tubular acidosis and the potassium enigma. *Semin Nephrol.* 2006;26:471-478.
Choi MJ, Ziyadeh FN. The untility of the transtubular potassium gradient in the evaluation of hyperkalemia. *J Am Soc Nephrol.* 2008;19:424-426.

Costanzo LS. *Physiology*. Philadelphia: Saunders Elsevier; 2010.

Funder JW, Carey RM, Fardella C, et al, and the Endocrine Society. Case detection, diagnosis, and treatment of patients with primary aldosteronism: an endocrine society clinical practice guideline. *J Clin Endocrinol Metab*. 2008;93:3266-3281.

Michalkiewicz E, Sandrini R, Figueirido B, et al. Clinical and outcome characteristics of children with adrenocortical tumors: a report from the international pediatric adrenocortical tumor registry. *J Clin Oncol*. 2004;22(5):838-845.

Morgan DB. Body water, sodium, potassium and hydrogen ions: some basic facts and concepts. *Clin Endocrinol Metab*. 1984;13(2):233-247.

Ng L, Libertino JM. Adrenocortical carcinoma: diagnosis, evaluation and treatment. *J Urol*. 2003;169:5-11.

Pérez Riera AR, Ferreira C, Filho CF, et al. The enigmatic sixth wave of the electrocardiogram: the U wave. *Cardiol J*. 2008;15(5):408-421.

R. Michelle Koolaee

A 57-Year-Old Female With Cavitary Lung Lesions

A 57-year-old female presents to the emergency department with 3 months of a progressive nonproductive cough, dyspnea, and subjective fevers. She denies any hemoptysis or rashes and has not traveled recently. She lives in Arizona, where she works as a schoolteacher. Her past medical history is significant for hypertension, for which she takes daily amlodipine. On physical exam, her blood pressure is 118/70 mm Hg, pulse rate is 90/min, respiration rate is 28/min, and oxygen saturation is 86% on room air. There are diffuse expiratory rhonchi on lung exam. The remainder of the exam is normal. A chest radiograph (CXR) reveals numerous bilateral large nodules and masses, with possible cavitation (see Fig. 53.1).

What are some causes of cavitary lung lesions?

There are various infectious and noninfectious causes of radiographic cavitary lung lesions, which are summarized in Table 53.1. *Mycobacterium tuberculosis* generally has the highest prevalence of cavities among persons with pulmonary disease of any infection because this pathogen causes extensive caseous necrosis (which leads to cavity formation). Lung abscess is another relatively common bacterial cause of cavitary lung lesions; this is usually polymicrobial. The most common noninfectious cause is pulmonary embolism with infarction; cavitary lesions occur as a result of pulmonary infarction and subsequent necrosis. Cavitary lung lesions in rheumatologic illness are relatively uncommon, with the exception of granulomatosis with polyangiitis (GPA), where this is a frequent finding.

In general, when should you consider systemic vasculitis as a diagnosis?

Vasculitis is defined by inflammatory infiltrate within the vessel walls, which can lead to compromise of vessel integrity, and subsequent tissue ischemia and necrosis. Affected vessels vary in size, type, and location. Vasculitis should be considered in situations where patients present with systemic symptoms along with either single or multiorgan disease involvement. There is no algorithmic approach to the vasculitides because disease manifestations are so variable. There are, however, classification criteria for most types of vasculitis proposed by the American College of Rheumatology. These criteria are most useful for clinical research purposes but may also often guide diagnostic evaluation.

BASIC SCIENCE PEARL   **STEP 1**

The classification criteria for vasculitides do not include all clinical characteristics of that particular disorder, only those that distinguish the disorder from other vasculitides. Thus, they should not be used exclusively for clinical diagnosis. All efforts should be made to confirm a diagnosis of vasculitis with tissue biopsy.

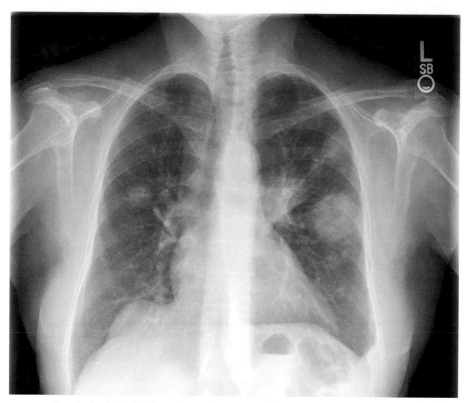

Figure 53.1   A chest radiograph reveals numerous bilateral large nodules and masses.

TABLE 53.1 ■ **Differential Diagnosis of Radiographic Cavitary Lung Lesions**

Infectious Causes

- Anaerobic bacteria
- Mycobacteria: *M. tuberculosis, M. avium, M. kansasii, M. malmoense, M. xenopi*
- Fungi: *Aspergillus, Coccidioides, Histoplasma, Blastomyces, Cryptococcus, Mucor, Pneumocystis carinii, Paracoccidioides brasiliensis*
- Other bacteria: *Staphylococcus aureus*, Enterobacteriaceae, *Pseudomonas aeruginosa, Legionella, Haemophilus influenzae* type B, *Nocardia, Actinomyces, Klebsiella pneumonia, Burkholderia pseudomallei, Rhodococcus equi*

Noninfectious Illnesses

- Pulmonary infarction
- Vasculitis (i.e., frequently in granulomatosis with polyangiitis)
- Sarcoidosis (rarely)
- Neoplasm (i.e., primary lung cancer, lymphoma, Kaposi sarcoma, lymphomatoid granulomatosis); metastatic disease from other primary sites is less likely to cavitate

- Rheumatoid arthritis (rheumatoid lung nodules may very rarely cavitate)
- Bronchiolitis obliterans organizing pneumonia
- Bronchiectasis
- Empyema with air fluid level

A detailed history and careful physical exam are essential in evaluating a patient with possible vasculitis. Also, be aware that the clinical manifestations of vasculitis can be mimicked by a number of other disorders (i.e., infection, malignancy, and other connective tissue diseases, to name a few). Although not sensitive or specific, some systemic symptoms of vasculitis may include fever, fatigue, neurologic dysfunction, respiratory dysfunction, renal insufficiency (with an active urine sediment), and abdominal pain.

What is the best way to elicit the cause of this patient's cavitary lung lesions?
Radiographic findings are rarely definitive in establishing a diagnosis. Culturing respiratory specimens for bacteria, mycobacteria, and fungi is an appropriate first step in evaluating the etiology of a cavity; a bronchoscopy is typically performed in order to elicit this information (provided that the patient is hemodynamically stable). Supplemental testing (i.e., antigen and antibody tests for specific infectious organisms) is useful when focusing on specific infectious etiologies. Clinicians should pursue a tissue diagnosis when clinically warranted.

> The results of laboratory testing are shown in Table 53.2. A computed tomography (CT) scan of the chest again demonstrates the cavitary lesions, which are scattered through the lungs within all lobes (see Fig. 53.2). There are no effusions or ground glass opacities.

BASIC SCIENCE/CLINICAL PEARL   **STEP 1/2/3**

Platelets are acute-phase reactants, therefore, they can be increased in response to various stimuli, including systemic inflammation or infection. On the wards, you may sometimes hear of platelets being referred to as the "poor man's sed rate"; both the sedimentation rate and the platelets may be elevated during an acute inflammatory response.

What is your differential diagnosis?
This is a 57-year-old female who presents with a nonproductive cough, dyspnea, subjective fevers, hypoxia, diffuse cavitary lung lesions, and a positive c-ANCA (antineutrophil cytoplasmic antibody)/proteinase-3 antibody (PR3-ANCA).

TABLE 53.2 ■ Laboratory Tests

Leukocyte count	18,000/µL (18 × 10⁹/L)
Hematocrit	35%
Platelet count	540,000/µL (540 × 10⁹/L)
Serum creatinine	1.1 mg/dL
Urinalysis	Normal
Erythrocyte sedimentation rate	76 mm/h
c-ANCA	Positive
p-ANCA	Negative
Antiproteinase-3 antibodies	Positive
Antimyeloperoxidase antibodies	Negative

ANCA, Antineutrophil cytoplasmic antibody.

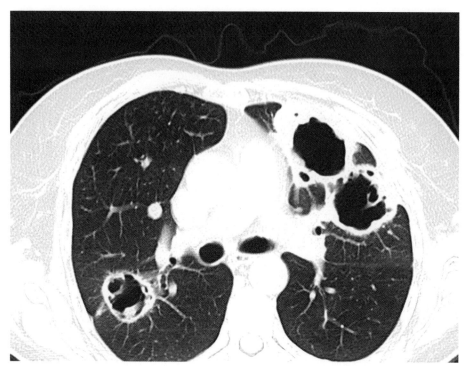

Figure 53.2 Computed tomography of the chest demonstrates numerous bilateral cavitary lesions within all lobes of the lung.

BASIC SCIENCE PEARL	STEP 1

Be aware of the pitfall of relying on immunofluorescence (IF) testing alone for the detection of ANCAs (i.e., c-ANCA, p-ANCA patterns), since IF testing is subjective and not specific for vasculitis. Positive IF testing should always be confirmed with antigen-specific enzyme-linked immunosorbent assay testing for myeloperoxidase (MPO) and PR3-ANCA.

Systemic vasculitis, particularly GPA, is highest on the differential diagnosis at this point. Antiproteinase-3 antibodies are highly specific for GPA in the appropriate clinical setting. GPA (formerly Wegener's granulomatosis) is a small vessel vasculitis (part of the ANCA-associated vasculitides) that typically produces granulomatous inflammation of the respiratory tracts as well as a necrotizing, pauci-immune glomerulonephritis in the kidneys. Although this patient does not have renal manifestations of disease, she definitely has the cavitary lung lesions that are typically seen in GPA. The other ANCA-vasculitides (microscopic polyangiitis [MPA], eosinophilic granulomatosis with polyangiitis [EGPA], formerly Churg-Strauss disease) are usually associated with antimyeloperoxidase antibodies (anti-MPO) and are less likely. Furthermore, EGPA is associated with adult-onset asthma, peripheral eosinophilia, and frequently neurologic dysfunction, none of which this patient has.

CLINICAL PEARL	STEP 2/3

GPA is believed to be far more common than MPA in Western countries. This ratio is inverted in Japan.

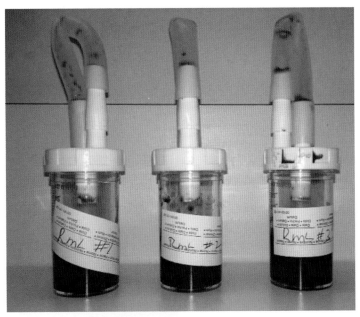

Figure 53.3   The diagnosis of diffuse alveolar hemorrhage is confirmed during a bronchoalveolar lavage when serial aliquots are progressively more hemorrhagic.

Despite the high likelihood of GPA, it is prudent to consider infectious etiologies as well. Not only can this patient's clinical manifestations of vasculitis mimic infection (i.e., fevers, cough, elevated inflammatory markers, cavitary lung lesions), but sometimes infections and vasculitis can occur simultaneously. Additionally, the therapy for GPA involves potent immunosuppressive therapy, which could have a potentially devastating outcome if infectious etiologies are not considered. As previously mentioned above, mycobacterial, fungal, and bacterial infections should be ruled out with appropriate cultures. The endemic region for coccidioidomycosis is in the South-western United States, most notably in California and Arizona, which would be particularly important to rule out in this case.

A bronchoscopy with bronchoalveolar lavage (BAL) is performed. During the procedure, lavage aliquots are progressively more hemorrhagic, confirming the diagnosis of diffuse alveolar hemorrhage (DAH) (see Fig. 53.3). Cultures from both the lavage fluid and tissue biopsy are negative for acid-fast bacilli and bacterial and fungal infection. Coccidioidomycosis antibody testing is negative (both immunoglobulin G [IgG] and immunoglobulin M [IgM]).

What are the respiratory manifestations of GPA?
GPA is a systemic necrotizing vasculitis that can affect both the upper and lower respiratory tracts.
   Upper respiratory tract manifestations include:
- Sinusitis (often patients present with chronic, recurrent sinus infections that are not responsive to antibiotic therapy)
- Nasal inflammation (symptoms frequently include nasal obstruction, bloody nasal obstruction, and nasal crusting)
- Inner ear inflammation

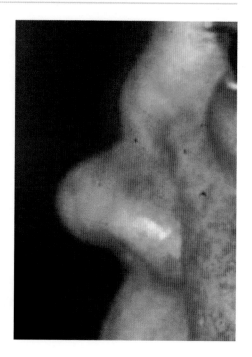

Figure 53.4   Saddle nose deformity in a patient with granulomatosis with polyangiitis. *(From Holle JU, Laudien M, Gross WL. Clinical manifestations and treatment of Wegener's granulomatosis.* Rheum Dis Clin North Am. *2010;36[3]:507-526.)*

If left untreated, persistent upper respiratory tract inflammation may lead to saddle nose deformity (see Fig. 53.4), nasal septal perforation, and even hearing loss.

Symptoms of lower respiratory tract disease include cough, dyspnea, pleuritic chest pain, and/or hemoptysis. DAH is a prominent and life-threatening manifestation of GPA, and requires prompt diagnosis and aggressive therapy. The symptoms of DAH may range in severity; some patients are less symptomatic whereas others may present with marked hemoptysis and acute respiratory failure. Multifocal nodules, infiltrates, and/or diffuse opacities are findings that can be seen on radiographic imaging. Subglottic stenosis is another manifestation of GPA. It can sometimes be the sole manifestation of disease and may be severe enough to necessitate tracheostomy.

CLINICAL PEARL   **STEP 2/3**

Stridor is a sign of severe subglottic obstruction and requires urgent evaluation.

How do you establish a diagnosis of ANCA-associated vasculitis, particularly in this case?

Because treatment of systemic vasculitis requires long-term potent immunosuppressive therapy (which itself carries a risk of toxicity), it is important whenever possible to confirm the diagnosis of systemic vasculitis with tissue biopsy. However, treatment should be initiated empirically if the suspicion is high for GPA (i.e., the presence of PR3-ANCA antibodies in a patient with classic upper airway manifestations, pulmonary infiltrates/nodules, and urinary abnormalities consistent with glomerulonephritis) and a biopsy cannot be performed in a timely manner.

A tissue biopsy is obtained from the most affected organ system (lung and kidney biopsies carry the highest diagnostic yield) and will show evidence of vascular inflammation (acute and/or chronic), vessel necrosis, and/or granulomas. Classic kidney biopsy findings of GPA include a necrotizing focal segmental or diffuse glomerulonephritis without significant immune deposits.

This patient has primarily lung involvement; typically lung tissue is obtained via a thoracoscopy or thoracotomy. This is because the tissue samples from a transthoracic or transbronchial biopsy, although less invasive, are often inadequate for a definitive diagnosis of GPA.

CLINICAL PEARL   **STEP 2/3**

Nasal/sinus and tracheal tissue biopsies, although less invasive, carry a very low diagnostic yield.

An open lung biopsy is performed and demonstrates prominent neutrophilic inflammatory infiltrate around arterioles and capillaries, associated with necrosis of the vessel walls and granulomatous inflammation in the surrounding tissue.

Diagnosis: Granulomatosis with polyangiitis with associated DAH

What are some other common manifestations of GPA?

Table 53.3 summarizes some systemic manifestations of GPA aside from pulmonary and renal disease. About half of patients with GPA have cutaneous manifestations. Other organ systems that may become involved include the eyes and nervous system and, less commonly, the heart, gastrointestinal tract, or genitourinary tract.

CLINICAL PEARL   **STEP 2/3**

Patients with GPA are at an increased risk of venous thromboembolic events. Venous inflammation, combined with the low-flow state in the venous circulation, may contribute to this phenomenon.

The patient receives a "pulse" dose of methylprednisolone 1000 mg daily for 3 days followed by prednisone 1 mg/kg daily in combination with intravenous (IV) rituximab. Her cough and dyspnea improve within a few days, and she is discharged home within a week with follow up.

TABLE 53.3 ■ **Some Other Manifestations of Granulomatosis With Polyangiitis**

Organ	Manifestation
Eye	Scleritis, uveitis, keratitis, retinal vasculitis, inflammatory retroorbital pseudotumor with extraocular muscle dysfunction and proptosis
Skin	Palpable purpura, ulcers, tender nodules, livedo reticularis
Nervous System	Mononeuritis multiplex, nerve abnormalities, central nervous system mass lesions
Heart	Pericarditis, myocarditis, conduction system abnormalities

How do you approach treatment for GPA?

In patients with organ-threatening or life-threatening manifestations (i.e., patients with deteriorating renal function or those with DAH), initial therapy involves aggressive immunosuppression with glucocorticoids along with either cyclophosphamide (oral or IV) or rituximab. A variety of prednisone tapering schemes have been employed, with the goal of taper within 6 to 9 months. There may be a role for plasma exchange in patients with either severe active and rapidly progressive renal disease or severe pulmonary hemorrhage. In patients with mild disease (i.e., without organ-threatening disease), methotrexate may be used as initial therapy. Following remission, maintenance therapy is initiated with either azathioprine or methotrexate and is usually given for 12 to 24 months.

CLINICAL PEARL **STEP 2/3**

ANCA titers do not reliably correlate with the timing of disease flares so they should not be serially monitored as a means of predicting flares.

The patient is tapered off of prednisone by 6 months and is maintained on azathioprine 150 mg daily. A follow-up chest CT demonstrates improvement in the size of the cavitary lesions.

BEYOND THE PEARLS

- EGPA has been reported as a rare complication of therapy with leukotriene-modifying agents (i.e., montelukast, zafirlukast) in patients with glucocorticoid-dependent asthma, usually in the setting of dose reduction of oral glucocorticoids.
- Much of the cocaine bought in the United States in recent years is contaminated with levamisole, an anthelminthic and immunomodulating agent. Levamisole-contaminated cocaine is associated with illness that can mimic ANCA vasculitides. Manifestations may include (but are not limited to) arthralgias, necrotic skin lesions, positive MPO-ANCA (less common PR3-ANCA), fevers, glomerulonephritis, and pulmonary hemorrhage.
- *Pneumocystis carinii (jiroveci)* pneumonia (PCP) can be a potentially fatal complication of immunosuppressive therapy for systemic vasculitis, particularly for those who receive cyclophosphamide and/or high-dose glucocorticoids. PCP prophylaxis with either trimethoprim-sulfamethoxazole or atovaquone is administered in this setting.
- Approximately 25% of cases of GPA are of a "limited" form, whereby disease is limited to the upper respiratory tracts and lungs (this does not include ANCA-associated DAH). Renal function is normal and constitutional symptoms are minimal or absent. ANCA testing may be negative in limited GPA.
- The diagnosis of GPA is confirmed by histopathologic evidence of necrotizing, granulomatous inflammation of affected tissue. Empiric immunosuppressive therapy is only initiated in cases where biopsy cannot be performed in a timely manner and the clinical suspicion for disease is high.
- Most GPA relapses occur within the first year after cessation of immunosuppressive therapy and may or may not affect the same organ system as the initial presentation (the incidence varies widely among studies and ranges from 11 to 57%).
- Acrolein is a urinary metabolite of cyclophosphamide; exposure to this compound may result in hemorrhagic cystitis. Mesna (2-mercaptoethanesulfonic acid) is an agent administered both before and after cyclophosphamide infusions and helps to reduce the risk of bladder toxicity by interacting with acrolein, resulting in an inactive compound.
- Clinicians should have a high index of suspicion for DAH in patients with GPA or MPA, as not all patients manifest with hemoptysis. Bronchoscopy with BAL is the best approach to excluding alveolar hemorrhage.

References

Gadkowski LB, Stout JE. Cavitary pulmonary disease. *Clin Microbiol Rev*. 2008;21(2):305-333.

Hogan SL, Falk RJ, Chin H, et al. Predictors of relapse and treatment resistance in antineutrophil cytoplasmic antibody-associated small-vessel vasculitis. *Ann Intern Med*. 2005;143(9):621.

Merkel PA, Lo GH, Holbrook JT, et al. Brief communication: high incidence of venous thrombotic events among patients with Wegener granulomatosis: the Wegener's Clinical Occurrence of Thrombosis (WeCLOT) Study. *Ann Intern Med*. 2005;142(8):620-626.

Nachman PH, Hogan SL, Jennette JC, et al. Treatment response and relapse in antineutrophil cytoplasmic autoantibody-associated microscopic polyangiitis and glomerulonephritis. *J Am Soc Nephrol*. 1996;7(1):33.

Emily Omura ■ John D. Carmichael

A 40-Year-Old Female With Weight Gain and Amenorrhea

A 40-year-old female presents for follow up of hypertension that started 2 years ago. She has been seen frequently in your clinic for titration of her antihypertensive medication and treatment of recently diagnosed hyperlipidemia and type 2 diabetes mellitus. During her visit she reveals that she is frustrated by weight gain that has occurred predominately over the past year. She reports regular menstrual cycles until the past year, when she notes increased time in between cycles and occasional spotting instead of regular periods. She is concerned that she may have early menopause because she is having changes in appetite, difficulty sleeping, and mood swings. She feels like these symptoms are getting worse, and she is frustrated that despite her increase in exercise and change in diet she is more fatigued and has experienced no weight loss.

How should you approach investigating whether a patient has common symptoms that are due to a secondary, treatable cause or are manifestations of lifestyle or genetic predispositions to metabolic abnormalities?

This patient has a past medical history and complaints that are very common to any internal medicine practice. Yet there are subtle clues within her history that should prompt more detailed questioning. The constellation of symptoms and the timing of their appearance is often crucial to making a diagnosis. Chronic diseases frequently present with symptoms insidious in onset and require a detailed history of these complaints and their associated conditions. The patient's concern about a recent and fairly sudden change in her health status is important to investigate. A unifying diagnosis can be made by gathering the information about the onset and progression of symptoms. This patient's recent history of hypertension and weight changes, which are findings consistent with the metabolic syndrome, and amenorrhea prior to the usual age of menopause are concerning for an endocrine disorder. More information regarding the onset of fatigue, previous endurance and physical activity, body habitus, timing of weight gain, and menstrual and obstetric history would be helpful in the evaluation for a potentially treatable underlying condition.

Upon further questioning, the patient states that she had three normal pregnancies and that her last was 4 years ago. She has gained 25 pounds in that time and has noted some hair growth on her chin and upper lip, which she has been waxing. She is concerned about her weight and reports that her legs feel weak and despite an increase in exercise, her waist is expanding.

CLINICAL PEARL   **STEP 2/3**

Many endocrine disorders can cause menstrual irregularities: hyperprolactinemia, hypothyroidism, hyperthyroidism, and polycystic ovary syndrome (PCOS). Other chronic medical conditions such as renal insufficiency, rheumatologic disease, and psychiatric diseases such as anorexia can also cause hypothalamic or functional amenorrhea.

TABLE 54.1 ■ Signs of Hypercortisolism

Central obesity (centripetal fat distribution of face ["moon facies"], supraclavicular and dorsocervical fat pads)

Signs of protein wasting: thin skin with violaceous striae on abdomen, flanks, breasts, hips; easy bruising; slow healing; and muscle wasting

Hypertension

Bone wasting leading to osteoporosis

Gonadal dysfunction and hyperandrogenism; menstrual irregularity; hirsutism

Mild to severe psychiatric disorders

Impaired immune defense mechanism with increased rate of infections

On physical exam she is in no distress, has a normal pulse rate and blood pressure of 132/85 mm Hg, body mass index (BMI) is 29 kg/m^2. There is some heavier hair growth underneath her chin and on the side of her face, which is very round and plethoric. She has no gross vision deficits and no thyromegaly; however, there is fullness to her supraclavicular subcutaneous tissue and her dorsocervical spine region, she has a skin exam remarkable for acanthosis nigricans, multiple bruises on extensor surfaces, and purple-red striae on her abdomen. Her waist circumference is 109 cm (the upper limit of normal for an adult female is 88 cm); however, her extremities appear thin with decreased proximal muscle strength bilaterally.

How does the physical exam help with your diagnostic evaluation?

This patient is presenting with signs and symptoms consistent with cortisol excess or Cushing's syndrome (see Table 54.1). The severity of hypercortisolism can be variable, and the symptoms can present in various degrees of severity and prevalence. Because many of the classic symptoms of Cushing's syndrome such as obesity, hypertension, menstrual irregularities, and mood disorders are common, and Cushing's syndrome is an uncommon disease, it is important to evaluate the patient looking for both specific and sensitive physical exam findings. These findings help form a degree of suspicion that is crucial to determine the need for screening for Cushing's syndrome and the interpretation of testing.

CLINICAL PEARL   **STEP 2/3**

Truncal obesity is the most common physical exam finding of Cushing's syndrome; however, it is not specific to this syndrome. The more specific findings in patients with Cushing's syndrome include proximal myopathy, facial plethora, and easy bruising.

What are some conditions that may mimic the physical exam findings of Cushing's syndrome?

Many effects of medications and medical conditions present with signs similar to Cushing's syndrome and can interfere with the proper interpretation of test results. These include alcohol abuse, renal insufficiency, estrogen-containing oral contraceptives, obesity, pregnancy, and depression. These so-called pseudo-Cushing's states make diagnosing Cushing's syndrome very challenging, as they can be associated with a normal physiologic increase in cortisol secretion causing false-positive test results.

It is crucial to obtain a detailed medication history in cases of suspected hypercortisolism. Any form of exogenous glucocorticoids can cause iatrogenic Cushing's syndrome. Intraarticular glucocorticoids injections, topical glucocorticoids, and inhaled glucocorticoids have all been implicated in cases of clinical symptoms associated with cortisol excess.

> The patient denies taking any medications other than her hydrochlorothiazide, metformin, simvastatin, and amlodipine. She denies using any herbal medications or hormonal contraceptive agents. She does not smoke or use any illicit drugs and only drinks alcohol on rare occasions. Although she has been unhappy with her recent health changes, she denies symptoms of depression.

Who should undergo testing for Cushing's syndrome?
Cushing's syndrome is rare, and the high prevalence of conditions that mimic Cushing's syndrome increases the risk of false-positive results. Therefore, it is important to establish a pretest probability of disease based on clinical history. Patients who are screened with a low pretest probability require multiple positive tests to establish the diagnosis, and positive tests should be viewed with skepticism with systematic sources for error excluded prior to further testing. In most cases, repeatedly normal screening results exclude the diagnosis of Cushing's syndrome.

Patients with unusual features for age, symptoms or signs that may be more specific for Cushing's syndrome (proximal myopathy, violaceous striae, facial plethora, easy bruising, osteoporosis at young age especially if male, weight gain with arrest of growth in pediatric populations), or the presence of suggestive symptoms in patients with incidentally discovered adrenal or pituitary adenomas are all appropriate patients for screening investigations. Indiscriminant testing of selected populations (i.e., patients with type 2 diabetes mellitus or obesity) have not yielded sufficient numbers of positive cases to become standard of care.

CLINICAL PEARL   **STEP 2/3**

Early in the disease process, patients with Cushing's syndrome lose the normal circadian rhythm of cortisol secretion. As a consequence, random measurements of adrenocorticotropic hormone (ACTH) and cortisol are of little diagnostic value. Nighttime cortisol measurement, either through sampling of saliva or serum, capitalizes on this loss of the normal physiologic nadir, and a high value measured at bedtime or midnight is a highly sensitive and specific sign of Cushing's syndrome.

What are other conditions that cause laboratory results consistent with hypercortisolism?
Prior to initiating screening, exclude or limit other causes of apparent hypercortisolism whenever possible. These conditions include:
- Pregnancy
- Depression and other psychiatric conditions
- Alcohol dependence
- Glucocorticoid resistance
- Morbid obesity
- Poorly controlled diabetes mellitus
- Physical stress
- Malnutrition
- Intense chronic exercise
- Hypothalamic amenorrhea
- Corticosteroid-binding globulin excess

Testing for abnormal cortisol secretion usually comprises three main methods:

- Suppression of cortisol secretion by dexamethasone (a synthetic steroid that does not interfere with the measurement of cortisol by assay methods).
- Collection of urinary cortisol to provide an integrated method of quantifying the degree of cortisol secretion over a period of time.
- Measurement of diurnal secretion usually by assessment of midnight or bedtime cortisol.

BASIC SCIENCE PEARL   **STEP 1**

The zona fasciculata in the adrenal gland is the only normal source of endogenous cortisol, which circulates bound predominately to corticosteroid-binding globulin, also known as transcortin. Cortisol has many functions such as maintenance of blood pressure through upregulation of alpha-1 receptors on arterioles and by increasing sensitivity to norepinephrine and epinephrine. Antiinflammatory and immunosuppressive actions include production of leukotrienes and prostaglandins, inhibition of leukocyte adhesion, reduction of eosinophils, and blocking of interleukin-2 production. Additionally, cortisol increases insulin resistance, enhances gluconeogenesis, and decreases bone formation through inhibition of osteoblast number and function.

What should the initial screening tests be for this patient?

Recommended screening methods for hypercortisolism include the use of at least two diagnostic tests: 24-hour urinary-free cortisol, late-night salivary cortisol, 1 mg overnight dexamethasone suppression testing, or in some cases, the 2-day low-dose dexamethasone suppression test. All of these tests are constructed to demonstrate the excess of cortisol secretion; however, the type of test must be chosen in the context of the patient's medications and clinical conditions. For example, renal insufficiency (glomerular filtration rate <60 mL/min) can result in falsely low urinary-free cortisol, and a midnight salivary cortisol may be more appropriate.

CLINICAL PEARL   **STEP 3**

There are several potential pitfalls for testing patients with possible Cushing's syndrome. Each test has both systematic and physiologic sources for error. Collection of urinary cortisol must be complete and verified by assessment of creatinine secretion. Increased urinary excretion of urine can falsely elevate cortisol secretion and renal impairment can falsely lower cortisol excretion. Several medications can interfere with dexamethasone testing through increased metabolism of dexamethasone or elevations in cortisol-binding globulin. Salivary cortisol testing is prone to contamination, and handling of the collection device must be done with care. It is important to recognize that the cutoffs employed by each test are set to maximize the sensitivity of the tests at the expense of specificity to assist in ruling out the disease in healthy patients.

When should referral be made to an endocrinologist?

A referral to an endocrinologist experienced in the interpretation of testing for cortisol excess and expertise in the diagnosis and management of patients with Cushing's syndrome is highly recommended in several situations. If initial testing is abnormal with no other apparent physiologic cause of hypercortisolism, then consultation with an endocrinologist can help with selection of a second test and subsequent workup, if needed. Those patients with normal test results with multiple progressing clinical features may benefit from a consultation with an endocrinologist. Furthermore, any patient with discordant tests may require several additional highly specialized tests for diagnosis. Similarly, patients who have been diagnosed based on positive screening and confirmatory testing often benefit from expert management.

TABLE 54.2 ■ Evaluation of Hypercortisolism

Hypercortisolism	
	ACTH Dependent
	Cushing's disease (ACTH secreting pituitary adenoma)
	Ectopic ACTH secretion
	ACTH Independent
	Adrenal adenoma
	Adrenal carcinoma
	Iatrogenic Cushing's syndrome

ACTH, Adrenocorticotropic hormone.

Initial screening for this patient results in a serum cortisol response of 8.5 ng/mL after 1 mg of dexamethasone administered at 11 PM. A 24-hour urinary free cortisol value of 248 mcg/24 hours returns well above the upper limit of normal (50 mcg/24 hours). She is then referred to endocrinology, who recommends a midnight salivary cortisol level for confirmation. Midnight salivary cortisol is then performed with a value of 6.2 nmol/L. Confirmation of the 24-hour urinary cortisol collection is ordered and results in another extremely elevated cortisol level of 308 mcg/24 hours.

What is the next step in management once hypercortisolism is confirmed?
Once hypercortisolism is confirmed, the next step in evaluation is to determine whether the cause is ACTH dependent or independent. A measurement of serum ACTH will guide workup and management (see Table 54.2).

BASIC SCIENCE PEARL	STEP 1

Corticotropin-releasing hormone (CRH) is produced in the paraventricular nucleus of the hypothalamus and circulates through a portal venous system to the pituitary to stimulate ACTH release from the pituitary corticotroph cells. ACTH in turn stimulates cortisol production and secretion from the adrenal zona fasciculata. Cortisol secretion by the adrenal gland circulates and causes negative feedback inhibition of both hypothalamic CRH and pituitary ACTH secretion, closing the long feedback loop.

Distinction between ACTH-dependent and ACTH-independent Cushing's syndrome is a very important step in the diagnosis and management of hypercortisolism. This distinction is generally made measuring plasma ACTH levels. In ACTH-independent forms of Cushing's syndrome, the circulating plasma ACTH is suppressed (usually <10 pg/mL). In ACTH-dependent forms of Cushing's syndrome, ACTH can be measured as low, normal, or elevated demonstrating an inappropriate responsive in ACTH to elevated levels of circulating cortisol. Occasionally patients with Cushing's syndrome of adrenal origin have ACTH levels between 10 and 20 pg/mL. In this situation or other ambiguous testing, a corticotropin-releasing hormone (CRH) stimulation test can be performed.

BASIC SCIENCE PEARL	STEP 1

States of hypercortisolism are defined as Cushing's syndrome; however, if the cause of cortisol excess is a functioning corticotroph pituitary adenoma, the diagnosis is termed Cushing's disease.

What is the corticotropin-releasing hormone stimulation test?

The CRH stimulation test, which can be performed alone or in combination with arginine vasopressin, desmopressin, or dexamethasone, is considered the most accurate dynamic noninvasive test for the differential diagnosis of ACTH-dependent Cushing's syndrome. Administration that shows a blunted ACTH response is observed in patients with ACTH-independent Cushing's syndrome, whereas a brisk response is seen in patients who have pituitary or ectopic excessive ACTH production. CRH is given either a weight-based dose (1 mcg/kg) or a fixed dose (100 mcg) and ACTH is monitored for a rise of 30 to 50% above baseline as a confirmation of ACTH-dependent disease. If ACTH-independent disease is confirmed, an adrenal computed tomography (CT) or magnetic resonance imaging (MRI) scan should be performed to investigate a possible adrenal lesion and help with further clarification of the etiology. CRH is also often administered as part of inferior petrosal sinus sampling, an invasive test to determine the site of ACTH secretion in cases of ACTH-dependent Cushing's syndrome. Petrosal sinus sampling is an endovascular procedure by which local concentrations of ACTH are measured in the right and left petrosal sinuses and are compared to peripheral concentrations of ACTH. The testing is performed as a baseline measurement and then in a timed test after the administration of CRH.

ACTH is measured in this patient and is found to be elevated at 53 pg/mL, a value consistent with ACTH-dependent disease. The patient undergoes a brain MRI with and without gadolinium contrast. She is found to have a 4-mm left-sided pituitary adenoma without evidence of invasion, which is highly suggestive of a diagnosis of Cushing's disease. She is scheduled for bilateral inferior petrosal sinus sampling and is found to have a baseline central to peripheral gradient of >2:1 before CRH administration and >3:1 after CRH administration, indicating a sufficient rise in ACTH in venous drainage of pituitary to indicate the origin of excess cortisol, with the majority of ACTH secretion found on the left side. She is subsequently scheduled for transsphenoidal resection with a neurosurgeon experienced in pituitary surgery. The pathologic specimen stains positively for ACTH with disruption of normal reticulin fibers, consistent with an ACTH-secreting pituitary adenoma.

Diagnosis: Cushing's disease

What percentage of patients with Cushing's disease have a normal brain MRI?

As many as 40% of patients with Cushing's disease will present with negative MRI findings on pituitary scans but will have clear evidence of ACTH-dependent Cushing's syndrome. In the setting of ACTH-dependent disease, if imaging does not reveal adenoma >6 mm, bilateral inferior petrosal sinus sampling (IPSS) stimulated by CRH or desmopressin should be performed to discover whether the ACTH production is pituitary in origin. A ratio of central to peripheral ACTH of more than 2:1 in the basal state or more than 3:1 after CRH stimulation is consistent with Cushing's disease.

CLINICAL PEARL   **STEP 2/3**

A stepwise approach to hypercortisolism is crucial; performing tests prior to clinical indication can result in invasive, unnecessary testing and potentially to intervention that is not indicated or therapeutic. It is vital that a patient has clear evidence of hypercortisolism and that the cortisol secretion is active at the time of IPSS. The IPSS will not aid in making the diagnosis of Cushing's syndrome, as healthy patients, patients with pseudo-Cushing's states, and patients with Cushing's disease will all have an elevated central to peripheral gradient during the IPSS.

What is the treatment for Cushing's disease?

Transsphenoidal surgery is the first-line treatment for Cushing's disease, with surgical cure rates ranging from 69 to 92%. Assessment of successful surgery is best measured by clinical and biochemical evidence of adrenal insufficiency after transsphenoidal surgery in the perioperative timeframe. Patients who are successfully treated with surgery require corticosteroid replacement for as long as 12 months or more in some cases while the hypothalamic-pituitary-adrenal axis recovers from prolonged suppression from pathologic cortisol secretion. Assessment of remission of disease can best be performed once a patient has been weaned off glucocorticoid replacement and should include measurement of urinary cortisol and salivary cortisol.

CLINICAL PEARL   **STEP 2/3**

Serum cortisol levels <2 µg/dL after surgery are associated with remission and low recurrence rate of approximately 10% at 10 years, whereas persistent serum cortisol levels >5 µg/dL for up to 6 weeks after surgery require further evaluation.

Patients require lifelong observation for recurrence, and treatment of recurrence includes a variety of multiple modes of therapy. Second surgery is efficacious in 50 to 70% of persistent disease; however, it is frequently associated with an increased risk of hypopituitarism, diabetes insipidus, and cerebrospinal fluid leak.

Radiation techniques have been widely used as treatment of Cushing's disease and include fractionated radiotherapy or stereotactic radiosurgery. Radiotherapy induces remission in the majority of cases; however, as many as 80% of patients subsequently develop new pituitary deficiencies.

Bilateral adrenalectomy can be used in either case of failure of pituitary surgery or when hypercortisolism is severe, necessitating a rapidly active treatment, with the expected outcome being lifelong adrenal insufficiency.

Medical treatments are aimed at decreasing synthesis and secretion of cortisol, blocking glucocorticoid receptors, or inhibiting ACTH secretion. The main drawback to medical therapy is that it only offers control not cure and can be accompanied by serious side effects. There are four indications for medical treatment: contraindication or refusal of surgery, lack of defined pituitary lesion, waiting for radiation techniques to be effective, or as part of multimodality approach in the rare case of pituitary carcinoma.

What are some specific medical treatments for Cushing's disease?

- Ketoconazole is an antifungal agent with steroidogenesis inhibitor effects and is effective in 50% of cases (although is associated with many gastrointestinal [GI] side effects).
- Metyrapone is a pyridine derivative that blocks cortisol synthesis by inhibition of 11-beta hydroxylase; side effects include hypokalemia and hyperandrogenism.
- Mitotane is an inhibitor of cortisol secretion, is effective in 50% of cases, and frequently induces adrenal atrophy; however, it is associated with many GI side effects.
- Etomidate is an intravenous (IV) anesthetic agent that inhibits cortisol synthase by inhibiting CYP11B1 with 11-beta hydroxylase activity. It is used only in severe and refractory cases.
- Mifepristone is a progesterone receptor antagonist with cross-reactivity with the glucocorticoid receptor at high concentrations and is effective at controlling clinical signs of Cushing's syndrome. It is indicated for the treatment of diabetes that is secondary to Cushing's syndrome and has been shown to improve other associated symptoms and signs. Side effects include endometrial hyperplasia and bleeding, hypokalemia, and symptoms of adrenal insufficiency in some cases.

- Cabergoline is a dopamine agonist that can be used in Cushing's disease as corticotroph adenomas can express dopamine receptors; studies have demonstrated response rates of up to 25%.
- Pasireotide is a somatostatin receptor ligand that reduces ACTH and cortisol secretion. It is associated with a risk of worsening hyperglycemia, as well as gastrointestinal side effects that are commonly seen in other somatostatin analog medications.

BEYOND THE PEARLS

- False-positive rates for the overnight dexamethasone suppression test are seen in 50% of women taking the oral contraceptive pill because of increased cortisol-binding globulin (CBG) levels, in which case urinary free cortisol is a more appropriate test.
- A 24-hour urine free cortisol (UFC) level fourfold greater than normal can be diagnostic for Cushing's syndrome.
- Many drugs may interfere with the diagnosis of Cushing's syndrome. Medications that accelerate dexamethasone metabolism by induction through CYP34A or that impair dexamethasone metabolism by inhibition of CYP34A (itraconazole, diltiazem) falsely decrease or increase test results. Agents that increase CBG and may falsely elevate cortisol results (estrogens and mitotane) and some medications inappropriately increase UFC results (carbamazepine, fenofibrate). Drugs that inhibit 11-beta HSD2 (licorice carbenoxolone) also interfere with testing.
- In patients with Cushing's disease, 85 to 87% may present with either a microadenoma or a negative MRI at the time of diagnosis.
- Multiple endocrine neoplasia (MEN I): Cushing's disease can be part of MEN 1a due to mutations of the menin gene. It is a rare syndrome transmitted in an autosomal dominant manner that associates hyperparathyroidism, endocrine tumors, and pituitary adenomas. Most of the pituitary tumors are somatotroph or lactoproph in origin, but corticotroph adenomas have been described in 5 to 10% of cases.
- Ectopic ACTH syndrome (i.e., bronchial, thymic, pancreatic carcinoids, medullary thyroid carcinoma) makes up around 7% of Cushing's syndrome.
- Nelson syndrome is the rare complication of bilateral adrenalectomy in which there is pituitary tumor progression with elevated ACTH levels as a result of losing negative feedback.
- Hypokalemic metabolic acidosis can be seen as a result of excess mineralocorticoid effects in patients with Cushing's syndrome, usually in patients with ectopic ACTH syndromes.
- Consider hypercortisolism in the pediatric patient with decreasing height percentile (short stature), normal thyroid function, and weight gain. Genetic causes of ACTH-independent Cushing's disease (McCune Albright and Carney syndromes) can also present in childhood.
- Up to 7% of surgically resected pituitary adenomas that are thought to be nonfunctional are silent corticotroph adenomas by pathology and are morphologically indistinguishable from adenomas associated with Cushing's disease. However, these patients do not have biochemical or clinical evidence of cortisol excess.

References

Boscaro M, Arnaldi G. Approach to the patient with possible Cushing's syndrome. *J Clin Endocrinol Metab.* 2009;94(99):3121-3131.

Castinetti F, Morange I, Conte-Devolx B, Brue T. Cushing's disease. *Orphanet J Rare Dis.* 2012;7:41.

Melmed S, Polonsky KS, Larsen PR, Kronenberg HM. *Williams Textbook of Endocrinology.* Vol. 1. 12th ed. Philadelphia: Elseveier; 2011:479-544.

Nieman L, Biller B, Findling J, et al. The diagnosis of Cushing's syndrome: an Endocrine Society Clinical Practice Guideline. *J Clin Endocrinol Metab.* 2008;93(5):1526-1540.

Tritos NA, Biller BMK, Swearingen B. Management of Cushing disease. *Nat Rev Endocrinol.* 2011;7(5): 279-289.

A 58-Year-Old Male With Chest Pain

A 58-year-old male with a history of type 2 diabetes mellitus and hypothyroidism presents with a chief complaint of 2 days of intermittent chest pain.

What do you consider in your differential diagnosis of the chest pain in this patient?
A broad differential diagnosis should be undertaken with a chief complaint of chest pain (see Table 55.1). Particular attention should always be focused first toward life-threatening causes of chest pain, then other serious (but not immediately life-threatening) causes, then finally less ominous causes.

What other historical elements can you use to elicit the history in a patient with chest pain?
With some of the life-threatening causes of chest pain, it is important to note that "pain" might not be the patient's chief complaint. Patients often describe a stabbing, crushing, pressurelike, or tearing sensation. Therefore, sometimes using alternate words to ask a history, including "chest discomfort," may be useful. Asking the patient if he or she has current chest pain is helpful for triage. Always obtain the usual elements, including prior events, onset/timing, location, severity, intensity, and alleviating and aggravating factors, as well as baseline functional status and exercise capability/limitations. It is important to undertake a complete medication history, family history, and social history and to elicit historical evidence of features that are characteristic for life-threatening causes of chest pain. Table 55.2 lists historical features of life-threatening causes of chest pain.

After asking the patient salient features of conditions that are life-threatening, one can then investigate other causes of chest pain. A general review of systems will oftentimes elicit the relevant symptoms seen in these disorders. Specific questions to ask include those related to fever, weight loss, cough, edema, abdominal pain, food association, joint pain, rash, weakness in extremities, and psychiatric screening.

The patient indicates he has never had this chest pain before. He was mowing his lawn when the chest pain first occurred. He rates the pain as 6 to 8 out of 10, lasting a few minutes at a time, with at least five episodes before presentation. He says the pain is pressurelike and points to his sternum when describing the area of the pain. It is exacerbated by walking around his home and improves when resting. It is nonradiating in nature. He takes metformin 500 mg twice a day and levothyroxine 25 mcg daily. He has a 30-pack-year smoking history and uses no illicit drugs or alcohol. He is an only child. His mother and father are both alive, in their 80s, and both have hypertension. He denies fever, cough, joint pain, or weight changes.

What physical exam clues can you use with a chief complaint of chest pain?
Table 55.3 lists physical exam findings with select causes of chest pain.

TABLE 55.1 ■ Causes of Chest Pain (Potentially Life Threatening in Bold)

Cardiac

- Coronary disease (stable angina, vasospasm and vasculitis, **coronary dissection infarction/ischemia with acute coronary syndromes**)
- **Cardiac tamponade**
- Pericarditis
- Pericardial effusion
- Congestive heart failure, stress cardiomyopathy
- Myocarditis
- Valvular diseases (notably AS and MVP)

Pulmonary and Vascular

- **Pulmonary embolism**
- **Pneumothorax**
- **Aortic dissection**
- Pleurisy (idiopathic, infectious, and autoimmune)
- Pulmonary hypertension
- Pneumonia, pneumonitis
- Chronic lung disease, acute bronchitis
- Pleural effusion, especially with empyema
- Malignancy

Gastrointestinal

- **Esophageal rupture,** esophagitis (erosive and infectious), esophageal spasm, achalasia, esophageal foreign body, esophageal diverticulum
- Gastroesophageal reflux disease
- Peptic ulcer disease, gastric obstruction, gastric malignancy
- Biliary stone diseases
- Pancreatitis

Musculoskeletal

- Costochondritis
- Muscular strain (esp. intercostal and pectoralis)
- Bursitis
- Rib fracture
- Referred cervical pain

Other

- Mediastinal masses (lymphoma, thymoma, teratoma)
- Psychiatric diseases (anxiety, panic disorder, somatization, malingering)
- Herpes zoster
- Chronic pain

AS, Aortic stenosis; *MVP,* mitral valve prolapse.

TABLE 55.2 ■ Historical Features of Life-Threatening Causes of Chest Pain

Condition	Clinical Hints/Findings
Myocardial Infarction/Ischemia	Prior history, risk factors, location in the retrosternal/left side, worse with exertion, alleviated with rest or nitroglycerin.
Aortic Dissection	Severe tearing pain radiating to back. May also present with strokelike symptoms (i.e., weakness in lower extremities). Can also present with symptoms from complications, including pleural effusion and ischemia.
Pneumothorax	Sudden dyspnea and chest pain that is pleuritic in nature.

Continued

TABLE 55.2 ■ **Historical Features of Life-Threatening Causes of Chest Pain—cont'd**

Condition	Clinical Hints/Findings
Cardiac Tamponade	Shortness of breath, weight loss (in a patient with malignancy-associated tamponade), fevers (in a patient with infectious or autoimmune disease-associated tamponade)
Pulmonary Embolism	Sudden dyspnea and chest pain that is pleuritic in nature. May have nonproductive or productive cough with hemoptysis. Risk factors include immobility, malignancy, smoking, oral contraceptive pills (OCPs), and inherited thrombophilias.
Esophageal Rupture	Sudden tearing pain. Recent straining, coughing, ingestion of caustic substances. History of reflux, carcinoma. Patients may also have back pain, referred shoulder pain, or abdominal pain.

TABLE 55.3 ■ **Physical Exam Findings With Select Causes of Chest Pain**

Condition	Clinical Hints/Findings
Myocardial Infarction/Ischemia	May have S3 (as seen in patients with acute heart failure) or S4 (as seen in patients with underlying coronary artery disease or hypertension) on exam. Murmur from onset of valvular disease or wall rupture. May also present with signs of low-output (hypotension, altered mental status) or volume overload (crackles, jugular venous distention, edema).
Aortic Dissection	Blood pressure difference in arms, murmur of aortic insufficiency, objective weakness in lower extremities, decreased pulses in lower extremities. Complications include hypotension, and exam findings consistent with pleural effusion and ischemia.
Pneumothorax	Decreased breath sounds, hyperresonance to percussion. Can see tracheal deviation with tension pneumothorax.
Cardiac Tamponade	Jugular distention, decreased breath sounds, hypotension, pulsus paradoxus.
Pulmonary Embolism	Tachycardia, tachypnea, hypoxia. Can have signs of deep vein thrombosis (DVT) and pleural effusion. Loud P2, fixed split S2.
Esophageal Rupture	Tachycardia, palpable subcutaneous emphysema, Hamman's sign (audible crunch with heart sounds).
Pulmonary Hypertension	Loud P2, fixed split S2, heave, eventual right-sided heart failure (jugular venous distention, pulsatile liver, edema).
Congestive Heart Failure	Jugular venous distention, hepatojugular reflux, S3, S4, crackles, exam evidence of pleural effusion, may hear wheezing, pulsatile liver/hepatomegaly/ascites, dependent edema, pulsus alternans.
Pericarditis	Friction rub. May be tachycardic and febrile. Lymph node, joint exam, and skin exam may reflect causes (i.e., autoimmune diseases, infection, malignancy, uremia). Kussmaul's sign (increased jugular venous distention or lack of decrease with inspiration) if constrictive.
Pneumonia	Fever, bronchial breath sounds, rhonchi, dullness to percussion, friction rub, signs of effusion.
Aortic Stenosis	Lack of normal carotid upstroke, systolic crescendo–decrescendo murmur which is loudest at the right upper sternal border that radiates to supraclavicular/carotid region. S4 may be present, and heart sounds may be paradoxically split or reveal the absence of A2 heart sounds.

Physical exam reveals a blood pressure of 148/92 mm Hg, with a pulse rate of 82/min. He is afebrile and his oxygen saturation is 97% on room air. He has no jugular venous distension, and his pulse rate is regular with no murmurs or rubs appreciated. Lung exam reveals normal breath sounds with no adventitious features. There is no abdominal pain, lower extremity edema, or rashes.

Does this patient have angina?

The definition of angina is chest pain or discomfort that may be pressurelike, a sensation of fullness or squeezing; it can be felt in the chest, jaw, shoulder, back, or arm. The pain is usually less than 5 minutes in duration. In a patient presenting with chest pain, and when angina is suspected, it is useful to classify the chest pain into anginal categories depending on historical information (see Table 55.4).

CLINICAL PEARL   **STEP 2/3**

Chest pain can be atypical in female patients or in those with diabetes. Women often complain of epigastric pain when presenting with angina. Other symptoms commonly seen with underlying coronary artery disease (CAD) including fatigue, diaphoresis, dizziness, dyspnea, nausea/emesis, and lightheadedness/syncope. Even some patients with underlying coronary disease or an acute cardiac event may present with atypical chest pain or even noncardiac chest pain.

What are the risk factors for coronary artery disease?

Table 55.5 lists the risk factors for underlying CAD.

The patient has risk factors for coronary artery disease (smoking, diabetes), and his description of the chest pain contains all three components for angina, so he is presenting with typical angina. Consider myocardial ischemia and infarction in this setting, specifically one of the acute coronary syndromes.

TABLE 55.4 ■ **Anginal Classification**

Components

1. Location and duration: retrocardiac or substernal
2. Aggravating factors: exertion or emotional stress
3. Alleviating factors: rest or nitroglycerin

Typical: 3/3 components	Atypical: 2/3 components	Noncardiac: 0-1/3 components

---

TABLE 55.5 ■ **Risk Factors for Underlying Coronary Artery Disease**

- Race, gender, age
- Obesity
- Sedentary lifestyle
- Diabetes mellitus
- Smoking
- Hypertension
- Dyslipidemia (typically high LDL and low HDL)
- Family history of premature coronary artery disease (first-degree male <55, female <65)

TABLE 55.6 ■ **Estimated Risk of Coronary Artery Disease**

	Typical Angina		Atypical Angina		Nonanginal	
	Male	Female	Male	Female	Male	Female
30-39 Years	59	27	29	10	18	5
40-49 Years	69	37	38	14	25	8
50-59 Years	77	47	49	20	33	12
60-69 Years	84	58	59	28	44	17

Given historical components, what is this patient's pretest probability of underlying coronary artery disease?

The pretest probability for underlying CAD is useful for risk stratification in the outpatient setting and can guide the need for noninvasive testing. It also provides you with a tool to consider if CAD is the likely cause of the patient's presentation with chest pain. Table 55.6 lists estimated risks for CAD.

It is useful to divide patients into probability based on features:
- Low probability:
  - Asymptomatic men and women regardless of age
  - Women <50 years old with atypical angina
- Intermediate probability:
  - Men of all ages with atypical angina
  - Women ≥50 years old with atypical angina
  - Women 30 to 50 years old with typical angina
- High probability:
  - Men ≥40 years old with typical angina
  - Women ≥50 years old with typical angina

The patient has a high probability of underlying CAD given his age with typical chest pain. Using Table 55.6, his pretest probability of underlying CAD is approximately 77%. This is likely higher given his risk factors. You should continue to be concerned about an acute coronary syndrome.

CLINICAL PEARL　　　　　　　　　　　　　　　**STEP 2/3**

The above chart for risk stratification is helpful but not always characteristically accurate. As mentioned previously, certain patients can present atypically even when they have underlying ischemia. In addition, patients may not have typical angina with some of the acute coronary syndromes. Therefore, consider risk factors in estimating the underlying risk in addition to these factors. Other historical elements, such as previous infarctions, stents, and bypass grafting, also should be obtained.

CLINICAL PEARL　　　　　　　　　　　　　　　**STEP 2/3**

Always consider underlying coronary disease in a patient with diabetes or a smoker presenting with chest pain.

How do you classify the acute coronary syndromes?

The acute coronary syndromes include the following:
- ST segment elevation myocardial infarction/acute coronary syndromes (STEMI) including new left bundle branch block (LBBB)

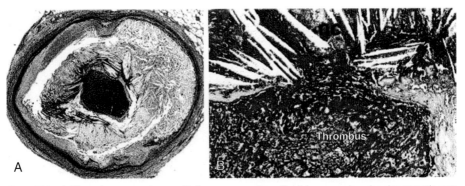

Figure 55.1   A, View of coronary plaque with fibrous cap rupture. **B,** High-power view showing necrotic core and thrombus. *(From Virmani R, Burke AP, Farb A, et al. Pathology of the vulnerable plaque.* J Am Coll Cardiol. *2006;47[suppl 8]:C13-C18.)*

- Non-ST segment elevation acute coronary syndromes (NSTE-ACS), which includes non-ST segment elevation myocardial infarction and unstable angina.

What is the pathophysiology of the acute coronary syndromes?

All acute coronary syndromes involve some obstruction of coronary flow. ST-elevation syndromes are due to complete occlusion of an epicardial blood vessel leading to myocardial necrosis in most cases. The non-ST segment elevation syndromes are due to a temporary vessel occlusion in patients, most commonly from a ruptured plaque or plaque erosion (Figs. 55.1 and 55.2). When vessel occlusion is severe and persistent, causing necrosis, it leads to non-ST elevation myocardial infarction, whereas patients with unstable angina have more mild narrowing over a short period of time without necrosis. With this being said, both non-ST elevation myocardial infarction and unstable angina are considered along the same spectrum of disease and are not distinguishable clinically.

CLINICAL PEARL   **STEP 2/3**

Not all coronary artery disease is atherosclerotic. Coronary dissection, coronary embolism (especially from malignancy and infections), vascular disorders (autoimmune, idiopathic, and drug mediated such as cocaine), coronary aneurysms, and extension of aortic dissection are all causes.

BASIC SCIENCE PEARL   **STEP 1**

Thrombosis occurs from plaque rupture, plaque erosion, and calcified nodules (rare). With plaque rupture, the lipid-rich necrotic core and overlying ruptured fibrous cap come into contact with platelets and inflammatory cells, which leads to luminal thrombosis. A cascade occurs with platelet adhesion and aggregation due to vWF-fibrinogen-glycoprotein IIb/IIIa. In addition, there is further damage due to interruption of vasodilator production, including nitric oxide (NO).

How would you initially workup this patient?

Workup should be guided by the specific causes. Depending on risk factors and likelihood for a life-threatening cause, initial workup should include an electrocardiogram (ECG), chest radiograph (CXR), and cardiac biomarkers (i.e., troponin).

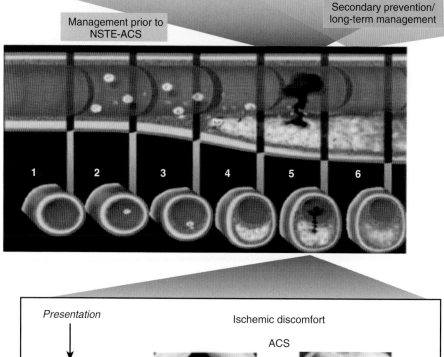

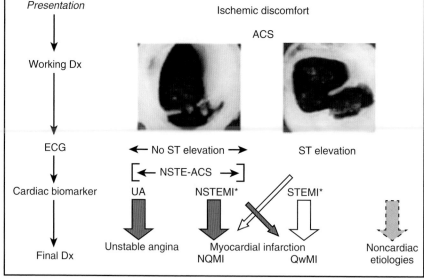

Figure 55.2 **Top,** Progression of plaque formation from (1) normal, (2) extracellular lipid in subintima, (3) fibrofatty stage, (4) weakened cap, (5) disruption of cap, and (6) thrombus resorption. **Bottom,** Graphic showing progression of findings as well as flow reduction in different entities of acute coronary syndrome. *, Conditions with elevated cardiac biomarkers; *ACS,* acute coronary syndrome; *ECG,* electrocardiogram; *ED,* emergency department; *NQMI,* non-Q wave myocardial infarction; *NSTEMI,* non-ST segment elevation myocardial infarction; *NSTE-ACS,* non-ST segment elevation acute coronary syndromes; *QwMI,* Q-wave myocardial infarction; *STEMI,* ST segment elevation myocardial infarction. *(From Amsterdam EA, Wenger NK, Brindis RG, et al. 2014 AHA/ACC Guideline for the Management of Patients with Non-ST-Elevation Acute Coronary Syndromes: a report of the American College of Cardiology/American Heart Association Task Force on Practice Guidelines. J Am Coll Cardiol. 2014;64[24]:e139-e228.)*

TABLE 55.7 ■ **Causes of Elevated Troponins**

- Myocardial necrosis
- Decreased clearance from renal failure
- Pulmonary embolism
- Congestive heart failure exacerbations
- Myocarditis
- Cardiac infiltration (i.e., amyloidosis)
- Cardiac tachyarrhythmias (esp. supraventricular tachycardia [SVT])
- Direct cardiac injury (cardioversion/defibrillator/surgery/ trauma)
- Severe sepsis
- Burns
- Severe asthma
- Brain injury, stroke, seizures

The ECG is helpful because it can show ST elevation (STEMI, pericarditis, aneurysm), ST depression (ischemia), Q waves (underlying CAD, hypertrophic obstructive cardiomyopathy), arteriovenous (AV) conduction abnormalities (ischemia), arrhythmias, and signs of atrial and ventricular enlargement. The ECG can also provide clues to pulmonary embolism (tachycardia, S1Q3T3) and pulmonary hypertension (right bundle branch block [RBBB], tall R waves, and T wave inversion in V1 and V2).

CXR is usually used to rule out causes (such as infection, effusion, pneumothorax, rupture) and provide clues to underlying pathology. You may see a widened mediastinum with pleural effusion with aortic dissection and a widened cardiac silhouette with cardiomyopathy or pericardial effusion/tamponade. Heart failure manifests with this silhouette and other findings (such as pulmonary edema, cephalization), whereas these other lung findings are usually absent (i.e., "clear lungs") in pericardial effusion or tamponade. Enlarged pulmonary vasculature can be seen in patients with pulmonary hypertension. Free air under the diaphragm may suggest esophageal perforation. Radiologic findings of pulmonary embolism may be seen, including pleural effusion or the rarer findings of Hampton's hump (a wedge-shaped infarct) or Westermark sign (oligemia on the side of the embolism), although these are rare.

Cardiac biomarkers should be sent when there is a concern for myocardial ischemia or infarction. It is important to be aware of conditions that can falsely raise markers as well as their time to positivity, peak, and duration of positivity to relate them to clinical presentation. This is particularly important as some patients with cardiac ischemia may present in a delayed nature, especially patients with a more atypical presentation. Troponin I and troponin T are very sensitive and specific and are the most widely used. They rise within 2 to 4 hours, peak in 8 to 12 hours, and can stay elevated for up to 10 days. The main disadvantage with troponin is that levels stay positive for a long time, so they cannot be used reliably postinfarction, and in this case, creatine kinase MB (CK-MB) or myoglobin levels are usually obtained. CK-MB is not as specific as troponin levels but rises in 4 to 6 hours and peaks in 10 to 24 hours, lasting a total of 36 hours. Myoglobin is also nonspecific but rises very quickly (2 hours). Keep in mind that there are many causes for elevated troponins besides cardiac necrosis (see Table 55.7).

Given the patient's presentation, you should order other routine labs, including complete blood count (CBC), complete metabolic panel (with attention to renal function, electrolytes, glucose, and transaminases), and a fasting lipid panel. Further workup depends on clinical suspicion. You could order a D-dimer or computed tomography (CT) angiogram of the chest if you are concerned about pulmonary embolism. A chest CT is used to diagnose aortic dissection. Blood cultures should be drawn in cases of suspected pneumonia. An echocardiogram can be used to evaluate valvular diseases, to assess left ventricular function, and to investigate a pericardial effusion as well as hemodynamics for tamponade.

> **CLINICAL PEARL**   **STEP 2/3**
>
> Remember to obtain old ECGs for comparison. With reoccurrence of symptoms or new features to the chest pain, obtain a repeat ECG and consider repeat workup for other causes if directed by symptoms.

The ECG and CXR for this patient are shown in Figures 55.3 and 55.4. Troponin I and troponin T are within the normal range. CBC and metabolic panel, including electrolytes and renal function, are normal.

Given his ECG, what are your concerns?

He is presenting with typical angina symptoms and has risk factors for underlying CAD. In the setting of an ECG that does not have ST elevation and normal cardiac biomarkers, unstable angina is the concern.

How do you diagnose unstable angina?

Unlike STEMI and NSTEMI, which have ECG changes and biomarkers that help guide diagnosis, unstable angina is a historical diagnosis that necessitates a high degree of suspicion. Besides the symptoms consistent with angina, key findings include:

- Previous angina that is becoming more severe, more frequent, or longer in duration (especially >15 to 20 minutes)
- Changes in the quality of previous angina (i.e., it feels different to the patient)
- New onset angina
- Angina at rest or with minimal exertion
- Angina not relieved with rest or nitroglycerin

With this being said, non-ST elevation MI and unstable angina are considered similar with regards to their pathophysiology. Therefore, their diagnostic evaluation and treaments are similar too.

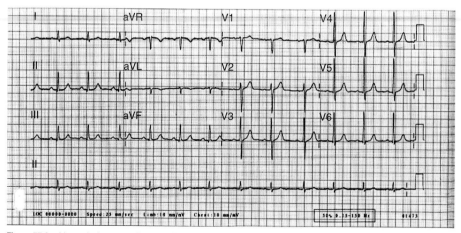

Figure 55.3 Normal electrocardiogram (ECG) in patient. *(From Davey P. How to read an EKG. Heart: The Foundation Years. 2008;4[3]:124-128.)*

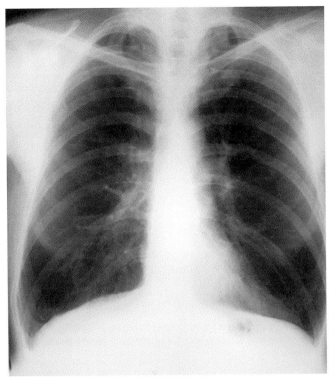

Figure 55.4 Chest radiograph showing hyperinflated lungs and flattening diaphragm. *(From Grichnik K, Hill S. The perioperative management of patients with severe emphysema.* J Cardiothorac Vasc Anesth. *2003;17[3]:364-387.)*

What is your immediate approach to this patient?

Admission is required for unstable angina. Based on risk of mortality and stability, the decision to admit to a monitored setting or coronary care unit (CCU) can be made. It is important to assess for hemodynamic stability and any complications of the syndrome, including decompensated heart failure or arrhythmias.

Patients with suspected non-ST segment elevation acute coronary syndromes should be given immediate treatment, including:

- Oxygen to those patients with respiratory distress or saturation ≤90%.
- Sublingual nitroglycerin with continual pain. This should be done every 5 minutes for a maximum of three doses, at which time intravenous (IV) nitroglycerin can be considered if severe disease is present.
- Oral beta blockers (avoid if the patient has evidence of low-output states, an ECG with advanced heart block or PR interval >0.24 seconds, severe reactive airway disease, or decompensated heart failure).
- IV morphine sulfate if pain persists despite other antianginal medication (nitrates and beta blockers).
- Antiplatelet therapy:
  - Aspirin therapy (preferable nonenteric and chewable at 162 mg to 325 mg dosing) unless there are contraindications. If patients do not tolerate aspirin but can take antiplatelet therapy, clopidogrel can be given.

- In the absence of contraindications, if an invasive approach to management is to be taken (i.e., angiography with intervention) you can use a $P2Y_{12}$ inhibitor (either clopidogrel or ticagrelor) and consider the use of a glycoprotein (GP) IIb/IIIa inhibitor (eptifibatide or tirofiban) in addition to dual antiplatelet therapy.
- Anticoagulation therapy:
  - Enoxaparin, therapeutic unfractionated heparin, fondaparinux (in combination with other medications), or bivalirudin (in select patients) should be given until percutaneous coronary intervention (PCI) is performed.
- High-intensity statin therapy

CLINICAL PEARL   **STEP 2/3**

Do not administer nitrates if the patient has received a phosphodiesterase inhibitor within the past 24 to 48 hours.

CLINICAL PEARL   **STEP 2/3**

Contraindications to aspirin therapy include serious active bleeding, active peptic ulcer disease or severe gastritis, or severe uncontrolled hypertension.

BASIC SCIENCE PEARL   **STEP 1**

GP IIb/IIIa inhibitors act by interfering with platelets binding to fibrinogen, inducing impaired platelet aggregation similar to patients with Glanzmann's thrombasthenia.

The patient is given chewable aspirin 325 mg, atorvastatin 80 mg, sublingual nitrogen 0.4 mg, metoprolol tartrate 50 mg oral and enoxaparin 80 mg subcutaneous.

What is this patient's risk of mortality?

Once a patient is diagnosed with either NSTEMI or unstable angina, you can use the Thrombolysis In Myocardial Infarction (TIMI) risk score or Global Registry of Acute Coronary Events (GRACE) score, which not only predict mortality but provide an approach to further workup and treatment of the patient.

Components to calculate the TIMI score assign 1 point each to the following (see Table 55.8):

T: Two or more episodes of chest pain
H: History of CAD with at least 50% stenosis
R: Risk factors for CAD (at least three including family history, hypertension, dyslipidemia, diabetes mellitus, smoking)
E: ECG changes of ST segment at least 0.5 mm
A: Age >65
A: Aspirin use within 7 days
T: Troponin elevation

The GRACE score is used to predict in-hospital mortality as well as 6-month mortality (see Table 55.9).

The patient's TIMI score is 1 (two or more episodes of chest pain), so he has a 14-day risk of about 4.7%. His GRACE score is 72, giving him an in-hospital risk of 0.5% and a 6-month risk of 1.6%.

TABLE 55.8 ■ Thrombolysis in Myocardial Infarction (TIMI) Score for NSTEMI/Unstable Angina

TIMI Risk Score	All-Cause Mortality, New or Recurrent Myocardial Infarction, or Severe Recurrent Ischemia Requiring Urgent Revascularization Through 14 Days After Randomization (%)
0-1	4.7
2	8.3
3	13.2
4	19.9
5	26.2
6-7	40.9

The TIMI risk score is determined by the sum of the presence of seven variables at admission; 1 point is given for each of the following variables: ≥65 years of age; ≥3 risk factors for coronary artery disease; prior coronary stenosis ≥50%; ST deviation on electrocardiogram; ≥2 anginal events in prior 24 hours; use of aspirin in prior 7 days; and elevated cardiac biomarkers.
(From Amsterdam EA, Wenger NK, Brindis RG, et al. 2014 AHA/ACC Guideline for the Management of Patients with Non-ST-Elevation Acute Coronary Syndromes: a report of the American College of Cardiology/American Heart Association Task Force on Practice Guidelines. *J Am Coll Cardiol.* 2014;64[24]:e139-e228.)

TABLE 55.9 ■ Risk Stratification for NSTEMI/Unstable Angina

Score	Features	Comments
TIMI	≥65 years of age; ≥3 risk factors for coronary artery disease; prior coronary stenosis ≥50%; ST deviation on electrocardiogram; ≥2 anginal events in prior 24 hours; use of aspirin in prior 7 days; and elevated cardiac biomarkers	Sum of number of features (1 point each)
PURSUIT	Age by decade, gender, worst Canadian Cardiovascular Society anginal class in previous 6 weeks, signs of heart failure, ST segment depression	Weighted score based on different point total (range, 0-14) for each feature
GRACE	Age, pulse rate, systolic blood pressure, creatinine level, Killip class, cardiac arrest, elevated markers, ST segment deviation	Weighted score based on different point total (range, 0-91) for each feature

GRACE, Global Registry of Acute Coronary Events; *PURSUIT,* Platelet Glycoprotein IIb/IIIa in Unstable Angina: Receptor Suppression Using Integrilin Therapy; *TIMI,* Thrombolysis In Myocardial Infarction.
(From Wiviott SD, Giugliano RP. Non-ST-segment elevation acute coronary syndromes. In: Antman EM, Sabatine MS, eds. *Cardiovascular Therapeutics: A Companion to Braunwald's Heart Disease.* 4th ed. Philadelphia: Elsevier; 2013:153-177, Table 9-1.)

What is the next approach to management?
There are two treatment strategies to pursue in the management of this patient: the invasive strategy and the ischemia-guided strategy. The choice of strategy is guided by many factors, including the scoring systems just described.
- **Invasive Strategy:** Used in patients with high-risk features, including a TIMI ≥2 or GRACE score ≥109. These patients receive treatment as above with aspirin, a P2Y$_{12}$ inhibitor, an anticoagulant, as well as a GPIIb/IIIa inhibitor in high-risk patients (i.e., troponin positive). In addition, coronary angiography is performed. Depending on findings, PCI or coronary artery bypass grafting (CABG) may be undertaken.

- **Ischemia-Guided Strategy:** Use in patients with low-risk scores (TIMI 0-1 or GRACE <109) without high-risk features. These patients receive treatment as above with aspirin, a P2Y$_{12}$ inhibitor, and an anticoagulant (in addition to other medications as outlined above). A noninvasive evaluation is performed (i.e., stress testing). Invasive evaluation with coronary angiography is undertaken only if the patient fails medical therapy by demonstrating refractory angina or symptoms with minimal activity, demonstrates new ECG changes, develops hemodynamic instability, or stress testing demonstrates ischemia. At this point, guided by findings, PCI or CABG may be undertaken.

Upon discharge, patients should be started/continued on treatment depending on the findings during the hospitalization course. Patients should receive aspirin therapy, consideration for a long-term P2Y$_{12}$ inhibitor, statin therapy, beta blockade, an angiotensin-converting enzyme (ACE) inhibitor as well as nitrates for symptoms as needed (with consideration of a long-acting nitrate and other agents for angina including ranolazine, nondihydropyridines, and short-acting dihydropyridines). Patients should be counselled on smoking habits (and enrolled in cessation if they are willing) and given information on diet and exercise.

Given the patient's lower TIMI and GRACE scores, an ischemia-guided strategy is undertaken and the patient is admitted to the medical wards with telemetry monitoring. An exercise ECG stress test is ordered for the next morning. However, 4 hours after admission he develops worsening chest pain. The ECG shows new ST segment depression. Cardiac angiography is performed due to the change in clinical status, and PCI with stenting is performed. The patient is admitted to the CCU for observation. He is continued on aspirin, clopidogrel, metoprolol, and atorvastatin. Lisinopril is started and he is discharged 72 hours after admission in stable condition with follow up.

Diagnosis: Unstable angina with low-risk TIMI and GRACE scores on presentation

---

BEYOND THE PEARLS

- The choice of using troponin I and troponin T is usually dependent on laboratory availability in each clinical setting. Overall, troponin I is less standardized and troponin T is more elevated in renal failure.
- Even though most patients presenting with NSTE-ACS have underlying CAD, an oxygen supply/demand mismatch can cause NSTE-ACS or lower the threshold for NSTE-ACS to occur in a patient with CAD. These include increased demand (infections, thyrotoxicosis), decreased supply (anemia or hypoxemia), or decreased coronary blood flow from hypotension or tachyarrhythmia.
- Statin therapy in patients that present with NSTE-ACS has decreased the rate of recurrent myocardial infarction, mortality from CAD, need for revasculation, and stroke.
- When treating a patient with suspected NSTE-ACS, if there is concomitant compensated heart failure, consider use of the beta blockers metoprolol succinate or carvedilol, which portend a mortality benefit.
- Patients with NSTE-ACS who have an early invasive approach to treatment should continue on a P2Y$_{12}$ inhibitor (either clopidogrel or ticagrelor) for up to 12 months.
- In patients who initially undergo an invasive strategy, timing is based on a variety of factors. Immediate coronary angiography (within 2 hours) is performed with refractory symptoms, evidence of heart failure, new or worsening mitral regurgitation, hemodynamic instability, or arrhythmias such as ventricular tachycardia (VT) or ventricular fibrillation (VF). Most other patients undergo early invasive (within 24 hours) coronary angiography especially with a GRACE score >140. A select group of patients (including those with

BEYOND THE PEARLS—cont'd

GRACE score between 109 and 140, renal insufficiency, recent PCI, or prior CABG) undergo delayed coronary angiography (between 25 and 72 hours).
- Fibrinolytic therapy has no role in the treatment of NSTE-ACS.
- According to guidelines, there are considerations in specific patient populations, including an early invasive strategy for patients ≥65.
- Patients with recent cocaine or methamphetamine use should not be given beta blockers if they demonstrate signs of acute intoxication (hypertension, tachycardia, euphoria). In these patients, benzodiazepines ± nitroglycerin can be given.
- Do not routinely transfuse patients with NSTE-ACS to a hemoglobin level >8 g/dL.
- In patients receiving chemotherapy or immunosuppressive agents, obtain a consultation with the prescriber, as certain agents (i.e., gemcitabine, fluorouracil [5-FU], sorafenib, sunitinib) can contribute to CAD.
- The use of short-acting dihydropyridines (such as nifedipine) can increase the risk of cardiac events and should be avoided.
- Attempt to avoid the use of nonsteroidal antiinflammatory drugs (NSAIDs) in patients with CAD, as studies have shown increased risk of reinfarction, rupture, heart failure, and death.
- Indications for CABG include patients with left main disease, two or three vessel disease with involvement of the left anterior descending artery (LAD), and left ventricular dysfunction, as well as diabetics with multivessel disease, especially with left ventricular dysfunction.
- Prior to discharge, patients should also be referred to a cardiac rehabilitation program, undergo annual influenza vaccination, and be considered for pneumococcal vaccination.

References

Amsterdam EA, Wenger NK, Brindis RG, et al. 2014 AHA/ACC guideline for the management of patients with non-ST-elevation acute coronary syndromes: a report of the American College of Cardiology/American Heart Association Task Force on Practice Guidelines. *J Am Coll Cardiol*. 2014;64(24): e139-e228.

Antman EM, Cohen M, Bernink PJ, et al. The TIMI risk score for unstable angina/non-ST elevation MI: a method for prognostication and therapeutic decision making. *JAMA*. 2000;284(7):835-842.

D'Ascenzo F, Biondi-Zoccai G, Moretti C. TIMI, GRACE and alternative risk scores in acute coronary syndromes: a meta-analysis of 40 derivation studies on 216,552 patients and of 42 validation studies on 31,625 patients. *Contemp Clin Trials*. 2012;33(3):507-514.

Diamond GA, Forrester JS, Hirsch M, et al. Application of conditional probability analysis to the clinical diagnosis of coronary artery disease. *J Clin Invest*. 1980;65(5):1210-1221.

Goodman SG, Steg PG, Eagle KA, et al. The diagnostic and prognostic impact of the redefinition of acute myocardial infarction: lessons from the Global Registry of Acute Coronary Events (GRACE). *Am Heart J*. 2006;151:654-660.

Lee TH, Goldman L. Evaluation of the patient with acute chest pain. *N Engl J Med*. 2000;342(16): 1187-1195.

Sabatine MS, McCabe CH, Morrow DA, et al. Identification of patients at high risk for death and cardiac ischemic events after hospital discharge. *Am Heart J*. 2002;143(6):966-970.

Swap CJ, Nagurney JT. Value and limitations of chest pain history in the evaluation of patients with suspected acute coronary syndromes. *JAMA*. 2005;294(20):2623-2629.

Virmani R, Burke AP, Farb A, et al. Pathology of the vulnerable plaque. *J Am Coll Cardiol*. 2006;47(suppl 8):C13-C18.

Monisha Bhanote ▪ Daniel Martinez

A 70-Year-Old Male With Iron Deficiency Anemia

A 70-year-old male presents to establish care with you, his new primary medical doctor (PMD), because he recently moved into the area. He says that he has iron deficiency anemia and has been taking iron pills for the past 3 years. Otherwise, he has no allergies, no past surgeries, no family history of cancer, heart disease, or strokes, and no smoking, alcohol, or drug use. He says that he had a colonoscopy at the time of diagnosis of his anemia because he was having bright red blood per rectum. The gastroenterologist removed two benign polyps and noted moderate internal hemorrhoids. He eats a high-fiber diet now and denies any constipation or bright red blood per rectum for the past 3 years. However, he is still dependent on taking iron supplementation to keep up his hemoglobin levels.

On physical exam, his temperature is 37 °C (98.6 °F), pulse rate is 74/min, blood pressure is 145/85 mm Hg, respiration rate is 14/min, and oxygen saturation is 99% on room air. He is well nourished and well developed. He has pink conjunctiva, moist mucus membranes, no jugular venous distention, normal heart and lung sounds, and a soft, nontender abdomen. There is no clubbing, skin rash, joint swelling, or peripheral edema. He wants to know if he can finally stop his iron.

Does the patient still need iron supplementation?

In the absence of a malabsorptive pathology or extreme malnutrition, iron deficiency anemia is generally caused by chronic blood loss of some time. It is typical for the source of bleeding to be from a gastrointestinal source. Referring this patient for a colonoscopy because of his symptoms of bright red blood per rectum in the setting of iron deficiency anemia was the correct decision at the time. However, the presence of one source of bleeding does not itself rule out the possibility of other sources of bleeding. Generally speaking, patients with an iron deficiency anemia should receive both a colonoscopy and an upper endoscopy to rule out other sources of bleeding such as a gastric or duodenal ulcer. This is especially the case when the patient is still iron dependent after his polyps are removed and his hemorrhoids are treated with a high-fiber diet. When the source of bleeding has been removed, a patient's iron stores should replenish in a few months of oral iron supplementation. Failure to do so should have prompted the PMD to evaluate further sources of occult bleeding.

You discuss with the patient that if he has no further sources of bleeding, he really should not need to be taking iron anymore. The fact that he has still needed iron to keep up his hemoglobin level is concerning for an alternative source of chronic bleeding. You refer him back to gastroenterology for an upper endoscopy.

While waiting for this appointment, he develops 2 days of nausea, vomiting, and crampy epigastric abdominal pain and goes to the local emergency room. He denies any fevers, chills, hematemesis, melena, or hematochezia. On physical exam, his temperature is 37.5 °C (99.5 °F), pulse rate is 110/min, blood pressure is 160/90 mm Hg, respiration rate is 18/min, and oxygen saturation is 99% on room air. He is in moderate discomfort but in no acute distress. His conjunctiva are pink and mucus membranes are moist. He is tachycardic but has no murmurs or extra heart sounds. His lungs are clear to auscultation. His abdomen is soft, with some mild to moderate epigastric tenderness to palpation. He has no rebound, guarding, or signs of peritonitis.

What are some considerations of abdominal pain in this patient?
The differential diagnosis for new-onset abdominal pain is very wide, and a good way to think about common causes is by considering the potential organs involved. In the left upper quadrant, the pancreas can be involved by pancreatitis and the stomach can be involved by a peptic ulcer or a mass. In the right upper quadrant, the hepatobiliary system can be involved by cholecystitis, cholangitis, or biliary colic. In the left lower and right lower quadrants, the small intestines and colon can be involved with diverticulitis, appendicitis, bowel obstruction, inflammatory bowel disease, and colonic masses. The possibility of bony metastasis or metastasis to other organs should be considered in a patient with a previously diagnosed malignancy. Another rare consideration is aortic dissection or ruptured aneurysm in the right clinical setting. If any of these are reasonable suspicions based on his clinical presentation, it is appropriate to order a computed tomography (CT) scan of the abdomen/pelvis with intravenous (IV) contrast. (The addition of oral [PO] contrast can also help evaluate the bowel better for a small bowel obstruction.)

Given the patient's tachycardia and new and acute epigastric pain, basic labs and a CT scan of the abdomen and pelvis with IV and PO contrast is ordered. White blood cell (WBC) count is 8000 cells/μL, hemoglobin is 14 g/dL, and mean corpuscular volume (MCV) is 82 fL/cell. The patient's CT scan is done quickly, and the radiologist evaluates the results. A 3.6-cm submucosal mass is found in the stomach (see Fig. 56.1). There is no evidence of pancreatitis, cholecystitis, appendicitis, or small bowel obstruction. He does have sigmoid diverticulosis, but there is no evidence of diverticulitis. No lymphadenopathy is appreciated.

CLINICAL PEARL   STEP 2/3

Diverticulosis is uncommon under the age of 40; however, more than 50% of individuals older than 70 have diverticulosis.

What is the differential diagnosis of a gastric submucosal mass?
Submucosal masses can be benign or malignant, and the differential diagnosis of a submucosal mass can be divided into mesenchymal versus nonmesenchymal lesions (see Table 56.1).

CLINICAL PEARL   STEP 2/3

Gastrointestinal stromal tumors (GISTs) can show local invasion and metastasis to the liver, omentum, or peritoneum; however, imaging does not typically show lymph node enlargement, which is more commonly seen in gastric adenocarcinomas or lymphomas.

CLINICAL PEARL   STEP 2/3

GISTs are the most common mesenchymal neoplasms of the gastrointestinal tract.

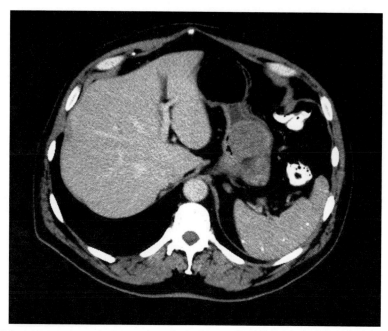

Figure 56.1   Axial contrast enhanced computed tomography (CT) image of a gastrointestinal stromal tumor in the fundus of the stomach. *(From http://commons.wikimedia.org/wiki/File%3ACT_image_of_a_GIST _tumor_in_the_gastric_cardia.jpg.)*

TABLE 56.1 ■ Differential Diagnosis of Submucosal Lesions in the Stomach

Mesenchymal	Nonmesenchymal
Gastrointestinal stromal tumor (GIST)	Heterotopic pancreas
Leiomyoma	Hamartoma
Schwannoma	Cysts/pseudocyst
Lipoma	Carcinoid
Granular cell tumor	
Vascular tumors	

CLINICAL PEARL   **STEP 1**

GISTs arise from the interstitial cells of Cajal, which are involved in pacemaker activity and regulate peristalsis.

The CT scan shows no evidence of active bleeding or infection, and his vital signs improve with moderate pain control. The patient is therefore discharged with follow-up with his gastroenterologist for an upper endoscopy and possible endoscopic ultrasound–guided fine needle aspiration (EUS-FNA). During the upper endoscopy, the stomach shows a protruding mass with intact overlying mucosa (see Fig. 56.2). The patient then proceeds to have a EUS-FNA without complications. The patient receives unfortunate news that the biopsy results confirm the presence of a spindle cell neoplasm. Due to the scant amount of tissue obtained during the EUS-FNA, there were limitations when it came to discerning the specific type of spindle cell neoplasm and its malignant potential.

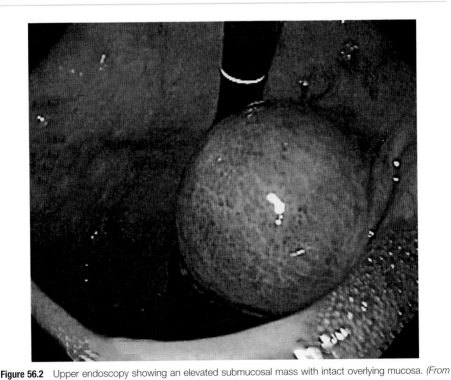

Figure 56.2 Upper endoscopy showing an elevated submucosal mass with intact overlying mucosa. *(From* http://commons.wikimedia.org/wiki/File%3AGIST_2.jpg.*)*

CLINICAL PEARL   **STEP 2/3**

The most common sites of GISTs include the stomach (60%), jejunum and ileum (30%), duodenum (5%), and colon (5%).

What are the benign and malignant histologic features of gastric stromal tumors?

GISTs are divided into four main tumor types: benign (cellular spindle cell tumor), malignant (spindle cell sarcoma), and benign epithelioid and malignant epithelioid tumors (see Table 56.2). Although confirmation of a spindle cell neoplasm was made by EUS-FNA, due to insufficient material for further testing, the type of neoplasm was not confirmed. Surgery is generally performed in lesions >3 cm and those with EUS features of malignancy.

The patient is referred to a surgeon for resection and pathologic staging of this gastric mass. He follows up with a surgeon and proceeds to a partial gastrectomy (see Fig. 56.3) without complications. The histology shows a spindle cell proliferation underlying the benign gastric mucosa (see Fig. 56.4). The mass is thoroughly sampled and shows a cellular spindle cell tumor forming tight fascicles (Fig. 56.5A) with at least 7 mitoses per 50 high power fields (see Fig. 56.5B). Immunoperoxidase stains are performed for a confirmatory diagnosis.

What are the common immunoperoxidase stains used to differentiate different spindle cell neoplasms?

The most common immunoperoxidase stains used to differentiate between different kinds of mesenchymal spindle cell neoplasms include CD117 (c-kit), CD34, SMA (smooth muscle actin),

TABLE 56.2 ■ **Histologic Features of Spindled and Epithelioid Gastrointestinal Stromal Tumors (GISTs)**

Features	Benign Spindled GIST	Malignant Spindled GIST	Benign Epithelioid GIST	Malignant Epithelioid GIST
Cellularity	High	High	Low	High
Nuclear atypia	None to minimal	Minimal to marked	None to minimal	Minimal to marked
Mitotic figures (per high power field [HPF])	Typically <2/50 HPF	Usually >5/50 HPF	Typically <2/50 HPF	Usually >5/50 HPF
Mucosal invasion	Absent	May be present	Absent	May be present
Tumor cell necrosis	Usually absent	Often present	Absent	Often present

Desmin, and S100. Leiomyomas are more commonly positive for SMA and Desmin, whereas Schwannomas are S100 positive. GISTs are positive for CD117 (c-kit) 95% of the time and CD34 70% of the time.

CLINICAL PEARL   **STEP 2/3**

The most sensitive marker for GISTs from all sites is CD117 (c-kit), with strong, diffuse, and pancytoplasmic staining.

CLINICAL PEARL   **STEP 2/3**

CD117 (c-kit) can be positive in other tumors including mastocytoma, seminoma, pulmonary small cell carcinoma, and granulocytic sarcoma.

Confirmatory immunoperoxidase stains CD117 (c-kit) and DOG1 are performed on this patient's specimen (see Fig. 56.6).

Diagnosis: GIST (malignant spindle cell sarcoma type), based on histology and confirmatory stains

---

What are risk factors for aggressive behavior in a GIST?

Several features consistently correlate with clinical outcome; however, not all tumors follow the rules. The National Institutes of Health developed a consensus to the diagnosis and prognostication on the basis of morphologic features. Using two criteria, size and mitotic figures, the tumors can be divided into four risk categories: very low risk, low risk, intermediate risk, and high risk (see Table 56.3).

What are additional treatment options that may be considered in GISTs?

Surgery is the primary treatment for all resectable tumors. However, if the tumor is large yet resectable, then neoadjuvant treatment with imatinib may be considered. Imatinib can decrease

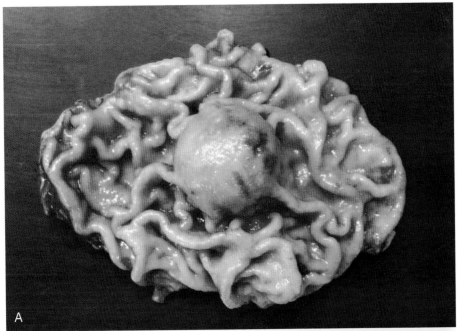

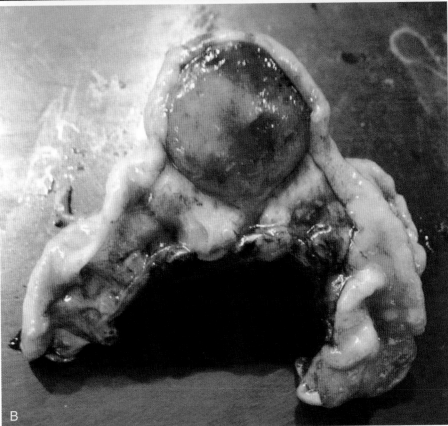

Figure 56.3 **A,** Gross photograph of partial stomach resection showing a 3.6-cm mass protruding into the stomach upon opening and with overlying minimal mucosal ulceration. **B,** The cut surface of the submucosal mass is pink-tan and focally soft.

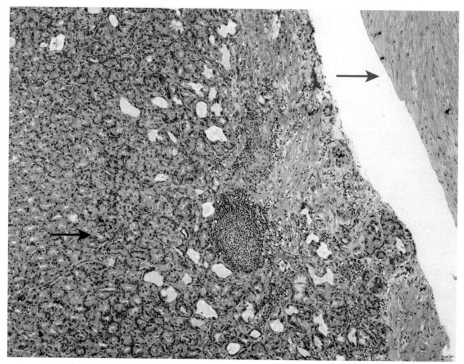

Figure 56.4 Histologic section of mass showing overlying benign gastric glands *(left, black arrow)* and adjacent spindle cell proliferation *(right, blue arrow)* representing the bulging mass (hematoxylin and eosin [H&E]).

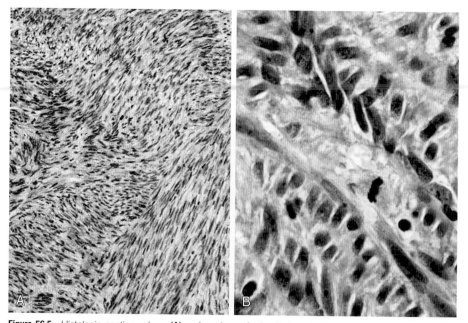

Figure 56.5 Histologic sections show **(A)** a densely packed spindle cell tumor arranged in fascicles with nuclear pleomorphism and hyperchromasia and **(B)** at higher power a mitotic figure can be appreciated (hematoxylin and eosin [H&E]).

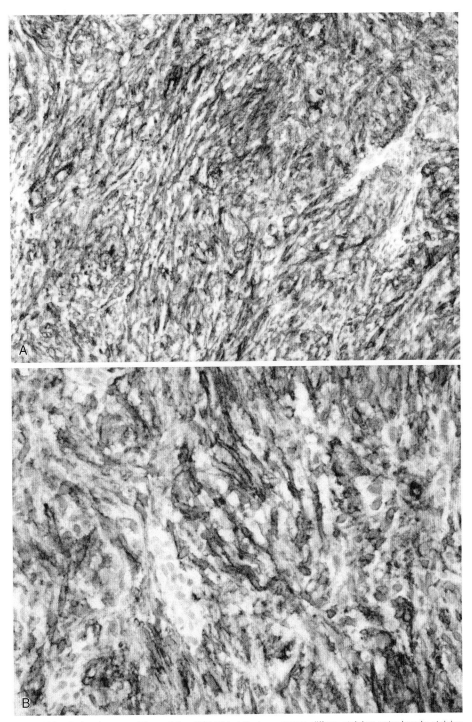

Figure 56.6 **A,** Immunoperoxidase stains CD117 (c-kit) show strong diffuse staining cytoplasmic staining while **(B)** DOG1 shows diffuse membranous and cytoplasmic staining.

TABLE 56.3 ■ National Institutes of Health Proposed Approach for Defining Risk of Aggressive Behavior

Risk	Size (cm)	Mitotic Figures (per 50 HPF)
Very low risk	<2	<5
Low risk	2-5	<5
Intermediate risk	<5 5-10	6-10 <5
High risk	>5 >10 Any size	>5 Any mitotic rate >10

the size of the mass prior to surgery, thereby increasing the possibility of negative margins without significant morbidity. Even with complete resection, 50% of patients can develop recurrence or metastasis. Adjuvant therapy with imatinib for 36 months has been found to be beneficial in patients with intermediate or high risk of recurrence. In patients who have received neoadjuvant imatinib, continuation for 2 additional years following surgery is recommended. Imatinib is also indicated in patients with unresectable, metastatic, or recurrent disease.

CLINICAL PEARL   **STEP 3**

Mutational analysis can be helpful in planning therapy because different mutations of CD117 (c-kit) and platelet derived growth factor receptor alpha (PDGFRA) may affect prognosis and response to therapy.

CLINICAL PEARL   **STEP 2/3**

Imatinib (Gleevec®) is an orally administered drug that inhibits both CD117 (c-kit) tyrosine kinase mutations and PDGFRA mutations.

CLINICAL PEARL   **STEP 2/3**

The most common side effects associated with imatinib include fluid retention, diarrhea, nausea, fatigue, muscle cramps, abdominal pain, and rash.

Continued surveillance is recommended in any patient diagnosed with either benign or malignant GISTs due to their unpredictable nature. The most intense follow-up is within the first 3 to 5 years because a majority of GISTs recur in this time.

After the pathologic diagnosis and staging from surgery, the patient is referred to an oncologist. He is started on adjuvant imatinib and tolerates it well. He continues to follow up with the oncologist for surveillance for the next few years without evidence of recurrence.

BEYOND THE PEARLS

- Hereditary syndromes associated with GISTs are neurofibromatosis type 1 (NF1), Carney's triad, familial GIST syndrome, and Carney Stratakis syndrome.
- 10 to 15% of GISTs lack CD117 (c-kit) or PDGFRA mutations; these include pediatric GISTs and GISTs seen in neurofibromatosis 1.
- Pediatric GISTS are biologically distinct, occur more commonly in girls and young women, and lack the oncogenic activating tyrosine kinase mutations in both CD117 (c-kit) and PDGFRA.
- DOG1 is a calcium-dependent, receptor-activated chloride channel protein expressed in GIST; this expression is independent of mutation type and can be used in the diagnosis of CD117 (c-kit)-negative tumors.
- DOG1 may be a more sensitive and specific marker than CD117 (c-kit) for GISTs.
- Tumors lacking CD117 (c-kit) or platelet derived growth factor receptor alpha (PDGFRA) mutations will not respond to targeted therapy (imatinib mesylate, sunitinib malate).
- Resistance to imatinib can develop. If this occurs, increasing the dosage is the first step; however, with continued resistance, the use of other kinase inhibitors (i.e., sunitinib) is recommended.
- Regorafenib (Stivarga®) was FDA (U.S. Food and Drug Administration) approved in 2013 for advanced GISTs that cannot be surgically resected or for those that no longer respond to imatinib.

References

Burkill GJ, Badran M, Al-Muderis O, et al. Malignant gastrointestinal stromal tumor: distribution, imaging features, and pattern of metastatic spread. *Radiology.* 2003;226(2):527-532.

Fletcher CD, Bermann JJ, Corless C, et al. Diagnosis of gastrointestinal stromal tumors: A consensus approach. *Hum Pathol.* 2002;33:459-465.

Miettinen M, Lasota J. Gastrointestinal stromal tumors: review on morphology, molecular pathology, prognosis, and differential diagnosis. *Arch Pathol Lab Med.* 2006;130(10):1466-1478.

Nishida T, Hirota S. Biological and clinical review of stromal tumors in the gastrointestinal tract. *Histol Histopathol.* 2000;15(4):1293-1301.

Odze RD, Goldblum JR. *Surgical Pathology of the GI Tract, Liver, Biliary Tract, and Pancreas.* 2nd ed. Philadelphia: Saunders Elsevier; 2009.

Pappo AS, Janeway KA. Pediatric gastrointestinal stromal tumors. *Hematol Oncol Clin North Am.* 2009;3(1):15-34.

Rammohan A, Sathyanesan J, Rajendran K, et al. A gist of gastrointestinal stroma tumors: a review. *World J Gastrointest Oncol.* 2013;5(6):102-112.

Yamamoto H, Oda Y. Gastrointestinal stromal tumor: recent advances in pathology and genetics. *Pathol Int.* 2015;65:9-18.

Walter Chou ▨ Aarti Chawla Mittal ▨ Raj Dasgupta ▨
Stanley Silverman

A 56-Year-Old Male With Cough and Shortness of Breath

A 56-year-old male with a history of type 2 diabetes mellitus presents with 3 days of fever, chills, and productive cough with thick green sputum. In the past day, he has become increasingly short of breath, with severe dyspnea on exertion. Previously, he was in good health, with no limited function.

What is likely to be the cause of his cough and shortness of breath?
Although the differential diagnosis for cough and shortness of breath is broad, a few key points in the history narrow it down for us. We become more suspicious of pneumonia given that the patient has fevers and a productive cough. If the patient had heart failure and another source of infection (i.e., a urinary tract infection), this could lead to a decompensation of his heart failure causing his fever, cough, and shortness of breath. Other things to consider are an acute exacerbation of an underlying pulmonary disease such as asthma or chronic obstructive pulmonary disease (COPD).

What studies should you order?
The first thing that comes to mind is a chest radiograph (CXR). Labs include a basic metabolic panel and a complete blood count (CBC) with differential. For the fever workup, you would also obtain blood cultures, sputum culture, and a urinalysis with microscopy.

On physical exam, the patient's blood pressure is 126/74 mm Hg, pulse rate is 124/min, respiration rate is 36/min, temperature is 38.4 °C (101.2 °F), and oxygen saturation is 82% on room air.

What do you want to do now?
All of these vital signs, except for the blood pressure, are very concerning. The most immediately worrisome ones are the high respiration rate (tachypnea) and low oxygen saturation (hypoxia). The first thing that needs to be done is to place the patient on supplemental oxygen. You also want to order an arterial blood gas (ABG) to evaluate the acid-base status and confirm the hypoxemia.

Figure 57.1 is the oxygen-hemoglobin dissociation curve. It shows how blood (specifically hemoglobin) binds and releases oxygen molecules. Each hemoglobin molecule can reversibly bind four oxygen molecules. The curve is in a sigmoid shape because binding the first molecule to hemoglobin is difficult. After the first one is bound, the structure of hemoglobin changes, and binding each successive oxygen molecule becomes easier. The binding is based on the partial

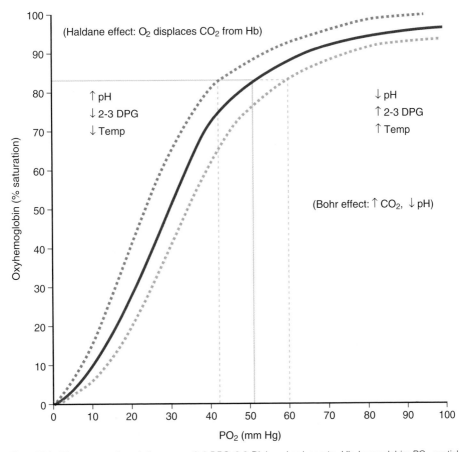

Figure 57.1 The oxygen dissociation curve. *2-3 DPG,* 2,3-Diphosphoglycerate; *Hb,* hemoglobin; *PO$_2$,* partial pressure of oxygen.

pressure of oxygen. In the alveoli, the partial pressure is very high, so oxygen is bound easily. In the tissues, the partial pressure varies depending on the clinical situation. If the curve is shifted to the right, it means that the oxygen is not tightly bound and is unloaded more readily. This occurs during periods of increased tissue oxygen consumption (e.g., in elevated temperatures and with acidosis). Similarly, if the curve is shifted to the left, there is a reluctance to release oxygen from hemoglobin (e.g., with alkalosis).

CLINICAL PEARL   **STEP 2/3**

Room air is 21% oxygen, which is equivalent to a fraction of inspired oxygen (FiO$_2$) of 21%. If a patient is requiring additional oxygen, there are many different ways that it can be given. Intubation is the invasive way, which will be discussed below. There are many noninvasive options:
- **Nasal cannula:** A double-pronged thin tube that sits in the patient's nostrils. This can deliver 1 to 6 liters per minute (lpm) of additional oxygen (25 to 40% FiO$_2$). Each additional 1 lpm of supplemental oxygen is approximately equal to an additional 4% of FiO$_2$.

Continued

CLINICAL PEARL—cont'd

- **Simple face mask:** A large mask that covers the mouth and nose. This can deliver 5 to 8 lpm of oxygen (28 to 50% FiO_2).
- **Nonrebreather mask:** A simple facemask with a reservoir bag attached. This is used to deliver from 10 to 15 lpm of supplemental oxygen (60 to 100% FiO_2).
- **Positive pressure ventilation:** Includes noninvasive modes such as bilevel positive airway pressure (BiPAP) and endotracheal intubation.

CLINICAL PEARL   **STEP 2/3**

Liebermeister's rule is the linear association between pulse rate and temperature. For each 1 degree Celcius in body temperature above normal, the pulse rate increases by 8 beats per minute. An exception to this rule is called the Faget sign, also known as sphygmothermic dissociation, where there is no increased pulse rate in response to a fever. This is seen in bacterial infections in which the bacteria have an intracellular life cycle. Examples include yellow fever, typhoid, tularemia, brucellosis, Colorado tick fever, legionella pneumonia, mycoplasma pneumonia, and salmonella.

The patient is placed on a nonrebreather mask at 15 lpm of supplemental oxygen. The ABG on room air prior to the nonrebreather mask reveals a pH of 7.32, partial pressure of carbon dioxide (PCO_2) of 34 mm Hg, partial pressure of oxygen (PO_2) or 48 mm Hg, and bicarbonate of 18 mEq/L.

How do you interpret this arterial blood gas?
Looking at the pH first lets you know that this is an acidosis. Now let's see if its metabolic, respiratory, or both. Respirations are driven by the level of carbon dioxide in the blood, which is normally around 40 mm Hg. The patient has a level just slightly below that. Remember that carbon dioxide is an "acid," so lower levels are due to a respiratory alkalosis. Next, look at the bicarbonate, which is a base, or alkali. The patient has a bicarbonate level of 18 mEq/L, whereas a normal level is 24 mEq/L. Overall, the patient has a metabolic acidosis, but his body is trying to compensate with a respiratory alkalosis. Lastly, look at the PO_2 in the blood. Normal PO_2 on room air is in the range of 95 mm Hg. On room air, the patient's PO_2 is extremely low, thus indicating that he is severely hypoxemic. It's a good thing you have already placed him on supplemental oxygen.

Figure 57.2 shows the patient's CXR.

How do you interpret the patient's CXR?
This is an upright CXR that is of good penetration and not rotated. Looking at the lung fields, we see bilateral patchy opacities, worse at the bases than the apices, and sparing the periphery. The heart does not look large, and there are no obvious masses.

Does this change your differential?
Although the infiltrates seen on the CXR could be pulmonary edema due to congestive heart failure, the fact that the heart is a normal size makes this less likely. Given the history of fevers and productive cough, pneumonia seems the most likely diagnosis. The patient's CXR also raises the possibility of acute respiratory distress syndrome (ARDS).

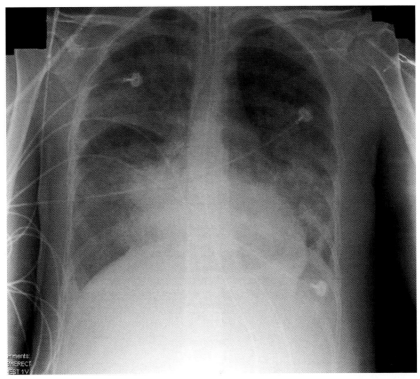

Figure 57.2   Chest radiograph of acute respiratory distress syndrome (ARDS). *(From* https://en.wikipedia.org/ wiki/Acute_respiratory_distress_syndrome#/media/File:AARDS_X-ray_cropped.jpg, *Samir modified by Delldot at English Wikipedia.)*

What is ARDS?

ARDS is a very serious cause of hypoxemia. When the body undergoes either direct injury to the lungs (i.e., pneumonia) or systemic inflammation (i.e., sepsis), there can be an inflammatory cascade that gets triggered in response to the injury or stress. This causes inflammation of the tiny vessels in the lungs, which disrupts their integrity and causes leaking of a cytokine-filled, protein-rich fluid into the alveoli. This has a twofold effect on disturbing gas exchange:
1. The protein in the fluid deactivates surfactant, leading to collapse of the alveoli.
2. Many of the alveoli that are not collapsed are filled with fluid rather than gases.

BASIC SCIENCE PEARL   STEP 1

Surfactant is made by type 2 alveolar cells in the lungs. It is a lipoprotein with both hydrophilic and hydrophobic properties that help it reduce surface tension, keeping the alveoli from collapsing and thereby facilitating gas exchange. Fetuses begin to produce surfactant between 24 and 28 weeks of gestation but do not make enough to prevent alveolar collapse until about 35 weeks.

CLINICAL PEARL   STEP 2/3

ARDS can have multiple etiologies, but the most common causes are trauma (to the head, chest, or body), sepsis, pneumonia, pancreatitis, blood product transfusion reaction, fat embolism, burns, or smoke inhalation.

How do you diagnose ARDS?

Four basic criteria must be met to be diagnosed with ARDS:

- Acute onset of 1 week of less
- Partial pressure of oxygen in arterial blood (PaO_2)/fraction of inspired oxygen (FiO_2) ratio <300
- Classic chest findings: bilateral opacities consistent with pulmonary edema
- CXR findings not due to decompensated heart failure; this can be based clinically or via some objective measure (e.g., a transthoracic echocardiogram or pulmonary artery catheter)

   Having these criteria, along with a cause, should make diagnosing a patient with ARDS relatively easy.

Does the patient meet the criteria for the diagnosis of ARDS?

Yes. For starters, he has the characteristic radiographic findings and a PaO_2/FiO_2 ratio (48 mm Hg/0.21 = 228) less than 300. The patient has no history of any cardiac disease or heart failure, so the pulmonary edema seen on the CXR is unlikely to be cardiogenic in origin. Additionally, per the history, he has been having symptoms for only about 3 days. Our patient likely has ARDS secondary to pneumonia.

> **Diagnosis:** Acute respiratory distress syndrome secondary to pneumonia

How would you classify his ARDS?

The classification system for ARDS is divided into three categories based on the PaO_2/FiO_2 ratio:

Mild: PaO_2/FiO_2 from 201 to 300
Moderate: PaO_2/FiO_2 from 101 to 200
Severe: PaO_2/FiO_2 less than 100

The patient's PaO_2/FiO_2 ratio is 228, so he is classified as having mild ARDS.

How is ARDS treated?

There have been numerous studies and trials to evaluate effective treatments for ARDS. The most important treatment for ARDS is to treat the underlying cause. In this case, pneumonia is the underlying cause of ARDS, and appropriate treatment for the patient's pneumonia should be initiated. For many years, the treatment of ARDS involved supportive care and treatment of the underlying cause. Regardless of the underlying cause of ARDS, there are now treatment strategies that have been proven to decrease mortality in ARDS, especially in those patients who require mechanical ventilation.

   The ARDS Network is a research network formed by the National Institutes of Health (NIH) to study the treatment of ARDS. The ARDS Network is responsible for one of the major breakthroughs in ARDS treatment: low tidal volume ventilation, also referred to as lung protective ventilation. This is widely used for the treatment of ARDS that requires mechanical ventilation for respiratory support.

CLINICAL PEARL   **STEP 2/3**

Low tidal volume ventilation intentionally uses lower ventilated tidal volumes based on the patient's predicted body weight. Note that predicted body weight is different from ideal body weight. The initial tidal volume should be 6 milliliters (mL) per kilogram (kg) of predicted body weight.
   Predicted body weight (kg):
- Males: 50 + 0.91 (height in centimeters − 152.4)
- Females: 45.5 + 0.91 (height in centimeters − 152.4)

What is the goal of low tidal volume ventilation?
The goal of low tidal volume ventilation is to reduce barotrauma and volutrauma to the lungs. Volutrauma refers to overdistention of alveoli from large tidal volumes, which can worsen lung injury in ARDS. The plateau pressure, which is measured at the end of inspiration, is a surrogate for the lung's static compliance. Tidal volume is titrated by 1 mL/kg of predicted body weight to keep the plateau pressure below 30 cm of water to minimize pressure-related injury to the lungs. As a consequence of lower tidal volumes, patients can develop a respiratory acidosis due to hypercapnia or elevated carbon dioxide levels in the blood. The concept of "permissive hypercapnia" means that we accept a respiratory acidosis in order to use low tidal volume ventilation. In ARDS, we allow acidosis to a lower pH than usual, to as low as 7.15. Below this pH, we should either increase the tidal volume or use a buffer such as sodium bicarbonate to increase the pH. When adequate oxygenation and ventilation cannot be achieved by conventional volume controlled ventilation, we sometimes use other modes of ventilation such as pressure-control ventilation or inverse-ratio ventilation, also known as airway pressure-release ventilation (APRV).

Does a patient's position during mechanical ventilation matter in ARDS?
Traditionally, mechanically ventilated patients are positioned lying supine. Prone positioning, or lying chest down, decreases the overall chest wall compliance and allows for a more uniform distribution of ventilation to perfusion in the lung. This helps improve gas exchange without increasing the pressures experienced by the lung, thus making it useful in ARDS. It is important to note that this is not the standard of care at this time. Prone positioning is very labor intensive for nursing staff. It is recommended that prone positioning be done in facilities highly experienced in prone positioning, as there are several complications that can occur. The daily changing of positions from supine to prone can lead to accidental disconnection of equipment, including intubation tubes and central lines. Dependent edema, especially of the face, is normal with prone positioning.

CLINICAL PEARL   **STEP 2/3**

Contraindications to prone positioning include spinal instability, elevated intracranial pressure, multiple unstable fractures, pregnancy, massive hemoptysis, or recent facial, tracheal, or sternal surgery or trauma.

Does the amount of IV fluids given to patients with ARDS affect their outcomes?
The question of the amount of IV fluids to give to patients with ARDS is an important one, given that the pathophysiology of ARDS involves fluid accumulation and leakage into the alveoli. It has been shown that a conservative fluid management strategy improves the number of ventilator-free days and intensive care unit-free days in patients with ARDS without causing more organ failure. Although improved mortality was not demonstrated, lower amounts of IV fluids and judicious use of diuretics likely improves patient outcomes with ARDS.

Is there anything else we can do to help treat ARDS?
A study published in the *New England Journal of Medicine* showed that early paralysis with cisatracurium, a neuromuscular blocker, in those presenting with severe ARDS improves 90-day adjusted mortality and ventilator-free days. According to the study, cisatracurium given within 48 hours of identification of severe ARDS for 48 hours improves outcomes. It is thought that early paralysis reduces patient–ventilator asynchrony, which reduces both alveolar overinflation and collapse. Early paralysis may also decrease inflammation, both systemically and in the lung.

It is important to note that neuromuscular blockade has shown benefit only in those with severe ARDS. There can be serious side effects of neuromuscular blockade, including critical illness myopathy. Early use of paralytics is not currently standard of care for ARDS. Often, it is utilized when more traditional measures such as low tidal volume ventilation are insufficient or when there is significant patient–ventilator asynchrony.

> The patient is treated with antibiotics for his pneumonia. His respiratory status worsens, with hypoxia and respiratory distress despite supplemental noninvasive oxygen with a nonrebreather mask. He is intubated for respiratory failure and transferred to the intensive care unit, with low tidal volume mechanical ventilation and conservative fluid management to help protect his lungs. His pneumonia resolves, he is extubated, and is eventually discharged home.

BEYOND THE PEARLS

- ARDS has a high mortality rate (>40% in some studies).
- Low tidal volume ventilation has been shown to reduce mortality in ARDS. The tidal volumes should be based on a patient's *predicted body weight* not actual body weight. So, if a patient is 5 feet 10 inches (or 178 cm), his tidal volume should be based on his predicted body weight of 73 kg (per the body mass index), not the 110 kg that the patient may actually weigh.
- The definition of ARDS was revised in 2012 with the Berlin definition. Previously, ARDS was defined by the American-European Consensus Conference (AECC) in 1994 with two categories: acute lung injury ($PaO_2/FiO_2 \leq 300$ mmHg) and acute respiratory distress syndrome ($PaO_2/FiO_2 \leq 200$ mmHg).
- The use of corticosteroids to reduce systemic inflammation has theoretic benefits in ARDS, but studies have been inconclusive or contradictory. At this time there is no major consensus on the use of corticosteroids in ARDS.
- Driving pressure is the ratio of ventilated lung to respiratory system compliance, or plateau pressure minus positive end-expiratory pressure (PEEP) in a patient with no independent respiratory effort. New studies suggest that minimizing driving pressure may benefit patient outcomes more than low tidal volume ventilation by individualizing respiratory parameters to each patient rather than predicted lung volumes.

References

Amato MBP, Meade MO, Slutsky AS, et al. Driving pressure and survival in the acute respiratory distress syndrome. *N Engl J Med.* 2015;372(8):747-755.

Brower RG, Matthay MA, Morris M, et al. Ventilation with lower tidal volumes as compared with traditional tidal volumes for acute lung injury and the acute respiratory distress syndrome. *N Engl J Med.* 2000;342(18):1301-1308.

Gattinoni L, Taccone P, Carlesso E, et al. Prone position in acute respiratory distress syndrome: rationale, indications, and limits. *Am J Resp Crit Care Med.* 2013;188(11):1286-1293.

Guérin C, Reignier J, Richard J-C, et al. Prone positioning in severe acute respiratory distress syndrome. *N Engl J Med.* 2013;368(23):2159-2168.

Meduri GU, Golden E, Freire AX, et al. Methylprednisolone infusion in early severe ARDS: results of a randomized controlled trial. *Chest.* 2007;131(4):954-963.

Papazian L, Forel J-M, Gacouin A, et al. Neuromuscular blockers in early acute respiratory distress syndrome. *N Engl J Med.* 2010;363(12):1107-1116.

Ranieri VM, Rubenfeld GD, Thompson BT, et al. Acute respiratory distress syndrome: the Berlin definition. *JAMA.* 2012;307(23):2526-2533.

Rosenberg AL, Dechert RE, Park PK, et al. Review of a large clinical series: association of cumulative fluid balance on outcome in acute lung injury: a retrospective review of the ARDSnet tidal volume study cohort. *J Intensive Care Med.* 2009;24(1):35-46.

Steinburg KP, Hudson LD, Goodman RB, et al. Efficacy and safety of corticosteroids for persistent acute respiratory distress syndrome. *N Engl J Med.* 2006;354(16):1671-1684.

Villar J, Sulemanji D, Kacmarek RM. The acute respiratory distress syndrome: incidence and mortality, has it changed? *Curr Opin Crit Care.* 2014;20(1):3-9.

Wiedemann HP, Wheeler AP, Bernard GR, et al. Comparison of two fluid-management strategies in acute lung injury. *N Engl J Med.* 2006;354(24):2564-2575.

Zambon M, Vincent J-L. Mortality rates for patients with acute lung injury/ARDS have decreased over time. *Chest.* 2008;133(5):1120-1127.

Daniel Martinez

A 55-Year-Old Male With Diabetes on an Angiotensin-Converting Enzyme (ACE) Inhibitor

A 55-year-old male with type 2 diabetes mellitus presents to his primary care doctor for a routine checkup. His diabetes is well controlled on metformin, but he has been found to be hypertensive on the last few clinic visits (blood pressures of 140 to 150/70 to 80 mm Hg). He is started on benazepril and told to go to the lab in 1 to 2 weeks to check a basic metabolic panel. He is busy at work, forgets to go to the lab, and a month passes by. He begins to feel nausea, fatigue, palpitations, shortness of breath, and a "pins and needles" sensation peripherally, so he presents to the local emergency room.

How do you manage these symptoms in the emergency room setting?

A thorough history and physical exam is the cornerstone of effective medical treatment. However, it is not always appropriate to delay workup and treatment until a formal history and physical exam has been completed. This is often the case in the emergency room setting where the top priority is to rule out life-threatening conditions. In the appropriate clinical setting (such as a middle-aged male with diabetes), a patient who presents with cardiac symptoms such as palpitations or chest pain should be evaluated with a STAT electrocardiogram (ECG), serial cardiac enzymes (i.e., troponin levels), and basic labs such as a basic metabolic panel and complete blood count.

Labs are drawn and are still pending. The ECG is done and is brought to you for interpretation (see Fig. 58.1).

How do you read the patient's ECG?

The ECG shows a regular pulse rate (around 70 beats/minute), regular rhythm, and normal axis. However, the P waves are difficult to appreciate. This makes it difficult to interpret whether the patient is in normal sinus rhythm or not. There is a widened QRS complex (greater than three small boxes) and peaked T waves. The Q-T intervals are normal (less than half the distance between the R-R intervals). There are no ST segment changes, Q waves, or T wave inversions to suggest new or old cardiac ischemia.

The most clinically relevant aspect of this ECG is the widened QRS complex. It indicates that there is an abnormal slowing of the electrical conduction through the heart during systole. This can be seen in a bundle branch block, ventricular paced rhythm (because the bundle of

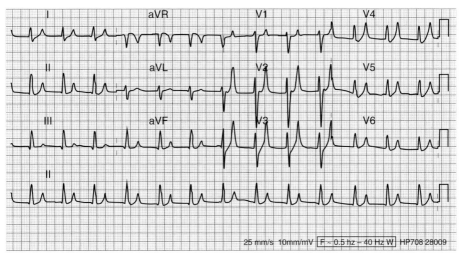

Figure 58.1   ECG in a patient with hyperkalemia, demonstrating a widened QRS complex (greater than three small boxes) and peaked T waves.

His is bypassed), or electrolyte abnormality causing action potential slowing. There are no findings of a bundle branch block in this ECG, so that is less likely. The absence of P waves initially suggests a ventricular-paced rhythm. However, the normal QRS axis and upright T waves throughout the ECG point against this. Taken together, these findings more likely suggest a severe electrolyte abnormality. However, an ECG interpretation should always be done with consideration of the clinical picture as a whole.

While you are reading the ECG, the nurse urgently approaches you stating that his labs show a potassium level of 7 mEq/L.

What are the ECG changes found in hyperkalemia?

Potassium is a key component of the action potentials that propagate the electrochemical signal throughout the heart. Thus, changes in its serum concentration can dramatically affect an ECG. Most medical students and residents remember the peaked T waves seen in hyperkalemia; however, this is not the most important change seen because it is generally associated with moderate levels of hyperkalemia. More important to remember are the ECG changes found as hyperkalemia worsens to dangerously high levels. At this point, an ECG can show a widened QRS complex, prolonged PR interval, absence of P waves, and finally a sine wave ECG morphology. Because these ECG findings are seen at more extreme levels of hyperkalemia, they are the most clinically important to remember.

What are the clinical manifestations of hyperkalemia?

Patients with mild hyperkalemia are often asymptomatic. However, as hyperkalemia worsens, patients can present with nonspecific symptoms of fatigue, weakness, nausea, and abdominal pain. They can also have more severe symptoms such as paresthesias, muscle weakness/paralysis, and cardiac palpitations.

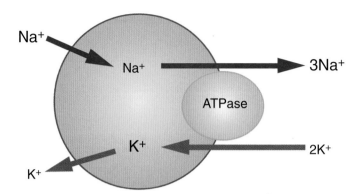

Figure 58.2   Schematic demonstrating the Na-K ATPase pump. For each molecule of ATP used, it transports three sodium ions out of the cell and two potassium ions into the cell.

CLINICAL PEARL   **STEP 2/3**

Hyperkalemia is common in patients with diabetes because they are at risk for kidney injury and are often on an ACE inhibitor, both of which can cause hyperkalemia. Patients with uncontrolled diabetes can also develop diabetic neuropathy, which can mimic the paresthesias seen in hyperkalemia. Thus, it is important not to discount a patient's paresthesias as simply a result of neuropathy as this may be an important clue for detecting life-threatening hyperkalemia.

How do you emergently treat hyperkalemia?

Untreated hyperkalemia is extremely dangerous because of its pronounced effects on cardiac electrophysiology. It affects the resting membrane potential, action potential velocity/duration, and electrical propagation through the heart. The first step in the emergent treatment of hyperkalemia is to stabilize the cardiac membrane by mitigating the adverse electrophysiologic effects of potassium. This is done by giving intravenous (IV) calcium. Calcium gluconate 10 mL of 100 mg/mL given intravenously over 2 to 3 minutes is a typical dose. (Calcium chloride also can be used but generally at lower doses.) This treatment helps to reverse the ECG changes described above but works only for about 30 to 60 minutes. Thus, it is also important to lower potassium levels shortly after membrane stabilization. Also, it is important to remember that IV calcium is relatively contraindicated as a treatment for hyperkalemia that is caused by digoxin toxicity.

Digoxin toxicity is a unique scenario. Although hyperkalemia is often seen because the Na-K adenosine triphosphatase (ATPase) enzyme is impaired by digoxin, the hyperkalemia itself is generally not what would kill the patient. Primary treatment of the hyperkalemia itself is not the first step to take. Instead, fragment antigen-binding (Fab) fragments (antibodies against digoxin) should be administered promptly when digoxin toxicity is diagnosed. This also helps correct the hyperkalemia because the Na-K ATPase enzymes begin to work again (see Fig. 58.2).

CLINICAL PEARL   **STEP 1**

Understanding how the Na-K ATPase functions is important for understanding the physiology and pathophysiology of many organ systems (see Fig. 58.2). It is an enzyme located in the plasma membrane of cells, and it utilizes energy for adenosine triphosphate (ATP) in the active transport of ions against their concentration gradients. For each molecule of ATP used, it transports three sodium ions out of the cell and two potassium ions into the cell. This maintains the high intracellular concentration of potassium and high extracellular concentration of sodium.

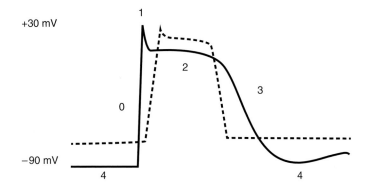

Figure 58.3 The effects of hyperkalemia on the resting membrane potential in a nonpacemaker cardiac cell.

CLINICAL PEARL   **STEP 2/3**

Digoxin is still in use today to treat congestive heart failure (CHF) and some tachyarrhythmias, and toxicity is not uncommon given its narrow therapeutic index. It is important to remember that digoxin only provides symptomatic relief and does not have a significant mortality benefit in CHF; this is a very common test question. Alternatively, beta blockers and ACE inhibitors do provide a mortality benefit in CHF.

BASIC SCIENCE PEARL   **STEP 1**

Understanding the pathophysiology of hyperkalemia in the cardiac action potential helps to solidify an understanding of cardiac physiology itself. Potassium has a high resting membrane permeability. Thus, its intracellular and extracellular concentrations significantly contribute to the resting membrane potential of the cardiac cell (generally at about −90mV in the heart; see Fig. 58.3). An abnormally high extracellular potassium concentration abnormally elevates the resting membrane potential (e.g., −80mV). This elevation brings the resting membrane potential dangerously closer to the threshold potential (−75 mV). Giving IV calcium helps to combat this effect by concurrently elevating the threshold potential as well (−65 mV). This helps to maintain the appropriate 15-mV gap between the resting and threshold potentials.

How you do lower serum potassium levels?

There are three ways to lower serum potassium levels. The first is to remove potassium from the body itself via gastrointestinal (GI) or renal systems, the second is to shift potassium directly into the body's cells, and the third is hemodialysis.

If a patient is clinically stable without symptoms or ECG changes, it is appropriate to give either kayexalate or a loop diuretic to promote potassium loss from the body. Kayexalate is a sodium/potassium exchanger in the intestines and serves to promote GI potassium loss. It only functions when patients are having regular bowel movements, and thus the addition of laxatives can be helpful. Kayexalate is actually contraindicated in patients with ileus as it can cause bowel necrosis. Loop diuretics block sodium and potassium reabsorption in the kidney and thus promote renal potassium loss (see Fig. 58.4). This is preferred in patients who are clinically volume overloaded and already require diuresis as a treatment modality.

Second, if a patient is clinically unstable and requires rapid lowering of serum potassium, it is appropriate to shift potassium directly into cells utilizing various potassium-linked transporters. These transporters include insulin (often 10 units of regular insulin with dextrose 50 [D50] as

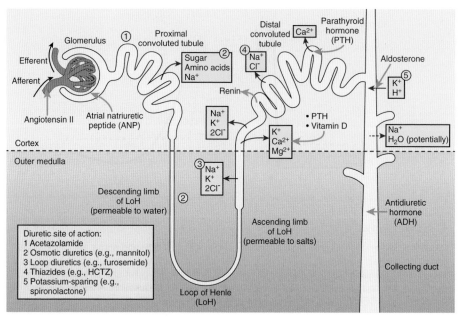

Figure 58.4   A graphic depiction of the typical nephron illustrating which electrolytes are reabsorbed and secreted at various parts of the nephron and which hormones are responsible for regulating this movement. It also illustrates the mechanism of action of each of the diuretic medications by pointing out where and how they act upon the nephron. *HCTZ,* Hydrochlorothiazide. *(From* http://www.pathophys.org/wp-content/uploads/2013/02/MPR-nephron.png.)

an IV push), beta-2 agonists (generally albuterol [10 to 20 mg nebulized], which is about four times higher than the typical dose), and bicarbonate. These treatments work very well in the acute setting but do not actually remove potassium from the body. If no further treatment is used, potassium will return to the original dangerous levels. Thus, these treatments should always be followed by an additional method of potassium removal.

Finally, hemodialysis can be employed in certain circumstances. If a patient has a pathology that causes massive cell death and rapid potassium release from cells (such as rhabdomyolysis, severe burns, severe sepsis, or tumor lysis syndrome), kayexalate and/or diuretics may not act fast enough for adequate potassium removal. These patients may require hemodialysis to aid in potassium removal and other metabolic abnormalities. Further, those with contraindications to kayexalate and diuresis may benefit from hemodialysis for potassium removal.

The patient is given 10 mL of calcium gluconate, and the repeat ECG normalizes; he is also given insulin/D50 and kayexalate. During this time, the patient also discloses that he has been short of breath while walking only a few blocks and has been waking up at night out of breath as well. He also reports that his chronic back pain has been worse, and he has been taking ibuprofen four times a day. On exam, the patient is afebrile with a blood pressure of 105/66 mm Hg, pulse rate of 79/min, respiration rate of 26/min, and oxygen saturation of 88% on room air. There is jugular venous distension in his neck, crackles in his lungs, and 2+ bilateral lower extremity edema in his legs. These findings are consistent with new onset CHF. He is then given furosemide 40 mg IV push. The basic metabolic panel results are as follows: sodium is 132 mEq/L, chloride is 94 mmol/L, carbon dioxide is 18 mmol/L, blood urea nitrogen (BUN) is 35 mg/dL, and creatinine is 3.2 mg/dL. A review of his medical record reveals a baseline creatinine of 0.8 mg/dL.

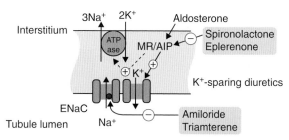

Figure 58.5   A graphic depiction of a principal cell in the distal nephron illustrating how it functions to reabsorb sodium and secrete potassium into the urine. It also illustrates that this action is under direction positive control of aldosterone and that spironolactone functions by blocking aldosterone and thus sodium reabsorption. *ENaC, Epithelial sodium channel. (From Waller DG, Sampson AP. Medical Pharmacology and Therapeutics. 4th ed. Philadelphia: Elsevier; 2014:213-223, Fig. 14.2.)*

What are the causes of hyperkalemia?

It is important to understand the causes of a patient's hyperkalemia because it is necessary for understanding how to manage it in the long term. The causes of hyperkalemia can be divided into three major categories:
- increased intake of potassium,
- transcellular shifts of potassium, or
- decreased excretion of potassium from the kidneys.

Dangerous levels of hyperkalemia are generally not caused solely by an increased intake of potassium-rich foods. Typically, a patient also has a secondary pathology, such as end-stage renal disease (ESRD), combined with an increased intake of potassium. Thus, it is important to educate patients on which foods are rich in potassium when they are at risk for developing hyperkalemia.

Transcellular shifts of potassium can cause very high levels of potassium in the serum without actually causing an increase in total body potassium. Thus, correcting the cause of the transcellular shift is more important and effective than simply trying to remove potassium from the body. Causes of such a transcellular shift include acidemia, insulin deficiency, beta blockers, massive cell death, digoxin intoxication, or succinylcholine use. Treatment should be aimed at treating the underlying cause.

The first step in excretion of potassium from the kidneys is filtration and delivery of potassium to the tubules; thus, any cause of decreased glomerular filtration rate (GFR) can cause hyperkalemia. This is commonly seen in ESRD or any cause of oliguric/anuric acute kidney injury. This also includes any cause of decreased effective arterial volume causing prerenal acute kidney injury (such as in CHF exacerbation, third spacing in cirrhosis, hypovolemia, or sepsis). Treating the underlying cause and improving GFR help to correct hyperkalemia. This can mean diuresis in CHF exacerbation to optimize cardiac function, IV fluid resuscitation in hypovolemia/sepsis, or even IV albumin in cirrhosis.

The second step in excretion of potassium from the kidneys is secretion of potassium by the principle cells of the distal tubules (see Fig. 58.5). The amount of potassium secreted is controlled mainly by aldosterone. Thus, anything that mitigates the effects of aldosterone can cause hyperkalemia. Any cause of decreased renin secretion causes a decrease in aldosterone and hyperkalemia (hyporeninemic hypoaldosteronism, diabetes, nonsteroidal antiinflammatory drug [NSAID] use). Also, any cause of decreased aldosterone synthesis in the setting of a normal renin state can also cause hyperkalemia (ACE inhibitors, angiotensin receptor blockers, primary adrenal insufficiency). Finally, medication that directly inhibits the effects of aldosterone causes hyperkalemia (trimethoprim, pentamidine, potassium-sparing diuretics, or cyclosporine).

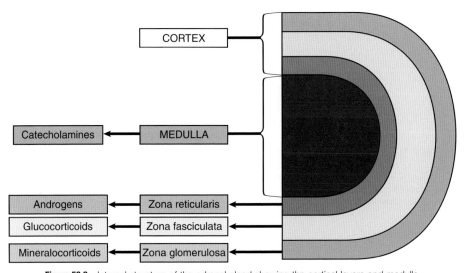

Figure 58.6   Internal structure of the adrenal gland showing the cortical layers and medulla.

BASIC SCIENCE PEARL   **STEP 1**

Hyperkalemia can be found in Addison's disease when there is a primary disorder of the adrenal glands and they are not able to secrete sufficient mineralocorticoids. However, this is not the case in secondary adrenal insufficiency (decreased secretion of adrenocorticotropic hormone) because the adrenal glands function normally and are still responsive to the renin-angiotensin system (see Fig. 58.6).

BASIC SCIENCE PEARL   **STEP 1**

In complicated patients with multiple etiologies of hyperkalemia, it can be useful to measure the transtubular potassium gradient $(U_K/P_K)/(U_{osm}/P_{osm})$ to determine whether the kidneys are playing a role in the patient's pathophysiology. There are no universally accepted cutoff points for this calculation, but there are loosely accepted ranges. In a patient with hyperkalemia, a normally functioning kidney should be actively secreting potassium, and this ratio is generally greater than 10. In that situation, the kidneys are not contributing to the hyperkalemia. However, an abnormally functioning kidney will not be actively secreting potassium, and this ratio is generally less than 7. In that situation, the kidneys are contributing to the hyperkalemia by failing to secrete it.

What are the causes of hyperkalemia in this patient?

The etiology of this patient's hyperkalemia is multifactorial. The patient was in a CHF exacerbation and on high-dose NSAIDs. This caused decreased renal perfusion, acute kidney injury, and hyperkalemia. The patient was also started on an ACE inhibitor, which indirectly inhibits aldosterone and causes hyperkalemia. ACE inhibitors can also decrease renal GFR, resulting in hyperkalemia.

The patient is admitted to the intensive care unit and placed on a furosemide drip; he symptomatically improves over the next few days. After he is nearly euvolemic he is transferred to the floor, and his kidney function returns to baseline. A transthoracic echocardiogram is performed, which shows global hypokinesis of the left ventricle (ejection fraction 40%), and a nuclear medicine stress test is performed, which shows no inducible ischemia. Because the patient's hyperkalemia was not caused solely by an ACE inhibitor, he is restarted on benazepril, a beta blocker, and a loop diuretic prior to discharge. He follows up with his primary care physician 1 week after discharge, and he is now asymptomatic with a normal basic metabolic panel.

Diagnosis: Hyperkalemia secondary to congestive heart failure and acute kidney injury

BEYOND THE PEARLS

- Although generally not clinically relevant, calcium gluconate is often preferred over calcium chloride because it is less likely to produce tissue necrosis if it extravasates.
- Hyperkalemia changes the action potential such that repolarization of the cell happens very quickly (see Fig. 58.3). This is thought to be the reason why we see the classic peaked T waves on ECG.
- The Na-K ATPase was first discovered by Jens Christian Skou in 1953. He was studying the mechanism of action of local anesthetics at the time. He received the Nobel Prize for this discovery in 1997.
- There are old case reports from the 1950s that administering IV calcium for hyperkalemia during digoxin toxicity causes death, and it is generally not recommended.
- Patients with hypertension are often asked to lower their salt intake. Sometimes they do so by replacing their table salt with salt substitute, which commonly is potassium chloride. This practice can cause dangerous serum potassium levels if the patient has kidney disease or is on an ACE-inhibitor or a potassium-sparing diuretic. Be sure to ask patients about this.

References

Choi MJ, Ziyadeh FN. The utility of the transtubular potassium gradient in the evaluation of hyperkalemia. *J Am Soc Nephrol.* 2008;19:424-426.
Costanzo LS. *Physiology.* Philadelphia, PA: Saunders Elsevier; 2010.
Dellinger PR. Management of severe hyperkalemia. *Crit Care Med.* 2008;36:3246-3251.
Morgan DB. Body water, sodium, potassium and hydrogen ions: some basic facts and concepts. *Clin Endocrin Metab.* 1984;13(2):233-247.
Parham WA, Mehdirad AA, Biermann KM, Fedman CS. Hyperkalemia revisited. *Tex Heart Inst J.* 2006;33:40-47.
Skou JC. Nobel lecture: the identification of the sodium pump. *Biosci Rep.* 1998;18(4):155-169.

Christopher J. Graber

A 34-Year-Old Male With Generalized Weakness

A 34-year-old male is admitted to the hospital with a 1-month history of gradually increasing generalized weakness. Over the week prior to admission, he notes fevers up to 38.9 °C (102 °F), a dry cough, and increased shortness of breath. Initial vital signs are notable for a temperature of 38.9 °C (102.1 °F), pulse rate of 102/min, blood pressure of 110/68 mm Hg, and respiration rate of 25/min with an oxygen saturation of 85% on room air. The physical exam is notable for scant white patches on the oropharyngeal mucosa and the pulmonary exam is notable for fine inspiratory crackles. Laboratory findings are notable for a white blood cell (WBC) count of 2,300/μL, hemoglobin 10.0 g/dL, platelets 179,000/μL, and creatinine 1.0 mg/dL. An arterial blood gas is obtained that reveals a pH of 7.44, partial pressure of carbon dioxide (PCO_2) of 32 mm Hg, partial pressure of oxygen (PO_2) of 58 mm Hg, and bicarbonate (HCO_3) of 23 mEq/L. A chest radiograph (CXR) is notable for diffuse bilateral interstitial infiltrates. The patient is started on intravenous (IV) trimethoprim-sulfamethoxazole and methylprednisolone, and direct fluorescence antibody testing of a sample from bronchoscopy reveals organisms morphologically consistent with *Pneumocystis jirovecii*. A human immunodeficiency virus (HIV) antibody test sent on admission comes back positive. On hospital day 2, a CD4 count and HIV viral load are sent; these subsequently return at 88 cells/mm^3 and 142,000 copies/mL, respectively.

The patient improves clinically, and trimethoprim-sulfamethoxazole and glucocorticoid therapy are switched to oral formulations on hospital day 7. By hospital day 10, the patient is stable for discharge. He asks you about antiretroviral therapy (ART) for his HIV infection: when should he start and what regimen should he start?

Diagnosis: *Pneumocystis jirovecii* pneumonia in the context of newly diagnosed HIV infection

What aspects of the patient's social history would influence the decision to initiate ART?
Obtaining a detailed social history is critical in determining the right time for ART initiation and devising the appropriate regimen. It is particularly relevant to know the patient's risk factor(s) for HIV acquisition and whether the patient still engages in those risk factors, as the patient is highly infectious in his currently untreated state. Substance abuse may represent a significant barrier to ART compliance and should be investigated, with treatment referral as appropriate. An assessment of the patient's current living situation and social support will also help you assess the patient's ability to be compliant with ART.

The patient notes that he only has sex with men and he uses condoms "occasionally." He notes having approximately 10 different partners in the past 3 months but has recently started a "serious" relationship with a new partner who is HIV-negative. He does not use IV drugs but snorts methamphetamines at parties 1 to 2 times per month. He lives with a roommate who is supportive and has visited him in the hospital. The patient's family is aware of and supportive of the patient's sexuality.

What are the benefits and risks of starting ART now in this patient?

There are several potential benefits to starting ART at this time. Some of the best data to support earlier ART initiation in the context of presentation with an opportunistic infection (OI) come from a randomized clinical trial in which HIV-infected patients who were not taking antiretroviral therapy at the time of OI presentation were randomized to start antiretroviral therapy either within 2 weeks of starting OI treatment or to defer antiretroviral therapy until OI treatment was complete. Patients in the early ART arm started a median of 12 days into their OI treatment, compared to 45 days in the deferred arm. Patients in the early ART arm had a lower rate of and longer time to death or progression of disease, with no increase in adverse events or loss of virologic response.

There are a few caveats to this trial: most (63% of) patients in the trial had *Pneumocystis* pneumonia as their presenting OI; a much smaller proportion had cryptococcal meningitis or mycobacterial disease, two conditions for which the decision-making for when to start therapy may be more complex, owing to potential severity of the immune reconstitution syndrome that may develop and the potential for drug–drug interactions, among other factors. Overall, however, it appears that starting ART sooner rather than later can have a long-lasting effect on immune restoration and may help modulate more subtle effects that HIV infection has on other comorbidities.

CLINICAL PEARL   **STEP 2/3**

Immune reconstitution inflammatory syndrome (IRIS) is a paradoxical worsening of preexisting infectious processes that can follow initiation of effective ART. It is brought on by an increased inflammatory response from CD4 cells that are reconstituted with ART. It may be particularly severe in patients treated with early ART in the setting of cryptococcal meningitis.

IRIS typically requires treatment for underlying opportunistic infection, but glucocorticoids may be given for severe disease. The overall goal in IRIS is to "weather the storm" and continue ART as possible.

Another potential benefit of starting ART now is that it can serve as an impetus to engage in regular HIV care upon discharge. In the United States, despite near-universal availability of ART, several gaps exist in the continuum of care between time of HIV infection, diagnosis, engagement in care, retention in care, receipt of ART, and adherence to ART in what is commonly referred to as the "HIV care cascade" (see Fig. 59.1). It has been estimated that only about one quarter of all HIV-infected patients in the United States are adherent to ART and have undetectable viral load. However, if patients can be effectively adherent to ART and maintain an undetectable HIV viral load long term, they can expect to have a relatively normal lifespan, particularly if ART is started at higher initial CD4 counts.

CLINICAL PEARL   **STEP 2/3**

HIV-infected patients who start ART at higher CD4 counts can have an essentially normal lifespan. A study based on British cohort data estimates that a 35-year-old male started and maintained on ART when his CD4 count is above 200 cells/mm^3 has a life expectancy of 77 to 78 years, essentially the same as for an HIV-uninfected individual. This estimate drops to 71 years for starting ART when CD4 is below 200 cells/mm^3.

Starting ART now also has the benefit of reducing transmission of HIV from the patient to other people. Although this phenomenon is best described in a trial of mostly heterosexual HIV-discordant couples, in which treatment of the HIV-infected partner reduced HIV transmission

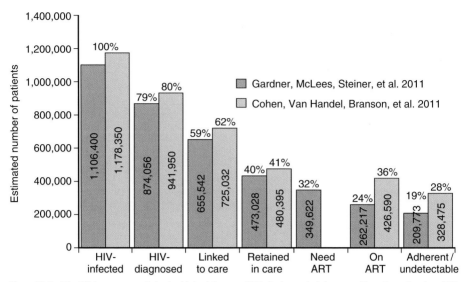

Figure 59.1 The HIV care cascade in the United States. *ART,* Antiretroviral therapy. *(Data from Gardner EM, McLees MP, Steiner JF, et al. The spectrum of engagement in HIV care and its relevance to test-and-treat strategies for prevention of HIV infection.* Clin Infect Dis. *2011;52:793-800; Cohen SM, Van Handel MM, Branson BM, et al. Vital signs: HIV prevention through care and treatment—United States.* MMWR Morb Mortal Wkly Rep. *2011;60:1618-1623.)*

by 96%, there is evidence to support that ART reduces HIV transmission in other settings as well.

There are potential barriers to successful adherence to ART that should be addressed as best as possible at the time of ART initiation, including mental health disease, substance abuse, unstable housing, and food insecurity. Patients may not fully understand their treatment regimen. Perhaps most importantly, patients are not likely to be adherent to ART if they are not motivated to do so, so exploring this motivation is critical prior to ART initiation.

Regardless of the timing of ART initiation, prophylaxis against OI (based on CD4 count) should be started promptly (see Table 59.1).

Is there a CD4 cell count threshold that should determine when ART should be started?

The optimal CD4 cell count at which to start ART has been controversial throughout the history of the HIV epidemic. In the early days of the epidemic, ART was not as effective, more toxic, and far more inconvenient to take than the options available today, so the risks and adverse effects of ART had to be balanced with its benefits. Now, as ART is highly effective, less toxic, and more convenient, it is easier to show the benefits of starting ART at higher CD4 cell counts than before. Randomized controlled trial data now support the benefits of starting ART at a CD4 count of 500 cells/mm³. Guidelines from the United States Department of Health and Human Services (as of the April 2015 update) recommend offering ART to all HIV-infected individuals to reduce the risk of disease progression and transmission, regardless of CD4 count.

What antiretroviral medications are currently used in devising an ART regimen?

As of 2015, the following categories of medications are available to be considered as components of ART: nucleoside(-tide) reverse transcriptase inhibitors (NRTIs), nonnucleoside reverse transcriptase inhibitors (NNRTIs), protease inhibitors (PIs), integrase strand transfer inhibitors

TABLE 59.1 ▓ **Prophylaxis for Opportunistic Infection According to CD4 Count**

Opportunistic Infection	When to Start Prophylaxis	Prophylaxis Options
Pneumocystis pneumonia	CD4 <200 cells/mm^3 or 14%, or patient presenting with oropharyngeal candidiasis	TMP-SMX, dapsone (check *G6PD*), atovaquone, aerosolized pentamidine
Toxoplasma encephalitis	CD4 <100 cells/mm^3 with IgG+	TMP-SMX, atovaquone, dapsone plus pyrimethamine plus leucovorin
Disseminated mycobacterium avium complex (MAC) infection	CD4 <50 cells/mm^3 (after ruling out active MAC disease)	Azithromycin 1200 mg weekly
Histoplasma	CD4 <150 cells/mm^3 with high risk of occupational exposure or area of hyperendemicity	Itraconazole 200 mg daily
Penicillium marneffei	CD4 <100 cells/mm^3 with prolonged stay in rural northern Thailand, Vietnam, or southern China	Itraconazole 200 mg daily or fluconazole 400 mg daily

IgG, Immunoglobulin G; *TMP-SMX,* trimethoprim-sulfamethoxazole.

(INSTIs), C-C chemokine receptor type 5 (CCR5) coreceptor antagonists, and fusion inhibitors (not commonly prescribed). Relative advantages and disadvantages of agents commonly prescribed as of early 2015 are described in Table 59.2.

BASIC SCIENCE PEARL   STEP 1

It is useful to conceptualize ART mechanisms of action according to how HIV initially enters a host cell, integrates into its genome, then replicates itself. CCR5 coreceptor inhibitors and fusion inhibitors block HIV entry into host cells. Nucleoside, nucleotide (tenofovir), and nonnucleoside reverse-transcriptase inhibitors block conversion of viral RNA into DNA that later integrates into the host chromosome, a process inhibited by integrase strand transfer inhibitors (typically just called integrase inhibitors). Protease inhibitors block proteolytic cleavage of precursor proteins that are assembled to make intact virions.

How is an ART regimen constructed?

The most well-studied ART regimens combine two NRTIs with a medication from another class, most typically an INSTI or protease inhibitor. Occasionally, patients will have contraindications to receiving some NRTIs and may be placed on combinations that spare this class, but these regimens are not well studied and should only be prescribed by or in consultation with an HIV specialist. Protease inhibitors (and the integrase inhibitor elvitegravir) typically need to be taken with a "booster" medication (either ritonavir or the newer cobicistat) that increases drug levels via cytochrome p450 enzyme effects. As of mid-2015, there are four one-pill-daily regimens that have been coformulated that combine two NRTIs with a medication from another class: ATRIPLA® (tenofovir, emtricitabine, efavirenz), COMPLERA® (tenofovir, emtricitabine, rilpivirine), STRIBILD® (tenofovir, emtricitabine, elvitegravir, cobicistat), and TRIUMEQ® (abacavir, lamivudine, dolutegravir).

TABLE 59.2 ■ Commonly Prescribed Antiretroviral Agents in the United States

Agent	Advantages	Disadvantages	Notable Interactions
Nucleoside(-tide) Reverse Transcriptase Inhibitors (NRTIs)			
Tenofovir	Once-daily dosing; active vs. hepatitis B; multiple coformulations	Can cause or exacerbate renal insufficiency (less with new alafenamide formulation)	Should not be used with unboosted atazanavir (lowers atazanavir levels); ledipasvir may raise levels
Abacavir	Once-daily dosing	Need to check HLA-B5701; possible small increase in cardiovascular risk	Should not be used in patients with decompensated cirrhosis
Lamivudine	Once-daily dosing; active vs. hepatitis B; multiple coformulations	Low genetic barrier to resistance (but resistance lowers viral fitness)	None
Emtricitabine	Once-daily dosing; active vs. hepatitis B; multiple coformulations	Low genetic barrier to resistance (but resistance lowers viral fitness)	Structurally similar to lamivudine (never give both)
Zidovudine	Efficacy when combined with tenofovir for resistant viruses	Twice-daily dosing; can cause macrocytic anemia; myalgias	Avoid coadministration with ribavirin (anemia)
Nonnucleoside Reverse Transcriptase Inhibitors (NNRTIs)			
Efavirenz	Long track record of potency; coformulated in once-daily pill (ATRIPLA®)	Central nervous system side effects; possible increase in suicidality	Contraindicated with Viekira Pak, voriconazole; can decrease elvitegravir, atazanavir levels
Rilpivirine	Coformulated in once-daily pill (COMPLERA®); likely fewer central nervous system side effects than efavirenz	Lower efficacy at higher viral loads (not recommended for viral load >100,000 copies/mL)	Contraindicated with proton pump inhibitors (PPIs) (can give H2 blocker 12 hours before or 4 hours after), rifampin; avoid with Viekira Pak
Etravirine	May be an option for viruses resistant to other NNRTIs	Twice-daily dosing	Contraindicated with Viekira Pak, rifampin, tipranavir
Protease Inhibitors (PIs)			
Darunavir	Potent; high genetic barrier to resistance; can be given once-daily with ritonavir in patients without prior PI exposure	Should be given twice-daily with ritonavir for PI-experienced patients; gastrointestinal side effects, hyperlipidemia, and lipodystrophy (though much lower risk than older PIs)	Contraindicated with lovastatin, simvastatin, rifampin, Viekira Pak; multiple cytochrome p450 interactions
Atazanavir	Potent; high genetic barrier to resistance; can be given once-daily with ritonavir	Unconjugated hyperbilirubinemia (resembles Gilbert's syndrome), gastrointestinal side effects, hyperlipidemia, and lipodystrophy (though much lower risk than older PIs)	Contraindicated with high-dose PPI (can give low-dose PPI or H2 blocker 12 hours apart), lovastatin, simvastatin, rifampin, Viekira Pak; multiple cytochrome p450 interactions

TABLE 59.2 ■ Commonly Prescribed Antiretroviral Agents in the United States—cont'd

Agent	Advantages	Disadvantages	Notable Interactions
CCR5 Coreceptor Inhibitor			
Maraviroc	Useful option when virus is resistant to other classes	Need to check tropism of virus (to ensure it uses CCR5 coreceptor)	Dosing depends on other medications in regimen that are cytochrome p450 CYP3A inducers or inhibitors
Integrase Strand Transfer Inhibitors (INSTIs)			
Raltegravir	Potent; few side effects	Twice-daily dosing	Increase dose when given with rifampin
Elvitegravir	Potent; few side effects; once-daily dosing in STRIBILD® combination pill	Avoid in patients with glomerular filtration rate <70 mL/min	Cobicistat booster in STRIBILD® contraindicated with lovastatin, simvastatin, rifampin
Dolutegravir	Potent; few side effects; highest genetic barrier to resistance of all INSTIs	Should be dosed twice-daily in patients with possible resistance to other INSTIs	Avoid with etravirine (lowers dolutegravir levels) unless ritonavir-boosted PI also in regimen; give twice-daily with efavirenz or rifampin

---

BASIC SCIENCE/CLINICAL PEARL   **STEP 1/2/3**

Ritonavir was initially used as a standalone protease inhibitor but was poorly tolerated (nausea, diarrhea) at a dose of 400 mg twice daily (the dose at which it had a significant antiretroviral effect). However, it was noted to be an extremely potent cytochrome p450 3A4 inhibitor, such that when it was given at lower doses, it increased drug levels of other protease inhibitors, thus allowing them to be dosed less frequently. Now, ritonavir is commonly given at a much lower dose (typically 100 mg) to "boost" more modern protease inhibitors. Ritonavir-boosted protease inhibitors are still associated with gastrointestinal side effects but at a much lower rate and severity than with higher-dose ritonavir. Ritonavir should not be used to boost other antiretroviral medications, however, as there is at least a theoretical risk that it can lead to protease inhibitor resistance when given without another protease inhibitor because the dose used to boost has incomplete antiretroviral effectiveness.

More recently, cobicistat, a potent cytochrome p450 3A4 inhibitor that lacks intrinsic protease inhibitor activity, has been developed and that avoids this issue. As such, it can not only be combined with protease inhibitors but integrase strand transfer inhibitors as well.

What antiretroviral combinations are recommended in initial therapy for HIV, and what would make one prescribe one over the other?

The Department of Health and Human Services (as of April 2015) recommends five different regimens as first-line options in the initial treatment of HIV infection, regardless of starting viral load (see Table 59.3), though other regimens may be considered depending on patient characteristics.

TABLE 59.3 ■ Recommended Antiretroviral Therapy Regimens for the Initial Therapy of HIV Infection (as of April 2015)

Integrase Inhibitor-Based	Abacavir/lamivudine/dolutegravir (coformulated as TRIUMEQ®) (for HLA-B5701-negative patients)
	Tenofovir/emtricitabine plus dolutegravir
	Tenofovir/emtricitabine/elvitegravir/ cobicistat (coformulated as STRIBILD®) (for patients with creatinine clearance >70 mL/min)
	Tenofovir/emtricitabine plus raltegravir
Protease Inhibitor-Based	Tenofovir/emtricitabine plus darunavir/ ritonavir

The first issue to consider is whether there are any medical contraindications to any regimen; checking a complete blood count (CBC), basic electrolytes including indices of renal function, and liver function tests prior to starting ART can be helpful in this regard. Tenofovir (in its current formulation as tenofovir disoproxil fumarate) has the potential to cause renal toxicity and should be avoided in patients with significant renal impairment, although a newer formulation of tenofovir (tenofovir alafenamide fumarate) will soon be available where it is anticipated that the association with renal insufficiency will be much less because of its ability to preferentially concentrate in lymphoid tissue such that a lower systemic dose can be given. The cobicistat booster should also be avoided in patients with a glomerular filtration rate less than 70 mL/min. Abacavir should not be prescribed in patients with the HLA-B5701 genotype due to their risk of having a hypersensitivity reaction, so HLA-B5701 testing should be sent for patients for whom abacavir is being considered.

BASIC SCIENCE/CLINICAL PEARL   **STEP 1/2/3**

Hypersensitivity to abacavir was a significant issue early in its use as a treatment option for HIV. This hypersensitivity would typically manifest within the first 6 weeks of taking abacavir, characterized by fever, myalgias, and gastrointestinal symptoms that would resolve upon discontinuation of the drug but could evolve into a more severe, even fatal, syndrome if abacavir was later restarted. It was discovered in 2002 that there was a strong association between this hypersensitivity reaction and having the human leukocyte antigen B (HLA-B) locus 5701, which is present in 3 to 6% of persons of European descent. It is now recommended that abacavir only be prescribed to patients who are negative for the HLA-B5701 locus. This screening is one of the first examples of pharmacogenomic testing.

Zidovudine should be avoided in patients with significant anemia. NRTIs in general have been associated with lipoatrophy (facial wasting most commonly), but those that have the strongest association with lipoatrophy—stavudine and didanosine—are no longer commonly used. Efavirenz, the most common side effect of which is vivid dreams, should be avoided in patients with significant psychological disturbances, as it has been linked to increased suicidality. Efavirenz and protease inhibitors can cause or exacerbate hepatotoxicity; consideration should be given to prescribing them in the setting of decompensated liver disease. Protease inhibitors have also been associated with lipodystrophy (buffalo hump, central adiposity, peripheral symmetric lipomas), although these effects are less common with the newer, most commonly used agents (i.e., darunavir and atazanavir).

The next issue to consider is whether the patient is likely to have infection with an HIV strain that may exhibit resistance to some antiretroviral medications. An HIV genotype (in which relevant genes of the predominant circulating HIV strain are sequenced to predict resistance to antiretroviral medications) should be obtained for all patients who are naïve to ART or in treatment-experienced patients for whom antiretroviral resistance is suspected (most commonly an elevated viral load in the setting of partial compliance with ART). The main reason why obtaining a genotype is recommended in all ART-naïve patients is that, although they will not have had the opportunity to engender resistance via partial compliance with therapy, they may have acquired a virus that is already resistant to some antiretroviral medications. A genotype often takes a few weeks to return, so in settings (such as the case above) where it may be particularly prudent to start ART sooner rather than later, an ART regimen that has a high genetic barrier to resistance (e.g., a protease inhibitor-based regimen) can be started, with subsequent streamlining to a simpler regimen later when the genotype results return. Occasionally, other resistance tests may be indicated.

CLINICAL PEARL   STEP 3

Although the HIV genotype relies on algorithms that predict antiretroviral resistance based on mutations that are found in the virus reverse transcriptase, protease, and integrase genes, an HIV phenotype directly measures antiviral activity in the presence of the specific drugs measured. It is more labor intensive and expensive, and as such is less commonly done. It can be helpful, however, in predicting antiviral activity when multiple resistance mutations are present (particularly in the protease gene).

When maraviroc, a CCR5 coreceptor inhibitor, is considered for use, a tropism test must be done to ensure that the patient's virus uses this coreceptor. When a virus uses the C-X-C chemokine receptor type 4 (CXCR4) receptor instead (or uses both), maraviroc should not be used.

Drug–drug interactions should also be considered, particularly among medications that inhibit or induce certain cytochrome p450 enzymes. Certain medications (atazanavir, rilpivirine) have impaired absorption at higher gastric pH and should not be taken concurrently with proton pump inhibitors (but can typically be spaced 12 hours apart from a histamine-2 antagonist). Notable drug–drug interactions of ART components are listed in Table 59.2.

Finally, patient convenience and lifestyle issues should play a role in determining optimal ART. A one-pill-daily regimen promotes compliance and should be offered when not contraindicated otherwise. Whether or not ART is best taken with food may also affect patient preference and compliance.

How should patients started on ART be monitored?

HIV viral load should be monitored 2 to 8 weeks following initiation of ART. Typically, the goal is to see a two-logarithm drop in viral load at 4 weeks. If this is seen, viral load can be checked again every 3 months, with the expectation that by 6 months, viral load should be near or at undetectable levels. Once an undetectable viral load is achieved, viral load should be monitored every 3 to 6 months. Occasionally, after an undetectable viral load is achieved, "blips" of viremia will occur, in which viral load will increase to low levels (typically less than 200 copies/mL). These blips are typically of limited clinical significance on their own, but if the viral load increase becomes more sustained and at higher levels (particularly above 1000 copies/mL), investigation into compliance and possible ART resistance should be undertaken.

Traditionally, CD4 monitoring has typically been performed in parallel with HIV viral load testing but likely does not need to be as closely followed. Although CD4 counts should typically be checked at the same time as viral load when initiating or modifying ART or when viremia develops while on ART, if a patient maintains a consistently suppressed viral load after 2 years on ART, current guidelines recommend only checking the CD4 count yearly if it has been in the 300 to 500 cells/µL range and only optionally if the CD4 count has been consistently greater than 500 cells/µL.

Indices of renal and liver function should also be monitored periodically, and lipid panels should also be routinely obtained in patients on regimens that affect lipids, particularly protease inhibitors and efavirenz. Semiannual to annual screening for proteinuria should also be considered in patients on tenofovir-based regimens.

BEYOND THE PEARLS

- The majority of HIV-infected persons in the United States are not on successful long-term treatment, so improving the HIV "care cascade" by getting more HIV-infected patients diagnosed, engaged in care, and treated is a critical public health goal.
- ART not only benefits the HIV-infected patient taking it but also prevents transmission to HIV-uninfected individuals.
- Recommended ART regimens for treatment-naïve patients consist of two NRTIs combined with an agent from another class, typically an ISTI or protease inhibitor; there are several factors to consider when determining which regimen to initiate.
- HIV viral load should be undetectable within 6 months of starting ART; failure to do so should prompt inquiries into noncompliance with ART and/or possible resistance.
- For a patient who maintains a consistently suppressed viral load after 2 years of ART and has CD4 count >500 cells/mm^3, there is not an absolute need to continue checking CD4 counts in the absence of any intercurrent event that would be expected to lower it (e.g., chemotherapy).
- HIV-infected patients should not receive live-virus vaccines (varicella, zoster, measles, mumps, and rubella [MMR]) if CD4 <200 cells/mm^3. Zoster vaccination is of unclear benefit for patients with higher CD4 counts but could be considered if CD4 is consistently in the 350 to 500 cells/mm^3 range or higher.
- All newly infected HIV-positive individuals should be screened for latent tuberculosis with either a protein purified derivative (PPD) skin test or interferon gamma release assay. Patients should be retested annually if they are at ongoing high risk of exposure (incarceration, residence in a congregate setting, active drug use, known contact with active tuberculosis).
- All newly infected HIV-positive individuals should be screened for sexually transmitted diseases (particularly gonorrhea and chlamydia at all potential exposure sites and syphilis), with retesting at least annually if they remain sexually active (more frequently if they engage in unsafe sexual practices).
- One patient (dubbed "the Berlin Patient") had a clinical cure of HIV by, as a part of his treatment for acute leukemia, receiving a bone marrow transplant from a donor who had a mutation in the CCR5 coreceptor such that HIV could not bind to it. Although this strategy is not viable for the vast majority of patients with HIV infection (as the risks of bone marrow transplantation are far greater than those of ART), it has opened up new avenues of research. It must be noted, however, that CCR5 is not the sole coreceptor that HIV uses to get into cells; a minority of viruses are able to use the CXCR4 receptor.
- Think of acute HIV infection in any patient with risk factors for HIV acquisition who presents with an acute febrile illness with lymphadenopathy, sore throat, rash, myalgia/arthralgia, and/or headache. Depending on the specific test used and the time after seroconversion, an HIV antibody may not be reliable in diagnosing these patients, and an HIV viral load should be pursued.
- Consider *Penicillium marneffei* infection in HIV-infected patients with CD4 counts <100 cells/mm^3 who either live in southeast Asia or have recently traveled there and present with fever, lymphadenopathy, hepatosplenomegaly, and/or a papular rash.

R. Michelle Koolaee

A 65-Year-Old Male With Muscle Weakness

A 65-year-old male presents for evaluation of weakness in bilateral hips and shoulders. He is an avid gardener and has noticed that the weakness has significantly limited his ability to garden as well as to keep up with his wife during their morning walks. He has a history of type 2 diabetes mellitus, obesity, and hypercholesterolemia. His medications include atorvastatin, metformin, and low-dose aspirin. He has a 20-pack-year smoking history but did quit 15 years ago.

What questions are helpful to ask in anyone who complains of weakness?
The etiologies of weakness are very broad but can be narrowed down with the proper history. First, determine the location of the weakness (i.e., is the weakness focal or diffuse? Proximal versus distal? Ascending versus descending?). Inflammatory myopathies typically involve proximal more than distal muscles. Some neuromuscular diseases (i.e., Guillain-Barre syndrome) are characterized by an ascending pattern of weakness. Electrolyte and metabolic disturbances may present with more generalized weakness. Second, be sure to ask the duration of symptoms. Acute focal weakness, for instance, suggests etiologies such as stroke, infectious myopathies, and medication/toxin-related myopathies. Last, note the presence of constitutional symptoms such as fevers and unintentional weight loss; they can help determine whether the weakness is related to a paraneoplastic process.

On further questioning, the patient states that the weakness has been progressively worsening for the past 6 months and is associated with subjective fevers and a 15-pound weight loss during this period. He also mentions that he has noticed some dryness and scaling around his fingers, in addition to some patches of discoloration on his hands.

What are the critical "red flags" to be aware of in someone with symptoms of myopathy?
Proximal muscle weakness with associated skin changes raises an early suspicion for inflammatory myopathy, which should prompt you to ask some critical questions. These are highlighted in Table 60.1.

The patient has no dysphagia but does note dyspnea on exertion after 1 to 2 blocks, which is a dramatic change over the past few months. This is associated with a dry cough. On physical exam, his temperature is 36.4 °C (97.5 °F), blood pressure is 106/66 mm Hg, pulse rate is 60/min, respiration rate is 16/min, and oxygen saturation is 90% on room air. He is able to speak in full sentences without respiratory distress. There are bibasilar fine inspiratory rales on lung exam. Erythematous, violaceous, clumped papules over the extensor surfaces of the metacarpophalangeal (MCP) joints and proximal interphalangeal (PIP) joints are present. On nailbed exam, there is

TABLE 60.1 ▪ Critical Questions to Ask in Patients Where There Is Concern for Inflammatory Myopathy

Question	Reasoning
Do you have shortness of breath?	The diaphragm is a muscle that can be involved in inflammatory myopathies as well as some neuromuscular diseases. If severe, these patients can require mechanical ventilation. There should be a low threshold for inpatient admission for management of these respiratory issues, particularly if the symptoms are acute and severe.
Do you have difficulty swallowing?	Dysphagia can be a sign of oropharyngeal muscle weakness, which increases the risk for aspiration. This requires evaluation by a speech and swallow specialist and often warrants more aggressive immunosuppressive therapy.
Smoking history? Fevers? Unintentional weight loss? Age of the patient?	These questions risk-stratify the patient for a malignancy-associated process. Inflammatory myopathies are associated with a higher incidence of malignancy.

periungual erythema and evidence of drop-out of nailfold capillary loops, as well as enlarged, dilated nailfold capillaries. There are also areas of dried, cracked skin at the lateral surface of most digits of the hand, particularly the second digits bilaterally. Bilateral proximal upper and lower extremity weakness is noted (with more weakness in the lower extremities); there is tenderness of the MCP and PIP joints bilaterally without synovitis.

CLINICAL PEARL   **STEP 2/3**

One quick way to assess quadriceps muscle strength is to have the patients sit in a chair with their arms across their chest; then, ask them to perform squats in and out of the chair without using their arms (this isolates the quadriceps muscles, which are commonly affected in inflammatory myositis).

How do you examine the nailfold capillaries, and when is this of value?
Nailfold capillaroscopy represents a way to analyze microvascular abnormalities in patients with autoimmune disease, with abnormalities seen classically in patients with scleroderma, dermatomyositis (DM), and mixed connective tissue disease (MCTD). Nailfold capillary loops are normally in a homogenous distribution just beneath the cuticle. Abnormal patterns include dilated and distorted nailfold capillary loops, loss of surrounding loop structures, and cuticle overgrowth. See Figure 60.1 for images of normal and abnormal nailfold capillary loops.

There are three ways to examine the nailfold capillaries. A microcirculation microscope is a sophisticated instrument (resembling a traditional microscope) that transfers the image to a television monitor and can be used to measure the cross-section area of the microvessel, as well as the speed and the quantitative amount of blood flow. There are also portable capillaroscope devices that offer increased magnification and a strong light in order to view microvasculature. The most easily accessible and cost-effective means of viewing nailfold capillaries is through the use of the light of an ophthalmoscope (at around 20× magnification). Place some surgical lubricant on the nailfold capillary, just underneath the cuticle, and look through the ophthalmoscope to the nail (as you would normally use the ophthalmoscope), only in much closer proximity.

Initial laboratory and radiographic tests are provided in Table 60.2.

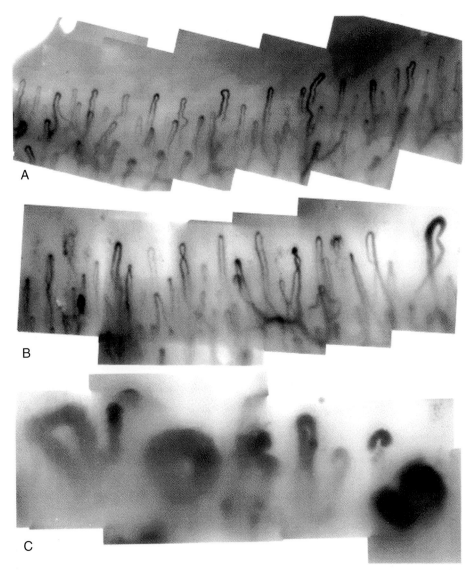

Figure 60.1 Nailfold microscopy showing **(A)** normal appearances, **(B)** some slightly widened capillary loops, suggestive of an underlying connective tissue disease, and **(C)** grossly widened capillary loops and areas of loop dropout in a patient with systemic sclerosis. (Magnification ×300.) *(From Herrick AL, Hutchinson C. Vascular imaging. Best Pract Res Clin Rheumatol. 2004;18[6]:957-979.)*

What is your differential diagnosis at this point?

This is a 65-year-old male presenting with progressive proximal muscle weakness, hypoxia with an interstitial radiographic pattern, rash, and elevated serum muscle enzymes. His chronic dyspnea on exertion, dry cough, hypoxia, lung exam with inspiratory rales, and interstitial pattern on chest radiograph are very suspicious for an underlying interstitial lung disease (ILD); computed tomography (CT) imaging of the lungs would be indicated to further evaluate the lung parenchyma.

TABLE 60.2 ■ **Initial Laboratory Tests**

Complete blood count	Normal
Creatine kinase level	812 units/L
Aldolase	14 units/L (elevated)
Erythrocyte sedimentation rate	82 mm/h
Serum creatinine	0.6 mg/dL
Aspartate aminotransferase	340 units/L
Alanine aminotransferase	412 units/L
Thyroid-stimulating hormone level	Normal
Chest radiograph	Mildly increased reticular markings at the periphery; no focal consolidation

TABLE 60.3 ■ **Common Skin Findings in Dermatomyositis**

Skin Finding	Description
Heliotrope eruption	Erythematous or violaceous rash around the eyes; can be accompanied by eyelid edema
Gottron's papules	Palpable erythematous to violaceous rash on the extensor surface of the MCP and PIP joints
"Mechanic's hands"	Dirty-appearing, dry, and fissured skin around the lateral and dorsal surface of the digits and of the palms; resembles those of a manual labor worker
Nailfold abnormalities	Dilated and tortuous nailfold capillaries alternating with capillary dropout; cuticular overgrowth; periungual erythema
Sun-exposed poikiloderma (including on the upper back ["shawl sign"] and anterior chest ["V sign"])	Poikiloderma refers to areas of hypopigmentation and hyperpigmentation, telangiectasias, and epidermal atrophy in sun-exposed areas; often pruritic; can be macular or papular; can appear violaceous in color
Calcinosis cutis	Deposition of calcium underneath the skin; presents as firm subcutaneous nodules that may or may not be painful

MCP, Metacarpophalangeal; *PIP,* proximal interphalangeal.

CLINICAL PEARL   **STEP 2/3**

Serum aspartate aminotransferase (AST) and alanine aminotransferase (ALT) are muscle enzymes that are very often abnormal in patients with inflammatory myositis.

An inflammatory myositis is highest on the differential at this time, particularly DM, given the skin findings. In addition, ILD is a common feature of the inflammatory myopathies, which also include polymyositis (PM) and inclusion body myositis (IBM). The erythematous papules on the MCPs and PIPs, with fissuring of the digits of the hands, are likely Gottron's papules and "mechanic's hands," respectively. Nailfold capillary abnormalities and periungual erythema are typical for DM as well. A summary of skin changes seen in DM are noted in Table 60-3. Figures 60.2 and 60.3 demonstrate Gottron's papules and the "shawl sign." IBM classically presents in older men (mean age is approximately 60 years), may also involve weakness in the distal muscle groups, and often only have moderate elevations of muscle enzyme levels (<10-fold the upper

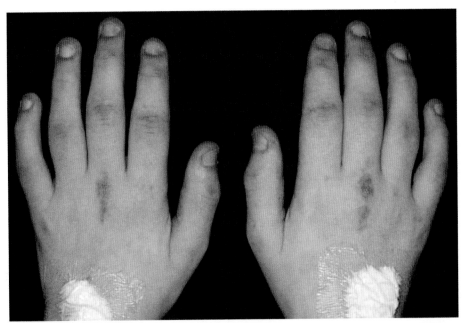

Figure 60.2   Gottron's papules over the extensor aspects of the small joints of the hands. *(From Hawley DP, Foster HE. Paediatric musculoskeletal examination: a case-based review.* Paediatr Child Health. *2011; 21[12]:527-533.)*

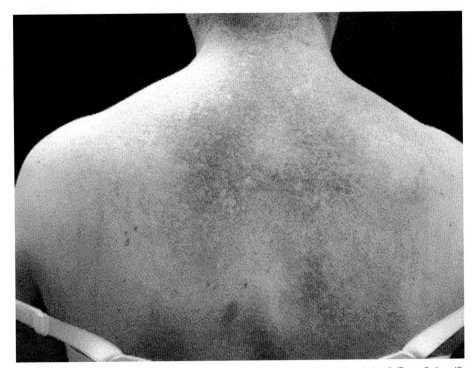

Figure 60.3   Poikiloderma on the upper aspect of the back is typical of the "shawl sign." *(From Callen JP, Wortmann RL. Dermatomyositis.* Clin Dermatol. *2006;24[5]:363-373.)*

limit of normal). The antisynthetase syndrome is a clinical subset of patients with inflammatory myositis (DM or PM), characterized by features which may include aggressive myositis, interstitial lung disease, mechanic's hands, Raynaud's phenomenon, and fever. Affected patients have antibodies to aminoacyl-transfer ribonucleic acid (tRNA) synthetase enzymes.

A paraneoplastic myositis should also be considered in this patient with a smoking history and unintentional weight loss. All patients with DM or PM should undergo an age-appropriate malignancy screening workup. Given the additional history of smoking, further imaging modalities should be considered.

Myositis with ILD may also be features of other connective tissue diseases, such as systemic lupus erythematosus (SLE), MCTD, or scleroderma. Although sometimes the photosensitive rashes seen in SLE may appear similar to that of DM, a negative antinuclear antibody (ANA) test makes these diagnoses far less likely. MCTD is characterized by features that may include myositis, ILD, Raynaud's, swollen hands, and antiribonucleoprotein (RNP) antibodies; it too would be unusual without a positive ANA. It is incredibly unusual to have scleroderma without Raynaud's phenomenon and a negative ANA test, not to mention the lack of sclerodactlyly.

Drug-induced myopathy can mimic the symptoms of inflammatory myositis and include drugs such as colchicine, glucocorticoids, alcohol, statins, antimalarials, antipsychotics, and certain antiretrovirals. Autoimmune necrotizing myopathy is a rare disorder that can present similarly to DM or PM, but that demonstrates necrotic muscle fibers on muscle biopsy, in contrast to DM or PM. Necrotizing myopathy has also been described in relation to statin use; unlike statin-induced myopathy, symptoms persist following withdrawal of drug therapy. The patient's history of statin use makes both statin-induced myopathy and necrotizing myopathy possibilities; the skin findings, however, are very classic for DM. Statin therapy should be withheld.

BASIC SCIENCE PEARL   **STEP 1**

Statins upregulate 3-hydroxy-3-methylglutaryl-coenzyme A reductase (HMGCR), and anti-HMGCR autoantibodies have been found in patients with statin-associated necrotizing myopathy.

Hypothyroidism can mimic the features of inflammatory myositis and should always be checked in anyone with symptoms of myopathy; normal thyroid function tests in this patient make this an unlikely diagnosis. Infectious etiologies are also less likely in this case, given the chronicity of the patient's symptoms. These include viral (i.e., human immunodeficiency virus [HIV], hepatitis B virus [HBV], hepatitis C virus [HCV]), bacterial (i.e., Lyme, pyomyositis), and parasitic infections.

Also very unlikely is the possibility of an inherited metabolic myopathy, which includes disorders of carbohydrate and lipid metabolism, such as carnitine deficiency. They are characterized by acute intermittent episodes of weakness, particularly after exercise.

Lastly and unlikely as well are the neuromuscular diseases, which can present with proximal muscle weakness; these include amyotrophic lateral sclerosis (ALS), muscular dystrophies, and myasthenia gravis. Rashes and ILD are atypical for these diseases, among a number of clinical features that differ from PM and DM. For instance, ALS often presents with distal rather than proximal weakness; muscular dystrophies have different histologic characteristics on muscle biopsy; myasthenia gravis is distinguished from myositis by the presence of facial muscle weakness, normal muscle enzymes, and antiacetylcholine receptor antibodies.

What is the difference between myopathy and myositis?

Myopathy is a generalized term for muscle disease derived from the Greek language (*myo* meaning muscle and *pathos* meaning suffering). *Myositis* refers specifically to inflammation of the muscle, as seen in PM, DM, IBM, and pyomyositis (due to bacterial infection of the skeletal muscles).

What type of diagnostic workup should be performed immediately?
This patient is hypoxic and short of breath, with an abnormal chest radiograph (CXR). This should be addressed immediately. His breathing is not labored, so there is no issue of airway compromise at this time. However, inpatient admission is reasonable given the degree of hypoxia. A CT scan of the chest should be ordered to evaluate for parenchymal lung disease but will concurrently evaluate for malignancy (given his smoking history and weight loss). If he had dysphagia, a speech and swallow evaluation would be indicated urgently to assess his risk for aspiration.

BASIC SCIENCE/CLINICAL PEARL   **STEP 1/2/3**

Always prioritize the "problem list" for each patient (particularly when he or she is an inpatient) and address first those issues that will lead to increased morbidity and mortality if not managed immediately.

Statin therapy is withheld and the patient is admitted to the hospital. A high-resolution CT scan of the chest shows an interstitial pattern of disease; this includes interstitial markings at the bases and at the lung periphery, traction bronchiectasis, and diffuse ground-glass opacities. There are no masses or lymphadenopathy.

What tests should be performed next to establish a diagnosis?
Muscle biopsy is the most important diagnostic test in order to establish a diagnosis; histopathologic findings can distinguish DM, PM, and IBM—not to mention the other forms of myopathy previously discussed. Often, magnetic resonance imaging (MRI) is ordered of the most affected muscle groups (in this case the bilateral thighs), which can show muscle edema, inflammation, fibrosis, and calcification. It can also help the surgeons localize the best area to biopsy, because myositis can often have a patchy distribution. MRI findings are nonspecific, however, and do not distinguish between the different forms of myopathy. Electromyography (EMG) is also performed, which can show characteristic changes of inflammatory myositis (again, this is nonspecific and would not establish the exact diagnosis). It does, however, help to distinguish inflammatory myositis from neuropathic disorders, such as ALS or myasthenia gravis.

BASIC SCIENCE PEARL   **STEP 1**

Skin biopsy in DM often reveals interface dermatitis, characterized by inflammatory cells at the dermo-epidermal junction. This is a nonspecific finding seen in many other connective tissue diseases, including SLE.

CLINICAL PEARL   **STEP 2/3**

Do not order an MRI in the same extremity that an EMG is performed; if you do, make sure the EMG is performed AFTER the MRI is done. An EMG can cause irritation in the muscle fibers and can lead to erroneous abnormalities on MRI.

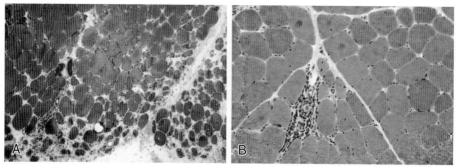

Figure 60.4 Biopsy in dermatomyositis. **A,** Low-power (original magnification ×100) view of a muscle biopsy from a patient with dermatomyositis. Note the marked variation in fiber size and the large number of atrophic myocytes, particularly at the periphery of the fascicles. **B,** High-power (original magnification ×200) view of inflammation around the vessels in the muscle biopsy of a patient with dermatomyositis. There are nearby atrophic cells and cells whose nuclei have moved away from the periphery of the cell (centralized nuclei). *(From Christopher-Stine L, Plotz PH. Inflammatory muscle diseases: In Rich RR, Fleisher TA, Shearer WT, et al., eds.* Clinical Immunology. *3rd ed. Edinburgh: Mosby; 2008:825-835.)*

MRI of bilateral thighs reveals diffuse areas of muscle edema and enhancement, most prominently at the rectus femoris muscles. EMG reveals increased insertional activity, spontaneous fibrillations, short-duration polyphasic motor unit potentials, and complex repetitive discharges, all compatible with an inflammatory myositis. A muscle biopsy is performed and reveals CD4+ inflammatory infiltrate in the perimysial region, along with perifascicular atrophy and fibrosis (see Fig. 60.4).

BASIC SCIENCE PEARL   **STEP 1**

IBM is characterized by filamentous inclusions and vacuoles seen on electron microscopy. These may sometimes be missed on muscle biopsy due to patchy disease involvement.

Diagnosis: Dermatomyositis

What is the role of autoantibody testing in this case?

Because the suspicion for a connective tissue disease–associated myositis is low, it is not necessary to order ANA testing at this time. There are several myositis-specific autoantibodies available for patients with inflammatory myositis, which may offer information regarding prognosis and pattern of disease involvement. They are costly tests to order (and not always available, depending on the location of practice), and so it is at the clinician's preference whether to order them. They should not be ordered haphazardly in an attempt to establish a diagnosis. It is the author's opinion not to order them unless they either change management or they offer prognostic information. There are many myositis-specific antibodies; the three most common categories are described in Table 60.4.

How would you approach treatment acutely?

The goals of therapy are to improve muscle strength and prevent respiratory compromise (due to diaphragm muscle involvement). Systemic glucocorticoids are the hallmark of therapy for management of acute weakness. There are no specific guidelines for dosing, but the general

TABLE 60.4 ■ **Myositis Specific Antibodies**

Antibody	Clinical Significance
Antiaminoacyl-tRNA synthetase (antisynthetase antibodies)	Most common are anti-Jo-1 antibodies; associated with antisynthetase syndrome (severe myositis, interstitial lung disease, polyarthritis, mechanic's hands, Raynaud's phenomenon, fever)
Antisignal recognition particle (SRP) antibodies	Associated with severe, aggressive, necrotizing myopathy
Anti-Mi-2 antibodies	Associated with dermatomyositis

approach includes higher doses at the onset in order to establish disease control, with a slower taper for a total duration of therapy between 6 and 12 months. The initial dose is typically with prednisone (or equivalent) of 1 mg/kg/day or pulse methylprednisolone 1000 mg per day for 3 days for patients who are severely ill (respiratory compromise or severe oropharyngeal muscle involvement causing aspiration). Intravenous immune globulin (IVIG) is also sometimes initiated acutely in patients with severe disease. The expense of this treatment is an important consideration in its long-term use.

What are some general treatment options for long-term therapy of DM?
Methotrexate and azathioprine are common glucocorticoid-sparing agents for DM. IVIG may be used to maintain remission as an outpatient. Physical therapy is critical to maintain muscle strength. Hydroxychloroquine and topical glucocorticoids may be used for patients with a refractory DM rash.

> The patient is started on prednisone 60 mg daily, and after a few days notes gradual improvements in his breathing, rash, and muscle strength. He is discharged home with arrangements for aggressive physical therapy, as well as with his primary care physician for age-appropriate malignancy screening given his new diagnosis of DM. At his follow-up visit with his rheumatologist, he is started on azathioprine.

BEYOND THE PEARLS

- Amyopathic DM (also called dermatomyositis sine myositis) comprises a subgroup of patients who have the cutaneous manifestations of DM without muscle involvement. The extent of malignancy risk is not clear in this subgroup; age-appropriate cancer screening tests should also be performed in these patients.
- Cancer can be diagnosed before, simultaneously with, or after the diagnosis of inflammatory myositis. The peak incidence of cancer diagnosis is within 2 years (before or after) of the diagnosis of inflammatory myositis.
- Muscle enzyme levels are not always significantly elevated in patients with inflammatory myositis, particularly in patients with advanced disease, where there is significant muscle atrophy.
- A rise in serum creatine kinase (CK) can occur prior to the onset of a myositis flare (before the patient has overt weakness); likewise, the clinical improvement in weakness can lag behind the improvements in CK levels (in this case, reassure patients that their weakness will likely improve).
- Serum aldolase is not a muscle-specific enzyme (i.e., it can be elevated in hemolytic states and liver damage), but in some patients it correlates better with disease activity and is more useful than the serum CK.

Continued

BEYOND THE PEARLS—cont'd

- Although further studies are warranted, recent data suggest that rituximab may have a role in treatment of refractory PM and DM.
- IBM is relatively resistant to glucocorticoids and other immunosuppressive therapy. Progression is very slow, and by 15 years, most patients are wheelchair bound or bedridden and require assistance with basic daily activities.

References

Buchbinder R, Forbes A, Hall S, et al. Incidence of malignant disease in biopsy-proven inflammatory myopathy. A population-based cohort study. *Ann Intern Med.* 2001;134(12):1087.

Oddis CV, Reed AM, Aggarwal R, et al. Rituximab in the treatment of refractory adult and juvenile dermatomyositis and adult polymyositis: a randomized, placebo-phase trial. *Arthritis Rheum.* 2013;65:314-324.

Targoff IN. Autoantibodies and their significance in myositis. *Curr Rheumatol Rep.* 2008;10(4):333-340.

Aarti Chawla Mittal ▨ Walter Chou ▨ Raj Dasgupta ▨
Joe Crocetti

A 43-Year-Old Female With Fevers

A 43-year-old female with a past medical history of insulin-dependent diabetes mellitus and hyperlipidemia presents to the emergency room with fevers up to 38.4 °C (101.1 °F) for the past 3 days. She also reports feeling weak and slightly dizzy when sitting or standing, which resolves when she lays down.

What are the potential causes of dizziness while sitting or standing that resolve when supine?

Orthostatic hypotension, or postural hypotension, is low blood pressure that causes symptoms only when the patient is in an upright position. This happens because when upright, there is pooling of blood in the lower extremities and splanchnic bed, which decreases venous return, thus dropping cardiac output and blood pressure. This is what causes the symptom of dizziness or lightheadedness when upright. Normally, the baroreceptors in the arteries near the heart and neck sense the low blood pressure, which provokes increased sympathetic tone, which increases pulse rate, peripheral vascular resistance, and cardiac output, thus limiting the symptoms. Depending on the cause and if the symptoms are severe, the hypotension can lead to syncope.

Etiologies for orthostatic hypotension are dehydration or problems with the cardiovascular, endocrine, or nervous systems. With the limited history, dehydration due to the patient's fever is the most likely cause.

The patient's vital signs are as follows: blood pressure 82/57 mm Hg, pulse rate 126/min, respiration rate 22/min, temperature 38.8 °C (101.8 °F), and oxygen saturation is 99% on room air. Cardiopulmonary and neurologic exam is normal. There is mild tenderness to palpation in the suprapubic area.

These vitals are concerning for what clinical syndrome?

All of the patient's vital signs are abnormal and worrisome, except the oxygen saturation. These findings point to the systemic inflammatory response syndrome (SIRS), which is a nonspecific cytokine-mediated inflammatory state involving multiple organ systems of the body. SIRS is usually a response to an infection but can also be caused by ischemia, burns, or trauma.

CLINICAL PEARL   **STEP 2/3**

The diagnostic criteria for the systemic inflammatory response syndrome (SIRS) requires two or more of the following:
- Fever >38 °C (100.4 °F) or <36 °C (96.8 °F)
- Pulse rate >90/min
- Respiration rate >20/min or $PaCO_2$ <32 mm Hg
- Leukocytosis >12,000/μL or leukopenia <4,000/μL, or >10% immature (band) formation

---

What is your differential diagnosis?

The differential diagnosis for this patient is very broad because SIRS is so nonspecific. Highest on the list is infection, as this is the most common cause of SIRS. Other possibilities also must be considered, such as pulmonary embolism, autoimmune disorders, pancreatitis, and substance abuse.

When questioned further, the patient endorses burning with urination and urinary frequency. She denies cough, chest pain, shortness of breath, headache, diarrhea, nausea, and vomiting.

What labs would you like to order and why?

Because the top differential diagnosis is infection and the patient complains of dysuria, it would be wise to start with a urinalysis and urine culture. To see if the patient has bacteremia, blood cultures should be ordered as part of the initial infectious workup.

CLINICAL PEARL   **STEP 2/3**

The correct way to obtain blood cultures is to order two sets (aerobic and anaerobic) drawn from a fresh peripheral stick for each set. The yield is best when cultures are drawn while the patient is febrile. It is NOT advisable to draw blood cultures from an indwelling intravenous (IV) or vascular catheter of any sort.

It is also wise to ask for a complete blood count (CBC) with a differential of the white blood cells. This will indicate whether the patient has any leukocytosis (or leukopenia) and bands. It is also possible to see whether the patient is anemic, which may explain her orthostatic hypotension. A basic metabolic panel will provide information regarding her general electrolytes, kidney function, and current glucose level.

Given the high suspicion for infection, along with the patient's hypotension, tachycardia, and tachypnea, it would also be prudent to order a serum lactate level. With her hypotension, the patient may not be adequately perfusing all of her organs and tissues. As cells become more hypoxic, they switch from aerobic to anaerobic metabolism for energy production. A by-product of the anaerobic pathway is a buildup of lactic acid (see Fig. 61.1).

An elevated lactate level in someone with infection is something to be very concerned about. All elevated levels, however, are not due to infection. Table 61.1 shows various mechanisms and causes of elevated lactate levels.

The urinalysis results come back and are shown in Table 61.2.

How do you interpret these data?

The presence of nitrites, leukocytes, bacteria, and white blood cells (WBCs) indicates that the patient has a urinary tract infection (UTI). It is important to note the quality of the sample, which can be evaluated by the number of epithelial cells seen. Zero epithelial cells per high-powered field is regarded as a "clean catch" and thus the rest of the findings in the urinalysis will not be secondary to bacteria and leukocytes from outside the urinary tract.

This is a patient with SIRS and a known source of infection.

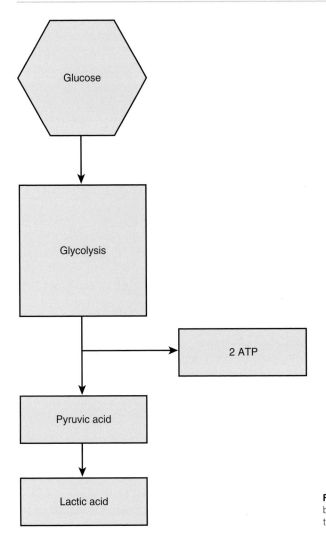

Figure 61.1 The anaerobic metabolic pathway. *ATP,* Adenosine triphosphate.

TABLE 61.1 ▨ **Causes of Elevated Serum Lactate**

Inadequate Oxygen Delivery	Inadequate Oxygen Utilization	Disproportionate Oxygen Demands	Decreased Clearance
Septic shock	SIRS	Shivering	Chronic liver disease
Severe hypoxemia	Total parenteral nutrition	Hypothermia	
Trauma	Thiamine deficiency	Seizures	
Severe anemia	HIV infection	Strenuous activity	
Volume depletion or dehydration	Medications (metformin, salicylates, antiretroviral agents, propofol, cyanide, lorazepam, isoniazid)		
Prolonged carbon monoxide exposure			

HIV, Human immunodeficiency virus; *SIRS,* systemic inflammatory response syndrome.

TABLE 61.2 ■ Urinalysis Results

Macroscopic	
Color	Amber
Specific gravity	1.030
Protein	+ (positive)
Glucose	+ (positive)
Ketones	0-10 mg/dL
Bilirubin	– (negative)
Blood	– (negative)
Nitrites	– (negative)
Leukocytes	+ (positive)
Microscopic	
Epithelial cells	0 per high powered field (HPF)
Bacteria	Many per HPF
WBC	Many per HPF
RBC	None
Casts	Coarse granular casts

RBC, Red blood cell; *WBC*, white blood cell.

What is the diagnosis?

SIRS plus an infection source (either identified or suspected) is defined as sepsis. Table 61.3 shows the diagnostic criteria for sepsis.

Diagnosis: Sepsis secondary to a urinary tract infection

How would you classify her degree of sepsis?

As you can see from Table 61.3, the diagnostic criteria for sepsis is very broad and encompasses patients who have limited organ dysfunction to patients with advanced organ dysfunction who are close to death. Given its large spectrum of severity, categories were established: sepsis, severe sepsis, septic shock, and refractory septic shock.

Severe sepsis is defined as sepsis-induced hypoperfusion or organ dysfunction as manifested in any of the following ways:
- Sepsis-induced hypotension
- Lactate above upper limit of normal
- Urine output <0.5 cc/kg/hour for more than 2 hours despite adequate fluid resuscitation
- Acute lung injury with partial pressure arterial oxygen (PaO_2)/fraction of inspired oxygen (FiO_2) <250 in the absence of pneumonia as infectious source
- Creatinine >2.0 mg/dL
- Bilirubin >2 mg/dL
- Platelets count <100,000 μL
- Coagulopathy (international normalized ratio [INR] >1.5)

Septic shock is defined as severe sepsis with hypotension, despite adequate fluid resuscitation necessitating vasopressor agents. Differentiating the degree of sepsis is important because it will help guide your management and treatment.

TABLE 61.3 ■ Diagnostic Criteria for Sepsis

General Variables

Fever >38.3 °C (100.9 °F)
Hypothermia <36 °C (96.8 °F)
Pulse rate >90 beats/minute or more than 2 standard deviations above normal for age
Tachypnea
Altered mental status
Significant edema or positive fluid balance (>20 mL/kg over 24 hours)
Hyperglycemia (plasma glucose >140 mg/dL) in the absence of diabetes

Inflammatory Variables

Leukocytosis (WBC count >12,000 μL)
Leukopenia (WBC count <4,000 μL)
Normal WBC count with >10% immature (band) forms
Plasma C-reactive protein >2 standard deviations above normal
Plasma procalcitonin >2 standard deviations above normal

Hemodynamic Variables

Arterial hypotension (SBP <90 mm Hg, MAP <70 mm Hg, or an SBP decrease >40 mm Hg)

Organ Dysfunction Variables

Arterial hypoxemia (PaO_2/FiO_2 <300)
Acute oliguria (UOP <0.5 mL/kg/hour for 2 hours despite adequate volume resuscitation)
Creatinine increase >0.5 mg/dL
Coagulation abnormalities (INR >1.5 or aPTT >60 seconds)
Ileus (absent bowel sounds)
Thrombocytopenia (platelet count <100,000 μL)
Hyperbilirubinemia (plasma total bilirubin >4 mg/dL)

Tissue Perfusion Variables

Hyperlactinemia (>1 mmol/L)
Mottling or decreased capillary refill

aPTT, Activated partial thromboplasin time; *FiO₂,* fraction of inspired oxygen; *INR,* international normalized ratio; *MAP,* mean arterial pressure; *PaO₂,* partial pressure of O_2 in arterial blood; *SBP,* systolic blood pressure; *UOP,* urine output; *WBC,* white blood cell.

This patient's hypotension alone (systolic blood pressure [SBP] <90 mm Hg) would be diagnostic of severe sepsis. To evaluate for septic shock or refractory septic shock, her response to treatment must be assessed.

How is sepsis treated?

The treatment of sepsis requires early identification of sepsis in combination with aggressive early initiation of treatments. These treatments include interventions to restore organ perfusion, such as intravenous (IV) fluids and vasopressors, and treatment of the underlying infection with antibiotics and source control, if needed. Once sepsis has been identified, an assessment of the patient's respiratory status should be performed. Patients in severe sepsis or septic shock often have increased work of breathing or inability to protect their airway due to depressed levels of consciousness. These patients may require intubation, sedation, and mechanical ventilation.

Does the patient need to be started on mechanical ventilation?

The patient is fully alert and oriented, with mild tachypnea and a normal pulse oximetry oxygen saturation. She does not require supplemental oxygen or mechanical ventilation at this time. Once the respiratory status is addressed, the patient should be evaluated for signs and symptoms of severe sepsis or septic shock.

As previously stated, severe sepsis occurs when there is evidence of end-organ hypoperfusion, such as hypotension, lactic acidosis, oliguria/anuria, acute kidney injury, acute lung injury, coagulopathies, elevated bilirubin, or thrombocytopenia. Once severe sepsis has been confirmed, immediate initiation of measures to increase intravascular volume and increase perfusion should be started. IV access should be obtained in any patient with suspected sepsis, and central venous access with a central venous catheter (CVC) may be necessary for those in severe sepsis or septic shock. An initial bolus of crystalloid fluids (such as 0.9% sodium chloride or lactated Ringer's solution) equal to 20 to 30 mL/kg should be given, with reassessment for response to further guide therapy.

What are the goals of therapy in sepsis?
Early goal-directed therapy (EGDT) uses objective physiologic parameters to guide fluid resuscitation in severe sepsis and septic shock within the first 6 hours of presentation. The emphasis is on early and aggressive management of sepsis during the first 6 hours, which has been shown to improve survival. Although recent studies have shown no mortality benefit with EGDT algorithms, early aggressive management of septic shock has been the key to improved survival. EGDT is still an objective, reproducible protocol recommended by several experts in the field, including the Surviving Sepsis Campaign; however, central venous pressure measurements and central venous oxygenation are not necessary for all patients.

CLINICAL PEARL   **STEP 2/3**

EGDT involves using physiologic parameters to drive the treatment of severe sepsis or septic shock in the first 6 hours of resuscitation. EGDT requires a central venous catheter to obtain certain parameters, such as central venous pressure (CVP) or central venous oxygenation saturation ($ScvO_2$).
Goal 1: CVP between 8 mm Hg and 12 mm Hg
Goal 2: Mean arterial pressure (MAP) ≥65 mm Hg or SBP ≥90 mm Hg
Goal 3: $ScvO_2$ ≥70%

Using EGDT, clinicians should first give intravenous crystalloid or colloid (e.g., albumin) fluid boluses to achieve a CVP of 8 to 12 mm Hg. Once this is achieved, the patient's blood pressure should be assessed, with the initiation of vasoactive agents such as norepinephrine if the mean arterial pressure (MAP) is <65 mm Hg or the SBP is <90 mm Hg. If the blood pressure is not at goal or there is still evidence of ongoing organ dysfunction, the clinician should decide whether to measure $ScvO_2$. If the $ScvO_2$ is <70%, the patient should receive red blood cell (RBC) transfusions until the hematocrit is ≥30%. If the $ScvO_2$ stays below 70% after the hematocrit, blood pressure, and CVP have reached the goal, an inotropic agent such as dobutamine should be started. In addition to the EGDT parameters, many clinicians use urine output and lactate as a marker of end-organ perfusion. The goal urine output is ≥0.5 mL/kg/hour, and lactate is ideally normalized. In EGDT, the physiologic parameters of interest should be continually reassessed, especially to note the effectiveness of interventions. Of note, to measure CVP and $ScvO_2$, a CVC positioned in the superior vena cava is required. Often, arterial catheterization is also performed to continuously monitor blood pressure.

In addition to hemodynamic optimization, early administration of antimicrobial therapy targeted at the likely source of infection is paramount. The Surviving Sepsis Campaign advocates antimicrobial therapy within 1 hour of identification of severe sepsis or septic shock. Appropriate cultures should be obtained before starting antimicrobial therapy if obtaining cultures does not delay antimicrobial treatment. If the patient's infection requires source control, the least taxing effective intervention should be pursued. For example, if the patient has an abscess requiring drainage, percutaneous drainage is preferred over surgical drainage in those with severe sepsis or shock.

The patient presents with dysuria and signs of systemic hypoperfusion. She is correctly assessed as having severe sepsis and is given an initial bolus of IV crystalloid solution of 30 mL/kg. She does not require mechanical ventilation at this time. Blood cultures and urine cultures are obtained, and IV antibiotics directed against urinary pathogens are started within the first hour of presentation. She still has an SBP <90 mm Hg despite initial fluid resuscitation, so early goal-directed therapy is started. A CVC is placed in her right internal jugular vein, and additional boluses of IV crystalloid are given. Her blood pressure and CVP reach goals after each bolus of IV crystalloids, so she does not require vasoactive medications. Her ScvO$_2$ is >70%, so she does not require RBC transfusions or inotropic medications. After 3 hours, she is normotensive with a normal pulse rate, and CVP, MAP, SBP, and ScvO$_2$ are at goal. She is admitted to the hospital with a diagnosis of severe sepsis from a urinary origin and has a complete recovery.

BEYOND THE PEARLS

- Due to the lack of specificity of the SIRS criteria, there are new approaches being developed for the evaluation of sepsis. In early 2016, the 3rd International Consensus Definitions for Sepsis and Septic Shock (Sepsis-3) proposed three new definitions:
    - Sepsis is defined as life-threatening organ dysfunction caused by a dysregulated host response to infection.
    - Organ dysfunction can be represented by an increase in the Sepsis-related Organ Failure Assessment (SOFA) score.
    - Septic shock is defined as a subset of sepsis in which particularly profound circulatory, cellular, and metabolic abnormalities are associated with a greater risk of mortality than with sepsis alone.
- The SOFA scoring system is used to determine the extent of a person's organ function or rate of organ failure. The score is based on 6 different organ system evaluations:
    1. Respiratory (PaO$_2$/FiO$_2$ ratio)
    2. Cardiovascular (mean arterial pressure)
    3. Hepatic (serum bilirubin level)
    4. Coagulation (platelet level)
    5. Renal (serum creatinine level or urine output)
    6. Neurologic systems (Glasgow coma scale)
- Procalcitonin (PCT) is a biomarker that exhibits greater specificity than other proinflammatory markers in identifying patients with sepsis. Levels may be useful to distinguish bacterial infections from nonbacterial infections and may help guide therapy and reduce antibiotic use, which can help with drug resistance.
- The ideal vasopressors for sepsis have been evaluated in numerous studies, with most showing no major differences in mortality or length of hospital stay. Some data support the use of norepinephrine rather than other agents as the first vasopressor in sepsis.
- The use of systemic glucocorticoids in refractory septic shock (hypotension despite fluid resuscitation and vasopressors) likely has benefit but has conflicting data that require more investigation.
- Hyperglycemia has been associated with poor outcomes in the critically ill. However, strict, intense control of serum glucose has been shown to be detrimental in critically ill patients.

References

Dellinger RP, Levy MM, Rhodes A, et al. Surviving Sepsis Campaign: international guidelines for management of severe sepsis and septic shock: 2012. *Crit Care Med*. 2012;41(2):580-637.

Djillali A, Sébille V, Charpentier C, et al. Effect of treatment with low doses of hydrocortisone and fludrocortisone on mortality in patients with septic shock. *JAMA*. 2002;288(7):862-871.

Havel C, Arrich J, Losert H, et al. Vasopressors for hypotensive shock. *Cochrane Database Syst Rev.* 2011;(5):1-79.

Laird AM, Miller PR, Kilgo PD, et al. Relationship of early hyperglycemia to morality in trauma patients. *J Trauma.* 2004;56(5):1058-1062.

NICE-SUGAR Study Investigators. Intensive versus conventional glucose control in critically ill patients. *N Engl J Med.* 2009;360(33):1283-1297.

Peake SL, Delaney A, Bailey M, et al. Goal-directed resuscitation for patients with early septic shock. *N Engl J Med.* 2014;371(16):1496-1506.

Rivers E, Nguyen B, Havstad S, et al. Early goal-directed therapy in the treatment of severe sepsis and septic shock. *N Engl J Med.* 2001;345(10):1368-1377.

Singer M, Deutschman CS, Seymour CW, et al. The Third International Consensus Definitions for Sepsis and Septic Shock (Sepsis-3). *JAMA.* 2016;315(8):801-810.

Sprung CL, Annane D, Keh D, et al. Hydrocortisone therapy for patients with septic shock. *N Engl J Med.* 2008;358(2):111-124.

Emily S. Gillett　　■　　Raj Dasgupta

A 54-Year-Old Male Who "Stops Breathing at Night"

A 54-year-old male patient with hypertension, type 2 diabetes mellitus, obesity, dyslipidemia, and coronary artery disease (CAD) status postcoronary artery bypass graft (CABG) presents to the sleep clinic because his wife is worried that he "stops breathing at night." He underwent CABG about 3 months prior to his appointment. He had initial difficulty sleeping after his surgery, but this has improved over time. He also found a supplement at a natural foods store that seemed to help.

How is insomnia defined? How would you assess this patient's insomnia?

Insomnia, defined as difficulty falling asleep or staying asleep, is a very common sleep complaint. Some studies estimate that up to 30% of the general population report chronic insomnia, while at least 10% of the general population report insomnia that is "distressing" or that significantly impairs their daytime functioning. Insomnia that occurs after a major life event, including a significant change in health status, a hospitalization, or a medical procedure, is called *adjustment insomnia* and is usually transient (lasting <3 months). However, in patients with cardiovascular disease, medication side effects must also be considered. In patients with congestive heart failure (CHF) or hypertension, diuretic therapy may lead to overnight awakenings related to nocturia. Cardiac patients are frequently prescribed beta blockers that depress sympathetic tone and thereby produce many positive effects from a cardiovascular perspective, but decreased sympathetic tone also decreases production of melatonin, a neurohormone that is critical for regulating the circadian sleep–wake cycle. For some of these patients, starting a melatonin supplement may help them fall asleep more quickly.

CLINICAL PEARL　　　　　　　　　　　　　　　　　　　　　　　　**STEP 2/3**

Many commonly prescribed medications can have deleterious effects on sleep, including selective serotonin reuptake inhibitors (SSRIs) and other antidepressants, antiepileptic medications, and stimulants prescribed to treat attention deficit hyperactive disorder (ADHD). When possible, adjusting medication dosages or timing, changing to a different class of medication, or discontinuing nonessential medications may have a significant impact on sleep quality.

The patient reports that he sleeps from 10 PM to 6 AM. He falls asleep quickly, usually in less than 5 minutes, sometimes on the couch while watching television. He typically awakens one or two times overnight to urinate. He returns to sleep quickly after using the bathroom. He denies excessive daytime sleepiness and has a normal Epworth Sleepiness Scale score of 6/24 (see page 270). He drinks about six cups of coffee each day and sometimes has an "energy drink" in the afternoon.

CLINICAL PEARL   **STEP 2/3**

Excessive daytime sleepiness may be masked by caffeine intake or by prescription stimulants such as methylphenidate (Ritalin®), dextroamphetamine/levoamphetamine (Adderall®), and modafinil (Provigil®). When evaluating any patient, it is always important to obtain a complete list of current medications and herbal supplements, to assess caffeine and alcohol intake, and to ask about tobacco and substance use.

The patient denies drowsy driving, falling asleep at the wheel, and motor vehicle collisions related to sleepiness. He does not nap.

CLINICAL PEARL   **STEP 2/3**

When assessing a patient who reports sleep-related difficulties, it is critical to assess safety concerns, including drowsy driving and if his or her occupation involves operating heavy machinery or vehicles involved in mass transit or the long-distance transportation of goods. All patients should be counseled to avoid driving and other high-risk activities when they are drowsy.

The patient is accompanied by his wife, who says that he does not move around much in his sleep and that she has not noticed any sleep talking (somniloquy) or sleep walking (somnambulism). He snores loudly every night, and has done so for about the past 10 years. The snoring is so loud that his wife sometimes has to sleep in a different room, especially on nights when they have had wine or cocktails earlier in the evening. She also reports that her husband "stops breathing" several times each night, and sometimes gasps or chokes. She thinks the pauses in breathing have recently become more frequent, even prior to his CABG.

What is your differential diagnosis for this patient's pauses in breathing during sleep?

There is a high prevalence of sleep disordered breathing in patients with cardiovascular disease, which includes coronary artery disease (CAD), hypertension, chronic heart failure, and atrial fibrillation. Obstructive sleep apnea (OSA) is the most common sleep-related breathing disorder in both the general public and patients with cardiovascular disease. Alcohol ingestion may reduce upper airway tone, worsening snoring and sleep disordered breathing in patients with OSA. However, patients with cardiac disease also exhibit a higher prevalence of central sleep apnea due to dysregulation of respiratory control mechanisms.

BASIC SCIENCE PEARL   **STEP 1**

There are multiple respiratory control centers in the human body whose outputs are integrated to determine respiration rate and effort:
- *Peripheral chemoreceptors,* found in the carotid bodies and aortic arch, are most sensitive to decreases in arterial partial pressure of oxygen (PaO_2), but will also increase ventilation if the arterial partial pressure of carbon dioxide ($PaCO_2$) rises significantly.
- *Central chemoreceptors* located in the medulla are most sensitive to changes in the acidity of the cerebral spinal fluid (CSF). An increase in the acidity of the CSF, due to an increase in localized hydrogen ion concentration (H^+), is often due to respiratory acidosis. Inadequate ventilation leads to an increase in $PaCO_2$, the excess carbon dioxide then crosses the blood–brain barrier where it is hydrolyzed by water to form H^+ and bicarbonate (HCO_3^-).

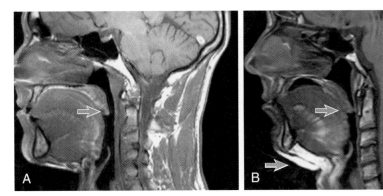

Figure 62.1   Normal versus apneic airway. Midsagittal magnetic resonance imaging (MRI) sections are shown for **(A)** a normal subject and **(B)** a subject with obstructive sleep apnea (OSA). *Orange arrows* indicate areas of the posterior neck and submental region where there is significantly more subcutaneous fat (areas of white signal) in the subject with OSA compared to the normal subject. *Blue arrows* indicate the posterior edge of the soft palate. In the subject with OSA, the soft palate appears to contact the posterior pharynx and occlude the airway. In the normal subject, the airway is patent. *(Adapted from* The Principles and Practice of Sleep Medicine, *Rapid Review of Polysomnographs, Figure 101-10.)*

When reviewing a sleep study, or polysomnogram, it is important to note the differences between obstructive and central respiratory events. Figure 62.1 shows the sagittal cross-sections from magnetic resonance imaging (MRI) studies of a normal individual and an obese individual with OSA. An increased amount of subcutaneous fat is one of several factors that can contribute to narrowing of the upper airway, increasing one's propensity to develop OSA. During obstructive respiratory events, respiratory effort persists against a narrowed or occluded upper airway. Due to increased effort, the movements of the rib cage and abdomen may become asynchronous, resulting in "paradoxical breathing" (see Fig. 62.2). In contrast, during central respiratory events, respiratory effort ceases and there is little to no apparent movement of the chest or abdomen (see Fig. 62.3).

Cheyne-Stokes respirations, a special form of periodic breathing, are sometimes seen in patients with heart failure. In Cheyne-Stokes respirations, there is a characteristic crescendo–decrescendo pattern to the depth or amplitude of a series of rapid breaths, followed by a respiratory pause/central apnea (see Fig. 62.4). This pattern is due to the inherent instability in these patients' respiratory control cycle, which is generated by a combination of increased chemoreceptor sensitivity and prolonged circulation time from the heart and lungs to respiratory control centers.

Cheyne-Stokes respirations are not always limited to sleep and may be seen during exertion, or even rest, in patients with advanced heart failure. Cheyne-Stokes respirations are also not pathognomonic for heart failure. They may be observed in patients with damage to the central nervous system due to stroke, traumatic brain injury, or tumor. The first step in treating Cheyne-Stokes respirations is to treat the underlying etiology (i.e., address uncompensated heart failure to optimize cardiac function). If Cheyne-Stokes respirations persist after optimizing medical therapy, noninvasive continuous positive airway pressure (CPAP) during sleep may be helpful.

What additional studies would you consider in patients with central sleep apnea in the absence of cardiac disease?

Other etiologies of central apnea exist, including medication use, neuromuscular disease, and lesions of the central nervous system (CNS) that alter central respiratory control. In patients with central sleep apnea but normal cardiac workup, one should consider brain MRI to assess for CNS

Obstructive apneas

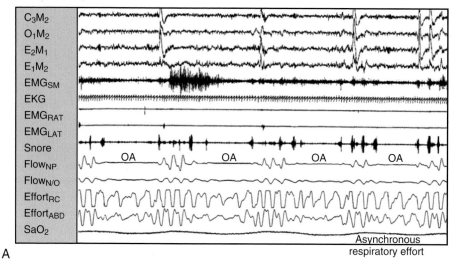

A

Obstructive hypopneas

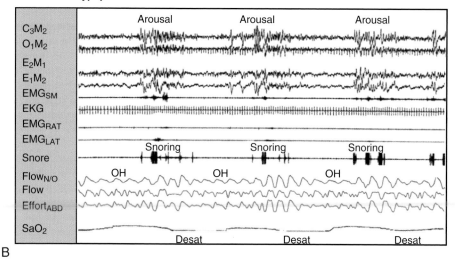

B

Figure 62.2 **Obstructive respiratory events during polysomnography. A,** Obstructive apnea events are marked OA. Obstructive apneas occur when there is ≥90% reduction in airflow but persistent respiratory effort. In some cases, there is asynchronous movement of the rib cage (RC) and abdomen (ABD), indicated in this figure by the broken lines. **B,** Obstructive hypopnea events are marked OH. Obstructive hypopneas require a significant reduction in airflow combined with an oxyhemoglobin desaturation event ("desat") and/or an arousal. (Adapted from The Principles and Practice of Sleep Medicine, Rapid Review of Polysomnographs, supplemental figures W182 and W184.)

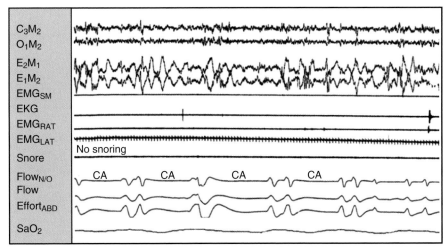

Figure 62.3 Central respiratory events during polysomnography. Central apneas (CA) are marked. Note the absence of airflow (FLOW) as well as the absence of respiratory effort in both the rib cage (Effort$_{RC}$) and abdomen (Effort$_{ABD}$) during each event. *(Adapted from* The Principles and Practice of Sleep Medicine, *Rapid Review of Polysomnographs, supplemental figure W186.)*

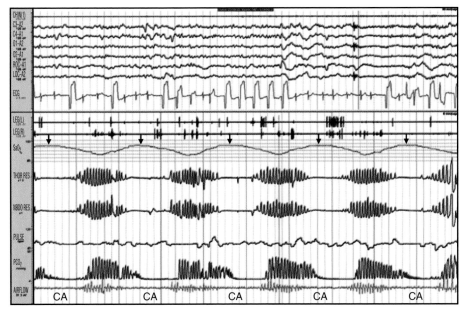

Figure 62.4 Cheyne-Stokes respirations. This respiratory pattern involves periods of rapid breathing alternating with apneic pauses/central apneas (CA). The depth of the breaths has a crescendo–decrescendo pattern. The SaO$_2$ peaks in the middle of the apneic pauses *(see black arrows)*. This patient is also noted to have an abnormal electrocardiogram with a combination of narrow and wide complex beats. *(Adapted from* The Principles and Practice of Sleep Medicine, *Cardiac Rhythm Abnormalities, supplemental figure W85.)*

lesions (including Arnold–Chiari malformation), pulmonary function testing that includes maximal inspiratory pressure to assess neuromuscular weakness, and arterial blood gas to determine whether a patient is hypercapnic.

CLINICAL PEARL   **STEP 2/3**

Patients with central apnea may be separated into those with and without hypercapnia. Chronic hypercapnia:
- Elevated $PaCO_2$ but normal serum pH because respiratory acidosis is buffered by metabolic compensation and elevated serum bicarbonate.
- Usually due to chronic respiratory insufficiency.
- Patients may have decreased responsiveness to incremental increases in $PaCO_2$.
- Neuromuscular disease leads to respiratory muscle weakness, decreased alveolar ventilation, and chronic carbon dioxide retention.
  - Seen in Duchenne's muscular dystrophy, amyotrophic lateral sclerosis (ALS), and other progressive neuromuscular conditions.
- Long-acting opioids, such as methadone, lead to hypercapnia by suppressing the central respiratory drive.
  - "Biot's breathing," a very irregular pattern of alternating tachypnea and apnea, may be seen with chronic opiate use and some central nervous system abnormalities.

Normocapnia:
- Patients with normal $PaCO_2$ may have central apneas due to an exaggerated ventilatory response to small increases in $PaCO_2$.
- When ventilation is increased too greatly, it can drive the $PaCO_2$ under the "apneic threshold" below which the drive to breathe is temporarily lost.
- Instability of the respiratory control system is due to increased chemoreceptor sensitivity and delay in feedback to respiratory control centers due to poor circulation.
- This mechanism of central apnea is seen during Cheyne-Stokes respirations.

CLINICAL PEARL   **STEP 2/3**

It is important to recognize the difference between acute respiratory failure and chronic respiratory failure/insufficiency.
- In acute respiratory failure, there is an uncompensated respiratory acidosis and low pH.
- Acute respiratory failure has many different causes.
- Excessive doses of opiates, or appropriate doses of opiates combined with additional respiratory depressants, such as alcohol or benzodiazepines, may lead to acute bradypnea (slow respiration rate) or apnea.
  - These patients lose their central respiratory drive.
  - In patients with pinpoint pupils and respiratory arrest, do not hesitate to give naloxone. This can be a life-saving intervention.
- In patients with pulmonary disease, acute respiratory failure may be due to an acute illness and can require a significant increase in respiratory support, including intubation and mechanical ventilation.

The patient reports that he currently weighs about 60 pounds more than he did in college when he was an avid runner and cyclist. His activities became more limited after he sustained a lower back injury about 15 years ago. He denies shortness of breath on exertion, such as when climbing stairs. He also denies orthopnea and sleeps with one pillow. On physical exam, the patient's body mass index (BMI) is 31.7 kg/m², blood pressure is 152/94 mm Hg, pulse rate is 65/min, respiration rate is 12/min, and oxygen saturation is 97% on room air at rest. His neck circumference is 20 inches. There are no abnormalities on cardiac auscultation with normal S1 and S2, and no audible murmurs or gallop. Radial and posterior tibial pulses are 2+, and there is trace lower extremity edema at the ankles. Jugular venous distention appears within normal limits.

Screening tools for OSA include the STOP-BANG questionnaire (see page 269). This patient has several risk factors for OSA, including history of snoring, observed apneas, hypertension, large neck circumference, male gender, and age >50 years old.

> An overnight polysomnography study is ordered. The patient has loud, continuous snoring and frequent obstructive apneas and hypopneas associated with oxyhemoglobin desaturations as low as 68% from a baseline oxygen saturation of 93% on room air. His apnea hypopnea index (AHI) during the first half of the night is 35 events/hour. Sleep is fragmented, and the patient awakens frequently after respiratory events. His Central Apnea Index is normal at 0.3 events/hour. Due to the severity of his OSA, the patient is started on CPAP during the second half of the night. His breathing during sleep improves with CPAP 12 cm of water.

Diagnosis: Severe obstructive sleep apnea (OSA)

This patient has some signs of CHF, such as trace lower extremity edema, but his cardiac symptoms appear well controlled with his current medication regimen. His polysomnography study demonstrates severe OSA without a significant degree of central apneas or evidence of Cheyne-Stokes respirations. In adults, mild OSA is defined as an AHI from 5 to 14.9 events/hour, moderate OSA is an AHI from 15 to 29.9 events/hour, and severe OSA is ≥30 events/hour. This patient's OSA improves with CPAP therapy.

CPAP is the first-line intervention for moderate to severe OSA. Untreated OSA contributes to an increased risk of future cardiovascular events, including stroke, and can also contribute to the development of uncontrolled hypertension and arrhythmias, such as atrial fibrillation. It is especially important to start CPAP treatment in patients with significant cardiac conditions, hypertension, and other comorbidities. Interestingly, in the general population, the risk of sudden cardiac death is at its lowest from 12 AM to 6 AM. In patients with OSA, however, the relative risk of sudden cardiac death from 12 AM to 6 AM is about 2.5-fold higher. Therefore, treating OSA may also reduce the risk of sudden cardiac death during sleep.

Clinic follow up with patients is essential to be sure that their CPAP continues to be effective and that the patients continue to use their machines. For patients who are unable to tolerate CPAP therapy due to claustrophobia or other factors, additional treatment options for OSA include referral to an otolaryngologist for consideration of surgical interventions, or fitting with a specialized dental device that advances the mandible forward to open the airway during sleep.

BEYOND THE PEARLS

- Beta blockers decrease sympathetic tone and may lead to difficulty with insomnia due to decreased production of melatonin. This may be a more significant problem for those patients taking nonselective beta blockers, such as propranolol and nadolol. Melatonin supplementation may be helpful for these patients.
- Melatonin is a weak hypnotic making it less likely to have deleterious side effects, such as a "hangover effect," but this property also makes it less effective for some people with significant insomnia.
- Melatonin is a naturally produced neurohormone. Melatonin tablets are therefore classified as dietary supplements and are not closely regulated by the Food and Drug Administration. Different melatonin preparations may have different levels of purity, and the indicated quantity of active ingredient may not always be accurate.
- Ramelteon (Rozerem®) is a synthetic melatonin receptor agonist with similar activity to melatonin. It is sometimes prescribed for sleep-onset insomnia and may have fewer side effects than other common sleep aids, most of which interact with the gamma-aminobutyric acid (GABA) receptor complex.

Continued

BEYOND THE PEARLS—cont'd

- Tasimelteon (Hetlioz®), another melatonin receptor agonist, was recently approved for treatment of non-24, a common circadian rhythm disorder in patients who are totally blind.
- "High altitude periodic breathing" is a pattern of periodic central apneas seen in normal individuals when they are transitioning from sea level to the mountains. It is most severe during sleep. Tachypnea is a natural physiologic response to lower atmospheric oxygen content, but increased minute ventilation decreases $PaCO_2$ close to the apneic threshold, resulting in periodic central apneas.
- Individuals with sleep-disordered breathing may have more symptoms at high altitude and require increased respiratory support.
- Some patients with Cheyne-Stokes respirations respond to simple CPAP while others require adaptive or automatic servo-ventilation (ASV) machines that use complex algorithms to modulate air pressure dynamically on a breath-to-breath basis. Although very successful in normalizing the respiratory pattern during sleep, safety concerns have recently emerged regarding the use of ASV in patients with low left ventricular ejection fractions. At this time, the mechanism leading to increased mortality risk in a subset of patients is not clear, but possibilities include that ASV use leads to negative hemodynamic effects, proarrhythmogenic effects, or loss of as yet uncharacterized benefits of central sleep apnea that are lost with treatment. Physicians have been advised to discuss the risks and benefits with all of their patients currently using ASV. We hope to better understand the mechanism underlying these results in the near future.
- Hypoglossal nerve stimulators are designed to advance the tongue forward in synch with respiratory efforts during sleep and were recently approved as an option for treatment of OSA in patients with significant OSA who do not tolerate CPAP and who meet certain selection criteria.

References

Ayas NT, Patil SP, Stanchina M, et al. Treatment of Central Sleep Apnea with Adaptive Servoventilation in Chronic Heart Failure. *Am J Respir Crit Care Med.* 2015;192:132-133.

Gami AS, Howard DE, Olson EJ, et al. Day-night pattern of sudden death in obstructive sleep apnea. *N Engl J Med.* 2005;352:1206-1214.

Linz D, Woehrle H, Bitter T, et al. The importance of sleep-disordered breathing in cardiovascular disease. *Clin Res Cardiol.* 2015;104:705-718.

Roth T. Insomnia: definition, prevalence, etiology, and consequences. *J Clin Sleep Med.* 2007;3(suppl 5):S7-S10.

Scheer FA, Morris CJ, Garcia JI, et al. Repeated melatonin supplementation improves sleep in hypertensive patients treated with β-blockers; a randomized controlled trial. *Sleep.* 2012;35(10):1395-1402.

Schweitzer PK. Drugs that disturb sleep and wakefulness. In: Kryger MH, Roth T, Dement WC, eds. *Principles and Practice of Sleep Medicine.* 5th ed. St. Louis: Elsevier/Saunders; 2015:544-560.

Stoschitzky K, Sakotnik A, Lercher P, et al. Influence of beta-blockers on melatonin release. *Eur J Clin Pharmacol.* 1999;55(2):111-115.

Wijdicks EF. Biot's breathing. *J Neurol Neurosurg Psychiatr.* 2007;78(5):512-513.

Woodson BT, Gillespie MB, Soose RJ, et al. Randomized controlled withdrawal study of upper airway stimulation on OSA. *Otolaryngol Head Neck Surg.* 2014;151(5):880-887.

INDEX

Page numbers followed by f indicate figures; t, tables; b, text in boxes.

Anti-topoisomerase I (anti-Scl-70) antibodies, associated
with diffuse systemic scleroderma, 195
Anti-VEGF, for diabetic macular edema, 146
Aorta, coarctation of, in secondary hypertension,
371*t*
Aortic dissection, 459*t*-460*t*
Aortic sclerosis, 407*b*
Aortic stenosis, 460*t*
  causes of, 410-411
  confirmatory diagnostic test for, 411-412
  murmur associated with, maneuvers in, 408-409, 409*b*,
    409*t*
  physical exam findings of, 408, 408*b*
  prognosis of, implications on, 409, 410*f*
  risk factors for, 410-411
  symptoms of, 409-410, 411*f*
  syncope in, mechanism of, 410*b*
  systolic heart murmur and, 278
  treatment of, 412, 413*b*
Aortic valve vegetation, 55-56, 55*b*, 55*f*
Aortic valves
  bicuspid, 411, 412*f*
  replacement of, 412
Apnea
  central, 271
  obstructive, 271
APRV. *see* Airway pressure release ventilation (APRV)
Aqueous humor, flow of, 253, 254*f*
ARBs. *see* Angiotensin receptor blockers (ARBs)
ARDS. *see* Acute respiratory distress syndrome (ARDS)
ARDS Network, 486
Arginine vasopressin, 101*b*
Arousal, in obstructive sleep apnea, 268
ART. *see* Antiretroviral therapy (ART)
Arterial blood gas, 484
Arterial insufficiency, 258-259
Arterial thrombosis, in deep vein thrombosis, 177*b*
Arthritis
  acute, 133
  chronic, 65, 66*t*, 133
  crystalline, 295*t*
  crystals in, 404, 405*f*
  inflammatory. *see* Inflammatory arthritis
  noninflammatory, 295*t*
    inflammatory arthritis *versus*, 68*t*
  polyarticular, acute, 397-406, 405*b*
    differential diagnosis of, 397
    physical exam for, 398, 398*b*
    test for, 398
  septic. *see* Septic arthritis
  in systemic lupus erythematosus, 137*b*
Arthrocentesis, 65
Articular cartilage, 296*b*
  function of, 296*b*
  premature damage of, in long-distance runners,
    298*b*
AS. *see* Ankylosing spondylitis (AS)
Aseptic meningitis, 114
  differential diagnosis of, 115*t*
Aspartate aminotransferase (AST), serum, 510*b*
Aspiration, pneumonia and, 165*b*
Aspirin
  for acute myocardial infarction, 27
  diabetic retinopathy and, 146*b*
  STEMI and, 30
  therapy, 467
    contraindications to, 468*b*
  for type 2 diabetes mellitus, 205
AST. *see* Aspartate aminotransferase (AST)

Asthma
  chronic cough and, 386*t*
  GERD and, 233*b*
Atazanavir, 502*t*-503*t*
Atonic paralysis, 269
ATP. *see* Adenosine triphosphate (ATP)
Atrial fibrillation, 93*b*
  electrocardiogram of, 158, 159*f*, 162*b*-163*b*
  electrocardioversion for, 161, 162*b*-163*b*
  etiologies of, 159
  hospitalization for, criteria for, 160
  imaging studies for, 160
  laboratory evaluation for, 160
  medications for, 160
  pathophysiology of, 159
  pharmacologic cardioversion *versus* rate control for, 161
  rhythm control for, 160-161
  signs and symptoms of, 158
  stroke prevention and, 162, 162*t*
  treatment options for, 162
  types of, 158-159
Atrial Fibrillation Follow-up Investigation of Rhythm
    Management (AFFIRM) trial, 160-161, 162*b*-163*b*
ATRIPLA®, 501
Attention deficit hyperactivity disorder (ADHD),
    obstructive sleep apnea and, 271*b*
Atypical pathogens, causing pneumonia, 167
Auscultation
  cardiac, 54*b*
  dynamic, 279
Autoantibody testing, 514
  role of, in diffuse systemic scleroderma, 195-196
  for systemic lupus erythematosus, 136, 139
Autoimmune illness, 242*b*
Autoimmune necrotizing myopathy, 512, 512*b*
Autologous hematopoietic stem cell transplantation, for
    diffuse systemic scleroderma, 198*b*
Avascular necrosis (AVN), systemic lupus erythematosus
    and, 139*b*
Avian influenza, 166
AVN. *see* Avascular necrosis (AVN)
Axonotmesis, 155*b*
Azathioprine, for dermatomyositis, 515
Azithromycin, 33

B
B cell activating factor, in systemic lupus erythematosus,
    137*b*
B lymphocyte stimulator (BLyS), in systemic lupus
    erythematosus, 137*b*
Babesiosis, 428-429
  diagnosis of, 429*b*
  laboratory testing results in, 429*t*
Bacillary angiomatosis, 33
Back, electrical sensation running down, 315-316
Baclofen, 318
Bacterial meningitis
  acute, 111, 111*b*, 120*b*-121*b*
  cause of, 111-113
  community acquired, 117
  complications of, 120*b*-121*b*
  CSF profile for, 118, 119*t*
  CSF testing for, 116, 118*t*
  diagnosis of, 119
  diagnostic test for, 116
  differential diagnosis of, 113-115
  empiric antibiotic therapy for, 114*t*, 117-118, 117*b*
  imaging for, 116, 116*t*, 117*b*
  increased intracranial pressure in, 117*b*